The
IMMUNOLOGIC REVOLUTION
Facts and Witnesses

Edited by

Andor Szentivanyi
Herman Friedman

University of South Florida College of Medicine
Tampa, Florida

CRC Press
Boca Raton   Ann Arbor   London   Tokyo

Library of Congress Cataloging-in-Publication Data

The immunologic revolution : facts and witnesses / edited by Andor
  Szentivanyi and Herman Friedman.
     p.   cm.
   Includes bibliographical references and index.
   ISBN 0-8493-4722-X
   1. Immunology--History.   I. Szentivanyi, Andor.   II. Friedman,
  Herman, 1931-
   [DNLM: 1. Allergy and Immunology--history--essays.   QW 511.1 I33
  1993]
  QR181.5.I45   1993
  616.07'9--dc20
  DNLM/DLC
  for Library of Congress   93-32559
                                                     CIP

No claim to original U.S. Government works
International Standard Book Number 0-8493-4722-X
Library of Congress Card Number 93-32559
Printed in the United States of America   1 2 3 4 5 6 7 8 9 0
Printed on acid-free paper

FOREWORD

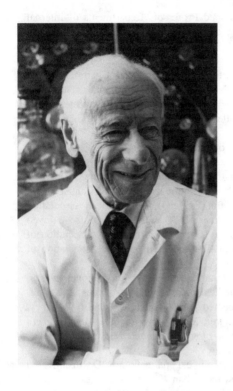

This book is dedicated to Dr. Michael Heidelberger, considered a founder of modern immunochemistry and immunology. Dr. Heidelberger was an enthusiastic supporter of the idea for this book. When the suggestion was first made that there should be a volume of essays concerning the founding of modern immunology by some of the most prominent immunologists in the world today, including reminiscences by some of those who were major participants in the "immunological revolution" this century, Dr. Heidelberger suggested a number of prominent immunologists as authors. Furthermore, Dr. Heidelberger was the first to submit a manuscript for this book and did so in an enthusiastic and unique manner. His manuscript was presented to us in **handwritten** form. A few months after the decision was made to proceed with this project, this handwritten manuscript was presented to the editors, close to his 100th birthday. Unfortunately, Dr. Heidelberger, who lived a very long life, passed away prior to the publication of this book. The American Association of Immunologists honored Dr. Heidelberger with a symposium at their annual meeting in honor of his 100th birthday and there were many celebrations of his birthday at his university in New York City and elsewhere. We believe it is appropriate to dedicate this book in his honor, since many prominent biomedical scientists in immunology today received their training and encouragement in this field from Dr. Heidelberger over many decades. He leaves a lasting legacy to all of biomedical science. Until the very end of his life, he continued to perform experiments in his laboratories and was an active investigator. The first chapter of this book is written by Dr. Heidelberger in the manner requested from all authors, i.e., a reminiscence of how the author became an "immunologist" and remembrances of other investigators who stimulated the development of this field.

The editors also wish to acknowledge with much thanks the assistance of Ms. Ilona Friedman, who served as the editorial coordinator for this book. The editors are also very pleased to acknowledge the assistance of Ms. Christine Abarca, Ms. Judy Flynn and Ms. Michelle Friedman for editorial and secretarial assistance during various phases of this book project.

THE EDITORS

Andor Szentivanyi, M.D., D.Sc. is University Distinguished Professor, Departments of Internal Medicine and Pharmacology and Therapeutics at the University of South Florida College of Medicine in Tampa, Florida.

Dr. Szentivanyi received his M.D. degree in 1950 from the University Medical School of Debrecen in Debrecen, Hungary. During his academic career Dr. Szentivanyi has served as Chairman of the Department of Medical Microbiology at Creighton University School of Medicine in Omaha, Nebraska; and at the University of South Florida in Tampa, Florida, he served in the capacities of Chairman of the Department of Pharmacology and Therapeutics, Dean of the College of Medicine, Director of the Medical Center, and Vice President for Medical Affairs.

Dr. Szentivanyi is currently a member of the Federation of American Societies for Experimental Biology, American Society for Pharmacology and Experimental Therapeutics, American Society for Clinical Pharmacology and Therapeutics, International Association of Asthmology, and the Society for Leukocyte Biology. He is a fellow of the American College of Clinical Pharmacology, American Academy of Allergy, American College of Allergists, Royal Society for Health (England), and American Association for Clinical Immunology and Allergy. In the course of his career Dr. Szentivanyi has also enjoyed memberships in the Association of Medical School Pharmacology Chairmen, American Association of Immunologists, American Medical Association, Southern Medical Association, and the Association of American Medical Colleges.

Dr. Szentivanyi is the recipient of 3 honorary degrees, more than 20 national and international awards, and 5 honorary memberships and 5 honorary fellowships in medical societies and academies. Dr. Szentivanyi has been honored to sit on the editorial boards of respected journals such as *Annals of Allergy, Allergologia et Immunopathologia, Clinical Immunology Newsletter, Revista Argentina de Asma, Alergia e Inmunología, EOS - Journal of Immunology and Immunopharmacology, Immunopharmacology Reviews,* and *Journal of Investigative Allergology and Clinical Immunology.*

In the fields of basic neurosciences, immunology and basic and clinical pharmacology, Dr. Szentivanyi has presented over 60 invited lectures at international meetings, more than 40 invited lectures at national meetings and approximately 50 guest lectures at universities and institutes in the United States and abroad. He has published more than 400 research papers, authored 3 books and has edited 14 books. He is the discoverer of the immune-neuroendocrine circuitry and author of the beta adrenergic theory of the atopic abnormality in bronchial asthma. Dr. Szentivanyi's current major research interests include the immunopharmacology of asthmatic and allergic inflammation.

Herman Friedman, Ph.D., is Professor and Chairman of the Department of Medical Microbiology and Immunology at the University of South Florida College of Medicine, Tampa, Florida. He received his A.B. and A.M. degrees from Temple University in Philadelphia, Pennsylvania, in 1953 and 1955. He then received his Ph.D. degree in microbiology and immunology from Hahnemann University College of Medicine in 1957, also in Philadelphia. He served as Head of the Department of Microbiology and Immunology at the Albert Einstein Medical Center in Philadelphia for nearly 20 years, and was Professor in the Department of Medical Microbiology and Immunology at Temple University School of Medicine at the same time. He relocated to Tampa, Florida in 1978, where he was appointed to the faculty at the University of South Florida.

He is currently a member of many U.S. and international biomedical societies, including the American Association of Immunologists, the American Society for Microbiology, the Association of Medical Laboratory Immunologists, the Clinical Immunology Society, etc. He is a fellow of several biomedical societies, including the N.Y. Academy of Sciences and the American Academy of Allergy and Clinical Immunology. He has served on many advisory committees for the National Institutes of Health, including being a member of the bacteriology and mycology study section for 8 years and the study section on immunology of the National Institute on Drug Abuse. He was also a charter member of the AIDS Basic Science study section of NIH for 4 years, as well as a member of the Advisory Committee for Microbiology and Virology of the American Cancer Society.

He received the Outstanding Alumnus Award from Hahnemann University, as well as the Distinguished Scientist Award from the University of South Florida College of Medicine. He also received the Becton Dickinson Award in clinical microbiology and immunology from the American Society for Microbiology, which has a membership of 40,000 microbiologists. He was instrumental in the founding of the Diagnostic and Clinical Immunology Division of the ASM and received the Distinguished Service Award from that Division. He was head of the clinical immunology program for the American Academy of Microbiology for approximately 12 years. He also was one of the organizers of the Association of Medical Laboratory Immunologists. He served as President of the Reticuloendothelial Society and was President of both the Eastern Pennsylvania and the Florida Branch of the American Society for Microbiology. He was a Foundation for Microbiology Visiting Lecturer several times. He has been a guest lecturer at many universities in the United States and abroad. He was a Visiting Professor several times at universities in several countries, including Israel, Japan, China, Peru and Germany.

He has been co-editor of the 4 editions of the Manual of Clinical Immunology, published by the ASM. He has been on the editorial board or Section Editor for many journals and was the co-editor of the Clinical Immunology Newsletter for 10 years. He has published over 500 peer reviewed journal articles and an equal number of abstracts for presentation at national and international scientific meetings. He has served as chair of many scientific sessions at such meetings over the last 30 years. He has also organized and served as chairman of over a dozen international scientific symposia. He is the editor/co-editor of over 55 books, including many proceedings of international symposia he organized and chaired.

His main research interests are in the area of immune responses to microorganisms, including bacteria, fungi and viruses, and the effects of microorganisms, especially retroviruses, on the immune response system. He is also involved in studying the effects of environmental agents, such as drugs of abuse, bacterial products, and immunomodulators on the immune response mechanism. His research is supported by many grants from national agencies such as the National Institutes of Health.

CONTRIBUTORS

ALAIN E. BUSSARD, Ph.D.
Hybridoma Data Bank, CERDIC, St. Paul de Vence, France

B. CINADER, Ph.D., D. Sc.
University of Toronto, Toronto, Ont., Canada

HENRY N. CLAMAN, M.D.
University of Colorado School of Medicine, Denver, CO

ERWIN DIENER, Ph.D.
University of Alberta Faculty of Medicine, Edmonton, Alberta, Canada

HERMAN FRIEDMAN, Ph.D.
University of South Florida College of Medicine, Tampa, FL

GÜNTHER GILLISSEN, M.D., Ph.D.
University of Aachen Faculty of Medicine, Aachen, Germany

ROBERT A. GOOD, M.D., Ph.D.
All Children's Hospital, St. Petersburg, FL

MICHAEL HEIDELBERGER, Ph.D. (Deceased)
New York University Medical School, New York, NY

PANAYOTIS LIACOPOULOS, M.D. (retired)
Paris, France

FELIX MILGROM, M.D.
State University of New York School of Medicine, Buffalo, NY

J.F.A.P. MILLER, M.D., Ph.D., S.Sc.
The Walter and Eliza Hall Institute of Medical Research, Melbourne, Australia

Sir GUSTAV NOSSAL, M.D., Ph.D.
The Walter and Eliza Hall Institute of Medical Research, Melbourne, Australia

ZOLTAN OVARY, M.D.
New York University School of Medicine, New York, NY

MAXWELL RICHTER, M.D., Ph.D.
University of Ottawa School of Medicine, Ottawa, Ont., Canada

NOEL R. ROSE, M.D., Ph.D.
The Johns Hopkins University School of Hygiene and Public Health, Baltimore, MD

JOSEPH G. SINKOVICS, M.D.
Cancer Institute, St. Joseph's Hospital, Tampa, FL

ABRAM B. STAVITSKY, Ph.D., V.M.D.
Case Western Reserve University, Cleveland, OH

KURT STERN, M.D.
The Lautenberg Center for General and Tumor Immunology, Hebrew
University/Hadassah Medical School, Jerusalem, Israel

JAROSLAV STĚRZL, D.Sc.
Institute of Microbiology, Czech Academy of Science, Prague, Czech
Republic

ANDOR SZENTIVANYI, M.D., D. Sc.
University of South Florida College of Medicine, Tampa, FL

DAVID W. TALMAGE, M.D.
University of Colorado School of Medicine, Denver, CO

DAVID W. WEISS, Ph.D., D. Phil. Med.
The Lautenberg Center of General and Tumor Immunology, Hebrew
University/Hadassah Medical School, Jerusalem, Israel

JOSEPH M. YOFFEY, M.D., D.Sc.
Hebrew University/Hadassah Medical School, Jerusalem, Israel

PREFACE

Neither a scientific, polemic, nor a historical analysis, this volume describes the origins, the underlying forces and trends, the principal events, findings, the vital participants, their associates, and witnesses, from the standpoint of their perspectives and vision of the immunological revolution of this century.

It hopes to extend the reader's perspective beyond the confines of simplistic formulas that have been used many times to explain this development. Thus, these chapters written by the participants as well as the witnesses are based on broad knowledge, insight, and personal experiences in this phase of the development of immunobiology. Thus emerges a rare and penetrating view of the immunological revolution.

Andor Szentivanyi, M.D., D.Sc.
Herman Friedman, Ph.D.

CONTENTS

Chapter 1

THE PRECIPITIN REACTION, MICROBIAL AGGLUTINATION, COMPLEMENTFIXATION, AND RELATIONS BETWEEN CHEMICAL STRUCTURE AND ANTIGEN-ANTIBODY INTERACTION

Michael Heidelberger

How and why did I, whose scientific training and early research were mainly in organic and analytical chemistry[1,2,3,4,5] become an immunochemist? It was the place, the then Rockefeller Institute for Medical Research (R.I.), it was the influence of several books[6,7,8,9] and it was the shining personal examples of two extraordinary men, Karl Landsteiner and Oswald T. Avery. Having painted in a background, I shall proceed with what I still believe to be the **facts** and **witnesses** although some readers may consider my memory to be presently somewhat hazy.

It was in 1922 that Karl Landsteiner, a famous European immunologist, arrived to assume membership at the R.I. He had already worked on the immunology of hemoglobin, and having heard that I was at that time in D.D. Van Slyke's group isolating crystalline equine oxyhemoglobin with intact oxygen-carrying capacity[10] Landsteiner proposed that we continue his study jointly if material and time were available. I jumped at this rare privilege which created problems in some other instances of collaboration because Landsteiner always insisted on doing the most important experiments himself. As I was only a beginner this worked well and I learned my first immunological techniques from a great master.[11,12]

During my two years with the oxyhemoglobin group, Oswald T. Avery, chief microbiologist of the R.I. Hospital's pneumonia group, often came into the laboratory with a small vial of grayish material to ask when I would begin work on it. "The whole secret of bacterial specificity is in this little vial," he affirmed. Accordingly, when the hemoglobin team was developed (1922), there began one of the most exciting periods of my scientific career.

Back in 1917 Dochez and Avery had described a "soluble specific substance" (SSS) of Pneumococcus.[13] This was secreted into the culture medium, it precipitated antisera of the homologous pneumococcal serological type, and could be found in the urine and blood of heavily infected patients with Pn pneumonia. Avery's small sample had been partially purified by Glenn Cullen, but available methods of purification and analysis demanded much larger amounts. Of the three known "fixed types," Avery advised beginning with type 2—type 1, he said, had the smallest capsules (presumably of SSS) and although type 3 had the largest, it was considered *Streptococcus mucosus* by some microbiologists. Our early methods of purification and isolation[14,15,16,17,18] were later improved.[19,20]

With increasing purity SSS 2 showed less and less nitrogen. This surprised us, as only proteins were assumed to possess immunological activity. "Could it be a carbohydrate?" said Avery. And so it turned out to be. We identified

D-glucose (D-glc)[*][15] and an acid, later shown to be D-glucuronic acid (D-glcA), and missed L-rhamnose (L-rha) entirely,[21,22] as we had to work with relatively little material, and paper chromatography and its column counterpart had not yet been invented. Only in 1975 was the structure of SSS 2 rigorously shown to be:[23]

$$\rightarrow3)\alpha\text{L-rha}(1\rightarrow3)\alpha\text{L-rha}(1\rightarrow3)\beta\text{L-rha}(1\rightarrow4)\beta\text{D-glc}(1\text{--DglcA}(1\rightarrow6)\alpha\text{Dglc}(1\uparrow_n^{\bullet\bullet}$$

Our next attempts were with SSS 3, which was easier to purify, was a much stronger acid, and was levorotatory in polarized light, unlike SSS 2. SSS 3 contains only D-glc and DGlcA and is a polymer of what we called an aldobionic acid. These are now known as aldobiuronic acids, enormous tonnages of which were later found widely distributed in the hemicelluloses and gums of plants but were originally isolated from a few grams of SSS 3.[24,25] The repeating unit of SSS 3 is cellobiouronic acid and each unit is joined to the next as follows:[26,27]

$$\dagger3)\beta\text{D-glcA}(1\rightarrow4)\beta\text{D-glc}(1]_n$$

Avery and I finally tackled type 1. Its SSS behaved like a polypeptide and was actually described as such by others. It was a strong acid and weak base with about 5% of nitrogen, and contained much galacturonic acid (GalA).[20] Without the use of alkali a more nearly native "A-substance" was isolated by Enders and Pappenheimer.[28] It contained an immunologically important labile-OAcetyl group.[29] The structure, has been determined[30] but the

$$\dagger3)\alpha2,4,6\text{-trideoxy-4-NH}_2\text{D-GalNHAc-}(1\rightarrow4)\alpha\text{D-GalA}(1\rightarrow3)\alpha\text{D-GalA}(1]_n$$

position of the OAc is still unknown (see also.[31]

The chemical differences of SSS (henceforth S) 1, 2, and 3 thus established a new class of substances with immunological activity and furnished a firm basis for the understanding of pneumococcal (Pn) type-specificity. Structures of a score of PnSs are now known (out of about 80) and vaccines containing in a single dose the PnS of many serological types are now available. Strangely enough, the polysaccharidic vaccines did not show the "antigenic competition" observed after injection of multiple protein antigens by early immunologists such as Hektoen.

As it turned out, *Streptococcus hemolyticus*, group A, was shown to have a type-specific "M" protein[32] and a group-specific polysaccharide[33,34,35] so that too wide a generalization was inappropriate; nevertheless, important additional polysaccharides were found: among *Streptococci*, another 80 or so among *Klebsiella*, and a huge number in *Escherichia coli* and *Salmonella*. Polysaccharides also determine the specificities of mammalian blood groups and of glycoproteins and glycopeptides of widely different forms of life.

In 1928 I became the first full-time chemist in a Department of Medicine, this time at the College of Physicians and Surgeons (P and S) of Columbia University, thanks to Walter W. Palmer, Professor of Medicine, who had been

---

[*]In this chapter the abbreviations for sugars are capitalized only when the sugar is immunodominant. All sugars are in the pyranose form unless stated otherwise.

on a sabbatical in Van Slyke's group while I was there. In the meantime, I had been reviewing much of what was known, or thought to be known of immunology. Kraus had announced a "precipitin reaction" in 1897:[36] the formation of a precipitate when proteins (antigens) which had earlier been injected into animals were added to serum taken after some days. This rapidly gave rise to the proposal of conflicting mechanisms for insolubilization.

Were the antibodies formed by the animal "denatured" by the antigen or was a complex formed which contained both antigen and antibody? The latter explanation was soon established independently by von Dungern and Braun. The former immunized rabbits with crab blood and found that one of its components (later shown to be the Cu-protein hemocyanin) caused the immune precipitate to turn blue on exposure to air. Braun used casein, a phosphoprotein of milk and showed that the precipitate with antibody contained more P than the amount of serum taken. But what fractions of the complex mixture of proteins in serum were antibodies? A long series of investigations showed that antibodies usually appeared in the so-called globulin fraction, but were they really globulins or substances of unknown nature "adsorbed" to globulins?

Up to the 1930's there had still been no definitive answer, nor was it known whether or not the agglutinins which bound bacteria together in the sera of immunized animal were the same antibodies that caused precipitation of soluble antigens. A dispute also arose over complement and its fixation, which had become an important and ubiquitous diagnostic test for syphilis and other widespread diseases. It seemed to me that immunology could never become a real science nor its disputes be resolved until the merely relative, supposedly quantitative but actually qualitative methods of titration in use could be supplanted by microchemical analyses giving the actual weight of antibodies in an antiserum, and until an antibody could be isolated in analytically pure form in order to determine its chemical nature. The standard procedure for estimating the "titer" of a serum was to set up a long series of small tubes each containing 0.5 ml saline. To the first tube was added 0.5 ml of the serum to titrated. The contents of this tube were drawn up two or three times into a pipette, and 0.5 ml of the "mixture" was transferred to the second tube and the process repeated down the line, often with the same pipette (there were no NIH nor NSF grants in those early days). Not only were mixtures often incomplete, but residues of the first dilutions could easily be carried along into the weaker ones. Moreover, the tube at which precipitin, agglutinin or complement fixation titers faded out could only be read subjectively and with difficulty. The result at best could only be whether or not a given serum was two or three or n times stronger or weaker than the standard used. Nor was there any indication of the actual quantity of antibody being measured. Therefore, the long overdue rectification of this intolerable state of immunology became my chief priority at P and S.

"Bill" Palmer had secured a half million dollars from Edward S. Harkness to establish the Harkness Research Fund, making it possible to equip two laboratories and attract a remarkable co-worker, Forrest E. Kendall, a young Ph.D. (chemistry) who had lost a hand in a threshing machine on his father's farm. During the eight years we worked together, the hand was never missed.

1928 was a good time to begin such studies, for there was earlier work on which to lean. Hsien Wu and his co-workers[37,38] had used a microKjeldahl method for estimating nitrogen for a similar purpose, but with dubious results.

However, if antibodies turned out to be actual globulins, as seemed likely, microKjeldahls would suffice. Moreover, we had nitrogen-free antigens, Pn S2 and PnS3, which precipitated homologous antibodies so that we did not have to worry about the amount of antigen N precipitated. In addition, Lloyd Felton had partially purified anti-Pn equine sera by pouring them into 10-20 volumes of slightly acidulated water and collecting the antibodies which came down with the precipitate of so-called euglobulins. These were redissolved in 0.9% NaCl solution buffered to ~pH 7.4 with Na_2HPO_4 (for detailed report see references.[39,40] Initial results, giving the amounts of precipitable N by difference (total N on the supernatant before and after addition of PnS 2 or S 3) showed that the composition of the precipitate varied with the relative proportions of antibody and antigen, and that there was an equivalence zone in which neither antigen nor antibody could be found in the supernatant (see Table VI in reference.[41] This meant that both antigen and antibody were precipitated quantitatively within the limits of error of the method. Later we used the whole serum, equine or rabbit, and with proper washing of the precipitate obtained identical results. It was also possible to extend the method to protein-antiprotein systems, at first with the help of a colored protein to distinguish between antigen N and antibody N in the precipitate,[42] then to move on to a colorless protein-antiprotein system,[43] and finally to the establishment of a quantitative theory of precipitin reaction[40] from which useful predictions could be made and tested for verification. The theory was based on the analytical findings and on the chemical and physical evidence that both antigen and at least the large equine antibody[44,45] were multivalent with respect to each other. Soon after our publication of 1929, John R. Marrack, author of the influential *Chemistry of Antigens and Antibodies*[46] arrived in New York as ship's doctor, mainly to tell us of his reservations as to our use of the law of mass action in explaining the precipitation. This visit established a permanent friendship and made us adopt a more rigorous use of the mass law.[40]

While all this was going on, our first graduate student, Elvin A. Kabat, arrived in the laboratory. He had graduated with honors from the City College of New York and earned a stipend as our laboratory assistant, quickly running microKjeldahls accurately and acquiring familiarity with our work. "Why don't you apply this to bacterial agglutination?" he asked. As Kendall and I had our hands full with precipitins we said, "We'll help *you* do it," which we did. This work showed that agglutination of *Pneumococcus* was actually a precipitin reaction at the surfaces of the cells, that the same theory sufficed[47,48] and that for a single antigen-antibody system precipitins and agglutinins were identical.[49] These data confirmed Zinsser's "unitarian" hypothesis[50] which had lacked quantitative backing.

There were also radically different guesses and theories as to the activity and nature of complement, a blood constituent which was both an enhancer of immunity and a widely used diagnostic tool, requiring rivers of guinea pig blood,** its most prolific source. Jules Bordet and his co-workers argued that complement (alexin) was merely an unstable colloidal state of fresh serum[7] while Paul Ehrlich and his group insisted that it was an actual substance.[5]

**In 1951 at the Central Drug Research Laboratories in Lucknow, India where the assistant Director, D.L. Shrivastava, was having trouble with guinea pigs, I suggested elephant blood as a larger source of complement. A sample was procured but the serum was completely inactive: as far as I know the reason for this has never been investigated.

Kendall and I thought that the precipitin reaction with PnS2 or 3 and rabbit anti-S2 or 3, which "fixed" complement, ought to decide the ongoing dispute. With adequate controls, we found that fresh guinea pig serum slowed down precipitation but added nitrogen to precipitates that had been given more time,[51,52,53] proving that complement was a protein or proteins, and that Ehrlich's views were more nearly correct than the Bordet hypothesis.

At the same time a similar conclusion was reached independently by Pillemer, Ecker, Oncley, and Cohn who isolated the so-called first component, relatively free of the other three known at that time.[54] We were also able to propose a theory of complement fixation[55] which, I believe, is still considered acceptable.

During this period, Torsten Teorell, a young Swedish physiologist, came to the laboratory for a tew months. He had been working with W.J.V. Osterhout at the R.I. and was passionately devoted to the biological effects of ions, so that he was an ideal person to study the effects of varying salt concentrations on the precipitin reactions with which we were occupied. Over a large range, increased concentrations of NaCl resulted in decreased precipitation of antibody by PnS2 and 3 but as long as antibody was in excess all of the polysaccharide added was in the precipitate.[56] It suddenly dawned upon us that this might lead to the isolation of analytically pure antibody by precipitating a large quantity of Felton's antibody solution in slight excess with PnS3 in 0.9% saline, washing the precipitate several times with 0.9% saline, and then extracting antibody in 5M saline. In the first batch there was only 70% antibody (up from the 40% originally present) and it took two years of study and modification before the final analytically 100% antibody was obtained--the last link in the chain of evidence that proved antibodies to be proteins[57] and provided a firm basis for the further development of immunology as a true science.

Confirmation by entirely independent physical chemical techniques, of the protein nature of antibodies and the accuracy of our analytical method, resulted from Elvin Kabat's studies of purified antibody preparations with Svedberg's ultracentrifuge[58] and Tiselius' electrophoresis apparatus[59] while on a Rockefellar Foundation fellowship in Uppsala. Our analytically pure bovine anti-Pn S3 behaved like a typical macroglobulin on electrophoresis and in the ultracentrifuge, and partially purified rabbit anti-egg albumin was entirely in the gamma-globulin fraction. Electrophoretic runs were made on the antibody solution before and after analysis and physical-chemical calculations corresponded exactly with the analytical values.[58]

In an effort to initiate interest in the more biological aspects of immunology I approached August Krogh, who was considered at that time the leading physiologist of the western world, and asked if he would be interested in finding out which cells of the animal body actually manufactured these remarkable immunologically specific globulins. The Danish physiologist was too busy with his studies of kidney function to branch out in this new direction, but cellular immunology soon had its beginning in Denmark and Sweden where the stimulus of the certainty of the nature of antibodies prompted Mogens Björneboe[60,61] and Astrid Fagraeus[62] to become the pioneers in that field.

Practical consequences of the introduction of the new truly quantitative techniques soon became evident. After Horsfall, Goodner, and MacLeod reported better clinical results[63] with the antibodies of relatively low molecular weight in rabbit anti-Pn sera than with the commonly used equine sera in which antibodies were mainly macroglobulins, we were joined by Joseph C. Turner, M.D. to attempt a newer regimen avoiding the necessity for dialysis and its delays and possibilities for contamination. Working with sterile equipment and reagents, we separated most of the anti-Pn of types 1, 2, and 3 rabbit sera by precipitation at 45% saturation with 37°C saturated Na^2SO^4 and inactive proteins were squeezed out, and was taken up in water made faintly alkaline with Na^2HPO^4 and run through a Berkefeld filter. Patients were typed as rapidly as possible and then infused i.v. with 600 mg of the appropriate antibody. Half an hour later a nurse brought me a sample of the person's blood and I tested the serum with PnS. The 600 mg given usually provided an excess and was sufficient for a cure, but one patient with pneumonia following a type 3 Pn mastoid infection required five such injections before an excess of antibody could be shown and recovery ensued. We had no serum sickness and no mortality as far as I was informed.[64] This proper and effective use of purified specific antibody had barely begun when therapy with penicillin supplanted it, but I believe many lives could still be saved if there were a bank of anti-Pn rabbit globulin available for quick usage. A good preparation was originally on the market, but its expense cause people to delay use of a second or third vial (no tests for excess antibody were made) often with fatal results.

At the Babies' Hospital of P and S, Hattie Alexander was using rabbit antisera for the treatment of *H. influenzae* b meningitis in infants. We assisted her with analyses of sera obtained from rabbits with varying doses and modes of injection, thereby raising the content of antibody almost tenfold and reducing the mortality to nearly zero.[65]

During the Great Depression following World War I, under Felton's leadership, a massive experiment to test a pneumococcol polysaccharide vaccine was carried out by Ekwurzel and co-workers. Thousands of members of the Civilian Conservation Corps were injected with vaccine and several camps were left out as controls. No conclusions could be drawn because the healthful outdoor activities of the corps resulted in too few pneumonia cases to be significant. Further study of the utility of an anti-Pn vaccine was required during World War II when a persistent epidemic of pneumonia was under scrutiny in an aviation camp at Sioux Falls by a group led by Colin MacLeod.

Even though the four year medical course was compressed into three, I had no difficulty acquiring almost 100 student volunteers to undergo bleedings and injections for a thorough test of vaccine containing 50 to 70 µg of each of the capsular polysaccharides of Pn types 1, 2, and 5, three of the types responsible for many of the cases at the camp. Complement was removed from the students' sera by precipitation with egg albumin and rabbit anti-egg albumin. Analysis of the supernatants was by a modification of our earlier method with the help of Catherine MacPherson[66,67] and Marie DiLapi,[68] organized so that it was possible to get duplicate values of four sera for anti-C (antibodies to the group-specific Pn polysaccharide) or anti-S1, 2 or 5 each day (see Table III in Heidelberger et al.[69] As our samples of the polysaccharides were less pure than those in today's commercial vaccines we injected only one-third of the dose initially and the rest two days later if the first dose was well tolerated. This avoided any severe reactions which might have occurred with the entire dose at once. The responses were irregular and unrelated to any previous history of pneumonia, but in most instances there was an increase over the pre-bleeding content for at least one Pn type and occasionally for all three. One student even manufactured enough antibodies to reach a level comparable to that of an average hyperimmune rabbit. But were our subjects immune? This could not be tested with living virulent pneumococci, but a paper by Barry Wood appeared at just the right time.[70] It showed that rats infected with type 1 pneumococci could be saved 12 hrs later by 0.02 ml of a rabbit anti-Pn 1 but not by 0.002 ml. Fortunately, Wood was able to spare a few ml of the antiserum, which I analyzed and could calculate that 0.02 ml gave a concentration in the blood of the cured rats of about three times as much anti-Pn S as the average anti-S in the sera of our volunteers. It seemed reasonable to assume that if three times the student response could cure an already sick animal, one-third as much might prevent infection, and this opinion I reported to the Surgeon General of the Army.

As the pneumonia epidemic was seriously interfering with teaching aviation cadets how to shoot down and bomb the enemy, the Surgeon General ordered a test of the vaccine under MacLeod's expert direction. The camp's population was randomly separated into two lines of about 8500 each. One line received 1 ml of vaccine containing 50-70 µg each of S1, 2, 5, and 7, the four Pn types causing about 60% of the pneumonias. The results are shown in Table III of MacLeod et al.[71]

After two weeks not only were there no more cases in the immunized group due to the types in the vaccine but the unvaccinated group was partially protected as well, because it was found that the vaccinated personnel no longer were carriers of these four types of Pn. As a further control, pneumonias due to Pn types not in the vaccine were roughly equal in both groups. One could conclude that henceforth any pneumococcal epidemic in a closed population could be stopped after two weeks by vaccination with the appropriate Pn Ss, many of which are now commercially available.

Other wartime projects also yielded practical results. An attempt to vaccinate against malaria between relapses was a failure,[72] but by-products with the help of Manfred Mayer were the realization that complement fixation in this disease could involve three separate reactions[73] and that the relatively few red cells parasitized in *Plasmodium malarii* infections could be concentrated 150-fold electromagnetically.[74] This facilitated diagnosis but was expensive.

In 1942 articles by W.O. Kenyon and co-workers appeared on the oxidation of cellulose.[75,76] Since Pn S3 is a polymer of cellobiouronic acid (D-GlcA and D-glc) and Pn S8 contains 50% of the same substance,[77] our theory of the precipitin reaction made it likely that oxidized cellulose would precipitate anti-Pn3 and anti-Pn 8. I wrote for samples, neutralized some of the strongly acid material and got immediate heavy precipitates in equine antisera to both types. At lunch in the faculty dining room at P and S, a surgeon remarked that they were using pads of oxidized cellulose as hemostatics and also because the pads could be left in wounds and would eventually dissolve and disappear. I asked for a few cc of such patients' blood or urine and by addition of small amounts of anti-Pn 3 or 8 it was possible to tell almost the exact hour when the pads were gone. With Gladys Hobby we tried to immunize mice against type 8 pneumococci with solutions of oxidized cellulose but were unsuccessful,[78] probably because oxidation with the NO^2 used had reduced the molecular size of the material, as indicated by the lack of viscosity of its solutions.

Other by-products of the work on precipitins were quantitative inhibition tests with sodium isomaltobiouronate and anti-Pn2[79] which pointed toward the formula for S2 found later; also inhibition tests with the same antiserum and anti-Pn23 showing differences between L-rha and D-rha;[80] and even inequalities of inhibition by the stereoisomers R and S of pyruvic acid linked as a ketal to a polysaccharide.[81]

Another almost immediate application of our work eventually grew into a major project. Avery's far-reaching intuition had convinced him that not only would other microorganisms contain immunologically active polysaccharides, but that analogous sugar polymers might even occur "free in nature" as he put it. Meanwhile, there had been an epidemic of pneumonia in guinea pigs due to a gram-negative Friedländer's bacillus (now designated *Klebsiella* type 2). We isolated its capsular substance,[82] a polysaccharide closely enough related to Pn S2 for mutual agglutination, precipitation, and even a degree of mouse protection between the antisera and these microbes belonging to biologically unrelated, but chemically related strains. The actual chemical structures of the polysaccharides were determined much later.[22,83] That of the *Klebsiella* type 2 capsular substance was found to be as follows:[82]

$$\rightarrow3)\beta D\text{-glc}(1\rightarrow4)\beta D\text{-man}(1\rightarrow4)\alpha D\text{-glc}(1]\alpha D\text{-GlcA}(1^{13}n$$

Among Avery's "free in nature" substances we soon found that gum arabic cross-reacted with anti-Pn 2, particularly after knocking off with acid[84] the labile arabofuranose groups that blocked access of antibodies to glcA which then became lateral end groups as in PnS2.[22] Serological properties of other plant gums were studied simultaneously in Marrack's laboratory and ours.[85,86] Many new products began to flow into our lab at P and S so that one almost had to concentrate on a major study of relations between chemical structure and immunological specificity. This was made more urgent by the proposal during World War II to use dextrans and/or synthetic polyglucoses as blood substitutes. Many crossreacted heavily in anti-Pn sera,[87,88,89,90,91,92] so that severe reactions seemed possible during or after their transfusion in occasional patients.

As a consequence of our quantitative theory of precipitin reaction one could predict that if a polysaccharide of unknown constitution contained one or more sugars in the same or similar linkage as in a Pn S of known structure, cross-precipitation would be likely: one could often tell by a qualitative test in a few minutes whether or not the unknown had non-reducing lateral end-groups of D-glcA or L-rha by testing with anti-Pn 2 or 23, respectively. To obtain this structural knowledge by the strictly chemical methods in use from the 1930's to 1960's or '70's would have required some weeks or months. Supplementation with quantitative analyses often led to more detailed information and predictions, as in the precipitation of anti-Pn3 or 8 by PnS8 or 3, respectively.[93,94] The structure of Pn S8 was not known until later, but not only could similarities in content of sugars be predicted, but also that linearity was to be expected rather than chain-branching. A detailed picture of the heterogeneity of anti-Pn3 and 8 was also obtained. We could show too, that D-glc and D-man,[95] as well as D-glcA and D-manA were similar serologically and could cause cross-reactions even though not fully exchangeable. Studies of other cross-precipitations among Pn types[96,97] also led to useful results as knowledge of the structures of more PnSs slowly became known and formed the basis for a tentative hypothesis for the prediction of reciprocal cross-precipitation.

As examples of other possibilities afforded by studies of cross-reactions we looked into the structural and immunological similarities and differences of the capsular polysaccharides of two widely different families of microorganisms, the 80-odd serological types of gram-positive pneumococci and the equally numerous serological types of gram-negative rods of *Klebsiella* (K1). Wolfgang Nimmich has isolated 81 of the capsular polysaccharides[98,99] and sent liberal samples for prolonged series of qualitative and quantitative tests. Many of the types were first recognized by microbiologists Sverre Dick Henriksen and Jorunn Eriksen. The latter and Stefan Stirm supplied rabbit antisera for our cooperative work, while Bengt Lindberg and his co-workers[100] and the G.G.S. Dutton and Stirm groups were responsible for the determination of many K1S structures.

Three generalizations may be made:

1. Many PnSs contain aminosugars, Kl capsular polysaccharides (K1Ss) never, so far.
2. Many K1Ss contain D-man; PnSs, none so far.
3. As in Rhizobiol polysaccharides, pyruvic acid in ketal linkage to two hydroxyls of a sugar is often present in K1s, seldom in PnS (only in types 4 and 27 so far.[101,102]

Strangely, although omnipresent in animal cells, pyruvic acid may make a sugar immunodominant.

Tables of the results of cross-precipitations and reciprocal data in anti-Pn are given in[95,96,100,101,102,103,104,105,106] data on anti-K1 in.[107]

REFERENCES

1. Metzger, F.J. and Heidelberger, M. J., *Am. Chem. Soc.* 31, 1040, 1909.
2. Bogert, M.T. and Heidelberger, M.J., *Am. Chem. Soc.* 31, 183, 1912.
3. Bogert, M.T. and Heidelberger, M. J., *Am. Chem. Soc.* 34, 183, 1912.
4. Willstätter, R. and Heidelberger, M., *Ber. Deut. Chem. Ges.* 46, 517, 1913.
5. Jacobs, W.A. and Heidelberger, M., *Proc. Natl. Acad. Sci.* USA 1, 226, 1915.
6. Ehrlich, P., *Studies on Immunity*, Wiley, New York, 1906.
7. Arrhenius, S., *Immunochemistry*, MacMillan, New York, 1907.
8. Bordet, J., *Traité de l'Immunité*, Masson, Paris, 1920.
9. Wells, H.G., *Chemical Aspects of Immunity*, 1st Edition, Chem. Catalog Company, New York, 1924.
10. Heidelberger, M., *J. Biol. Chem.* 53, 31, 1922.
11. Heidelberger, M. and Landsteiner, K. *J. Exp. Med.* 38, 561, 1923.
12. Landsteiner, K. and Heidelberger, M., *J. Gen. Physiol.* 6, 131, 1923.
13. Dochez, A.R. and Avery, O.T., *J. Exp. Med.* 26, 472, 1971.
14. Heidelberger, M. and Avery, O.T., *J. Exp. Med.* 38, 73, 81, 1923.
15. Heidelberger, M. and Avery, O.T., *J. Exp. Med.* 40, 301, 1924.
16. Avery, O.T. and Heidelberger, M., *J. Exp. Med.* 42, 367, 1924.
17. Avery, O.T. and Heidelberger, M., *J. Exp. Med.* 42, 367, 1924.
18. Heidelberger, M., Goebel, W.F., and Avery, O.T., *J. Exp. Med.* 42, 727, 1925.
19. Heidelberger, M., Kendall, F.E., and Scherp, H.W., *J. Exp. Med.* 64, 559, 1936.
20. Heidelberger, M., MacLeod, C.M., Markowitz, H., and Roe, A.S., *J. Exp. Med.* 91, 341, 1950.
21. Stacey, M., *Quart. Rev.* 1, 147, 1947.
22. Butler, K. and Stacey, M., *J. Chem. Soc.* 1537, 1955.
23. Kenne, L., Lindberg, B., and Svensson, S., *Carbohydr. Res.* 40, 69, 1975.

24.   Heidelberger, M. and Goebel, W.F., *J. Biol. Chem.* 70, 613, 1926.
25.   Heidelberger, M. and Goebel, W.F., *J. Biol. Chem.* 74, 613, 1927.
26.   Hotchkiss, R.D. and Goebel, W.F., *J. Biol. Chem.* 121, 195, 1937.
27.   Reeves, R.E. and Reeves, G., *J. Biol. Chem.* 139, 511, 1937.
28.   Enders, J.F. and Pappenheimer, A.M., Jr., *Proc. Soc. Exp. Biol. Med.* 31, 37, 1933.
29.   Avery, O.T. and Goebel, W.F., *J. Exp. Med.* 58, 731, 1933.
30.   Lindberg, B., Lindqvist, B., Lönngren, J., and Powell, D. A., *Carbohydr. Res.* 78, 111, 1980.
31.   Guy, R. C. E., How, M. J., Stacey, M., and Heidelberger, M., *J. Biol. Chem.* 242:5106, 1957.
32.   Lancefield, R.C., *J. Exp. Med.* 47, 469, 1928.
33.   Schmidt, W.C., *J. Exp. Med.* 95, 105, 1952.
34.   Barkulis, S. S. and Jones, M. F., *J. Bacteriol.* 74, 207, 1957.
35.   McCarty, M. and Lancefield, R. C., *J. Exp. Med.* 102, 11, 1955.
36.   Kraus, R., *Weiner Klin. Wochenschr.*, 796, 1897.
37.   Wu, H., Cheng, L.-H., and Li, C.-P., *Proc. Soc. Exp. Biol.* Med. 25, 853, 1927.
38.   Wu, H., Sah, P.P.T., and Li, C.-P., *Proc. Soc. Exp. Biol. Med.* 26, 737, 1928.
39.   Felton, L.D., *J. Inf. Dis.* 37, 199, 1925.
40.   Heidelberger, M. and Kendall, F. E., *J. Exp. Med.* 50, 809, 1929.
41.   Heidelberger, M. and Kendall, F. E., *J. Exp. Med.*, 61, 563, 1935.
42.   Heidelberger, M. and Kendall, F. E., *J. Exp. Med.*, 62, 467, 1935.
43.   Heidelberger, M. and Kendall, F. E., *J. Exp. Med.*, 62, 697, 1935.
44.   Goodner, K., Horsfall, F. L., and Bauer, J. H., *Soc. Exp. Biol. Med.*, 44, 617, 1936.
45.   Heidelberger, M. and Pedersen, K. O., *J. Exp. Med.*, 65, 393, 1937.
46.   Marrack, J. R. *Chemistry of Antigens and Antibodies*, 2nd Edition, HMSO, London, 1938.
47.   Heidelberger, M. and Kabat, E. A., *J. Exp. Med.*, 60, 643, 1934.
48.   Heidelberger, M. and Kabat, E. A., *J. Exp. Med.*, 65, 885, 1937.
49.   Heidelberger, M. and Kabat, E. A., *J. Exp. Med.*, 63, 737, 1936.
50.   Zinsser, H., *J. Immunol.*, 18, 483, 1930.
51.   Heidelberger, M., *J. Exp. Med.*, 73, 681, 1941.
52.   Heidelberger, M. et al., *J. Exp. Med.*, 75, 695, 1941.
53.   Heidelberger, M., *J. Exp. Med.*, 74, 359, 1941.
54.   Pillemer, L., Ecker, E. E., Oncley, J. L., and Cohn, E., *J. Exp. Med.*, 24, 297, 1941.
55.   Heidelberger, M. Weil, A. J., and Treffers, H. P., *J. Exp. Med.*, 73, 695, 1941.
56.   Heidelberger, M., Kendall, F. E., and Teorell, T., *J. Exp. Med.*, 63, 813, 1936.
57.   Heidelberger, M. and Kabat, E. A., *J. Exp. Med.*, 67, 181, 1938.
58.   Kabat, E.A., *J. Exp. Med.*, 69, 103, 1939.
59.   Tiselius, A. and Kabat, E. A., *J. Exp. Med.*, 69, 119, 1939.
60.   Björneboe, M. and Gormsen, H., *Nord. Med.*, 9, 891, 1941.
61.   Björneboe, M. and Lundquist, F. *J. Immunol.*, 55, 125, 1947.
62.   Bing, J., Fagraeus, A., and Thorell, B., *Acta. Physiol. Scand.*, 10, 282, 1945.
63.   Horsfall, F. L., Jr., Goodner, K., and MacLeod, C. M., *Science*, 84, 579, 1936.
64.   Heidelberger, M., Turner, J. C., and Soo Hoo, C. M., *Proc. Soc. Exp. Biol. Med.*, 7, 734, 1938.
65.   Alexander, H. E., Heidelberger, M., and Leidy, G., *Yale J. Biol. Med.*, 24, 16, 425, 1944.
66.   Heidelberger, M. and MacPherson, C. F. C., *Science*, 97, 405, 1943.
67.   Heidelberger, M. and MacPherson, C. F. C., *Science*, 98, 63, 1943.
68.   Heidelberger, M. and DiLapi, M., *J. Immunol.*, 61, 153, 1949.
69.   Heidelberger, M., MacLeod, C. M., Kaiser, S. J., and Robinson, B., *J. Exp. Med.*, 83, 303, 1946.
70.   Wood, W.B., Jr., *J. Exp. Med.*, 73, 201, 1941.
71.   MacLeod, C. M., Hodges, R. G., Heidelberger, M., and Bernhard, W. G., *J. Exp. Med.*, 24, 82, 445, 1945.
72.   Heidelberger, M., Coates, W. A., and Mayer, M. M., *J. Immunol.*, 53, 101, 1946.
73.   Heidelberger, M. and Mayer, M. M., *J. Immunol.*, 54, 89, 1946.
74.   Heidelberger, M., Mayer, M. M., and Demarest, C. R., *J. Immunol.*, 53, 325, 1946.
75.   Yackel, E. C. and Kenyon, W. O., *J. Am. Chem. Soc.*, 64, 121, 1942.
76.   Yackel, E. C., Kenyon, W. O., and Unruh, C. C., *J. Am. Chem. Soc.*, 64, 127, 1942.

77. Jones, J. K. N. and Perry, M. B., *J. Am. Chem. Soc.*, 79, 2787, 1957.
78. Heidelberger, M. and Hobby, G. L., *Proc. Natl. Acad. Sci.*, USA 28, 516, 1942.
79. Heidelberger, M., Roy, N., and Glaudemans, C. P. J., *Biochemistry*, 8, 4822, 1969.
80. Heidelberger, M. and Ashwell, G., *Atti. Accad. Naz. Lincei.*, 4, 44, 695, 1968.
81. Heidelberger, M., Kvarnström, I., Eriksen, J., Nimmich, W., and Dudman, W. F., *Proc. Natl. Acad. Sci. USA*, 77, 4244, 1980.
82. Heidelberger, M., Goebel, W. F., and Avery, O. T., *J. Exp. Med.*, 42, 701, 1925.
83. Gahan, L. C., Sandford, P. A., and Conrad, H. E., *Biochemistry*, 6, 2755, 1967.
84. Heidelberger, M., Avery, O. T., and Goebel, W. F., *J. Exp. Med.*, 49, 807, 1929.
85. Heidelberger, M., *Prog. Chem. Org. Nat. Prod.*, 18, 504, 1960.
86. Heidelberger, M., *Prog. Chem. Org. Nat. Prod.*, 42, 287, 1982.
87. Heidelberger, M. and Adams, J., *J. Exp. Med.*, 103, 189, 1956.
88. Heidelberger, M., *J. Exp. Med.*, 111, 33, 1960.
89. Heidelberger, M., Jahrmärker, H., Björklund, B., and Adams, J., *J. Immunol.*, 48, 419, 1957.
90. Heidelberger, M., Björklund, B., and Larner, J., *J. Immunol.*, 78, 431, 1957.
91. Heidelberger, M., Jahrmärker, H., and Cordoba, F., *J. Immunol.*, 78, 427, 1957.
92. Goodman, J. W. and Kabat, E. A., *J. Immunol.*, 84, 333, 347, 1960.
93. Heidelberger, M., Kabat, E. A., and Shrivastava, D. L., *J. Exp. Med.*, 65, 487, 1937.
94. Heidelberger, M. and Mayer, M. M., *J. Exp. Med.*, 75, 35, 1942.
95. Heidelberger, M. and Slodki, M. E., *Carbohydr. Res.*, 24, 401, 1972.
96. Heidelberger, M. and Tyler, J. M., *J. Exp. Med.*, 120, 711, 1964.
97. Heidelberger, M., *Infect. and Immun.*, 41, 1239, 1983.
98. Nimmich, W., *Zeitschr. Med. Mikrobiol. Immunol.*, 154, 147, 1968.
99. Nimmich, W., *Acta. Biol. Med. Germ.*, 26, 397, 1970.
100. Kenne, L. and Lindberg, B., in *The Polysaccharides*, G.O. Aspinall, ed., Volume 2, Academic Press, New York, 1983, chap. 6.
101. Heidelberger, M. and Nimmich, W., *J. Immunol.*, 109, 1337, 1976.
102. Heidelberger, M. and Nimmich, W., *Immunochemistry*, 13, 67, 1977.
103. Heidelberger, M. and Nimmich, W., *Ann. Immunol.*, (Inst. Pasteur) 128, 225, 1977.
104. Heidelberger, M., Nimmich, W., Eriksen, J., and Stirm, S., *Acta. Path. Microbiol. Scand. B.*, 86, 313, 1978.
105. Heidelberger, M. and Dutton, G. G. S., *Acta. Path. Microbiol. Scand. C.*, 90, 87, 1982.
106. Heidelberger, M. and Dutton, G. G. S., *Acta. Path. Microbiol. Scand. C.*, 90, 87, 1982.
107. Heidelberger, M, Nimmich, W., Eriksen, J., Dutton, G. G. S., Stirm, S., and Fang, C. T., *Acta. Path. Microbiol. Scand. C.*, 83, 397, 1975.

Chapter 2

DARWIN AND PASTEUR AND CAUSAL REALISM
ONE IMMUNOLOGIST'S VIEW OF THINGS

David W. Talmage

1858 was the year of the great Lincoln-Douglas debates that preceded the American Civil War and changed forever the face of American society. 1858 was also a banner year for the struggle of reason over tradition in the biological sciences. This was the year that Darwin and Wallace first published their concept of evolution through natural selection, and Pasteur demonstrated to the wine industry of France that fermentation was caused by a living organism. The significance of Darwin and Pasteur was not so much in the advances in scientific knowledge that they achieved as in the development of a new scientific philosophy, a new way of thinking about reality and the relative importance of reason, causality, chance and observation. It is my thesis that this was the beginning of the most recent step in the evolution of contemporary philosophy of science, a step that was both necessary for and a dominant factor in the explosion of knowledge that has occurred in the biological sciences in the last 130 years.

The human species is unique in that the knowledge gained in one generation is passed on to the next. Thus, knowledge has grown by innumerable small additions. But the way that knowledge is organized has changed only a few times in history. I can discern five distinct steps in this development, each step essential for those following. And each succeeding step has built on and continued to use the preceding accomplishments, a true evolution of human thought. These five steps are tool making, logic and reason, controlled observation, mathematics and causal realism.

I will try to show, using my own experience as an example, how each individual scientist climbs these five steps. Like the evolution of the species, in scientific philosophy ontogeny recapitulates phylogeny.

TECHNOLOGY

The foundation step of science is technology. The ability to make tools dates from the earliest prehistoric humans. At first tools were made of stone, then of bronze (3000 B.C.), glass (1500 B.C.), iron (1100 B.C.) and paper (105 A.D.). Agriculture and domestication of animals began in Mesopotamia and Egypt between 4000 and 3000 B.C. The inventions of the wheel, the lever, writing and numbers all occurred around that time.

I was exposed to technology at an early age with electric lights, showers, door knobs and bicycles. I was given wooden blocks to play with at the age of 4. I used them to build houses and experiment with numbers. I still remember the excitement when I discovered that two piles of 14 blocks added up to 28.

It is interesting that the zero to indicate an empty decimal place was not introduced until around 600 A.D. in India. The Arabs brought the zero to Spain where it was introduced into Europe around 1100 A.D. The decimal numbering system that evolved from that event has become today the one truly international language. It also may have been the technological discovery that sparked the explosion of modern science.

0-8493-4722-X/94/$0.00 + $.50

LOGIC AND REASON

The ancient Greeks worshipped reason and to them geometry was pure reason. In high school I was merely told that geometry would improve my mind, but the exhortation was unnecessary. I was fascinated by the story of Pythagoras and the classic theorem that bears his name. Starting with a few unquestioned axioms, it was possible to arrive at a firm conclusion by pure logic. Here was something you could hang your hat on.

The Pythagorean theorem does not involve observations or questions of cause. It is a generalization based on pure deductive reasoning. It is impossible to say why the square of the hypotenuse should equal the sum of the squares of the other two sides. That's just the way it is. Understand it and admire it. Geometry reached its greatest heights under Euclid around 300 B.C.

The concept of cause was probably introduced by Aristotle, the greatest of the Greek philosophers. Aristotle had an explanation for everything, but his explanations were derived from logic, which was permanent and could be trusted, not from observation, which was temporary and deceptive. Each cause must have a preceding cause and the ultimate cause was God. I was raised to believe that.

But it is difficult to concentrate on ultimate causes in today's world, and it was so in the world of my childhood. When the bicycle was broken it was because there was a hole in the tire or the chain was off the cogs. We live in a much more mechanical world than Aristotle did. We are overwhelmed by immediate causes and cannot be bothered by ultimate causes.

OBSERVATION

The idea that observation might be more important than logic probably stems from Copernicus and his time. Copernicus was 19 years old when Columbus by direct observation convinced his peers that the world was round. When asked by the Pope to straighten out the mess with the calendar, Copernicus decided to have a look at the heavens. He came up with the idea that the earth and the planets revolve around the sun and the result is what we know as modern science. As we shall see, scientists differ from each other in many ways, but they all share one common belief, namely that the ultimate test of theory and knowledge is observation.

Copernicus may have been influenced by an associate at the University of Padua named Girolamo Fracastoro. The latter was an astronomer and physician who proposed in 1538 that the planets revolve around a central fixed point. As a physician he observed the similarities in the symptoms of disease in the same epidemic and proposed the germ theory of disease with these words, "Contagion is an infection that passes from one thing to another....The infection is precisely similar in both the carrier and the receiver of the contagion....The term is more correctly used when infection originates in very small imperceptible particles."

I was introduced to the concept of contagion at the age of 8 when I came down with typhoid fever. In the absence of antibiotics the disease ran its course over several weeks. What impressed me at the time and what I remember from the incident is what my parents did after I was over the infection. They sealed up my bedroom with tape and fumigated it with some kind of gas. It was really important to get rid of all those imperceptible particles.

Fracastoro's ideas were based on a careful balancing of observation, reason and causality and the postulation of an objective reality behind the perceptible. The germ theory of disease did not make much progress over the next two centuries partly because of the absence of good microscopes and partly because the science of physics went off in a slightly different direction.

Tycho Brahe was the king's astronomer in Prague, and Johannes Kepler was his assistant. The king needed an astronomer for the same reason that Nancy Reagan did, in order to know the proper time for everything. Brahe took his job seriously and made very many observations of the positions of the planets over many years and accurately mapped the stars even though he did not have a telescope. And Kepler was a genius and with Brahe's observations he was able to plot the orbits of the planets in three dimensional space. His tools were observation and the reasoning of Euclidean geometry. Kepler discovered that the planetary orbits were ellipses with the sun at one focus. The earth was not even in the planes of the planetary orbits. Kepler discovered some other regularities like the fact that lines from the planets and earth to the sun swept out equal areas in equal times. Complementing this fact was the observation that the cute of the average distance of a planet from the sun was proportional to the square of the time for one full orbit. These were called Kepler's laws and greatly enhanced the acceptance of the Copernican model of the solar system. When I was ten I tried to work out the orbit of the moon to predict the next moon eclipse. This only required that lines be drawn on the inner surface of the sphere of the stars to represent the orbits of the sun and moon. I can appreciate the difficulty in solving the three dimensional orbits of the planets from accumulated point observations.

Galileo Galilei was a mathematician of Florence who applied technology to basic science even faster than we do today. In 1608 he heard that someone in Holland had invented a telescope. He immediately made one for himself and in 1609 he reported that he could see four moons circling around Jupiter. This not only confirmed the Copernican system firmly in his mind, but for many years these moons with their short but regular orbits became the celestial clock from which longitude was calculated. Galileo also worked out the mathematics of acceleration, supposedly by dropping objects off the leaning tower of Pisa. Galileo supported the Copernican system with the power of reason and observation. For his efforts he was placed under house arrest by the church.

MATHEMATICS

Isaac Newton's father died before he was born and he was raised by his maternal grandmother in Woolsthorpe, Lincolnshire, England. He was sent off to Trinity College, Cambridge in 1661 at the age of 19. Four years later he received his Bachelor's degree just before the college was shut down because of the Great Plague. One of his accomplishments while a student was the discovery of the binomial theorem. His main interests were in geometry and optics.

Newton spent two years on the farm in Lincolnshire while the Great Plague burned itself out. Nobody had the foggiest notion what caused it. But Newton did not waste his time. During those two years he laid the ground work for his discoveries of the law of gravitation and light refraction and the invention of the calculus.

About gravity he later wrote, "In the same year (1666) I began to think of gravity extending to the orb of the Moon...compared the force required to keep the Moon in her orb with the force of gravity at the surface of the earth and found them to answer pretty nearly." Newton knew that the average diameter of the moon's orbit was 60 times the diameter of the earth. Ptolemy had calculated the ratio as 59, but Copernicus and Huygens had made it 60. He also knew that an object (such as a cannon ball) released in a horizontal direction at the earth's surface at any velocity would drop 15½ Paris feet (approximately 15 English feet) in the first second. By his calculations, the moon in its orbit bent from a straight line exactly 15½ Paris feet in one minute. Thus the moon fell in one minute exactly the same distance the cannon ball fell in one second. Since the distance an object fell was known from Galileo to be proportional to the square of the time, he arrived at the idea that the force of gravity fell off as the square of the distance. It is interesting but fortuitous that the number of earth radii to the moon is the same as the number of seconds in a minute.

We might say that at this point Newton had a descriptive hypothesis. It took him 20 years to work out his "proof" for a universal law of gravitation. The most difficult part was to show by geometry that the force of gravity at the earth's surface and beyond was the same as if all the mass of the earth was at its center. In the process he perfected his calculus and extended the inverse square law to orbits of all the six planets and those of the nine known moons of Jupiter and Saturn. He did this by showing that all the observations of Kepler, Galileo and other astronomers fit exactly with the inverse square law of gravity and certain other assumptions such as the law of inertia and the equivalence of gravitational inertial masses.

One might object on logical grounds to the practice of making observations and generalizing them into laws. But in 300 years no exception nor even a fractional deviation from the inverse square law has ever been found. Newton was a strong believer in God and causality, and the two concepts were probably linked in his mind as the creator of order in the universe. However, Newton did not wish to become involved in religious controversy with Galileo's troubles with the church only a few years past. So he refrained from speculating about the cause of gravity and said, "I frame no hypotheses." He was content to make mathematical generalizations of his observations and those of others, and to leave the causes to God. However, Newton did make a causal analogy. Although he refused to speculate as to the cause of gravity, he proposed that whatever it was that made the apple drop to the earth also made the moon stay in its orbit. Newton had only four rules of reasoning in philosophy and the first two were as follows:

"I. We are to admit no more causes of natural things than such as are both true and sufficient to explain their appearances.
II. Therefore to the same natural effects we must, as far as possible, assign the same natural causes."

Newton's distaste for speculation led some philosophers of science to downgrade the usefulness of all hypotheses. The word developed a bad connotation to the point that the Scottish philosopher and mathematician Reid could write the following in 1785:

"Scientific discoveries have always been made by patient observation, by accurate experiments, or by conclusions drawn by strict
reasoning from observations and experiments, and such discoveries

have always tended to refute, but not to confirm, the theories and hypotheses which ingenious men have invented.

"As this is a fact confirmed by the history of philosophy in all past ages it ought to have taught man, long ago, to treat with contempt hypotheses in every branch of philosophy, and to despair of ever advancing real knowledge in that way."

Among the reasons given by Reid for avoiding hypotheses were that it would prejudice the impartiality of the scientist and would assume that the mind of man was capable of understanding the works of God.

In the nineteenth century causal hypotheses came under attack from another direction, the logical positivism of Comte and the Vienna school led by Ernst Mach. Comte was a French philosopher who claimed that human understanding of the universe had advanced through three "states": theological, metaphysical, and positive. Comte viewed positivism as the most advanced state in which one accepts only the objective evidence of the five senses. In retrospect Comte's views seem to be a reaction to the claims of the church that every cause had an earlier cause and God was the first cause. By eliminating causal hypotheses altogether Comte freed himself from the dominance of the church. Thus, the concept of God first prevented the use of causal hypotheses for fear of intruding on His domain, and then the revolt from God prevented its use for fear of giving Him too much credit.

Ernst Mach was a physicist and leader of the Vienna school of logical positivists. His work with the physics of sound led the adoption of the Mach unit of sound velocity. He refused to accept the concept of the atom because it could not be demonstrated objectively to his senses. He was a friend and mentor to Einstein and influenced him greatly by his refusal to accept Newton's concepts of absolute space and time. Mach thought that objectively all motion was relative to the total mass of the visible stars and this is still known as Mach's principle.

Newton's fondest hope was that his methodology of observation and mathematical generalization would solve the problems of mankind. What more important problem could there be than the plague that closed down universities. But significant progress was not made in this direction for 200 years. Could it be that his scientific philosophy, so brilliant at analyzing the orbits of the moons and planets, was not adequate for the complexities of biology? It is true that one factor delaying the advance of microbiology was the absence of a decent microscope. But why was the microscope so long in coming? Glasses had been widely used in Europe since the 14th century and Leeuwenhoek, a contemporary of Newton, had observed bacteria with a primitive scope in the 17th century. But nobody asked the right questions. If anyone had even suggested that the little bacteria were the cause of disease they would have been interfering with God's work. Apparently it was permitted to build telescopes and study the moons of Jupiter, but microscopes had to wait for a change in philosophy.

There was one important observation made in 1798 that must have stimulated a little change in attitude. This was the introduction of cowpox vaccination. Edward Jenner was a country doctor in England who had observed that milkmaids frequently escaped affliction with small pox. It was known that they contracted a much less severe disease on their fingers called cow pox. Without any idea of what caused the poxes (pustules), Jenner decided to test the notion that one disease (cow pox) could prevent the development of another disease (small pox). It was already known that a person who survived an attack of small pox would usually not suffer a second attack for the remainder of his life, and it was also known that small pox could be transmitted by taking pus from the pox of a small pox patient and scratching it into the skin of someone who had never had the disease. This practice, called variolation, had been used for some years because its 2-3% mortality was an acceptable risk compared to the 50% mortality and severe scarring of survivors seen during a small pox epidemic.

So Jenner took pus from the cow pox on the finger of a milkmaid and scratched it into the skin of an eight year old boy. The boy developed a pox at the site of application, but this healed within a couple of weeks without further spread. Then to test his hypothesis Jenner transferred pus from a small pox patient to the same boy and observed that he only developed a small bump. This was a very simple if courageous experiment and it is not clear that Jenner's hypothesis was causal, but it must have led to a lot of speculation as to the cause of this remarkable result. And it demonstrated that man could profitably intervene in what had been considered God's work. It also led very quickly to the control of the most deadly disease known to man.

CAUSAL REALISM

Pasteur devised a dramatic test of a causal hypothesis. It was known that bacteria growing in broth could be killed by boiling but the bacteria would return again in a few days if the container were left open to the air. The current theory was that bacteria were spontaneously generated from the ingredients in the broth and the oxygen in the air. Pasteur proposed an alternative cause of the contamination, namely that the bacteria came from the dust in the air. The controversy became very heated and the French Academy of Sciences proposed a test of Pasteur's hypothesis in the academy chambers. Pasteur built glass flasks that were sealed except for a long curved tube that let in the oxygen but no dust. The broth in the flasks was sterilized and left at the Academy for months without becoming contaminated. This ended the controversy of spontaneous generation.

But Pasteur's demonstration did a great deal more. It established the value of the causal hypothesis in the biomedical sciences. Thus while the physical sciences have grown more and more dependent on pure mathematics, biology has exploited the pragmatic value of causation. The purposes of this research are 1) to understand the causes of natural phenomena (basic science) and 2) to control natural phenomena for the benefit of mankind (applied science). This differs from the purposes of physical science which are 1) to describe natural phenomena with mathematical equations and 2) to predict past and future events.

The philosophers of science argue endlessly about the logic and validity of the scientific method. Most claim to be realists of one sort or another. I do not claim to be a philosopher, but as a practicing scientist it seems to me that the following are the basic assumptions of causal realism that were made by Darwin and Pasteur and are made by biologists today.

(1)   **All reproducible phenomena including those involving statistically significant variations are based on a reality that is defined as the cause, even though that reality is not known nor observable.** Pasteur was able to postulate that there were invisible living things in the dust of the air that

contaminated his broth even though he could not see them nor know what they were.

(2)   **It is useful to understand the immediate, probable cause of a phenomenon in general terms even if the exact, certain and ultimate causes seem unobtainable.** Darwin was content to determine the cause of species variation before understanding the origin of life.

(3)   **It is useful to propose and test for a common cause of related phenomena even if this cause is unknown.** Pasteur thought there was a relationship between fermentation of wine and the contamination of his broth and proposed that both were due to living microorganisms. It is important to note that this follows Newton's second principle and his analogy between the causes of the motion of the apple and the moon.

(4)   **The probable cause of a phenomenon may be obtained by exclusion.** The philosophers of the 18th century had said it was impossible to list all the possible causes, but Pasteur showed that it was possible to state the alternatives in sufficiently general terms that they covered all possibilities. Thus, either Pasteur's broth became contaminated through spontaneous generation or because bacteria came in from the outside.

(5)   **The best method to determine the cause of a natural phenomenon is through controlled quantitative experiments designed to distinguish between alternative hypotheses.**

Using these principles scientists have created an explosion of knowledge the likes of which the world has never seen. The first human pathogen, the gonococcus, was identified by Neisser in 1897. Ten more, including the tubercle bacillus and diphtheria were discovered in the next ten years. Viruses were discovered by Ivanovski in 1892 and blood group antigens by Landsteiner in 1900. DNA was discovered in 1872 by Miescher and proved to be the stuff that genes are made from in 1946 by Avery, MacCleod and McCarty. The genetic code was completed in 1966 and recombinant DNA first used in 1973.

APPLICATION TO IMMUNOLOGY

Immunology, like much of modern biology, grew out of the marriage between the quantitative techniques of the physical sciences and the pragmatic realism of physicians. Jenner was a country doctor; Pasteur was an industrial biochemist; Darwin went to medical school. Much of the research in microbiology and immunology has taken place in medical schools and with funds provided by the National Institutes of Health.

I finished medical school in 1944, and then spent nine months in a rotating internship in Atlanta, two years in military service in Korea and two more years in hospital training in St. Louis. I then had the good fortune to spend two years with Frank Dixon, who was a master at experimental design. Radioisotopes had just been introduced as a quantitative tool in medical research. Frank taught me how to label proteins with radioactive iodine and do experiments involving 50 rabbits. We exposed the rabbits to varying doses of X-radiation and injected them with labeled antigen. The production of antibodies three or four days later caused the antigen to be rapidly cleared from the blood stream and it was easy to establish that small doses of radiation that reduced only the blood lymphocyte count also inhibited the antibody response.

In 1952 I moved to the University of Chicago and made use of the opportunity to work with William Taliaferro who was an authority on cells of the immune system. One year after arriving in Chicago the Watson-Crick model of DNA was published and it soon became obvious that proteins were synthesized by ribosomes through the translation of a trip code residing in the DNA and transmitted to the cytoplasm by means of a messenger RNA. When Jerne came out with his natural selection model of antibody formation in 1955, it was clear that although the model was generally sound, it clashed with the new molecular biology in postulating the replication of protein molecules. It was an easy matter to substitute cell selection for molecule selection and advance the first cell selection theory of antibody formation in 1957. In this way the ideas of Darwin and Pasteur were finally unified.

APPLICABILITY TO PHYSICS

Causality and realism have long been controversial topics among physicists. It is significant that Einstein criticized quantum mechanics as incomplete because of its lack of causality. Yet Einstein's own theories of special and general relativity lack the degree of causal realism that would make them intelligible to biological scientists. They are rather mathematical equations that make accurate predictions of the results of experiments. But the cause of these results and the reality they represent are far from clear.

For example, it has been observed repeatedly that mass increases and time slows down in a particle traveling near the speed of light. A causal realist is forced to conclude that these effects are real (not just appearances) and must have a cause. For it was from observations of mass increase that Einstein derived the famous formula, $E = mc^2$ that led to the development of nuclear bombs and nuclear energy. Could anything be more real? And real time effects have been confirmed by clocks flown around the world on jets.

Much like Newton on the cause of gravity, Einstein is silent on the cause of his "relativistic effects." And the concept of symmetry in these effects, an essential part of "relativity," seem incompatible with the principles of causal realism. In the general theory, Einstein may have toyed with the idea of ascribing relativistic effects to motion relative to the mass of the universe, according to Mach's principle. He seems to have given up in the end, however, because it conflicted with the concept of symmetry.

The problem with quantum mechanics is even worse and it is doubtful if anyone can understand the reality represented by quantum equations. Thus, modern physics presents a serious dilemma to the causal realist. Either he must concede that the principles of causal realism are not generally applicable to all of nature or he must assert, as I do, that a mathematical description of nature is incomplete and inadequate as an explanation of reality.

REFERENCES

Adair, R.K.,   *The Great Design*, Oxford University Press, New York, 1987.
Barrow, J.D.,   *The World Within the World*, Oxford University Press, Oxford, 1988.
Bergmann, P.G.,   *The Riddle of Gravitation*, Charles Schribner's Sons, New York, 1987.
Burke, J.,   *The Day the Universe Changed*, Little, Brown and Company, Boston, 1985.
Burnet, F.M.,   A modification of Jerne's theory of antibody production using the concept of clonal selection, *Aust. J. Sci.* 20:67, 1957.

Clark, R.W.,   *Einstein: The Life and Times*, The World Publishing Company, New York, 1971.

Cohen, I.B.,   *Revolution in Science*, Harvard University Press, Cambridge, 1985.

Dubos, R.,   *The Unseen World*, Rockefeller University Press, 1962.

Feynman, R.P.,   *QED: The Strange Theory of Light and Matter*, Princeton University Press, Princeton, 1985.

Foster, W.D.,   *A History of Medical Bacteriology and Immunology*, William Heineman Medical Books, Philadelphia, 1970.

Friedman, M.,   *Foundations of Space-Time Theories*, Princeton University Press, Princeton, 1983.

Graves, J.C.,   *The Conceptual Foundations of Contemporary Relativity Theory*, The MIT Press, Cambridge, 1971.

Hawking, S.W. and Israel, W., Eds., *300 Years of Gravitation*, Cambridge University Press, Cambridge, 1971.

Holton, G.,   *Thematic Origins of Scientific Thought*, Harvard University Press, Cambridge, 1988.

Jerne, N.K.,   The natural selection theory of antibody formation. Proc. Natl. Acad. Sci. 41:849, 1955.

Morris, R.,   *The Nature of Reality*, McGraw-Hill Book Company, New York, 1987.

Newton, I.,   Mathematical Principles of Natural Philosophy, *Great Books*, 34:1, 1952.

Park, D.,   *The How and the Why*, Princeton University Press, Princeton, 1988.

Penrose, R. and Isham, C.J.,, Eds., *Quantum Concepts in Space and Time*, Clarendon Press, Oxford, 1986.

Parrish, H.J.,   *Victory with Vaccines*, E. and S. Livingstone, Edinburgh, 1968.

Russell, B.,   *A History of Western Philosophy*, Simon and Schuster, New York, 1964.

Talmage, D.W.,   Allergy and immunology, *Ann. Rev. Med.*, 8:239, 1957.

Talmage, D.W.,   A century of progress: Beyond molecular immunology, *J. Immunol. Suppl.* 141:85, 1988.

Will, C.M.,   *Was Einstein Right*, Basic Books, Inc., New York, 1986.

Chapter 3

FROM TRANSIMMUNOLOGY TO THE PRESENT PARADIGM

Alain E. Bussard

FOREWORD

In this chapter I will try to incorporate not only my intellectual evolution in science, as influenced by the great minds I have met and sometimes worked with, but also some facts of my life especially during the war and the resistance, inasmuch as they can interest the readers as a testimony about a fascinating period.

Great and dramatic events can act as litmus paper to reveal psychological traits which are usually hidden during more ordinary periods. This is true of scientists as well as for any other man.

Furthermore, politics, in general, influence the history of science not only for practical reasons (scientists banned together for political reasons, budgetary restrictions on science, war destruction of laboratories, etc.) but also for socio-psychological reasons. Without being a devotee of Marxism I must admit that the social environment of a scientist (especially during his youth) molds his mind and influences deeply his view over the world, and consequently, his scientific thinking.

This is why I will try to introduce some personal touch about the scientists I have met, some personal facts of my own history as well my remarks on what I see as the evolution of immunology.

This chapter will be somewhat different from some others inasmuch as it happens that I have been directly involved in some historical events in which great scientists such as, among others, P. Langevin, F. Joliot-Curie, J. Monod, were implied and whom I met and worked with, not only scientifically, but also in our activity of political resistance to Nazism.

Really this chapter will not concern itself so much with facts but with the emergence of ideas and hypotheses in immunology as well as the description of the authors of these theories, in their historical context.

I have been attracted to science ever since my youth. My father was a botanist and, though my mother was a writer, I was given a certain overview of scientific knowledge in that milieu of mixed culture. My elder brother was a "self-made" engineer (an "inventor") whose god was Thomas Edison and in whose glory I was educated. Endless discussions took place during family dinners concerning the respective values of rational and metaphysical approaches (my mother was a convinced Protestant while my father a typical agnostic) in trying to understand the world. In fact, the debate was centered around two views, one related to the spirit of geometry and other to the spirit of finesse, in pascalian terms. This was an extremely fruitful experience for a young mind and I have been influenced up to the present by the feeling that these two intellectual aspects are complementary and that they underlie a true understanding of the world.

My brother was a close friend of Stanislas Danysz, son of the great Polish immunologist Danysz, Chef de Service at the Pasteur Institute and well known as the discoverer of the "Danysz Effect" which regulates the proportions of

0-8493-4722-X/94/$0.00 + $.50

reacting toxin and antitoxin according to the number of steps used in the making of the mixture. As a child of nine or ten I was repeatedly taken to the Pasteur Institute and my first acquaintance with the lab came in the late twenties in the basement of the old Department of Rabies Vaccination where my brother was pursuing experiments on animal behavior. This familiarity later led me to consider the Pasteur Institute as a kind of second home for my family.

Another exposure to experimental science came through my father's lab. He was a plant physiologist involved in the study of seed germination; I was always amazed by the phenomenon of plant growth from a small seed sitting on simple wet blotting paper. It was fascinating to watch this blueprint become reality the same way, experiment after experiment.

My education took place at the Alsatian School, famous for its liberal education in both science and literary culture were held in high esteem, and I was greatly influenced by my year-long philosophy course taught by André Maublanc, a well known Marxist writer.

Our lives, as well as our thinking, were deeply influenced by the dramatic events taking place in France and in Europe during the fateful years preceding the Second World War: 1933-1940. The rise of Nazism in Germany and of fascist movements in France, the start of the Spanish Civil War and the establishment of a left-wing "Popular Front" in France involved many of my friends as well as myself: pure thinking in an ivory tower was unacceptable for us and during our years of intellectual formation we led a kind of "split life" between an intellectual approach to knowledge and the need to act on the political level.

I began my scientific career in 1939 when I was recruited as a technician by Paul Langevin, the well known French physicist, to work in the Ecole de Physique et Chimie of the city of Paris of which he was the director. My task was to study the possible changes of viscosity brought on by certain pathological states in the human serum, under the direction of a Mexican physiologist.

Such a frontal approach, with very little basic background then available on the structure of serum proteins was doomed to fail. It nevertheless provided me with the daily work experience and the atmosphere of a physics laboratory where experimental work led to hard facts which were later incorporated into conceptual analysis, which was of invaluable consequence to me. In addition, the extraordinary gentleness of Paul Langevin and his colleagues and their openness to discuss any new idea, as long as it was logical, was an unbelievable experience for me, and it molded my future career as a biologist deeply influenced by thinking in terms of physical and chemical reality.

The war broke out in 1939 and remained a "phony war" for many months while the French Army more or less slept behind what they perceived to be an invincible wall of fortifications. At that time I was travelling back and forth between Paris and an army hospital in Rheims where I was doing some esoteric work on the physical parameters of serum eventually modified by syphilis. Then everything fell apart in May 1940 and in a little less than three weeks the Panzer divisions had invaded France. I was then a soldier in the signal corps of the French Army and withdrew to the South of France with my regiment. During this journey I met the French physicist Frédéric Joliot-Curie whom I already knew from Langevin's laboratory, and we had a fascinating discussion on the world's future. In an enlightening prediction he prophesied that the U.S. and the U.S.S.R. would join the war against the Nazis and that, finally, Germany would be defeated! And that in June of 1940!

Back in occupied Paris I found that it was no longer possible to work at the Ecole de Physique et Chimie of which Paul Langevin, the director, was under police control outside Paris, in the city of Troyes.

I was directed to work with Robert Courrier, a well known French endocrinologist (co-discoverer of estradiol) to isolate and purify the gonadostimulin hormone from pregnant women's urine. My laboratory was in the new building of the Collège de France which was used for the preparation of physics lectures given by Frédéric Joliot-Curie. I was alone in this lab, which turned out to be very convenient later on for the preparation of chemicals such as the tear gas grenade which was to be used by the Resistance against the Nazis.

In October 1941 I was solicited to become a member of a clandestine organization fighting against the Germans and Pétain's French government: the FTP (Franc Tireurs et Partisans) and its civilian branch, the National Front. The group's founder was Jacques Nicolle, son of Maurice Nicolle was a great bacteriologist at the Pasteur Institute and the nephew of the famous microbiologist Charles Nicolle, Nobel prize winner in medicine and also a member of the Pasteur Institute. For security reasons the basic groups of this Resistance movement were divided into extremely small "cells" composed of three people and, at the cell's first meeting in October 1941 I discovered that our group included Jacques Nicolle, Frédéric Joliot-Curie and myself.

The group's activities were multiple during the occupation: diffusing the underground press, providing technical support to the Resistance network (developing undetectable radio networks, producing "invisible" radioactive ink undetectable using ordinary methods of detection, etc.), supplying vials of smoke bombs and irritating gas (Ti C14) to groups protecting the radios, and finally the gathering of intelligence on every sort of enemy activity which Frédéric Joliot-Curie gathered from the many civil servants in his acquaintance: policemen, railroad employees, etc.

One of our activity's original technical aspects concerned the fabrication of false papers, especially stamps, achieved through galvanoplastics. This enabled a perfect reproduction in several copies. Frédéric Joliot-Curie was a man of charming simplicity who proved to be a very reliable comrade. Already famous at the time, he could hardly lead a secret life and his contacts had to take very special precautions. Our connections were facilitated by the fact that we were working in the same research institution (the Collège de France) and our meetings could be passed off as professional ones, which they were in part.

The Germans and the Vichy authorities were aware of Joliot's convictions and even of his political involvements (he had been a member of a group of antifascist intellectuals), but they were unaware of his more direct participation in the Resistance. A sort of cat-and-mouse game arose between Joliot and the authorities who, thanks to his notoriety, did not dare interfere too directly with him (arresting him, for example), under the condition, of course, that he not be too obvious an opponent to Vichy or to the Nazis. On the other hand, Joliot had a German physicist in his lab who had been placed there as a rule by the occupation authorities in order to keep an eye on his research, sensitive research since it dealt with nuclear physics. In reality, this collaborator, son of the secretary of Foreign Affairs and himself close to the anti-Nazi German aristocracy, protected Joliot until the end of the war, and even managed to send Irène Joliot to Switzerland in January 1941 so that she could receive treatment in a sanitarium.

During this period I had gotten back into contact with J. Monod whom I knew from my stay at the Marine Biology laboratory in Roscoff (1937-1938). He was then an assistant at the zoological laboratory at the Sorbonne, secretly working for the Resistance.

When Marcel Prenant, professor at the Sorbonne and a historical Resistance figure in the armed struggle against the Germans, was arrested, I destroyed very compromising plans (of a military nature concerning Paris) which were hidden in the unimaginable jumble of laboratories and attics of the Old Sorbonne. Certainly the "laboratories" have always exerted, and still do today, a sort of fear and uneasiness upon policemen (even German ones then) who little desire to expose themselves to the risk. Policemen, simple people who are generally completely uncultured in the world of science, obscurely fear the dangers: radioactivity, microbes, viruses, etc. This salutary protection next exerted itself for us at the Ecole de Physique et Chimie, at the Collège de France, and at the Pasteur Institute.

My relationship with Jacques Monod become one of amicable fraternity during the occupation. We shared the same housing when more or less living underground, and his wife, secretly as well, took refuge at Vésinet because she was a member of the Lévy-Bruhl family. Jacques Monod was then a member of the General Staff of the FTP in charge of communications between that staff and the intelligence services of the Forces Françaises Libres in London. He was aided in this task by his brother Philippe Monod, who was a member of said intelligence services and living in Geneva where Monod often went secretly.

The liberation of Paris finally came in August 1944. I participated as a liaison for our intelligence network with the Second French Armored Division and led one of the armored sections from Rambouillet to Paris. Following the liberation of Paris I was detached to the First French Army to work in a scientific task force gotten under way by F. Joliot to perform diverse scientific missions: mine clearing, recovery of radium stolen by the Nazis, examining the research of German scientists, etc. On this occasion I had the opportunity to frequent or recruit French scientists with whom I was later associated in my scientific career. Labeyrie, Berthelot (of the Atomic Energy Commission), and above all, André Lwoff and Pierre Grabar of the Pasteur Institute. I finished the war in Innsbrück, Austria, in the latter's department and he suggested I work in his lab after my demobilization so that I could prepare a thesis in science, which I did in September 1945 at the Pasteur Institute in Paris.

The immunochemistry lab directed by P. Grabar at the Pasteur Institute was certainly, in 1945, the best (and practically the only) French immuno-chemistry laboratory and one of the best in the world. Before the war, Grabar, who was a chemical engineer by training, studied under M. Heidelberger for one year. Heidelberger influenced him deeply, and Grabar returned to France determined to apply the chemical and physico-chemical techniques he had learned to immunological problems.

Grabar's laboratory between 1945 and 1965 was extraordinarily vibrant and active with a constant flow of French and foreign scientists who went on to found modern immunology: from Gowans to Ouchterlony, from Fagraeüs to Terasaki, etc., not counting more recent ones such as E. Kabat who remained a bit like the laboratory's pillar. In addition, permanent collaborators such as A. M. Staub and J. Oudin, followed by C. Lapresle, assured the department's permanent framework.

The different qualitative aspects of the antigen-antibody reaction constituted in fact the laboratory's common research theme. Endowed with a considerable immunological background, possessing an enormous memory, and perusing the immunological and biochemical literature almost exhaustively, Grabar was an outstanding inspirer.

Having adopted the teamwork habit in the U.S., Grabar brought the custom of regular workshops in which, several times per week, we broached topics on the agenda or discussed his personal work or analyzed recently read articles, all of which was relatively new in the French university context.

My work concerned the human gonadostimulin hormone (placentary) considered to be a proteic antigen. Until then, the "antihormones" were considered as physiological entities, unassociated with defined substances, and the apparition of an antihormonal activity following the exogenous administration of the hormone had not yet entered the traditional field of immunology. Collip was the only one, shortly before my work, to have suggested that antihormones could be antibodies.

I was able to demonstrate that the human GSH acted as an ordinary antigen in the mouse and the rabbit, that its injection induced the apparition of specific antibodies which were immunoglobulins and lastly, above all, that the hormone was a specific component of the precipitate because this precipitate was hormonally active. This classic immunochemical exercise, quite common today, was possible only thanks to the technical and intellectual environment which then prevailed in P. Grabar's laboratory. An immediate practical consequence of my research was the development of an immunochemical pregnancy test which was patented in 1948. Since then many more efficient, more rapid, and less complicated tests have been proposed, but the principles behind the process were thus established as early as 1948.

This school of immunochemistry was very profitable for me, and it clearly established ties which link together chemistry and biology in general and more specifically in immunology. It was, in a manner of speaking, a reductionist school, but one which was tempered by the awareness that the animal is an extraordinarily complex system, a place often unsuspected interactions. Interactions take place throughout the entire organism but also at the immunocompetent cell level, to such a degree that we still ignore today the details of the interactions which come into play during the first phase of the immune response ("Cis" phase) because we are incapable of provoking a truly primary *in vitro* response.

Throughout this period the work relationship and discussions with J. Oudin, which were more and more frequent and elaborate, were to establish a profound friendship between us which lasted forty years. Oudin had a very strong personality which was both winning and complex. True to his friends, yet tempestuous towards any lack of intellectual integrity as well as towards the ownership of his ideas, one needed great devotion to remain his friend, devotion repaid by the joy one felt in keeping company with a great mind.

J. Oudin made three major experimental discoveries for immunology in the 1950's and 1960's: the immunochemical gel analysis (more an invention which revolutionized the study of complex antigenic systems), the allotypy and the idiotypy. These discoveries had been made possible by the fact that Oudin was completely lacking in an "esprit de système" and he questioned "all that was not established as evidence," which itself is the essence of the Cartesian method.

In the jumble of prejudices obstructing immunology in 1950, it was quite an achievement to be able to discard a number of dogmas. Oudin's procedure was entirely analytical and expanded in depth by isolating the phenomenon in question and the parameters which could obscure it. He was extremely distrustful of any synthesis which could collect these phenomena in a theoretical ensemble. This attitude, usually vindicated given the state of immunology at that time, could nevertheless irritate by its very excesses and led us into interminable debates. (This analytical spirit is terribly lacking today where any post-doctorate researcher thinks he can launch a new theory, especially in cellular immunology, in order to link together extremely debatable or uninterpretable facts. Thus meteoric reputations which die out as fast as they appear are established.)

My Doctorate ès Sciences thesis having been accepted by the Sorbonne in June 1950, I left to spend one year in the United States as a Rockefeller fellow at the University of Wisconsin (Madison). Since I had already acquired the foundations of the scientific spirit at the Collège de France and the Pasteur Institute, as well as the basics of immunochemical methodology under Grabar, I was then to discover the extraordinary enthusiasm and vitality of post-war American science. On the one hand I frequented extremely brilliant and winning minds working within that up-to-date university: J. Lederberg, Q. Luttinger (physics), E. Ackerknecht (history of medicine) but also historians, linguists, etc. On the other hand, my host laboratory included Mayer in endocrinology and his collaborator McShan and I also had contacts with the members of the laboratories in which I took classes (chemistry, physics: Williams; zoology: Wolfe) who influenced me deeply.

During the winter of 1950-1951 I began collaborating with E. Becker and O. Plescia on electrophoresis in the liquid vein (in William's laboratory) and on antigen-antibody soluble complexes in order to determine the antibody valence in those complexes. On this occasion I was able to appreciate E. Becker's intellectual qualities and rigor and he remains a close friend today. Throughout this period I became more and more interested in electrophoresis in the solid phase which was then only beginning, and especially in electrophoresis on paper. Thus, in a letter to J. Oudin in the spring of 1951, I proposed the combination of electrophoresis on paper (lengthwise) with the gel precipitation in a transversal direction. This was in fact the immunoelectrophoresis on which Grabar and Williams worked concurrently at the Pasteur Institute, which illustrates how similar ideas in science can appear separately and simultaneously to several researchers once a certain technological maturity has been attained. Oudin then answered me that it wasn't proper that I pursue this endeavor because he had heard of Grabar's attempts toward this end at the same time. This proves, if any proof is necessary, the extreme care with which Oudin preserved the priority of discoveries, even regarding those whom he did not like. In any case, my results were much less satisfying than Grabar's because I used an early stage of electrophoresis on paper followed by a second phase of double diffusion in gel, while Grabar's method combined two stages, both in gel.

Towards the end of my stay in the United States, the Rockefeller Foundation allowed me to travel and study in different American immunology centers. This was an unforgettable experience for me in that I met all the "big shots" in immunology at the time; prestigious forefathers or researchers in full maturity, some of whom became very close friends: from the admirable M. Heidelberger to F. Haurowitz, from M. Mayer to E. Kabat, from Pincus to H. Koprowski, etc. This list alone reflects the deplorable blindness of the Nobel Prize jury!

Upon my return to France I continued my research in a new field: immunochemistry of venoms at Garches Annex of the Pasteur Institute in P. Boquet's laboratory. I worked on the components of cobra venom and was able to demonstrate that lecithinase, a hemolytic element of the venom, was not the neurotoxin, a small protein which could diffuse itself through the pores of cellophane.

This stay at the Pasteur Institute in Garches had a great educational impact on me, imbued as I was with the qualities of American research: open-mindedness, transparence, willingness to teamwork; I rediscovered the French scene, with more solitary researchers, less communicative but also endowed with a broader culture, more universalist with a touch of academism, old-fashioned perhaps but full of charm.

On this occasion I met Marcel Raynaud whose work in toxin science and immunology was blooming with brilliant successes, and whose contributions to those disciplines were not perhaps recognized as they should have been. His was an encyclopedic mind; he was a hard worker, and he possessed an extraordinary knowledge of bibliography. He was also very preoccupied with social questions (see resistance, etc.). Very active in the Labor Union Movement, he exerted a heavy influence upon the transformations at the Pasteur Institute from 1965 until his death in 1974. He was close to the group which reformed the Pasteur Institute (E. Wollmann, J. Monod, A. Lwoff, and later F. Jacob) but nevertheless came into conflict with them when J. Monod wanted, in 1972, to inflict brutal transformations which failed to consider the human factors. During the 1950's the entire group of biochemists and microbiologists of the Pasteur Institute in Garches, including M. Raynaud, G. Cohen, J. Pagès, B. Nisman, H. Amos, Gowans, etc. was bursting with ideas and they found themselves enlisted in the first ranks of the movement which saw the transformation of microbiology or cellular biology into biochemistry, a movement which was in the process of shaking up the scientific world.

In 1953 I returned for a while to P. Grabar's department at the Pasteur Institute in Paris where two topics especially interested me: the technique of gel electrophoresis and the cellular aspect of antibody synthesis. On the first topic I was inspired by Oudin's work and by that of Ouchterlony who worked in his laboratory. Their theoretical analysis of the phenomena of immunoglobulin diffusion in gels, specifically in agar, roused me to study the diffusion phenomena which accompanied the electrophoretic migration of proteins in gels.

I attempted to apply a rigorous treatment to the phenomenon accompanying gel electrophoresis as Swenson had done for electrophoresis in the liquid vein; I specifically proposed the utilization of electrophoresis in agar in a quantitative manner in order to determine the pHi of proteins and their electrophoretic mobility, which was not very successful because electrophoresis was commonly used by physicians and biological analysis laboratories in a qualitative perspective. With the development of this work I invented a technique which simultaneously combined gel electrophoresis and immunological precipitation in gel, called electrosyneresis and which enjoyed some later success in immunochemistry under the name of "counter-electrophoresis."

Alongside this physico-chemical work, conducted especially with D. Perrin, grandson of the physicist Jean Perrin, I turned towards cellular immunology. I was encouraged in this direction by Astrid Fagraeüs who was then working in Grabar's laboratory. She was a pioneer in immunology and had identified the first antibody-producing cell: the plasmacyte. The B cell, not yet designated as so doing, had shown up for the first time! In the context of the time it was of great value to leave behind vague generalities concerning tissues involved in the immune response and to assign a definite function, that of antibody secretion, to a morphologically well-defined cell which was likely to survive (if not to be cultivated *in vitro*) outside the organism.

Whereas immunochemistry, at least since Landsteiner, spoke in terms of specific molecules, cellular immunology emerged from medical histology limbo to become an autonomous scientific discipline whose subjects were not longer theoretical abstractions but defined organic entities: tissues, cells, isolatable in the individual and able to pursue (at least for a certain amount of time) their activity.

This then oriented me toward the study of the immune response at the cellular level. I first approached the aspect of the immunological tolerance, recently brought into the mainstream of immunological thought by Ray Owen's work on dizygotic cow twins, by Hanan and Oyama, by Dixon and Maurer, and above all by Billingham, Brent and Medawar's publications on tolerance induction to allotransplants through the injection of lymphoid cells in neonates. In 1954 I entered the Cellular Biochemical Department, recently created by my friend J. Monod at the Pasteur Institute in Paris which was installed in the quarters vacated by M. Macheboeuf's death. I participated in the establishment of this new laboratory and was mainly to follow for ten years, above all as a witness, the prodigious adventure of the creation of molecular biology from my modest vantage point as an immunologist.

All the world's researchers who were important actors in this field poured into laboratories run by J. Monod, A. Lwoff, F. Jacob and E. Wollmann. This wonderful period of intense creativity has been described in numerous works, one of the most veracious and exciting being the *Eighth Day of Creation*. Thus I shall only dwell upon my participation in two simple immunochemical aspects of the work on the induction of the B-galactosidase synthesis. I would add that an extraordinary cheerfulness was permeating the lab during this time. Jokes, puns, spoonerisms in which J. Monod and G. Cohen were masters, were bubbling in the corridors where everybody met everybody and an atmosphere of continuous cheerfulness was reigning.

My friend, B. Cinader, with whom I was close since my stay at the Lister Institute in London in 1946 at Keckwick's laboratory, had come to demonstrate that immunological tolerance not only could be aroused by cells, but also by isolated molecules as well, the human serum albumin, for example. In addition, Cinader had introduced a quantitative test based on the comparison of the circulating tolerogen's half-life in the rabbit with the half-life of the autologous substances.

Employing these techniques, in 1956 I used known tolerogenous enzymes in order to follow inferred tolerance in the rabbit to these enzymes. This led me to study the enzyme-antienzyme reaction which, in brief, linked enzyme biochemistry to the antigen-antibody reaction allowing the establishment, though still very roughly, of the possible correlations between the active sites of enzymes and the epitopes recognized by the combining sites of the antibody molecule. One could likewise establish certain laws concerning the inactivation of the enzyme in the antigen-antibody complex (a rare case) or its non-inactivation (a relatively frequent case) which I had already exploited in a similar context, that of hormone-antihormone precipitate.

Immunochemical technology helped me with two pieces of work started by J. Monod and in collaboration with him in 1959 and 1960 on induced synthesis of B-galactosidase by *E. coli* or similar antigens having an analogous structure although devoid of enzymatic activity, and on the effect of uracil upon the synthesis of these proteins. Although completely outdated now after the introduction of the new tools of molecular biology, these results were able to serve as modest stones for constructing the edifice which Monod was to contribute to this molecular biology.

In this era of marvelous intellectual efflorescence where one rubbed shoulders in J. Monod's laboratory with the great names in molecular biology as well as in immunology (immunology not yet having been dissociated with microbiology) such as Melvin Cohn, Ed Lennox, Al Pappenheimer, who all became close friends of mine. Leo Szilard applied his physicist's penetrating mind to immunology and sought to elaborate a vast synthesis which would assemble disparate facts in that field in a general theory. The degree of our science's advancement and above all the uncertain reliability of many of its results did not allow for the sure establishment of such a theory, but Szilard had the merit of stirring up general ideas and of playing the role of a catalyst among the numerous biologists and immunologists whom he met and questioned with tireless patience and great intellectual brilliance.

Thus I discovered a new aspect of Jacques Monod's personality, who was by this time a scholar and scientific leader while I had known him as a comrade in the resistance and who was a bit like a big brother. I greatly admired his mind's acuteness, the clarity of his judgment and his intellectual dauntlessness which were, however, mingled with a certain irritation caused by his strongmindedness and his obvious "actor's" tendencies, all of which was clothed by the personal affection I felt for him and which, I believe, he felt in return.

The study of the immune tolerance which is central to any theory on the immune response led me naturally to study the latter in an attempt to use "in vitro" methods in examining the mechanisms of proteic synthesis of isolated cells which were used all round me in bacterial biochemistry. In the research on "de novo" antibody synthesis by "in vitro" tissues, thanks to the use of radioactive precursors (1960) on up to the study of antibody production by individual cells by Ingraham (1963), the manipulation of those cells by G. Nossal (1969), the discovery of massive antibody production by peritoneal cells (1966), the establishment of the genome of these peritoneal cells in a hybridoma permanently secreting said antibodies (1977), and finally the biochemical discovery of a new family of VH genes revealed by these autoantibodies (1985), I was guided by a single idea: to try to understand the generation of antibody diversity at the isolated cell level. Curiously the cellular approach which was nature and obvious to microbiologists since they have clones at their disposal was never very much in favor in immunology. Firstly due to technical reasons because tissue culture in mammals is difficult and has only been developed recently, the culture of these isolated cells is even more difficult and hazardous and finally because the speed of bacterial growth is approximately one hundred times faster than that of mammal cells. In addition the study of isolated cells, micromanipulation, photonic and electronic microscopy, etc., is still not widespread, today's researchers being hesitant to use new and delicate methods which are too rigorous and slow to permit hasty and numerous publications!

Furthermore, the dissection of the elements of the immune system into separate components has not until now allowed the reconstitution of the entire immune response, i.e., the primary response. Now we understand why since so many different cellular lines are involved: macrophages, B cells, various T cells, as well as specific factors and tissue structure about which we know practically nothing. Even today immunologists are compelled to repeat separate acts with few actors in a long and complicated play without knowing the show's general argument. On the contrary, molecular biologists have at their disposal almost all of the mechanisms which make up the machine they study, and from whence their advances proceed.

Newborn molecular biology's influence on immunology towards the end of the 1950's was considerable. While the central paradigm of molecular biology was established in 1953, in 1956 Burnet still supported an adaptive theory of antibody synthesis which was heavily influenced by Monod's work, although Jerne proposed a selective theory, it's true, in 1955, but one which implied a molecular "self-reproduction" of antibodies which seems strange to us today. Nevertheless as of 1957 Burnet, heavily influenced by the central dogma of molecular biology which stated that the flow of information only transmits itself irreversibly from the nucleic acids towards the proteins (message probably transmitted by J. Lederberg) and through Nossal's experiments in his laboratory, broadcasted his famous theory of clonal selection.

Since then that theory, practically accepted with no further research, can be considered as an essential paradigm, with the exception of a few "old timers" and experimentalists troubled by some "hard facts" which are very difficult to explain using that theory.

The (finished?) conflict between the instructive theory and the selective theory of antibody synthesis is apparently only a conflict between Lamarckism and Darwinism, since any theory on the generation of antibody diversity needs only to explain a somatic generation of the diversity and not an hereditary effect. This does not prevent the conceptual "things left unsaid" from maintaining (or rather from having maintained, since the conflict is hardly current any more) this theoretical debate; the theory of clonal selection is considered, without more ample research, as being in line with current Neo-Darwinian thought.

The study of tolerance being intimately tied to that of the immune response, I parallelly pursued both types of research, as much as possible, on the cellular level and this led me to participate in a meeting which was also, I believe, an important event in the formation of ideas in immunology. I refer to the meeting on the mechanisms of antibody production organized near Prague (in Liblice) by Sterzl in 1961. The best known immunologists of the time participated in this conference in which the flourishing Czech immunological school was the ferment. I was profoundly influenced by my contacts with Niels Jerne at this meeting. We had long and exciting discussions at a time when the latter was deeply preoccupied with "cis" cellular immunology (the early step in the immune response, or stimulation) and "trans" cellular and molecular immunology (antibody synthesis).

A penetrating mind, profoundly reductionist in his approach to biochemical problems due to his form of intellect but also to the styles of Cal-Tech and Delbrück, Jerne was particularly well armed to propose using simple mechanisms to explain G.O.D. He combined to the utmost a systematic mind of great brutality and an exceptional intellectual openness which did not care at all about social hierarchies nor the respectability of dogmas, etc. These were admirable assets in proposing broad explicative syntheses. As all great system creators, he neglected at will little embarrassing facts ("inconsistent") in order to see the entirety of the phenomena. This allowed him to establish a theory which combined tolerance, clonal selection, and antibody synthesis, a theory which is still valid today until an "idea-handler" in the future and with help from new technology and a pile of new facts can discard this theory or fuse it into a more general synthesis.

While pursuing his speculations on G.O.D., Jerne was absorbed by the problem of antibody production by a cell, as I was myself, and considered, due to his education as a microbiologist using amplification techniques such as that of lysis operated by the bacteriophage in a bacterial culture in agar, at least from what I assume since we spoke less about that methodological aspect than theoretical problems. The central dogma of another branch of science: molecular biology, rendered the instructionists' (initial!) position untenable: the antigen could not instruct antibody synthesis. This was very well analyzed by M. Cohn in several articles on G.O.D. (Generator of Diversity). Jacques Monod summarizes this idea (le Hasard et al., Nécessité, p. 125) in a provocative yet clear manner: "...the entire system, consequently, is totally, intensively, conservative, closed off and absolutely incapable of receiving any information whatever from the outside world..." And (p. 140) "But it has been established today that the antibody structure owes nothing to the antigen..." Thus the antigen, or rather that which I called the immunogen, disappeared from immunological thought.

Consequently, one understands that Jerne practically "evacuated" cis immunology from his diagram (see Fig. 1) in focusing his attention on the "black box." The Generation of Diversity (G.O.D.) either taking place through somatic mutations or through the rearrangement of the minigenes or even through both at the same time, which matters little to the basic conflict between instructive and selective theories.

The experimental counterpart to these theoretical conceptions needed to be investigated on the cellular level and specifically on that of the isolated cell. Oddly enough, rather little work was recorded in this field. Either the techniques of studying the lymphoid cell were a little forbidding or the researchers were quite happy with the heuristic base of clonal selection.

While Cohn and his collaborators first proved that the production of several antibodies by a single cell was possible, in a second phase Cohn dismissed the phenomenon, though not challenging the experimental protocol's value, due to the theoretical consequences which is entailed and returned to the selectionist camp, a remarkable example of intellectual agility. As for Nossal and Lederberg, they always found a single type of antibody per secreting cell. Ironically, if the demonstration of the pluriproductivity of a cell refutes clonal selection, the demonstration of the contrary does not confirm the theory, because a cell's virtual pluriproductivity is the only requirement for an instructive theory.

Cis-Immunology	BLACK BOX	Trans-Immunology

G.O.D.
(Generation of Diversity)

Figure 1.

In 1962 I organized a CNRS symposium at Royaumont on immunological tolerance. The majority of the immunologists who had most influenced immunological thought were assembled in the ideal atmosphere for intellectual confrontation: Royaumont Abbey. J.F.A Miller, Chase, Humphrey, Coons, Jancovic, Mitchison, Hasek, Weigle, Cinader, Koprowski, Dubiski, B. Waksman, Simonsen, Nossal, Karush, and Medawar, among others, freely discussed experimental and theoretical aspects of the tolerance phenomena and their possible influence on our conceptions of the mechanisms of immunity. I believe that this symposium had a profound influence upon all the participants, allowing them to form lasting relationships and doing much to reinforce this network of informal interactions between researchers so essential to the development of any growing science.

I continued my research at the isolated cell level, convinced that the new paradigm's final fate would be decided there. In 1963 J. Trefouël, director of the Pasteur Institute, allowed me to create an autonomous laboratory in the "temporary" quarters where I was to remain (on and off) until 1985! In 1962 I had the good fortune of being able to welcome J. Ingraham to my department for a second sabbatical year. He had invented a technique for detecting local hemolysis in gel (carboxy methyl cellulose) as early as 1958 which allowed the detection of antibodies produced by a single cell (rabbit in this case) and performed some encouraging experiments. J. Ingraham was a perfectionist researcher who surrounded himself with all possible controls and he was in the end too conscientious to reap all the benefits of his invention! He had in fact chosen cellulose as the cell support, aware of the anticomplementary activity of agar and conceived of a system which permitted microscopic observation and the long survival of the cells, instead of using agar and Petri dishes. All these laborious and meticulous preparations lasted, with a few intervals, nearly four years so that it was only in October 1962 that the first demonstrative preparations of hemolysis on plates took place and that Jerne, in November of that same year, showed us the photos of the technique he perfected with Nordin a few months earlier. Thus the technique of lysis plaques was attributed only to Jerne while Ingraham had had the idea earlier, a classic example of independent inventions in the history of sciences.

In my laboratory we were to develop Ingraham's technique which was superior to Jerne's for cytology, micromanipulations and sensitivity. Electronic (with J.H. Binet) and photonic (with A. Hannoun) cell microscopy, the study of the evolution of immunocyte cultures and the discovery of an astonishing polymorphism in B cells (with Hannoun) were our work's results.

The primary stimulation, *in vitro*, of isolated cells which was (and is still) the immunologist's Holy Grail, became my major preoccupation since I had the appropriate methodology at my disposal.

Thus in 1966 I discovered that peritoneal cells in non-stimulated mice produced high quantities of antibodies which were directed against the mouse's red blood cells. This phenomenon was a real challenge to the supporters of clonal selection because it was difficult to explain that in a lymphocyte population 1 to 10 percent of the cells were capable of one type of antibody synthesis and this without previous division.

Long and tedious work was necessary in order to establish the reality of this phenomenon which was so contrary to our dogmas. G. Nossal helped me a lot in this task when he worked in my laboratory in 1968. As usual, this true gentleman of science was teeming with ideas and worked relentlessly in the laboratory all in remaining socially available for all his friends and in enjoying every facet of exciting Parisian life with his family. He came up with the idea of transforming the lysis plaques system into a technique allowing micromanipulation which proved to be very successful for microcinematographic study of antibody production by isolated cells which I later pursued with J.C. Mazié. Thanks to these techniques we were later able to study allelic exclusion in antibody-secreting lymphoid cells in the rabbit.

The "peritoneal cell phenomenon" turned out to be a phenomenon of autoimmunity since a large number of these cells produced the antibodies which reacted with erythrocytes from the mice yielding these lymphocytes, provided the erythrocytes be treated beforehand with bromeline, a protease. It seems that the synthesis of these antibodies brought into play the expression of a set of previously unknown V_k genes of the germinal line. We proved this by establishing hybridomas (1976, J. Pagès) whose lymphoid component was a non-stimulated peritoneal cell. J.C. Jaton and his team in Geneva analyzed the molecular composition of monoclonal antibodies produced by these hybridomas.

It now seems clear that these peritoneal cells are the non-differentiated Ly-1 B cells which spontaneously become differentiated mainly during *in vitro* culture. The very high percentage of these cells possessing the corresponding structural information for autoantibodies without requiring previous cellular division presents a theoretical problem concerning the clonal selection hypothesis and so do numerous facts in blatant contradiction with the hypothesis. These facts were momentarily left unexplained and were generally ignored, thus providing the present paradigm's supporters with a restful intellectual crutch.

Until the discovery of a probable molecular mechanism which allows the explanation of how antigen orients antibody's stereocomplementarity during its synthesis, tomorrow's instructionist theory will not see the light of day. In the meantime the present paradigm will prevail by ignoring the major factual difficulty: the number of different possible antibodies is infinitely greater than the total number of existing clones!

Throughout the last twenty years of my activity in experimental immunology I was led to intervene in the social life of the international community of immunologists whose number continued to grow with that discipline's success.

Under D. Campbell's initiative (Dan was a delightful personality), I participated in 1964 with F. Karush and H. Isliker, in the launching of the first journal of immunochemistry called *Immunochemistry* and later renamed *Molecular Immunology* which enjoyed growing success. Convinced that, in the heart of the I.U.I.S. (International Union of Immunological Studies) the powerful and active European immunological community needed to organize itself, I organized the first European Congress of Immunology (Strasburg 1972) in my capacity as president of the Société Française d'Immunologie (founded by P. Grabar and M. Raynaud in 1965). This congress gathered together French, German, Swiss, Yugoslavian and Israeli immunological societies and was entirely successful. As a follow-up I managed to create, though not without several difficulties, the European Federation of Immuno-logical Societies (E.F.I.S.) in 1977 which has later vigorously expanded and of which I became president. Lastly, believing that a rapidly produced journal of brief communications could become the federation's mouthpiece, I launched the journal entitled *Immunology Letters* in 1979 which has expanded auspiciously.

In summary, this revolution in immunology was, for its participants, an exciting adventure. Molecular biology's entry into immunological thought and the analysis of antibody synthesis at the cellular and molecular levels brought immunology out of its purely phenomenological phase and into the mainstream of modern biochemistry. Lastly, in terms of human achievement rarely has a small, "integrated" group of colleagues, I would not hesitate to say friends, been able to combine factual discoveries with their corresponding theoretical conceptualization so quickly, intensely, and in such an atmo-sphere of excitement and liveliness. Participating in this advance was a fascinating adventure.

Today's immunological research is holding conquered ground. Shortly new advances will be made in light of new concepts which are now brewing in molecular physiology.

Chapter 4

LOOKING BACK ON THE INDUCTION PHASE OF THE IMMUNE RESPONSE

Jaroslav Sterzl

PROLOGUE

It is generally accepted that scientists are reluctant to write autobiographies partly owing to a professional "schizophrenia". On the one hand scientists fight for credit and priority on publishing results. On the other hand, they feel that they are a part of an anonymous enterprise which searches for the truth. They hesitate to write memoirs and witness accounts as too open an act of the ego.

In this contribution I am abandoning such hesitations for a very good reason: having been kept out of the mainstream of international contacts since 1968 I have the feeling that if I fail to take advantage of the offered chance to recall the events of 1953-1967, some aspects of the history of immunology could be lost.* Another reason is to describe the specifics of the externally imposed intellectual "self-made man" approach to immunology.

Most of the authors in this monograph who recall the events in immunology in the fifties, are pupils and successors of eminent immunologists (Heidelberger, Burnet, Marrack and others), microbiologists (Delbrück) or physical chemists (Pauling). By contrast, the geographical region where I was finding my way to the scientific work had spawned recently only a few world famous scientists such as the physical chemist Heyrovsky, the physiologist Laufberger and the microbiologist Málek.

I was born in 1925 in Czechoslovakia in Plzen in a teacher's family. When Czechoslovakia was occupied by the Nazis, my education during the last years of High School included a compulsory draft to dig trenches. However, like all my generation I had before me a firm goal—to prepare myself for further studies when the universities, closed by the Nazis, opened again. By that time I was already firmly determined to strive for a complex understanding of the phenomenon of life by studying medicine.

In 1944 I fell ill with diphtheria; by a lucky coincidence this enabled me to work in the autopsy center of the Plzen Hospital. At that time the laboratory performed not only autopsies, but also all laboratory examinations in microbiology, serology and histology. The medium containing ascites fluid was routinely used for the cultivation of *Mycobacterium tuberculosis*; in this medium the bacteria grew in the depth at the bottom of the test tube. This phenomenon stimulated me to study the oxido-reductive metabolism of the microbe which, up to then, had been conventionally classified as a strict aerobe.[1]

Joining the Institute of Medical Microbiology at the Charles University in Prague, I followed my interests in general microbiology, studying the

---

*Submitted treatise was prepared in 1987 for publication in this volume. After November 17, 1989 the political situation in the Czech Republic changed profoundly for the better. The Czech scientists who lost scientific contacts for the last 10 years, like me, are now trying to incorporate into the international scientific community again.

0-8493-4722-X/94/$0.00 + $.50

character of the bacterial nuclear material;[2] the action of oil-soluble vitamins, in particular retinol, as bacterial growth factors;[3] induction of mutants and the change of morphological shape in bacteria induced by colchicine;[4] the use of bacterial mutants for the study of disaccharide metabolic pathway;[5] the action of antihistamines on bacteria;[6] and related problems.

Having finished my medical studies I became more and more involved in the problem of the relationship between bacteria and the host cell metabolism. It was proven that, after infection and immunization with *Mycobacterium tuberculosis*, there is an increase in host cell bactericidal activity and resistance against the harmful effects of bacteria.[7]   During a one year stay in the biochemical laboratory of the Institute of Chemistry (1951) using chemical methods, I studied changes in lymphoid cell extracts after immunization with ovalbumin and hemoglobin. We failed to prove that immunization is followed by an increase in the proteolytic activity in the extracts and serum, or by appearance of new proteinases specific against protein antigens, i.e., Abderhalden's "Abwehrfermente".[8]   However, a gamma-globulin fraction bearing antibody activity was demonstrated in these extracts by chemical isolation and by paper electrophoresis.[9]

These studies already drew conceptually from the notion of the formation of antibodies as analogues of adaptive enzymes of bacteria.[10]

A milestone in my scientific career was the participation at the VIth International Congress of Microbiology in Rome. At that time immunology was an integral part of microbiology. I presented communications about the formation of antibodies via cellular nucleoprotein precursors, and about the effect of an anti-leukocyte serum on the immune response.[11]   The congress in Rome was a unique opportunity to meet several renown immunologists (J.R. Marrack, M. Heidelberger, P. Grabar, A.H. Coons, M.W. Chase, and others) as well as scientists with whom I became life-long friends (J.H. Humphrey, M. Simonsen). The meeting allowed me also to inform my colleagues about the work being done at the Department of Genetics in Prague, where Dr. M. Hašek, who was making an effort to "approach" mutually allogeneic individuals using embryonal parabiosis. He had achieved an immunological reactivity in parallel with that achieved by the Medawar group in England. The scientific contacts formed during the Rome meeting made it possible for us to organize the first international immunological conference in Liblice in November 1954; this represented a boost that gradually led to the formation of one of the world's centers of immunology in Prague in the late 50's.

THE NUCLEOPROTEIN PRECURSOR OF ANTIBODIES AND ITS TRANSFER TO NEWBORN RECIPIENTS

From the very beginning of immunological studies, the onset of the immune response, the period shortly after antigenic stimulation, was regarded as the decisive period. As an analogy to the growth phase of bacteria, this early phase—from the injection of an antigen (Ag) to the first detection of antibodies (Ab) in the serum—was named the latent phase, in contrast to the later logarithmic phase characterized by a steep increase in the quantity of the antibody.

Shortly after the discovery of antibodies[12] and their identification as serum globulins,[13] the first hypotheses were formed as to how the specific characteristics of Ab are achieved. The proposal that antitoxin is formed from the toxin itself [Buchner, 1893][14] was not long in coming. It was

Ehrlich's imaginative concept[15] of side chains on the cell which predicted the existence of cell binding sites as membrane receptors. Later, the binding sites were suggested to exist as serum natural antibodies—[16] a reverse shift when compared with the backbone of modern selective theories which shift attention from natural serum binding molecules[17] to cell receptors.[18,19,20]

Ehrlich's theory lost its appeal when Landsteiner in 1917[21] showed that antibodies are produced also against synthetic chemicals such as arsenilic acid. These findings again stressed and reviewed the former theory of instructive role of the antigen, advanced at the beginning of the century by Bail (1914; ref. 14). Breinl and Haurowitz[22] put forward a hypothesis that serum globulins acquire Ab specificity through changes in the amino acid sequence of their peptide chains; later Pauling[23] proposed the hypothesis that specificity is due to complementary folding of globulin chains to the shape of antigenic determinant groups.

The principal opponents of the instructive role of Ag were Burnet and Fenner.[10] They assumed that cells contain self-markers which make them recognizable and liable to be destroyed by their own cellular enzymes. If an antigen is injected, a new adaptive pattern is induced and becomes stabilized as a part of the genetic heritage of the cells, and it is transmitted to their descendants. If Ag acts on the developing embryo, the adaptive enzyme develops which deals with foreign Ag as with self components; no Ab response but rather immunologic tolerance develops. This notion integrated developmental biological and biochemical processes into immunological concepts.

The key role of nucleic acids in protein synthesis assumed an increasing importance.[24] A quantitative increase in nucleic acids in lymphocytes was determined during Ab induction.[25,26] Even the template hypothesis underwent innovation to include nucleic acids as part of the forming pattern.[27]

Under the impact of these ideas we started to study the role of nucleic acids in the Ab formation process. Extracts of the rabbit lymphatic tissue and bone marrow after immunization with ovalbumin were purified by ethanol fractionation according to Cohn (pH 6.9, ionic strength 0.1, saturation with ethanol 25%) and the Ab activity was present in the fraction containing nucleoproteins. Nucleic acid was isolated from the specific precipitate with antigen as an additional proof of existence of a tissue nucleoprotein precursor of Ab.[11,28]

To confirm the existence of the cell precursor already prior to the secretion of Ab into serum, cells from the spleen and bone marrow of rabbits immunized with *S. paratyphi B* were isolated shortly (1-72 hr) after immunization. The isolated cells were transferred intraperitoneally into newborn rabbits which, at least during the first 14 days of life, do not form Ab after immunization. During this negative period, antibodies produced solely by the transferred cells were detected in the serum of the newborn recipients, the production maximum being observed six days after transfer.[29] As stated by Solomon,[30] this was the first time that immunologically immature newborns were used as recipients simulating *in vivo* cultivation medium.

To determine the presence of Ab precursors in the form of nucleoproteins, the lymphatic cells from the immunized donor were fractionated according to Mirsky and the isolated nucleoprotein fractions were transferred into newborn rabbits.[31] The detection of Ab in the serum of the recipients was explained as maturation or purification of the transferred precursor. I appreciate now this careful interpretation because some readers of our communication understood it as a *de novo* induction of antibody formation, as a "transforming" action of nucleic acids. We were aware of what was later proven experimentally, viz., that RNA fractions could also stimulate the synthesis of serum gamma globulins.[32,33]

The action of nucleic acids in the induction of Ab response attracted renewed interest at the beginning of the '60's thanks to experiments on the action of RNA and DNA on mammalian cells,[34,35] and on the isolation of "immune" RNA from macrophages.[36] This marked the onset of the period of "immune nucleic acids." Some authors assumed that by introduction into the cells of nonimmunized individuals, nucleic acid fractions would exert a transforming action. The role of nucleic acids, especially RNA, in the immune response was critically evaluated at the conference organized by H. Friedman[37] which covered the informational action of nucleic acids, RNA-antigen complexes and the function of RNA as signal amplifier. On the basis of our own experiments we adhered to the latter opinion; namely, that an action of transferred nucleic acids has a nonspecific enhancing effect on the already pre-existing immune machinery. DNA and RNA isolated from lymphocytes of immunized adult pigs were incubated *in vitro* with lymphocytes of newborn piglets containing no background antibody-forming cells (AbFC). After an *in vitro* incubation with the "immune" nucleic acids the cells were transferred either as a free suspension, or enclosed in diffusion chambers inserted intraperitoneally into piglets; the presence of AbFC was determined after 48 hr by the plaque technique. In more than 20 experiments we never obtained a positive result, i.e., the development of detectable AbFC.[38]

Looking back from the present day level of knowledge, when the incidence of informational action of nucleic acids cloned for individual genetic marker and introduced intentionally into the cell is well established, we can understand the improbability of induction of Ab formation by heterogeneous nucleic acids mixed with lymphatic cells, not to mention the even riskier procedure—an injection of nucleic acid fractions into the whole animal.

The existence of nucleoprotein precursor as a stage of Ab formation fits with contemporary knowledge, but nascent antibody chain on polysomes in the form of ribonucleoprotein, precipitated by anti-Ig antibody, we believed only serves for isolation of specific mRNA.[39,40]

DEMONSTRATION OF INDUCTION PHASE BY TRANSFER OF ANTI-GEN-STIMULATED LYMPHATIC CELLS TO NEWBORN RECIPIENTS

In the '50's, induction of primary antibody response in tissue culture, measured serologically by means of an Ab increase in the culture medium, gave questionable results interpreted as being due to inadequate cultivation conditions for lymphocytes.[41,42,43] Successful transfer of lymphatic cells to newborns provided us with a tool for studying the induction of primary antibody response by *in vitro* stimulation of isolated cells, which were then transferred into newborn recipients. The cells were stimulated with bacterial antigens—*S. typhimurium* and *Br. suis*. Treatment with these Ag's allowed cells to pass through the induction phase and produce Ab during their short life period in the recipients.[44,45,46] The alloreaction of the recepient, however, curtailed their existence after four days.[47] This short life period did not permit the cells to respond to the protein Ag unless they were protected against the alloreaction by being transferred into cell-impermeable diffusion chambers. Surprisingly, in Dixon's laboratory the newborn recipients were found to be an inadequate medium for the transferred cells.[48] On inviting Dixon to Prague and comparing views and experimental protocols, we found a new friend and broadened our international contacts. It was at Dixon's prompting that the next year (1958) a group of the most renown immunologists travelling through Europe (Benacerraf, Dixon, Good, Miescher, Stetson, Thomas) visited our laboratory in Prague. The data we presented to them showed that the newborns were not inadequate; in fact, they react too actively to allow the cells to survive for a longer period of time. When chicken cells were transferred into 18 day old chick embryos they were not destroyed by the alloreaction and produced high titers of Ab in 80% of recipients; however, all recipients were killed by the transferred cells with signs of a graft-vs-host reaction. If the same cells were transferred into new-hatched chickens, the alloreaction stopped the function of the cells, and Ab were detected only in 10% of the recipients.[49] The ability of neonatal rabbits to support the existence of transferred cells was also confirmed by other experimental groups as was the ability of newborn rabbits to reject the transferred cells as fast as did the adults.[50,51] All doubts about the inadequacy of the newborns were dispelled by a clear demonstration that neonatal rabbits were capable of launching an allograft rejection more rapidly than adults.[52]

The studies with transfer of cells to newborns brought about a series of important findings. According to the original clonal selection, the inductive phase differs from the production phase only quantitatively, reaching the level of detection by multiplication of preformed cells; this view was opposed by the observation that during the induction phase qualitative changes occur before the onset of antibody production.[53] The cell transfer proved that the minimum quantity of immunocompetent units producing a detectable quantity of Ab is about 10^6 transferred cells. If 50×10^6 cells are mixed with antigen and transferred to newborn rabbits, the first Abs are detected on day 3 to 4 after transfer. Such an induction phase is limited only quantitatively, it could be shortened by increasing the number of cells transferred. Instead of 50×10^6, $500\text{-}1000 \times 10^6$ cells, i.e., a dose 10-20 times larger than standard, was used for the transfer in our experiments, but no shortening or elimination of the induction phase under these conditions was observed.

A significant step forward in cell transfers occurred when donor cells were injected into an isologous, lethally irradiated recipient.[54] This procedure formed a basis for cell transfers which made it possible to estimate the hemopoietic stem cells by the number of noduli formed in the spleen[55] and to elaborate the *in vivo* cloning of immunocompetent cells forming colonies or foci of hemolysin producing cells.[56,57,58]

The qualitatively distinct character of the induction phase was indicated also by its sensitivity to the action of cortisone[59] and to vitamin deficiency.[60] A more analytical approach, i.e., the transfer of isolated cells stimulated by Ag *in vitro*, was used to study the sensitivity to the metabolic inhibitor 6-mercaptopurine (6-MP) whose action on Ab formation had already been demonstrated.[61,62] If 6-MP was administered simultaneously with the cell, or within 24 hr after the cell transfer, the Ab response of the transferred cells was completely suppressed. If 6-MP was applied later than 72 hr after the transfer, when the antibody production begun, it was without effect. The action of 6-MP thus proved the qualitatively distinct character of the induction period; we were able to conclude that the period is characterized by *de novo* ribonucleic acid synthesis.[63]

THE EFFECT OF ANTIGEN DOSE AND QUALITY ON INDUCTION OF THE IMMUNE RESPONSE IN FETUSES AND NEWBORNS

Immunization of newborn rabbits just after birth with a bacterial antigen requires that large amounts of antigen be given in order to elicit the primary Ab response which was detected from the 14th day of life onwards.[64] This unexpected observation with bacterial Ag was confirmed and extended by Bellanti et al.[65] Moreover, if the primary response was induced in newborn rabbits by sheep erythrocytes (SRBC) or bacteriophages, the induction period was shorter and the levels of Ab produced were higher when more Ag was used.[66,67]

To exclude the possibility that the duration of the induction period is limited by the sensitivity of antibody detection, improved serological methods were developed for detection of minimum amounts of Ab. Different numbers of Ab molecules bound to Ag are needed for secondary manifestation; the presence of two IgM molecules have to be bound to the red cell to elicit hemolysis.[68] There is a linear relationship between the decreasing number of red cells and the number of molecules required for 50% SRBC hemolysis. Using 0.0001% SRBC instead of 2% suspension, and monitoring the hemolysis by directly counting red cells in a Bürker's chamber, 10^{-6} µg N/ml of antibodies was detected. Similarly, the bactericidal test using S-forms of gram-negative bacteria and the complement present in the sera of colostrum-free piglets (containing no traces of "natural" Ab) detected also antibody quantities of 10^{-5} to 10^{-6} µg N/ml.[69]

When these hemolytic and bactericidal tests were used to detect the onset of Ab formation in mice, rabbits, and sheep immunized with different antigens, Ab formation was never detected before 48 hr.[66,70] Reported cases of a very rapid onset of antibody formation[71] ought to be interpreted as the response of already pre-sensitized animals. Results with the induction of the primary response of Ab detected by sensitive serological techniques led to the conclusion that the negative period should be regarded as a stage qualitatively distinct from the phase when Abs are already produced.

Another aim of the use of newborns and fetuses for immunization was to shed light on the origin of the so-called "natural" antibodies.[72] Since in most species maternal Ab are transferred to the fetuses during the gestation period, we used the model of pig fetuses born by Cesarean section, kept under sterile conditions in the isolators and fed by artificial diet [germfree (GF)], colostrum-free piglets.[73] In pigs the six-layered placenta prevents the transfer of maternal immunoglobulins (i.e., antibodies).[74] The levels of an actively synthesized protein detected immunochemically in the serum of GF piglets, which cross-reacts with adult IgG were a mere 40 µg/ml.[75] The above-described sensitive serological tests detected no traces of Ab in the sera of GF piglets and isolated Ig fractions. Later, using tests at the cellular level, no background plaque-forming cells (PFC) were detected in the lymphatic tissues of GF piglets before immunization. The serum had no bactericidal activity against smooth strains of gram-negative bacteria (*E. coli, Salmonella*) unless specific Ab were added or antibodies were actively induced by immunization.[76]

However, the sera from precolostral piglets were bactericidal for the rough forms of the same gram-negative strains and this activity depended on the amount of the complement present.[77] Objections that traces of Ab could participate in this bactericidal action of the complement were ruled out later, when the bactericidal effect on rough strains was proved to be alternative pathway of complement activation by assembling eleven isolated complement components.[78]

The onset of immunocompetency during the ontogenetical development was studied by immunizing pig fetuses on different days of gestation. With bacterial antigens (*S. paratyphi, Br. suis*) the dose necessary for immunization was not reached because these antigens caused damage to the fetuses. Using high doses of SRBC or the ϕX 174 phage, agglutination, hemolytic and neutralizing Ab were determined as early as 5 days after fetal immunization. A typical secondary response was induced by injecting the SRBC antigen into a fetus on day 70 of gestation, detected by a challenging dose just after birth.[67,79] A stepwise maturation, attained by using different types of Ag for immunization (early response to bacteriophages or ferritin, and delayed responses appearing for the first time after birth to bacterial Ag) was described by Silverstein and Kraner.[80] The stepwise maturation of immunocompetency in sheep was recently confirmed on the molecular level.[81]

A new stimulus for an exact deliniation of the induction phase was brought about by the detection of individual AbFC by localized hemolysis, using the plaque technique.[82,83] Using a modified version of mounting the cells in agarose[84] we studied the onset of the Ab response.[85] In conventional (CONV) mice, a background number of AbFC (60 on average) was detected even before immunization with SRBC. The increase in AbFC (PFC) during the first 24-48 hrs was not significant; some authors found the latent phase to last as long as 36 hrs.[86]

In GF piglets in which no background AbFC are present before immunization, the induction period, during which no AbFC were detected, lasted 36 hrs; this negative period is followed by a rapid increase in the number of AbFC, first with a doubling time of 2.6 hrs, later with 3.3 hrs. This increase in cell numbers cannot be caused by cell multiplication (the generation time of lymphocytes is 12 hrs) and a direct differentiation was thus presumed, i.e, shift of the cells from the compartment of immunologically activated cells (IAC) into the AbFC pool. The need for high quantities of Ag to induce the primary response reflects a random chance of Ag meeting and hitting an immunologically competent cell (ICC; these cells are present in very low numbers—one per 10^6 lymphocytes). To induce the primary response in newborns, a 100 to 1,000 times higher dose of Ag is needed in comparison with the induction threshold in adults. The linear relationship between the quantity of the given Ag and the number of AbFC detectable in the primary response holds for the whole range of Ag doses. However, in the secondary response the antigen reaches the saturation level early; this indicates differences in binding capacity between the cells of the primary and the secondary response.[87]

Comparison of responses in newborns versus adults and in conventionally-reared animals vs. those kept in a GF environment showed that the Ag stimulation is decisive for expansion of the immune potential, which under the CONV conditions and during aging is induced by an inapparent immunization by intestinal microflora, by food and environmental Ag.

We studied the action of different doses of an antigen given as a primary stimulus followed one month later by a secondary dose challenging all groups of the primarily immunized animals. Primary doses which were near the threshold level had a priming effect which, on challenge, exhibited a zone of the secondary response. By increasing the primary doses, a low but definite number of AbFC in the primary response was detected; on challenging these high dose groups the zone of unresponsiveness, tolerance, was detected. On the basis of these observations it was concluded that cells activated by high doses of Ag passed, without proliferation, straight into a compartment of short-living AbFC. After their death, the specific cell clone is deleted and the state of unresponsiveness, tolerance, was considered as a result of exhaustive terminal differentiation.[88] The described exhaustive mechanism of unresponsiveness was in good agreement with the observations of other authors.[89,90,91,92]

Even on administering the whole scale of increasing doses of Ag to GF animals and challenging them secondarily we were unable to detect the low zone tolerance described in CONV mice by Mitchison.[93] The difference in conditions, namely, the use of CONV vs. GF animals, appeared to be decisive. We therefore conventionalized all GF animals after birth by a purposely given identical dose of Ag. These "conventionalized" animals were given increasing doses of Ag, from a very low dose to an excessive dose. The effect of different doses was tested one month later by challenging the animals with the same dose. Three regions of response were obtained: a low dose tolerance, a zone of secondary response and a high dose tolerance region.[94,95] The induction of low zone tolerance by the prior exposure of subimmunogenic dose was recently observed with T-independent antigen.[96]

The importance of the continuous presence of Ag during the induction phase was determined.[43] When spleen cells isolated from the donor shortly after immunization were transferred to newborn recipients, they did not produce Ab if no additional Ag was added. Cells cultivated in the presence of a limited quantity of an easily degradable antigen (SRBC) in diffusion chambers develop into AbFC only if an additional dose of Ag is supplied into the diffusion chamber 24 hrs later.[97] Comparable results were obtained on inducing Ab response in the Marbrook tissue cultures: if the soluble Ag isolated from the SRBC membranes was washed off 24 hrs after cultivation, the Ab response was significantly diminished, and was restored only by an additional dose of Ag. Removal of the Ag by an antiserum given simultaneously or 24 to 48 hrs after immunization suppressed the primary response but not the preparation for the secondary response.[98] The quantity of Ag, which is not sufficient for triggering the primary response, is still sufficient for processes connected with the preparation of the secondary response.[99]

These studies stressed the role of Ag as an inducer of a differentiation signal. The continuous presence of an antigen during the early steps of differentiation (24-48 hrs) is needed to ensure its continuous binding to the newly formed membrane Ig molecules. The continuous formation and shedding of membrane molecules in complexes with antigen (mIg-Ag) results in a kind of "pumping," amplifying in a feedback loop, the gene transcription process that gives rise to increasing amounts of the mRNA specific for newly formed Ig.

PROLIFERATION VS. DIFFERENTIATION OF THE ANTIGEN-ACTIVATED CELL DURING THE INDUCTION PHASE

As stated above, the induction phase was explained by the clonal selection theory as a quantitative increase in the number of pre-determined cells stimulated by Ag. Contact of an immunocyte with the corresponding antigenic determinants is followed by mitosis and proliferation, not immunoglobulin production.[100]

The notion of proliferation as the first step in Ab formation was in conflict with observations on protein synthesis which showed that RNA is the template which is catalytically active. When RNA synthesis is blocked, adaptive enzyme synthesis ceases.[101]

The dissociation between differentiation and proliferation was prompted by simple calculations. If one cell out of 10^6 lymphocytes reacts specifically with an antigen and then multiplies with a generation time of 12 hr, it does not generate sufficient number of cells to produce detectable levels of Ab after 3 days.[102] This calculation suggested that during the induction an amplification of the Ab synthesis machinery takes place in individual lymphocytes.

As mentioned before, the sensitivity of the early phase is distinct from that of the period when antibodies are already produced. Using the model of cell transfer we investigated the action of various types of inhibitors of Ab formation, and we concluded that none of the compounds inhibiting mitotic division (colchicines) and metabolic inhibitors of DNA synthesis (6-aza-thimine, 5-fluorouracil, alkylating agents) affect Ab induction under these conditions.[103,104]

Cells transferred to an allogeneic donor survive in recipients only a few days and do not exhibit signs of proliferation.[105] Therefore the Ab synthesis is not inhibited by DNA antagonists given during the induction phase, in contrast to the effective action of purine analogs (6-MP,6-TG).

To determine directly the proliferation activity of cells activated by Ag, ^{14}C-thymidine was administered at 5 h intervals to cover most DNA synthesis phases (S) through which a cell going through mitotic cycles has to pass. The labelling of individual terminal AbFC was estimated by autoradiography. Although the detection efficiency for thymidine incorporation was maximized by using ^{14}C-thymidine instead of ^{3}H-thymidine (the ß particles from ^{14}C have a longer range—60 µm—than those from ^{3}H) and by using a very thin layer for autoradiography (around 20 µm after fixation achieved by dropping a mixture of agarose + SRBC and lymphatic cells on a plate), only 25% of AbFC were found to be labelled at the earliest possible time (72 h after immunization). Between days 3 and 4 the labelling with ^{14}C-thymidine increased to 75% of AbFC.[70,106] These experiments showed that during the early stages the pool of AbFC is replenished mostly by direct differentiation without proliferation and only later does the increase in the number of AbFC result from proliferation.

In another set of experiments, when a high paralytic dose of pneumo-coccal polysaccharide III (100 µg) was injected and ^{14}C-thymidine was administered at 5 hr intervals during the first 7 days, only 50% of the AbFC which developed as a short-lasting wave were labelled. This contrasts with the situation when an immunogenic dose of Pn III (0.1 µg) was administered; nearly 100% of the AbFC were labelled.[95] These experiments demonstrated that the proliferation of IAC depends on the dose of Ag. It is in agreement with the recent findings that induction of tolerance is attendant on the decreasing ability of lymphocytes to proliferate in response to Ag.[107]

The dissociation of lymphocyte proliferation from differentiation was confirmed by current studies. The derepression on the gene level starts with an activation of protein kinases, and includes new mRNA synthesis; the DNA synthesis starts only later, 30 hr after antigenic stimulation. B cell proliferation and differentiation are two events dissociable by means of their initial induction requirements (quantity of antigens bound to the cells) and through the action of metabolic inhibitors with different target mechanisms.[108]

During the proliferation stage of IAC, the immune response changes not only quantitatively, but a shift also occurs between Ig isotypes. The existence of separate precursors for IgM and IgG cell lines was suggested.[109] On comparing the mechanisms of the switch between fetal and adult hemoglobins, we proposed the existence of a common precursor which, during proliferation following antigenic stimulation, switches to the expression of the new isotype.[97] This hypothesis was tested experimentally using a method permitting the detection of individual plaque forming cells producing not only IgM, but also IgG.[110] The proof of the switch in the proliferating IAC was achieved by cloning lymphocytes in lethally-irradiated recipients stimulated by Ag. In approximately 10% of lymphocyte clones the early IgM Ab producing cells later changed into IgG producers.[111] It is noteworthy that not only the isotype change but also new binding specificities were conclusively proved in the same cell line in the last years.[112,113]

MODELING OF THE INDUCTION PHASE

From the experiments determining varying sensitivity of individual stages to X-irradiation and 6-MP, the flow chart of individual steps in the differentiation sequence was inferred.[114,115] Similar conclusions were derived from other experimental data by Sercarz and Coons[116] who named the sequential cell stages X-Y-Z. At that time the attractive evolutionary hypothesis was acceptable provided that one lymphocyte stimulated by antigen expresses in the same cell line different immune profiles as a reflection of different stages of the immune cell differentiation.[117] The first step (X → Y) characterized by an increased binding capacity to the Ag[118] would have the functional manifestation of specific cell immunity (delayed hypersensitivity). The terminal step towards which the cell is shifted by Ag (Y → Z) would be an antibody producing cell. We adhered to this unitarian view too long[119] because we underestimated the diversification potential of the stem cell which—early on during the embryogenesis—separates into T and B cell progenitor lines with different functional prospects[120,121] and their mutual cooperative functions.[122,123]

Therefore in 1967 the life-story of the lymphocyte on the way towards antibody formation was described only as an antigen-dependent process, no attention being paid to the regulatory and feedback factors which have been in the center of interest in the last decade.[97]

A graphical model of the X-Y-Z sequence was described as follows: a minimum threshold number of Ag molecules is needed to activate the ICC (X) and transform it into the IAC (Y); the antigen is needed for at least 24 hr. During this period the IAC (Y) arises, characterized by morphological and metabolic changes and by an increased number of Ig receptors and binding capacity for the Ag and by recirculation dynamics.

The fate of the IAC is determined by the presence or absence of the Ag. If IAC escapes from the driving effect of Ag, IAC continues to proliferate and new isotype genes are activated (e.g., IgM → IgG). After 10-12 proliferation cycles the dividing capacity of the IAC ceases and it changes into a resting memory cell (MC). If during the dividing cycles IAC contacts with the Ag again, Ag acts as a stimulus for terminal differentiation, i.e., for AbFC (Z) formation.

The binding of a small amount of Ag to IAC which is not sufficient to move the cells towards terminal differentiation, accelerates its death and leads to its abortive differentiation. If the IAC is exposed to an excessive quantity of the antigen, the proliferation capacity of IAC is restricted and the IAC is transformed directly into AbFC without leaving the reserve of MC. The extinction of short-lived AbFC leads to the depletion of the clone activated by Ag which results in a state of inhibition (tolerance) caused by exhaustive terminal differentiation.

This verbal and graphical model was transformed into mathematical terms as an approach to test a complex and intricate theory. The mathematical model had the form of a non-homogeneous Poisson process and the Monte Carlo stochastic process was used for its verification. In order to obtain the sum of randomly distributed values, an attempt was made to record the random fate of at least 100 differentiating lymphocytes, but the demands for computer time were excessive.[124] Therefore, an analytically-solved system of differential stochastic equations was used which substantially reduced the working time demands. The results of the simulations showed remarkable agreement with the Ab response obtained experimentally.[125] The computation stimulated further laboratory experimental work.

EPILOGUE

My recollection of immunology covers the time span between the 6th Congress of Microbiology held in Rome in 1953 and the Cold Spring Harbor Symposium on Antibodies in 1967.

The events described above constitute a story of a search for scientific truth and have to be understood in this sense. The described results form, as any temporarily valid scientific truth, the sum of facts and of theoretical generalization which have not yet been—at the time of presentation—shown to be wrong. The readers, but ultimately the advance in science as a more objective judge, can decide which facts are to be maintained and incorporated into today's immunological knowledge and which will be valid in the future.

When the 1967 Cold Spring Harbor Symposium was closed many of the questions had not yet been answered including the following: "How does the genetic variability arise? What is the mechanism of phenotypic restriction? Can immunological information be transferred from one cell to another by subcellular entities? What are the receptors and the signals which allow the antigen to affect an immunocyte?"[126] During the last 20 years I witnessed the solution of most of the questions posed in 1967.

I should like to close by expressing my feeling that, should I never have been active in immunology, this science would not be quite the same, but it would be awfully hard to see the difference.

REFERENCES

1. Sterzl, J., On the respiration of *Mycobacteria tuberculosis*, *Biol. Listy* 28, 134, 1947 (in Czech).
2. Málek, I. and Sterzl, J., Les substances nucléaires du bacille tuberculeux, *Compt. Rend. Soc. Biol. (Paris)*, 142, 1053, 1948.
3. Sterzl, J., Growth effect of vitamins sojluble in oil in *Brucella abortus*, *Cas. lék. ces.*, 87, 1215, 1948 (in Czech).
4. Sterzl, J., Morphological variability of nuclear substance, *Nature*, 163, 28, 1949.

5. **Sterzl, J.,** Non-hydrolytic utilization of disaccharides by bacteria, *Cas. lék. ces.,* 88, 249, 1949 (in Czech).

6. **Sterzl, J. and Krecek, J.,** Competitive inhibition by histamine and thiamine of the metabolic influence of antihistamines on bacteria, *Nature,* 164, 700, 1949.

7. **Sterzl, J.,** Über immunbiologische Vorgänge im Verlaufe experimentell Herbeigeführter Tuberkulose, *Cs. Biol.* 1, 275, 1952 (in Czech).

8. **Sterzl, J.,** Proteolytische Aktivität der Sera und der Leukozyten von mit Eiweisskörpern immunisierten Tieren, *Cs. biol.,* 2, 138, 1953 (in Czech).

9. **Sterzl, J.,** Der Nachweis normaler und immuner gamma-globuline in den Leukozyten, *Cs. biol.* 1, 299, 1952 (in Czech).

10. **Burnet, F.M. and Fenner, F.,** *Production of Antibodies,* Macmillan, Melbourne, 1949.

11. **Sterzl, J.,** Nucleoprotein origin of antibodies, *in Atti del VI Congr. Intern. Microbiology,* Roma, Vol. II, 253, 1953.

12. **Behring, E. and Kitasato, S.,** Über das Zustandekommen der Diphtherieimmunität und der Tetanusimmunität bie Tieren, *Deutsch. med. Wochenschr.,* 16, 1113, 1890.

13. **Tizzoni, G. and Cattani, G. ,** Über die Eigenschaften des Tetanus-Antitoxins, *Zentralbl. Bakteriol. Mikrobiol. Hyg.,* (A)9, 685, 1891.

14. **Silverstein, A.M.,** History of immunology, A history of theories of antibody formation, *Cell. Immunol.,* 91, 263, 1985.

15. **Ehrlich, P.,** On immunity with special reference to cell life, *Proc. Roy. Soc. London* 66, 424, 1900.

16. **Sahli, H.,** Über des Wessen und die Entstehung der Antikörper, *Schweiz. med. Wochenschr.,* 50, 1129, 1920.

17. **Jerne, N.K.,** The natural selection theory of antibody formation, *Proc. Natl. Acad. Sci. USA,* 41, 849, 1955.

18. **Talmage, D.W.,** Allergy and immunology, *Ann. Rev. Med.,* 8, 239, 1957.

19. **Burnet, F.M.,** A modification of Jerne's theory of antibody production using the concept of clonal selection, *Aust. J. Sci.,* 20, 67, 1957.

20. **Burnet, M.,** *The Clonal Selection Theory of Acquired Immunity,* Cambridge University Press, 1959.

21. **Landsteiner, K.,** *The Specificity of Serological Reactions,* Harvard University Press, 1945.

22. **Breinl, F. and Haurowitz, F.,** Chemische Untersuchung der Präzipitates aus Hämoglobin und Anti-hämoglobin serum und Bemerkungen über die Natur der Antikörper, *Ztschr. Physiol. Chem.,* 192, 45, 1930.

23. **Pauling, L.,** A theory of the structure and process of the formation of antibodies, *J. Am. Chem. Soc.,* 62, 2643, 1940.

24. **Brachet, J.,** *Biochemical Cytology,* Academic Press, New York, 1957.

25. **Ehrlich, W.E., Drabkin, D.L., Forman, C.,** Nucleic acid and the production of antibody by plasma cells, *J. Exp. Med.,* 90, 157, 1949.

26. **Harris, T.N. and Harris, S.,** Histological changes in lymphocytes during the production of antibodies in lymph nodes of rabbits, *J. Exp. Med.,* 90, 169, 1949.

27. **Haurowitz, F. and Crampton, C.F.,** The mechanism of the immunological response, *Biol. Rev.,* 27, 247, 1952.

28. **Sterzl, J.,** *Defense Processes in the Organism,* Academia, Prague, 1954 (in Czech).

29. **Sterzl, J.,** The demonstration and biological properties of the tissue precursor of serum antibodies, *Folia Biol. (Prague),* 1, 193, 1955.

30. **Solomon, J.B.,** *Foetal and Neonatal Immunology,* North-Holland, Amsterdam, 1971.

31. **Sterzl, J. and Hrubesová, M.,** The transfer of antibody formation by means of nucleoprotein fractions to non-immunized recipients, *Folia Biol. (Prague),* 2, 21, 1956.

32. **Hrubesová, M., Askonas, B.A., Humphrey, J.H.,** Serum antibody and gamma globulin in baby rabbits after transfer of ribonucleoprotein from adult rabbits, *Nature,* 183, 97, 1959.

33. **Hoagland, M.B. and Askonas, B.A.,** Aspects of control of protein synthesis in normal and regenerating rat liver, *Proc. Natl. Acad. Sci. USA,* 49, 130, 1963.

34. **Niu, M.C., Cordova, C.C. and Niu, L.C.,** Ribonucleic acid-induced changes in mammalian cells, *Proc. Natl. Acad. Sci. USA,* 47, 1689, 1961.

35. **Szybalska, E.H., Szybalski, W.,** Genetics of human cell lines, *Proc. Natl. Acad. Sci. USA,* 48, 2026, 1962.

36. Fishman, M. and Adler, F.L., Antibody formation initiated *in vitro*, II. *J. Exp. Med.*, 117, 595, 1963.

37. Friedman, H., Ed., RNA in the Immune Response, *Ann. N.Y. Acad. Sci.* 207, 1973.

38. Sterzl, J., in *Molecular and Cellular Basis of Antibody Formation*, J. Sterzl et al., Eds., Publ. House Czech. Acad. Sci., Prague, 1965, p. 553.

39. Adams, J. M., Immunoglobulin messenger RNA, in *Progress in Immunology III*, T.E. Mandel, Ed., Austr. Acad. Sci., Canberra, 1977, p. 236.

40. Legler, M.K. and Cohen, E.P., Hybridization properties of immunoglobulin mRNA: failure to detect covalently associated IgG mRNA transcripts of reiterated and unique mouse DNA, *Proc. Natl. Acad. Sci. USA*, 74, 3528, 1977.

41. Parker, R.C., Studies on the production of antibodies *in vitro*, *Science*, 85, 292, 1937.

42. Sterzl, J. and Rychlíková, M., An attempt to produce antibodies in tissue cultures, *Folia Biol. (Prague)*, 4, 11, 1958.

43. Sterzl, J., Maintenance of the ability of cells cultivated in vitro to commence formation of antibodies, *Experientia*, 15, 1, 1959.

44. Sterzl, J., The production of antibodies by isolated spleen cells following contact with an antigen *in vitro*, *Folia Biol. (Prague)*, 3, 1, 1957.

45. Holub, M., Antibody production by lymphocytes after in vitro contact with bacterial antigen and transfer to newborn rabbits, *Nature*, 181, 122, 1958.

46. Trnka, Z., Antibody formation by isolated cells of hen spleen after mixing with antigen *in vitro* and transfer to chicks, *Nature*, 181, 55, 1958.

47. Sterzl, J., Presence of antigen - a factor determining the duration of antibody formation by transferred cells, *Nature*, 183, 547, 1959.

48. Dixon, F.J. and Weigle, W.O., The nature of the immunologic inadequacy of neonatal rabbits as revealed by cell transfer studies, *J. Exp. Med.*, 105, 75, 1957.

49. Sterzl, J. and Trnka, Z., Conditions essential for antibody formation by isolated cells after their transfer to newborn animals, *J. Hyg. Epid. Microbiol.*, 3, 405, 1959.

50. Harris, T.N., Harris, S. and Farber, M.B., Effect of injection of rabbit leucocytes into neonatal rabbits on subsequent lymph node cell transfer, *Proc. Soc. Exp. Biol. Med.*, 102, 495, 1959.

51. Harris, T.N., Harris, S., and Farber, M.B., Transfer of rabbit lymph node cells to neonatal recipient rabbits, *J. Immunol.*, 88, 199, 1962.

52. Najarian, J.S. and Dixon, F.J., Homotransplantation immunity of neonatal rabbits, *Proc. Soc. Exp. Biol. Med.*, 109, 592, 1962.

53. Sterzl, J., The inductive phase of antibody formation, in *Mechanisms of Antibody Formation*, M. Holub and L. Jarosková, Eds., Publ. House Czech. Acad. Sci., Prague, 1960, p. 107.

54. Makinodan, T., Perkins, E.H., Shekarchi, I.C. and Gengosian, N., Use of lethally irradiated isologous mice as *in vivo* tissue cultures of antibody-forming cells, in *Mechanisms of Antibody Formation*, M. Holub and L. Jarosková, Eds., Publ.Hous Czech. Acad. Sci., Prague, 1960, p. 182.

55. Till, J.E. and McCulloch, E.A., A direct measurement of the radiation sensitivity of normal mouse bone marrow cells, *Radiat. Res.*, 14, 213, 1961.

56. Kennedy, J.C., Siminovitch, L., Till, J.E. and McCulloch, E.A., A transplantation assay for mouse cells responsive to antigenic stimulation by sheep erythrocytes, *Proc. Soc. Exp. Biol. Med.*, 120, 868, 1965.

57. Playfair, J.H.L., Papermaster, B.W. and Cole, L.J., Focal antibody production by transferred spleen cells in irradiated mice, *Science*, 149, 998, 1965.

58. Sterzl, J., in *Thymus*, G.E.W. Wolstenholm and R. Porter, Eds., Ciba Foundation Symposium, Churchill, London, 1966, p. 103.

59. Berglund, K. and Fagraeus, A., Effect of cortisone on antibody formation, *Atti. VI. Cong. Intern. Microbiol., Rome*, Vol. 2, 231, 1953.

60. Axelrod, A.E. and Pruzansky, J., The role of vitamins in antibody production, *Ann. N.Y. Acad. Sci.*, 63, 202, 1955.

61. Sterzl, J. and Holub, M., The influence of 6-mercaptopurine on antibody formation, *Cs. Biol.*, 6: 75, 1957 (in Czech) and *Folia Biol. (Prague)*, 4, 59, 1958.

62. Schwartz, R., Stack, J. and Dameshek, W., Effect of 6-mercaptopurine on antibody production, *Proc. Soc. Exp. Biol. Med.*, 99, 164, 1958.

63. Sterzl, J., Inhibition of the inductive phase of antibody formation by 6-mercaptopurine examined by the transfer of isolated cells, *Nature*, 185, 256, 1960.

64. Sterzl, J. and Trnka, Z., Effect of very large doses of bacterial antigen on antibody production in newborn rabbits, *Nature*, 179, 918, 1957.

65. Bellanti, J.A., Eitzman, D.V., Robbins, J.B. and Smith, R.T., The development of the immune response. Studies on the agglutinin response to Salmonella flagellar antigens in the newborn rabbit, *J. Exp. Med.*, 117, 479, 1963.

66. Riha, I., Antibody formation in young rabbits immunized with erythrocytes, *Folia Microbiol.*, 6, 355, 1961.

67. Sterzl, J., Mandel, L., Miler, I., Ríha, I., Development of immune reactions in the absence or presence of an antigenic stimulus, in *Molecular and Cellular Basis of Antibody Formation*, J. Sterzl et al., Eds., Publ. House Czech. Acad. Sci., Prague, 1965, p. 351.

68. Humphrey, J.H. and Dourmashkin, R.R., Electron microscope studies on immune cell lysis, in *Complement*, G.E.W. Wolstenholm and R. Porter, Eds., Ciba Foundation Symposium, Churchill, London, 1965. p. 175.

69. Sterzl, J. and Kostka, J., Demonstration of small amount of haemolytic antibody using low concentrations of red cells in the reaction system, *Folia Microbiol.*, 8, 60, 1963.

70. Sterzl, J., Vesely, J., Jilek, M. and Mandel, L., The inductive phase of antibody formation studied with isolated cells, in *Molecular and Cellular Basis of Antibody Formation*, J. Sterzl et al., Eds., Publ. House Czech. Acad. Sci., Prague, 1965, p. 463.

71. Litt, M. , Primary antibody in guinea pig lymph nodes 10 mins after introduction of chicken erythrocytes, *Fed. Proc.*, 26, 752, 1967.

72. Boyden, S.V., Natural antibodies in the immune response, *Adv. Immunol.*, 5, 1, 1966.

73. Sterzl, J., Kostka, J., Mandel, L., Riha, I. and Holub, M., Development of the formation of gamma-globulin and of normal and immune antibodies in piglets reared without colostrum, in *Mechanisms of Antibody Formation*, M. Holub and L. Jarosková, Eds., Publ. House Czech. Acad. Sci., Prague, 1960, p. 130.

74. Sterzl, J., Rejnek, J. and Tiávnicek, J., Impermeability of pig placenta for antibodies, *Folia MIcrobiol.*, 11, 7, 1966.

75. Franek, F., Riha, I. and Sterzl, J., Characteristics of gamma-globulin, lacking antibody properties in newborn pigs, *Nature*, 189, 1020, 1961.

76. Sterzl, J., Kostka, J. and Lanc, A., Development of bactericidal properties against gram-negative organisms in the serum of young animals, *Folia Microbiol.*, 7, 162, 1962.

77. Sterzl, J., Pesák, V., Kostka, J. and Jílek, M., The relationship between the bactericidal activity of complement and the character of the bacterial surfaces, *Folia Microbiol.*, 9, 284, 1964.

78. Schreiber, R.D., Morrison, D.C., Podack, E.R. and Müller-Eberhard, H.J., Bactericidal activity of the alternative complement pathway generated from eleven isolated plasma proteins, *J. Exp. Med.*, 149, 870, 1979.

79. Tlaskalová, H., Sterzl, J., Hájek, P., Pospísil, M., Ríha, I., Marvanová, H., Kamarytová, V., Mandel, L., Kruml, J. and Kovárû, F., The development of antibody formation during embryonal and postnatal periods, in *Developmental Aspects of Antibody Formation and Structure*, J. Sterzl and I. Ríha, Eds., Academia, Prague, 1970, p. 767.

80. Silverstein, A.M. and Kraner, K.L., Studies on the ontogenesis of the immune response. in *Molecular and Cellular Basis of Antibody Formation*, J. Sterzl et al., Eds., Publ. House Czech. Acad. Sci., Prague, 1965, p. 341.

81. Perlmutter, R.M., Kearney, J.F, Chang, S.P. and Hood, L.E., Developmentally controlled expression of immunoglobulin VH genes, *Science*, 227, 1597, 1985.

82. Jerne, N.K and Nordin, A.A., Plaque formation in agar by single antibody producing cells, *Science*, 140, 405, 1963.

83. Ingraham, J., Identification individuelle des cellules productrices d'anticorps par une réaction hémolytique locale, *C.R. Acad. Sci.*, 256, 5005, 1963.

84. Bernovská, J., Kostka, J. and Sterzl, J., Haemolytic reaction in gels, *Folia Microbiol.*, 8, 376, 1963.

85. Sterzl, J. and Mandel, L., Estimation of the inductive phase of antibody formation by plaque technique, *Folia Microbiol.*, 9, 173, 1964.

86. Cerny, J., McAlack, R.F., Sajid, M.A., Fronton, J. and Friedman, H., Early accumulation of antibody plaque-forming cells in mouse spleens lacking a pre-existing immune background, *J. Immunol.*, 106, 1371, 1971.

87. Sterzl, J. and Jílek, M., Number of antibody-forming cells in primary and secondary reactions after administration of antigen, *Nature*, 216, 1233, 1967.

88. Sterzl, J., Immunological tolerance as the result of terminal differentiation of immunologically competent cells, *Nature*, 209, 416, 1966.

89. Benacerraf, B., in *Immunological Tolerance*, M. Landy and W. Braun, eds., Academic Press, New York, 1969, p.3.

90. Bell, E.B., Cellular events in protein tolerant inbred rat. II, *Eur. J. Immunol.*, 3, 267, 1973.

91. Chiller, J.M., Romball, C.G. and Weigle, W.O., Induction of immunological tolerance in neonatal and adult rabbits, Differences in the cellular events, *Cell. Immunol.*, 8, 28, 1973.

92. Howard, J.G. and Courtenay, B.M., Induction of B cell tolerance to polysaccharide by exhaustive immunization and during immunosuppression with cyclophosphamide, *Eur. J. Immunol.*, 4, 603, 1974.

93. Mitchison, N.A., Induction of immunological paralysis in two zones of dosage, *Proc. Roy. Soc.*, 161B, 275, 1964.

94. Sterzl, J., in *Immunological Tolerance*, M. Landy and W. Braun, Eds., Academic Press, New York, 1969, p. 25.

95. Sterzl, J., Síma, P., Medlín, J., Tlaskalová, H., Mandel, L. and Nordin, A.A., Induction of the primary response, preparation of the secondary response and tolerance, in *Developmental Aspects of Antibody Formation and Structure*, J. Sterzl and I. Ríha, Eds., Academia, Prague, 1970, p. 865.

96. Elkins, K.L., Stashak, P.W. and Baker, P.J., Prior exposure to subimmunogenic amounts of some bacterial lipopolysaccharides induces specific immunological unresponsiveness, *Inf. Immunity*, 55, 3085, 1987.

97. Sterzl, J., Factors determining the differentiation pathways of immunocompetent cells, *Cold Spring Harbor Symposium Quant. Biol.*, 32, 493, 1967.

98. Sterzl, J., Johanovská, and Milerová, J., Passive administration of antibodies during the primary immunization. The influence on the secondary response, *Folia Microbiol.*, 14, 351, 1969.

99. Hanna, Jr., M.G. and Peters, L.C., Requirement for continuous antigenic stimulation in the development and differentiation of antibody-forming cells: effect of antigen dose, *Immunology*, 20, 707, 1971.

100. Burnet, M., *Cellular Immunology*, Cambridge University Press, 1969.

101. Schweet, R.S. and Owen, R.D., Concepts of protein synthesis in relation to antibody formation, *J. Cell. Comp. Physiol.*, 50 Suppl 1, 199, 1957.

102. Sterzl, J., in *Cellular Aspects of Immunity*, G.E.W. Wolstenholm, Ed., Ciba Foundtion Symposium, Churchill, London, 1960, p. 163.

103. Sterzl, J., Effect of some metabolic inhibitors on antibody formation, *Nature*, 189, 1022, 1961.

104. Sterzl, J., The effect of immunosuppressive drugs at various stages of differentiation of immunologically competent cells, in *Immunity, Cancer and Chemotherapy*, E. Mihich, Ed., Academic Press, New York, 1967, p. 71.

105. Holub, M., Potentialities of the small lymphocyte as revealed by homotransplantation and autotransplantation experiments in diffusion chambers, *Ann. N.Y. Acad. Sci.*, 99, 477, 1962.

106. Sterzl, J., Jílek, M., Vesely, J. and Mandel, L., Differentiation of immunologically competent cell, in *Genetic Variations in Somatic Cells*, J. Klein, M. Vojtísková and V. Zeleny, Eds., Academia, Prague, 1966, p. 233.

107. Chace, J.H. and Scott, D.W., Activation events in hapten-specific B cells from tolerant mice, *J. Immunol.*, 141, 3258, 1988.

108. Sterzl, J., Pathways of immunocompetent B lymphocyte activation studied by inhibitors of the membrane signal and gene transcription, in *Highlights of the Modern Biochemistry*, A. Kotyk et al., Eds., VIP Publishers, Ziest, The Netherlands, 1989.

109. Bauer, D.C., Mathies, M.J. and Stavitsky, A.B., Sequences of synthesis of p-1 macroglobulin and p-2 globulin antibodies during primary and secondary responses to proteins, Salmonella antigens and phage, *J. Exp. Med.*, 117, 889, 1963.

110. Sterzl, J. and Ríha, I., Detection of cells producing 7-S antibodies by the plaque technique, *Nature*, 208, 858, 1965.

111. **Sterzl, J. and Nordin, A.A.,** The common cell precursor for cells producing different immunoglobulins, *in Cell Interaction and Receptor Antibodies in Immune Response,* O. Makela, A. Cross, T.U. Kusunen, Eds., Academic Press, New York, 1971, p. 213.

112. **Griffiths, G.M., Berek, C., Kaartinen, M. and Milstein, C.,** Somatic mutation and the maturation of immune response to 2-phenyl oxazolone, *Nature,* 312, 271, 1984.

113. **Manser, T., Wysocki, L.J., Gridley, T., Near, R.I. and Gefter, M.L.** , The molecular evolution of the immune response, *Immunol. Today,* 6, 94, 1985.

114. **Sterzl, J.,** Studies on inhibition of immune reactions, in *Allergology,* E.A. Brown, Ed., Pergamon Press, New York, 1962, p. 269.

115. **Sterzl, J.,** Development and mutual relations of specific immune reactions, in *Advances in Biological Sciences,* I. Málek, Ed., Academia, Prague, 1962, p. 149.

116. **Sercarz, E. and Coons, A.H.,** The exhaustion of specific antibody producing capacity during a secondary response, in *Mechanisms of Immunological Tolerance,* M. Hasek, A. Lengerova and M. Vojtísková, Eds., Academia, Prague, 1962, p. 73.

117. **Pappenheimer, A.M., Scharff, M. and Uhr, J.W.,** Delayed hypersensitivity and its possible relation to antibody formation, in *Mechanisms of Hypersensitivity,* J.H. Shaffer, G.A. Logrippo and M.W. Chase, Eds., Churchill, London, 1959, p. 417.

118. **Monod, J.,** Antibodies and induced enzymes, in *Cellular and Humoral Aspects of the Hypersensitive States,* H.S. Lawrence, Ed., Hoeber-Harper, New York, 1959, p. 628.

119. **Sterzl, J. and Silverstein, A.M.,** Developmental aspects of immunity, *Adv. Immunol.,* 6, 337, 1967.

120. **Roitt, I.M., Torrigiani, G., Greaves, M.F., Brostoff, J. and Playfair, J.H.L,** The cellular basis of immunological responses. A synthesis of some current views, *Lancet* ii, 367, 1969.

121. **Osoba, D.,** Cellular cooperation in the primary immune response. The need for a uniform terminology, *Eur. J. Clin. Biol. Res.,* 15, 929, 1970.

122. **Claman, H.N., Chaperon, E.A. and Triplett, R.F.,** Thymus-marrow cell combinations. Synergism in antibody production, *Proc. Soc. Exp. Biol. Med.,* 122, 1167, 1966.

123. **Mosier, D.E.,** Cell interactions in the primary immune response in vitro: a requirement for specific cell clusters, *J. Exp. Med.,* 129, 351, 1969.

124. **Jílek, M. and Sterzl, J.,** A model of differentiation of immunologically competent cells, in *Developmental Aspects of Antibody Formation and Structure,* J. Sterzl and I. Ríha, Eds., Academia, Prague, 1970, p. 963.

125. **Jílek, M. and Sterzl, J.,** Modeling of the immune processes, in *Morphological and Functional Aspects of Immunity,* K. Lindahl-Kiessling and M.G. Hanna, Eds., Plenum Press, New York, 1971, p. 333.

126. **Burnet, F.M.,** Cold Spring Harbor Symposium, personal communication, 1967.

Chapter 5

TOLERANCE AS A REGULATORY PROCESS COMMUNICATION IN THE IMMUNE SYSTEM AND BETWEEN MMUNOLOGISTS

B. Cinader

Throughout my scientific career, I selected my research targets to satisfy my curiosity about the structural relationships between molecules of self and of the outside world. This led me to analyze the specificity of antibodies against foreign enzymes. Thereafter, I investigated the effect on specificity of neonatal injection with foreign proteins (tolerance), particularly when the animal was later immunized with an antigen that was structurally related to the tolerance-inducing macromolecule. In a subsequent phase, we turned to age and strain differences in the regulation of the immune system.

With the clarity of hindsight, I can classify my work as an exploration of the body's communication with the molecular outside world. It began with a search for physically different types of macromolecules which could express antibody specificity against the same bacterial toxin. I sought to determine the effect on molecular communication of determinants, shared between external ("foreign") and internal ("autologous") macromolecules and how this regulation could be circumvented. The study of regulation was extended by an analysis of regulatory changes of aging. This could be defined in terms of molecular and cellular changes in communication. An exploration of this linguistic concept of biology was expressed in a series of volumes which I initiated, as Series Editor, with Marcel Dekker Inc. and continued with Cambridge University Press. Before I could engage on the pathway just outlined, I had to find my way through an obstacle course, with which I shall start the tale.

I decided to become a physician when I was about seven years old and thought of this in terms of a contribution to the well-being of mankind through service and study of function. This aspect of my interest was intensified when I was 11 years old and my parents provided me with a tutor who was to prepare me for the Bar-Mitzvah. He was a graduate student in Paul Kammerer's laboratory, and was always willing to spend part of the weekly session discussing some aspect of biology. On my 13th birthday, he presented me with Paul Kammerer's "Allgemeine Biologie".[1] This gift intensified my interest in cellular, social and chemical interactions in biology and strengthened my determination to study Medicine. My resolve was diverted when political events made me feel that my future should lie in preventing the next war, and I became active in the illegal anti-fascist movement of Austria.

At the age of 16, I was arrested and kept for some hours in solitary confinement, providing an opportunity for reflection and the realization that Medicine was indeed my life's goal. However, I remained an active member of the illegal Austrian anti-fascist youth movement and was profoundly affected by the rumors that reached us about Stalinist oppression and particularly about the Moscow trials. I persuaded my parents to let me visit Paris, and there I confronted the exiled Central Committee of the Austrian Communist Party with questions as to the events in the U.S.S.R. They refused to answer these questions: "it was inappropriate to ask them." I moved through France - from Trotskyites to Anarchists - in search of an alternative

0-8493-4722-X/94/$0.00 + $.50

left-wing, anti-fascist movement. In the process, I learned much that was new to me, from Picasso's paintings to Tribal Art. At the end of the summer, I returned to Austria with grave doubts that resistance to Hitler would find a morally or even a tactically adequate leadership. In spite of this, I continued my activity in the Austrian anti-fascist youth movement.

When I completed High School, I enrolled in my first year of Medicine at the University of Vienna, where my interests soon became focused on experimental biology as a result of a course I took on cancer research with Professor Wilhelm. I was occasionally allowed to help with simple laboratory procedures, carried out by his postdoctoral students. Another experience that steered me toward experimental science was participation in a seminar in Vienna's Institute of Psychoanalysis. Every year, three medical students were admitted to an Introductory Seminar Course. In 1937/38, I was among them, presumably because the total number of applicants did not exceed the number of vacancies. At any rate, it provided an interesting experience, and re-affirmed my decision to seek my future in a framework where I could test conclusions and validate them, i.e., in experimental biology and, particularly, in immunology.

My determination became increasingly important as Hitler's invasion of Austria forced me to leave Vienna before the end of my first year in Medical School and work in a factory in the East-end of London. I had to retrace the last few years of my education, so I studied English Matriculation via a correspondence course, and started my first year of University at Chelsea Polytechnic, which was then an External School of the University of London. Three days before the first University examination, the defeat of the Allies at Dunkirk caused fears that led to internment of enemy aliens. I had already been cleared by a tribunal which had been informed of my Austrian anti-fascist activities by the Austrian Socialist committee that was associated with the British Labour Party, but the perceived threat of a German invasion led British Authorities to set aside any differences between individual refugees from Germany and Austria, and we were all interned.

Internment, coming when it did, was a terrible blow to my hopes for the future. However, youthful optimism led me to believe that I might be released in time to take the examination, and so the luggage which I took to the Internment Camp consisted mainly of notebooks and texts - much to the astonishment of the soldiers of the Irish Guards who searched it. In fact, the examination took place in my absence and, a few days later, I found myself on a ship, the H.M.S. Dunera.

After a journey of nine weeks, I was placed on a train in Australia that raced for short stretches with kangaroos and emus, finally bringing its human cargo to Hay in New South Wales. I spent the next nine months in a succession of Australian internment camps, worked in the Medical Hut, was a member of our Camp Parliament and took a variety of courses in our emerging Camp University. At last, I was released and returned to war-scarred England. I took up the broken thread of my education and soon passed the intermediate B.Sc. in subjects that would permit me to continue in a Medical or a Science course.

When I obtained a scholarship from the International Student Service, I chose to take a degree in Chemistry with a subsidiary in Physiology at Queen Mary College, which had been evacuated to King's College in Cambridge. I wanted to begin creative work before "I was too old". Time - I thought - was running out on me. The two years in Cambridge were most stimulating, since

I attended not only courses prescribed by my College but much else that was offered in Cambridge.

My interest in immunology arose from my perception of communication and memory as the two central problems of contemporary biology. I felt that these issues could best be explored through the study of the regulation of the immune response. Before I could begin this study, one more hurdle had to be taken. When I completed my Bachelor's degree, my academic fate was decided, once again, by tribunal, but - this time - a tribunal that considered the fate of *all* graduating students. I was given a mandate to pursue "pure" research. However, I felt it was important that my research, for the time being, have relevance to the ongoing struggle with Germany, and should ultimately put me in a position to pursue my own objectives of research in immunology.

The first offer of a research position came in Cambridge, at Sir Eric Rideal's Institute of Colloid Science, where there was an opportunity to investigate the proteins of rubber latex. The intellectual atmosphere of the Colloid Institute was very attractive, but the work would take me in a direction I did not want to follow. After much soul searching, I decided not to accept this offer. I consulted the Director of the Biochemical Laboratory, Dr. Albert Charles Chibnall, who discussed my interests in a very understanding way, involved Dr. Malcolm Dixon in the conversation, and finally wrote a warm letter of introduction to Dr. Alan Drury, the Director of the Lister Institute. Dr. Drury suggested that I work on the freeze-drying of serum protein and vaccine preparations. This turned out to be a problem of vacuum and refrigeration engineering, two areas in which I was singularly unprepared to make a contribution. I worked with a young physicist, Claude Bradish. With his know-how and our common enthusiastic dedication, we managed to put together a makeshift assembly with which we could maintain the freeze-drying of a variety of proteins, which were isolated by Dr. Ralph Kekwick and Margaret Mackay. Fibrinogen foam was thus made eventually on a scale sufficient to supply the need of transplantation surgeons. These surgeons restored the burned faces and bodies of airmen, with the fibrinogen foam Bradish and I had freeze-dried for these procedures.

When the European war came to an end, I spoke to Dr. Alan Drury to see whether I could proceed with research towards my original goal. The Director pointed out that while he felt bound to allow me to do so, immunology was a bad choice for a career: antibiotics were making vaccination redundant and there was nothing of biological importance to be found. When I showed myself determined to continue in my chosen path, he brought me to Dr. Ralph Kekwick. It was agreed that I should examine physically separable entities of horse antitoxin against tetanus toxoid, and that I should take routine responsibilities for analytical runs in the ultra centrifuge and for electrophoresis.

My routine responsibilities for analyses with Svedberg's Ultracentrifuge and Tiselius' Elecrophoresis apparatus led to relationships with scientists in France. Alain Bussard, who had fought in the French Underground, was sent to the Lister Institute to acquaint himself with the latest scientific developments, and it became my task to introduce him to the new analytical tools. A shared interest in the immunology of biologically-active proteins, and our antifascist past, led to a lifelong friendship that soon extended to other scientists at the Institut Pasteur who shared our scientific outlook and political experiences, such as Jacques Monod and Marcel Raynauld.

During the two years of research towards my Ph. D., I was taught the relevant techniques and then left to my own devices. I soon found a rewarding collaborator in Dr. Bernard Weitz. We isolated and described the properties of two distinct immunoglobulins, which differ not only in molecular weight and electrophoretic mobility, but also in affinity for tetanus toxoid. Two years after I started this work, I received my Ph.D. and obtained a postdoctoral fellowship with Louis Pillemer in Cleveland, with the intent to isolate a hemolysin, with which I hoped to extend my analysis of molecular classes of antibody molecules. I succeeded in isolating and characterizing streptolysin S, but found it unsuitable for my long-term goals.[2] However, the period in the U.S.A. and the contact with Pillemer allowed me to learn much about molecular kinetics, purification of macromolecules and the sociology of science. I also learned a great deal from Pillemer about what makes scientists "tick". Gaining the esteem of other scientists was almost as important a driving force for most investigators as was their interest in gaining insight into a process of nature. Interactions with Pillemer continued after I left the U.S.A.: we both developed an interest in complement, though from very different viewpoints. His discovery of properdin,[3] which became a bandwagon for investigators in need of one, and the shattering effect on Pillemer when properdin was, temporarily, discredited, contributed to his premature death. This phase of his life would form an instructive chapter in the history of complement.

On returning to England in 1949, I was awarded a Beit Memorial Fellowship, and assigned my own laboratory, a shed in the courtyard of the Lister Institute. I continued in this space until 1956, and for the last three of these seven years was a grantee of the Agricultural Research Council. The Lister Institute was a wonderful place to work. Staff members shared a warm, interactive relationship as they pioneered research in nutrition, blood group chemistry, blood group genetics and bacterial genetics. Sadly, the scientific idealism that permeated the Lister Institute ultimately became its downfall. The staff of the Institute voted down a proposal that the Lister Institute should become the Medical Research Council's Institute, afraid that this could lead to governmental control and interference with freedom of research. This decision led to the demise of the Institute in the mid-seventies and the stately building, overlooking Chelsea Bridge and the Thames, was vacated and later converted into a private hospital.

In 1956, the unstable economic basis of the Institute made it impossible to obtain a permanent position there, and so I followed its director, Sir Alan Drury, to Babraham when he became head of the Department of Experimental Pathology in the Institute of the Agricultural Research Council in Babraham Hall, Cambridge. I was appointed a Principal Scientific Officer and thus obtained my first "permanent" position. However, I was soon attracted by other offers, one from the Institut Pasteur in Paris, one from the newly--founded Princess Margaret Hospital in Toronto, Canada and a dozen from various research centres in the U.S.A. I finally accepted the position in Toronto and arrived there in 1958.

The Princess Margaret Hospital provided an interesting and challenging milieu for pioneering research and provided the economic basis for continuation and extension of my research.

My position at the Princess Margaret Hospital, as Head of the Subdivision of Immunochemistry, involved a cross-appointment in the Department of Medical Biophysics of the University of Toronto. As an Associate Professor in the Departments of Biophysics and Clinical Biochemistry, I felt that the University in a "new" country ought to pioneer a structure for the discipline of Immunology and at last was able to persuade the authorities to initiate an organizational home for Immunology in an Institute of Immunology. I became its first Director, a position I retained from 1971 to 1980, when the Institute finally became a Department. My activities in the Institute of Immunology made it desirable that I should transfer my laboratory towards the geographic centre of the University. I made the move when a central Medical Sciences Building was erected in 1971. While the Director of the Institute of Immunology, I retained my appointment in the Princess Margaret Hospital.

I have summarized nine years of career development so that I can focus on describing my research objectives and scientific interactions without having to dwell on my geographic location or explain my professional status during this period.

Upon returning to the Lister Institute in 1949, I began to ask myself whether the response to toxin and to an enzyme would differ. I felt that enzymes, unlike toxins, might be expected to share determinants with those of isofunctional autologous macromolecules. I assumed that "universal" determinants would not induce an immune response. The catalytic site would constitute such a universal determinant, common to the donor and recipient of the enzyme; consequently antibodies would not be made against the catalytic site. In the following years, I explored this problem and found a number of mechanisms by which an enzyme could be inhibited by steric hindrance or activated by antibody-mediated configurational   alteration of the enzyme's catalytic site, without antibodies being directed against the catalytic site.

While pursuing my studies of antienzymes in terms of the assumed unresponsiveness to shared determinants, i.e. the evolutionary stable catalytic site, I became aware of Ray Owen's work,[4] published in 1954, on "immunogenic consequences of vascular anastomosis between bovine twins". When he examined the cause for the presence of excessive numbers of allelic products in dyzogotic cattle twins, he concluded that the precursors of red cells, belonging to one twin, had been transferred to the other twin and had continued throughout life to produce red cells with genetically-foreign antigens. The presence of these "foreign" antigens clearly indicated that the immune system had failed to reject the foreign red cells which it encountered in early life. The work on inhibition of enzyme by antibody had prepared me to extend our investigation from naturally-occurring unresponsiveness to the catalytic site to experimentally-induced unresponsiveness. The courage to attempt this project owed much to conversations with a very extraordinary scientist, Muriel Robertson. She was much-travelled, vivacious, intelligent, opinionated and one of England's pioneer women scientists. She had inhibited the antibody response of cattle by the injection of freeze-dried or acetone--dried *Trichomonas foetus* into newborn calves.[5]

In 1955, I began to search for the effect of specific tolerance on the specificity of the immune response. It seemed intuitively clear that induced unresponsiveness to a self-macromolecule would affect the response to structurally-related foreign antigens. To explore the cross-reactivity of tolerance, I injected newborn rabbits with human serum albumin and immunized the animal, some weeks later, with a p-azosulfonic derivative of the human serum albumin. The antibody, produced under these circumstances, was mainly directed against the chemically-modified portion of the albumin, i.e., against the part of the molecule against which unresponsiveness had *not* been induced. In addition, to my surprise, there was cross-reactivity with the protein determinants of the tolerogen.[6,7,8] We realized that "This appears to be a breakdown of the inhibition of the human response to H.A.".[6] Some years later, Weigle repeated our experiments, confirmed our results and described them as "termination of tolerance".[9]

In 1954, when I had completed the process of injecting newborn rabbits for this experiment, J.M. Dubert, my first postdoctoral fellow, arrived from Paris. He was sent by Jacques Monod, who had become Chef de Service, in succession to Michel Machebouef, and had found in his service a young immunologist, left behind by the "ancien regime". Monod suggested that he should come to me and participate in ongoing work on antienzymes. However, Jean-Marie Dubert found the experiments, which were waiting to be analyzed, sufficiently interesting to change his plans. He became an important contributor to their early completion.

When our paper was sent to the *British Journal of Experimental Pathology,* John Humphrey informed me that Peter Medawar was carrying out work that might be closely related to ours. He arranged for me to see Medawar, who was warmly welcoming and whose first response was one of amazement at my verbal report. He had been convinced that tolerance induction was dependent on the viability of the cell which brought antigens into the embryonic lymphocyte system. He was delighted to learn that there were molecular approaches to the investigation of tolerance. Soon, we recognized that different components of the immune response were involved in tolerance, as probed by cell-mediated response in transplantation or humoral response in antibody formation.

One year after this encounter, I was invited by Peter Medawar to participate in a meeting on tolerance that he was organizing in London under the aegis of the Royal Society. (A summary of the meeting was subsequently published in the Proceedings of the Royal Society, series B, 1956.) This meeting was, in many ways, an important event for all participants. For me, it was the first step into the personal network of international relations that is so important to the intellectual and tribal interaction of scientists. The symposium opened the door between people who saw the immune response from different viewpoints. It helped to define the difference between cell-mediated and humoral-immune response, and to illustrate viral interactions with the immune system. It also resulted in occasions for informal, relaxed discussions about the biological framework of immunology with Macfarlane Burnet, Ray Owen and other participants in this relatively small meeting. As a result of some of these experiences, I became fascinated with the sociology of science and societal forces which determine problem selection by scientists. This perspective was particularly stimulated by my encounter with Milan Hašek and the differing motivations that led the Czech and English groups to the work providing the conceptual background driving the Royal Society Meeting. In both groups, the social experiences of the scientist had an important influence on problem formulation: Medawar had been directed by the need to repair airmen's wounds to an intense interest in transplantation; Hašek had been deeply affected by his participation in the resistance to Hitler, Czechoslovakia's alliance with the U.S.S.R. and his acceptance of prevailing communist ideology, including their dogma on inheritance of acquired characteristics. I will make an attempt to convey the background of this part of the story of theory and experimental design.

The Lamarckian view of the inheritance of acquired characteristics had become discredited by the end of the 19th century, though it showed a remarkable capacity for resurrection. I have already referred to my youthful encounter with the book by Paul Kammerer who was a proponent of inheritance of acquired characteristics. One of these resurrections was staged by Michurin and Lysenko in the Soviet Union. It became one of the dark chapters of the 20th century, in which the integrity of science, or rather scientists, was endangered by mystical movements. Lysenko's dogma was mainly directed against genetics, but it had ramifications in other areas of biology, since it incorporated Pavlovian concepts of conditioning and applied them to immunology. In Czechoslovakia, which had just emerged from the night of Nazi oppression, the U.S.S.R. had come as the anti-fascist and pan-slavic liberator; all that it stood for was gladly accepted by a young group of intellectuals. Guided by Lamarckian ideas, Milan Hašek attempted to modify inheritance by presenting foreign tissues to birds. He did not succeed in creating a new heritable trait, but did succeed in transplanting skin and feathers from the donor of the cells. This experiment is probably the only instance of a fruitful outcome of a Lysenko-inspired endeavor! While Hašek was engaged in study of transplantation, Billingham, Brent and Medawar[10,11] did analogous experiments, influenced by Owen's discoveries, their own work on transplantation between cattle twins, and Burnet and Fenner's ideas. In England, there was "in the air" a strong general desire to advance clinical transplantation, as a consequence of the second World War experiences. Injuries of fighter and bomber airmen had created a need for facial reconstructive surgery and for concomitant transplantation. The resistance to allografts restricted possible strategies to autografting and heterografting became an important objective of applied research.

Hašek's visit to London precipitated his rejection of Lamarckian views and created many lifelong friendships. In the following decade of concepts and experimental development, we kept in touch through several symposia - some in Prague - and maintained close contacts during the tragic events in the political life of Czechoslovakia and in the personal life of Czech immunologists.

The invasion of Czechoslovakia by the Soviet army in 1968 was a bitter blow to many young Czech scientists who were members of the Communist Party and had wanted a socialist economic structure with a democratic political system. Invasion by the U.S.S.R. was, therefore, not only a blow against their nation but also against their faith as dedicated socialist intellectuals. Hašek was profoundly shaken by these events. We maintained contact through scientific and personal meetings throughout this crisis in his life, his expulsion from the Communist Party and his demotion from the directorship of his institute.

In the years after the symposium of 1956, I pursued the analysis of regulation of the antibody response by studies of neonatally-induced tolerance and of the modification of enzyme activity by antibody. When I moved to Toronto, the enzyme work was enriched by enthusiastic and able co-workers: from Australia, M. Branster and K.J. Lafferty; from Japan, T. Suzuki, and from Czechoslovakia, H. Pelichova. Extension of the analysis of the effects of tolerance on antibody specificity was carried out with a co-worker who joined me from Poland, Dr. S. Dubiski, and Dr. A. Wardlaw, a colleague who had come to Toronto from England at the same time I did.

Starting in 1954, I had examined the effect of down regulation on the response to subsequent immunization with a molecule that possessed some, but not all, the determinants to which tolerance had been induced. This experimental system provided a model for the circumstances which arise when an animal is naturally down-regulated to the determinants of its own macromolecules, i.e., to autologuous molecules, and encounters an environmental, but structurally-related, macromolecule. Self-tolerance would have a particularly striking regulatory effect if an animal were immunized with a molecule obtained from another individual of the same species. Such an isofunctional molecule might differ in some determinants from those of the immunized animal, whereas most other determinants would be the same in the donor and in the immunized individual. I had examined antibodies to enzymes as one example of this type. Molecular variation of this general type had been found among immunoglobulin molecules and had been designated allotype by Oudin.[12,13] In this situation, antibody elicited with antigens of the same species is directed against very few determinants of the antigen. The number of determinants which can evoke an immune response is related to the evolutionary distance between the donor of the antigen and the antibody, and is minimal when this distance is minimal (between individuals of the same species).

Landsteiner had recognized this phenomenon and had described it as immunological perspective.[14] We argued from our model experiments (1) that immunological perspective was mediated by tolerance to autologous molecules and (2) that there would be an exception to this correlation between cross-reactivity and evolutionary distance in a situation in which two animals of the same species differed by one possessing, and the other lacking, a particular macromolecule. In the latter case, the deficient animal would respond to determinants which are conserved in the evolution of the species and of the order, and hence are not normally immunogenic. To test this proposition, we immunized mice of various inbred strains with the serum obtained from other inbred mice, and screened the resulting antisera with sera obtained from species other than mice. One of the antisera, thus generated and tested, cross-reacted with the sera of many other mammals. It was directed against a murine antigen, which we designated MuBl. For once, an antiserum, obtained by immunizing an individual of a species with the serum of another individual of the same species, deviated in its reactivity from the rule of immunological perspective in that it reacted with the serum of many distantly-related species, from African elephant to sperm whale.[15]

It was clear that the mouse donor of this antibody lacked a macromolecule, present in the serum of other mice and of most other mammals; we soon discovered that a significant proportion of inbred mice lacked this molecule, MuB1. The cross-reactivity of the antibody elicited in the same species as the donor of the antigen confirmed our concept of the effect of autologous determinants on antibody specificity.

We were now intrigued by the question: what was the functional role of the MuB1 molecule? We proceeded to scan the literature for reported functional defects in inbred mice and to search for correlation between them and the molecular defect detected by our antibody. We finally found a correlation with a reported defect in the haemolytic complement system.[16] Crosses and back-crosses between animals which possessed and animals which lacked the antigen allowed us to establish that lack of MuB1 and complement defect did not segregate and, hence, that the molecular defect was causally linked with the complement defect. At this stage, several human complement components had been isolated by Muller-Eberhard and his colleagues. The fact that our mouse antibody cross-reacted with antigen of most mammalian species meant that it was possible to check the isolated human components for their ability to react with our murine antibody. The antigen detected by our murine antibody turned out to be C5.[17]

We had thus verified our view as to the effect of down regulation on the specificity of the immune response and had identified a molecular defect which affected a large proportion of inbred mice. We had established a criterion by which one can distinguish defects due to functionally-incompetent allelic product and defects due to failure to synthesize a particular macromolecule.[15,18,19] Various inborn errors of metabolism have since proven to be separable into disease entities, differing from one another in this respect.[20,21,22,23,24]

Our concern with regulation led Stanislaw Dubiski and me[25] to investigate the ability to turn off the synthesis of a particular type of immunoglobin by administering antibody, directed against a determinant (allotype) of an immunoglobulin, which we assumed to appear on the membrane of antibody-forming cells, following an original observation by Sheldon Dray.[26] To this end, we treated allotypically heterozygous newborn rabbits with an antibody directed against one of their two allotypic specificities, a determinant of the immunoglobin molecule, and saw persisting inhibition of the formation of immunoglobulins which carry this allotype. Since we had animals available which had a complement defect,[15] we could examine the involvement of a complement in the antibody-mediated inhibition and concluded that complement-lysis of a B cell-type was not involved in the persistent antibody-induced inhibition.[25]

In science, as in politics, it is a challenging task to identify limits of applicability of a concept. In science, we do so by testing the validity of predictions derived from the concept. In this context, it is interesting to examine research in which we encountered the limits of usefulness of the concept that specificity can be the outcome of the relation between autologous and foreign macromolecules. A prediction that followed from a hypothesis that had been fruitful in some contexts proved to be irrelevant when extended to mechanisms of inheritance of immune response.

The concept of down regulation (immunological tolerance) to self as a factor in the inheritance of the antibody response, was put forward in 1960.[27,28,29] It was tested in terms of responsiveness to alloantigens: crosses and back-crosses between MuB1 positive and MuB1 negative animals were immunized with MuB1-containing sera. Responsiveness was found to be recessive and to be inherited in a unigenic manner.[19] The response to an ethrocyte antigen EA-1 was a second instance of recessive inheritance. In this case, a cross-reactive autologous antigen was not known. If it existed, it should be possible to observe rapid elimination of antibody, directed against EA-1, when injected into a low responder. This prediction as to differences between rate of antibody removal in responder and non-responder mice, was not fulfilled; in this case, a link between autologous molecules and responsiveness could not be demonstrated.[30] A later experimental design appeared to lend support to autologous tolerance-mediation: responder mice were rendered neonatally tolerant by injection with spleen cells from hybrids between responders and non-responders. The injected animals lost the ability to respond to EA-1 ethrocyte antigen and thus lost the responsiveness of their untreated littermates.[31]

The question of whether tolerance to autologous macromolecules affects inheritance of immune responsiveness to alloantigens seemed to hinge on the dominant inheritance of unresponsiveness, i.e., on recessive inheritance of responsiveness. In fact, responsiveness, controlled by immune-response genes, proved to be dominant[32] and by 1970 it was clear that tolerance plays little role in the control of antibody responsiveness and is - at most - a minor perturbation on other types of genetic control.

Having dealt with "territorial" limits of working hypotheses, I would like to turn, briefly, to an episode I believe to be relevant to a discussion of factors which affect acceptance of alternative methods of therapeutic intervention. I have already shown how our work on specificity had been driven by the concept of autologous tolerance; it was also motivated by an interest in specificity in the context of immune response as therapy of tumors. We saw a particular challenge in the case where foreign transplantation antigens occur on a tumor, as may be the case in choriocarcinoma which has its origin in placental tissue and may thus express antigens encoded in the consort's genome. On this basis, we treated a patient by active immunization with her husband's antigens and finally with passive antibody against them. There was a steady decline in the amount of excreted chorionic gonadotrophins and in the number of pulmonary metastases.[33] Promising results were also obtained with other patients, except when there were metastases in the brain.[34] This difficult, but promising, immuno-therapeutic approach did not result in clinical trials since a more conveniently administered chemotherapeutic approach became available.

In the preceding paragraphs, I may appear to have given excessive attention to two endeavors that came to naught. I have done so because I am fascinated by the interaction of subconscious intuition with the rational rigor of verification which characterizes science. The intuitive component is as essential to scientific as to artistic creation. Scientists, as artists, have a style, which is visible in scientific problem formulation much more than in the resulting contribution to the collectively accepted body of results.

So far, we had dealt with regulation in early life. Next, I turned to investigation of regulatory changes in later life, motivated by a perception that the scientific basis should be prepared for health-care policy that needs to be in place when the next generation reaches old age. To this end, we have to find strategies by which we can identify individuals at risk from degenerative diseases of old age and use appropriate dietary, hormonal or pharmacological measures to delay or arrest the types of different age-related changes which precipitate different degenerative diseases. It seems reasonable to assume that if we can elucidate functional consequences of the polymorphism and multicentricity of age-related changes, we can identify markers for genes whose activation or inactivation contributes to initiation and progress of different degenerative diseases. Against this formulation of problems and goals, we chose prototype strains of inbred mice, selected for differences in onset and rate of progression in immunological aging. It was known that autoimmunity was a feature of aging. I selected mouse strain, so as to reflect an extraordinary degree of individual diversity to be found in outbred species where Darwinian selection would not eliminate mutations that manifest themselves after the peak of reproductive activity. In this respect, events of aging are distinct from other areas of "terrestrial" biology!

Our analysis of changes in different types of suppresser capacity and interleukins gave us models for the decrease as well as for the increase which can occur in various functional units when individuals age, and models for compartmentalization as well as for correlation of age-related changes in the concentration of different molecules.

Different cell populations in the same individual undergo age-related changes at rates and in directions that differ from one another. This might be the consequence of controlling genes which are activated in the final stage of steps in which an end cell develops from a precursor cell. We tested this assumption in terms of the consequences of interventions which alter the rate of age-related changes in a particular cell population and by investigating whether age-related changes in another cell population are affected in the same direction or in the opposite direction or not at all. If either of the first two of these three effects were observed, it could be concluded that a gene activated in the precursor cell is involved. In fact, we have tested interventions which change age-related progression in one cell population while those in another population are completely unaffected. In short, it appears as if different cells age under the control of different genes.

There are indications of controls which affect aging in many tissues i.e. there appears to be a general relation between the magnitude of a cell product and the rate at which this quantity decreases as the individual ages. My colleagues and I have described this relationship as economic correction.[35] It may reflect the processes which lead to selection of mice for the generation inbred strains. A strain will only be developed if vitally important responses, such as those dependent on receptor densities, do not decrease below a functionally adequate critical level; the relative quantity produced in youthful synthetic abundance will be functionally adequate, in spite of individual variation. On the other hand, the quantity in middle age, after decrease in cell output, can reach a level at which survival may be endangered. It is reasonable to assume that evolutionary selection will similarly affect the heterogeneity of the human population.

Having given an overview of our gerontological research, I shall now turn to its chronological development. It was fascinating to discover the exquisite polymorphism of aging processes; resistance to down regulation can be detected by the age of nine weeks in some strains, such as SJL,[36,37,38] while resistance occurs by the age of thirty-five weeks in animals of other strains, such as C57BL/6. In a third group of animals, resistance to tolerance could be observed if we selected a tolerogen, such as human myeloma protein IgG3, which has a low capacity for down regulation.[37] In short, resistance to down regulation is a general feature of aging; the polymorphism of the *rate* of progression is striking. One type of early resistance to tolerance induction is dominantly inherited.[39] In animals which show early resistance to down regulation, there is a gradual disappearance of a primary precursor pool from the thymus and depletion of a secondary precursor pool; this could be demonstrated by thymectomy and by inhibition of the immediate precursors of suppresser cells by treatment with cochicine or cyclophosphamide.[40]

Age-dependent changes in the suppresser capacity of the thymus can also be revealed by reconstituting irradiated SJL mice with thymus cells from donors of varying ages and lymphocytes from six to eight week old donors. Thymus cells from young donors are inhibitory and thymus cells from older donors enhance lymphocyte response. These changes are also reflected in the serum, where an ultrafilterable factor appears after immunization; the factor found in the serum of younger animals inhibits, while that from older animals enhances the response, if given to other animals undergoing immunization.[41] However, loss of suppresser capacity is not always responsible for the phenotype of age-dependent changes in the response to a tolerogen. One prototype strain, C57BL/6 shows sensitization by tolerogen with advancing age. When the C57BL/6 animal reaches the age of 30 to 40 wks, the tolerogen induces suppresser cells, though slightly fewer than in the younger animal. A small but significant proportion of B cells are stimulated to cell division by tolerogen. Another proportion of B cells are tolerized. The sensitized B cell subpopulation makes a large response when the status of the tolerized animal is tested by subsequent immunization. It is this set of B cells that determines the phenotype of resistance against tolerance induction, observed in the older C57BL/6 mouse.[42-45] In the following years, it became apparent from work with D. U. Ponnappan in my laboratory, and our collaboration with Dr. V. Gerber and Dr. K. Blaser in Bern that resistance against tolerance did not progress at the same rate for different isotypes and that isotype-specific regulation occurred at different rates in different strains.[46]

With post-doctoral fellows from many countries, but particularly from Japan and India, and with senior collaborators from Switzerland, France and Japan and from various departments of the University of Toronto, we examined the extraordinary polymorphism in age-related density of receptors, changes of subtypes of histones and error repair. Even the density of iso-functional receptors on different cell-types of the same individual changes at different rates. We found that aging rates can be modified differentially, by feeding diets differing in the ratio of polyunsaturated to saturated fatty acid. Clearly, aging is a multicentric, polymorphic developmental process. The polycentricity of aging processes and strategies by which the progression of some aspects of aging can be modified continue to fascinate and intrigue my colleagues and me. Aging of suppresser capacity for humoral and for cell-mediated immunity differ in the same strain in that one decreases while the other increases. The independence of these two regulatory changes during aging can be revealed by the reaction to a variety of interventions such as targeted passive antibody, drugs and diets, differing in the ratio of saturated to unsaturated fatty acid.[47,48,49]

This is one of the many examples of age-related changes which are compartmentalized i.e., appear to be under separate regional control. There are other types of changes in the concentration of different molecules which appear to be correlated with one another; we have found one situation in which this can be attributed to an increase in a cellular subpopulation that releases several different products. We discovered intriguing differences in the direction of age-related changes of interleukins, some increasing, others decreasing. We could show this to be due to demographic changes in sub-populations of T helper cells; Th1 decreasing, Th2 increasing as animals became older.[50] The age-related changes of several types of interleukins are correlated since they depend on increasing numbers of the Th2 cells which produce them.

I have referred, in earlier pages, to our interest in regulatory changes in terms of tolerance and antibody-mediated suppression of allotypes. We observed an intriguing age-related change in tolerance inducibility, to which I have already made reference; there was also a change in the ability of passive antibody to induce suppression. Antibody against a membrane molecule of T cells, CD4, can be immuno-suppressive for the humoral response of young, not of old, mice.[51]

Though the polycentricity and compartmentalization of aging is a feature that was important to our research design, we also discovered and analyzed some general features of age-related changes that were shared by different compartments. These included the already-mentioned relation between the molecular output in early age and the extent of decrease in output in later life, which we designated as economic correction.[52]

In parallel with the exploration in my laboratory of scientific problems, I attempted to contribute to the framework in which immunologists interact with one another and with the surrounding world. When I came to Canada in 1958, I began to explore the possibility of founding a Canadian Society for Immunology and, after some negotiations, succeeded in raising enough money to allow us to put on an International Symposium in Toronto in 1967. The focus for the symposium was problem formulation, to which I have already referred, and the proceeding finally appeared in 1968 as a book, *Regulation of the Antibody Response* , published by Charles C. Thomas, Springfield. This task completed, I began to talk with immunologists in other countries about the possibility of setting up an International Union. It was established in 1969.

As first President of the International Union, I helped create a number of committees involved in international activities, ranging from education to organization of international symposia, standardization and nomenclature. My activities in these areas grew out of my perception that certain needs had to be fulfilled for immunology to develop into its full flowering. Facilitation for international interaction between scientists was important, but, in addition, profound organizational changes had to take place in the institutions in which immunology was to develop.

Every new scientific discipline had, in the past, encountered obstacles in the rigidity of University structure. This had been so for biochemistry, which was held back by its organizational inclusion in physiology. Similarly, immunology was restrained by its organizational linkage with microbiology. Universities were founded in the Middle Ages to preserve and hand on what knowledge was left from the Roman and Hellenic period and therefore were in essence, rigid and conservative. By some chance or mischance, this conservative body became the forum for science, as it emerged in the early Renaissance. It resisted institutional adaptation of the continuous development of science into new areas of endeavor. Change can be brought about, but the process is slow and arduous. To create the climate which would favor separate University departments of immunology was one of the tasks of the I.U.I.S., our International Union.

Our new international body interacted with international organizations, such as the World Health Organization. Standardization at WHO was largely concerned with toxins and toxoids, but we now perceived the need to standardize many other types of substances, such as immunoglobins, allergens and, more recently, lymphokines. In education, we attempted to provide courses that would assist in technology transfer; one of the vehicles for this activity was an Institute in Amsterdam, founded by Dr. Karel Pondman, with an advisory board which I chaired. It linked training with the plans of the Home Institution of the trainee, monitored the employment of the returning student after his or her training in Amsterdam, assisted the Home Institution with reagents and equipment for the returning student and assisted trainees to form regional networks of mutual help. This format of interaction between the developed and the developing world arose from recognition that training had to be based on objectives and skills defined in the developing country. We had encountered many instances where failure to observe this practice has left gifted scientists unable to exercise their training in the developing country of their origin, forcing them to seek their career goals in the developed world.

In the last decade, we implemented a collaborative scheme between Thailand and Canada which incorporates the concept that objectives are to be defined in the developing country, with a second concept that there should be a linkage between academic research and industrial activities to promote economic developments in both participating countries. The creation of Thai Can Biotech Co., a firm marketing Canadian biotechnology products in Thailand, is intended to assure sustainability of Thailand's biotechnology research and to strengthen Canadian firms. The company will also assist the technological application of developments in Thailand's university laboratories while simultaneously promoting the impact of Canada's biotechnology industry. These activities were coordinated by Drs. Pornchai Matangkasombut and Stitaya Sirisinha in Thailand and by Dr. Tom Wegmann and myself in Canada. The Thai-owned company is directed by Preeya Sibunruang.

The "linguistics" of Immunology was the responsibility of the Nomenclature Committee, which worked toward international agreements as to the technical language that would be used between scientists. The Committee started its activities by accepting nomenclature for complement, human immunoglobins and the human HL-A system, in agreement with WHO and the Transplantation Society. Before accepting these recommendations, agreement of major investigators to this proposed nomenclature was sought. Further proposals, notably on the nomenclature of the complement system, on human and animal allotypes and cytotoxic lymphoid cells were considered by subcommittees. Progress in these areas was slow and occasionally frustrating. Nevertheless, the contribution of the Nomenclature Committee to the coherence of communication within the immunological community was significant, as anyone can attest who has struggled with "Immunogenese" prior to the work of this committee. I was involved in the activities of this committee throughout its existence and served as its chair from 1980 to 1983.

International Congresses were among the most important direct interactions between individual immunologists. The first Congress was organized by the oldest National Immunological Society, the American Society of Immunology, founded in 1913. The organizers of the Congress used a novel format; sessions of "free" papers and communications were replaced by workshops and discussion groups, a system that has been copied in all subsequent Congresses. The workshop discussions were summarized by the chairman of each workshop during an afternoon general session. A bronze medal of Paul Ehrlich - with a congress symbol on the reverse - was commissioned and brilliantly executed by Dora de Pedery Hunt for this Congress. The Second International Congress was to be held in 1974 in Berlin, but by the fall of 1972, it had become clear that opposition to this location would make it unsuitable. When I realized this, I flew to London in the summer of 1972 to discuss an alternative location with John Humphrey and his colleagues. With only two years' preparation time, the British Society undertook to organize the Second Congress. It was held in Brighton, England, July 21-26, 1974.

The Congress in Toronto was my own responsibility. We attempted to match our predecessors in the even-handed and international consultation by which topics were selected for Symposia and Workshops. We created the first Symposium on the History of Immunology, which set a precedent for future activities in this area. I also endeavored to present Congress participants with a broad image of Canadian culture.

To this end, a group of colleagues, led by Bruce N. Wilkie, sampled wines from all across the Niagara Peninsula and finally selected a red and a white wine which we put into bottles labeled with a design selected from an international competition. Dora de Pedery Hunt designed a medal depicting Landsteiner and I curated an exhibition of Canadian First Nations' art entitled, "The Birch Bark Sings", that opened as one of the many evening celebrations.

After successful Congresses in Sydney (1977), Paris (1980), Kyoto (1983), Toronto (1986), Berlin (1989) and Budapest (1992), we decided to close the circle and have the next Congress again in the U.S.A., this time in San Francisco.

My early inclination towards medicine and lifelong commitment to medical research motivated my enthusiasm for interactions with WHO. Among them was participation in the attempt to evolve effective fertility control, which came about almost by chance. A medical student who followed my lectures at the University of Toronto's Princess Margaret Hospital went on to become an obstetrician, training in Columbus, Ohio. There he met Vernon Stevens, who dreamed of vaccination against Chorionic Gonadotrophin, which would prevent implantation. Stevens felt the obstacle to this strategy was resistance against induction of antibody-formation with an autologous macromolecule. The Toronto medical graduate told him of my lectures on tolerance and tolerance breakdown. When Vernon visited us, we prepared derivatives and he persuaded the directors of the special fertility control programme of WHO to initiate a task force on Immunology. I was a member of this task force for many years and later a member of the Scientific and Technical Advisory Group to the special programme in Human Reproduction, S.T.A.G., which advised on the entire programme. Quite recently, I returned to the task force.

The concept of communication instructed both my biological investigations and organizational scientific interrelations. I felt that it would be useful to express the communication perspective in a series of books on the language of intercellular and intracellular communication[53,54] dealing with biology as molecular communication and disease as metabolic aberration or molecular deficiency in this communication. I formulated this concept in the introduction to volumes of these series: "Interlocking ligand-receptor networks of communication constitute an intercellular and intracellular language, in which molecules, e.g., growth factors, lymphokines and hormones, serve as words and convey messages through combination with membrane molecules, i.e., receptors. These signals can give rise to the production of other factors which can combine with receptors and thus form the sentences of the intercellular language. In the immune system, macromolecules of the external world cause distortions of the internal communication. The resulting change in the balance of molecular communication constitutes the immune response. Factors of the immune system interact with receptors of the immune as well as the neural system and so do factors of the neural system... Malfunction of a single step in cell communication results in disease."

In all the areas of research and organizational activities which I have described in the preceding pages, many gifted and influential people from all over the world participated. We shared the intellectual structure of scientific thinking, the ethical base and values of science, and the resulting mutual trust. Whether it was in the Soviet Union or in Peru, colleagues felt and expressed confidence and openness to a "member of the family". Remarkable numbers of these associates were not only outstanding scientists, but also excelled in other cultural activities from painting, to ornithology, to Noh Drama. Interaction with these citizens of the world was one of the pleasures of my being involved in international tasks as well as in the research in my laboratory.

Creative science and scientific culture were, and are, my motivation. The activities I have outlined, and others, including responding to the culture of First Nations,[55-59] and acting as president of the Royal Canadian Institute, resulted from the conviction that the future of *Homo Sapiens* lies in the application of the scientific method, not only to the interaction between human beings and nature, but also to the interaction between individuals.

ACKNOWLEDGEMENT

Thanks are due to Barbara Sutton for editorial criticism and improvements, and to Niall Byrne, Mary Crookston, Pauline Mazumdar and Rick Miller for their constructive criticism.

REFERENCES

1. **Kammerer, Paul,** *Allgemeine Biologie Dritte Verbesserte Auflage Deutsche Verlags-Anstalt Stuttgart, Berlin, und Leipzig,* 1925.
2. **Cinader, B., and Pillemer, L.,** The purification and properties of streptolysin S., *J. Exp. Med.,* 92, 219, 1950.
3. **Cinader, B. Professor Louis Pillemer,** *Nature,* 181, 234, 1958.
4. **Owen, R.D.,** Immunogenetic consequences of vascular anastomoses between bovine twins, *Science,* 102, 400, 1954.
5. **Kerr, W.R. and Robertson, M.,** Passively and actively accquired antibodies from *Trichomonas foetus* in very young calves, *J. Hyg.,* 52, 253, 1954.
6. **Cinader, B. and Dubert, J.M.,** Acquired immune tolerance to human albumin and the response to subsequent injections of diazo human albumin, *Brit. J. Exp. Path.,* 36, 515, 1955a.
7. **Cinader, B. and Dubert, J.M.,** Acquired immune tolerance to human albumin and the response to subsequent injections of diazo human albumin, *Proc. 3rd Cong. Int. Biochem.,* Brussels, 1-6 August, 1955, 14, 58, 1955b.
8. **Cinader, B. and Dubert, J.M.,** Specific inhibition of response to purified protein antigens, *Proc. Roy. Soc. (London) B,* 146, 18, 1956.
9. **Weigle, W. O.,** Termination of acquired immunological tolerance to protein antigens fllowing immunization with altered protein antigens, *J. Exp. Med.,* 116, 913, 1962.
10. **Billingham, R.E., Brent, L. and Medawar, P.B.,** Actively acquired tolerance of foreign cells, *Nature (London),* 172, 603, 1953.
11. **Billingham, R.E., Brent, L. and Medawar, P.B.,** "Enhancement" in normal homografts with a note on its possible mechanism, *Transplant Bull.,* 3, 84, 1956.
12. **Oudin, J.,** L'"allotypie" de certains antigènes proteidiques du sérum, Relation immuno-chimiques et génétiques entre six des principaux allotypes observés dans le sérum de lapin, *CR Acad. Sci. (Paris),* 242, 2489, 1960.
13. **Oudin, J.** in *The Rabbit in Contemporary Immunological Research,* S. Dubiski, Ed., Longman Scientific and Technical, Co-published in the U.S. with John Wiley & Sons, Inc., New York, 1987.
14. **Landsteiner, K.,** *The Specificity of Serological Reaction,* Rev. Ed. Cambridge, Mass., Harvard (reprinted 1962, New York, Dover Publications, Inc.), 1945.

15. Cinader, B., Dubiski, S. and Wardlaw, A.C., Distribution, inheritance and properties of an antigen, MuBl, and its relation to haemolytic complement, *J. Exp. Med.*, 120, 897, 1964.

16. Herzenberg, L.A., Tachibana, D.K., Herzenberg, L.A. and Rosenberg, L.T., A Gene locus concerned with haemolytic complement in Mus musculus, *Genetics*, 48, 711, 1963.

17. Nilsson, U. and Muller-Eberhard, H.J., Immunologic relation between human δ_{1F}-globulin and Mouse MuB1 (HC), *Federation Proc.*, Vol. 24, Issue 2 (Part 1) 620, 1965 Abst. 2706.

18. Cinader, B., Dubiski, S. and Wardlaw, A.C., Allotypy and Eniotipy, *Nature*, 210:1291, 1966.

19. Cinader, B., Koh, S.W. and Naylor, D., Tolerance-mediated inheritance of immune responsiveness, *Int. Arch. Allergy*, 35, 150, 1969.

20. Ottolenghi, S., Lanyon, W.G., Paul, J., Williamson, R., Weatherall, D.J., Clegg, J.B., Pritchard, J., Pootkrakul, S. and Boon, W.H., Gene deletion as the cause of thalassaemia, *Nature*, 251, 389, 1974.

21. Kan, Y.W., Dozy, A.M., Trecartin, R. and Todd, T., Identification of a nondeletion defect in x-Thalassemia, *N. Eng. J. Med.*, 297, 1081, 1977.

22. Tolstoshev, P., Mitchell, J., Lanyon, G., Williamson, R., Ottolenghi, S., Comi, P., Giglioni, B., Masera, G., Modell, B., Weatherall, D.J. and Clegg, J.B., Presence of gene for β-globin in homozygous βo thalassaemia, *Nature*, 259, 95, 1976.

23. Forget, B.G., Hillman, D.G., Lazarus, H., Barrell, E., Benz Jr., E.F., Caskey, C.T., Huisman, T.H.J., Schroeder, W.A. and Housman, D., Absence of messenger RNA and gene DNA for β-Globin chains in hereditary persistence of fetal hemoglobin, *Cell*, 7, 323, 1976.

24. Neal, W. R., Tayloe, Jr., D. T., Cederbaum, A. I., and Roberts, H. R., Detection of genetic variants of haemophilia B with an immunoabosorbent technique, *Brit. J. Haematol.* 26:63, 1973.

25. Cinader, B. and Dubiski, S., Suppression of murine allotypic specificities in animals with a complement defect and in animals with a complete hemolytic complement system, *J. Immunol.* 101, 1236, 1968.

26. Dray, S., Effect of maternal isoantibodies on the quantitative expression of the allelic genes controlling δ-globulin allotypic specificity, *Nature*, London 195, 785, 1962.

27. Cinader, B., Specificity and inheritance of antibody response: A possible steering Mechanism, *Nature* 188, 619, 1960.

28. Cinader, B., Dependence of antibody responses on structure and polymorphism of autologous macromolecules, *Brit. Med. Bull.* 19, 219, 1963.

29. Cinader, B. and Dubiski, S., Effect of autologous protein on the specificity of the antibody response: Mouse and rabbit antibody to MuB1, *Nature* 202, 102, 1964.

30. Gasser, D.L., Genetic control of the immune response in mice, I. Segregation data and localization to the fifth linkage group of a gene affecting antibody production, *J. Immunol.*, 103, 66, 1069.

31. Gasser, D.L., h-3 Linked Unresponsiveness to EA-1 and h-13 Antigens, in *The role of the Histocompatibility Gene Complex in Immune Responses*, D.G. Katz and B. Benacerraf, Eds., p 289, Academic Press, New York, 1976.

32. Benacerraf, B. and McDevitt, H.O., Histocompatibility-linked immune response genes, *Science*, 175, 273, 1972.

33. Cinader, B., Hayley, M.A., Rider, W.D. and Warwick, O.H., Immunotherapy of a patient with choriocarcinoma, *Canad. Med. Assoc. J.* 84, 306, 1961.

34. Rider, W.D. and Cinader, B., Immunotherapy for trophoblastic disease, (Abstract) *International Cancer Congress*, Tokyo, 1966.

35. Cinader, B., Compartmentalization (multicentricity) and interaction between sub-compartments, in *"Aging and Cellular Defense Mechanism"*, Proc. of the N.Y. Acad. Scies., 663, 294, 1993.

36. Fujiwara, M. and Cinader, B., Cellular aspects of tolerance. V. The *in vivo* cooperative role of accessory and thymus derived cells in responsiveness and unresponsiveness of SJL mice, *Cell. Immunol.*, 12, 194, 1974a.

37. Hosono, M., Cinader, B. and Ellerson, J., Tolerance induction as an index of age-related changes, *Imm. Comm.*, 6(3), 239, 1977.

38. Hosono, M. and Cinader, B., Resistance to tolerance-induction and age-dependent cellular changes in SJL mice, *Int. Arch. Allergy and Appl. Immunol.*, 54, 289, 1977.

39. **Fujiwara, M. and Cinader, B.,** Cellular aspects of tolerance, VII. Inheritance of the resistance to tolerance induction, *Cell. Immunol.* 12, 214, 1974b.

40. **Nakano, K. and Cinader, B.,** Accelerated age dependent decline in the T suppresser capacity of SJL mice, *Eur. J. Immunol.,* 10, 309, 1980a.

41. **Cinader, B., Paraskevas, F. and Koh, S.,** An age dependent decline in suppresser activity of SJL mice, *Cell. Immunol.,* 40, 445, 1978.

42. **Cinader, B., Amagai, T., Matsuzawa, T. and Nakano, K.,** Changements dépendants de l'âge du système immunitaire, in *Recherches biomédicales sur le vieillissement,* pp. 5-33, Cahiers de l'ACFAS 7, 1981a.

43. **Cinader, B., Amagai, T., Matsuzawa, T. and Nakano, K.,** Genetic programmes for the changes in immune responsiveness in adult life, in *Cellular and Molecular Mechanisms of Immunologic Tolerance,* T. Hraba and M. Hašek, Eds., pp. 187-199, Marcel Dekker, Inc., New York, 1981b.

44. **Amagai, T., Matsuzawa, T. and Cinader, B.,** The effect of Ribavirin and Rifamycin SV on age-dependent changes of the immune system during the adult life of SJL mice. *Immunol. Letters,* 4, 149, 1982.

45. **Amagai, T., Nakano, K. and Cinader, B.,** Mechanisms involved in age-dependent decline of immune responsiveness and apparent resistance against tolerance induction in C57BL/6 mice, *Scand. J. Immunol.,* 16, 217, 1982.

46. **Ponnappan, U., Cinader, B., Gerber, V. and Blaser, K.,** Antibody response and acquired tolerance of A/J mice: age and immunogen related isotype differences, *Scand. J. Immunol.,* 27, 419, 1988.

47. **Cinader, B., Clandinin, M. T., Hosokawa, T., and Robblee, N. M.,** Dietary fat alters the fatty acid composition of lymphocyte membranes and the rate at which suppressor capacity is lost, *Immunol. Lett.,* 6, 331, 1983.

48. **Cinader, B.,** Developmental change in the second half of life-strategies for modification of selected compartments of aging, *Immunol. Lett.,* 16, 193, 1987.

49. **Ponnappan, U., Cinader, B., and Clandinin, M. T.,** Effect of dietary fat on antibody response and on down-regulation, *Immunol. Lett.,* 18 (3), 205, 1988.

50. **Kubo, M. and Cinader, B.,** Polymorphism of age-related changes in interleukin production-differential changes of Th subpopulations, IL-2, IL-3, and IL-4, *Eur. J. Immunol.,* 20(6), 1289, 1990.

51. **Ponnapan, U., Dubiski, S. and Cinader, B. A.,** Effect of treatment with anti-CD4 on antibody response as a function of advancing age in C57BL/6 and SJL mice, *Aging, Immunol. and Infect. Dis.,* 3(3), 91, 1992.

52. **Cinader, B., Dubiski, S., Greenwood, C., Ponnapan, U. and Sauder, D.N.,** Economic Correction: Quantity and Age-related Rate of Change, in *Highlights of Modern Biochemistry,* A. Kotyk, J. Skoda, V. Paces and V. Kastka, Eds., pp. 1761-1768. VSP *Internat'l Science Publishers,* Zeist, 1989 and in *Mech. Aging Dev.* 48, 111, 1989.

53. **Cinader, B.** Series Editor: Receptors in Biology and Medicine: The Language of Intercellular Communication, Marcel Dekker, Inc., New York and Basel, 1983-1987.

   a. Multiple Dopamine Receptors, Milton Titeler, Ed.
   b. Structure and Function of Fc Receptors, Arnold Froese and Frixos Paraskevas, Eds.
   c. Cell Surface Phenomena, Alan S. Perelson, Charles DeLisi and Frederik W. Wiegel, Eds.
   d. Polypeptide Hormone Receptors , Barry I. Posner, Ed.
   e. Recognition and Regulation of Cell-Mediated Immunity, James D. Watson and John Marbrook, Eds.
   f. Insulin: Its Receptors and Diabetes, Morley D. Hollenberg, Ed.
   g. Parasite Antigens: Toward New Strategies for Vaccines, Terry W. Pearson, Ed.
   h. Adrenergic Receptors in Man, Paul A. Insel, Ed.

54. **Cinader, B.** Series Editor: Intercellular and Intracellular Communication, Cambridge University Press, Cambridge, U.K., 1986-1993.

   a. Hormones, Receptors and Cellular Interactions in Plants, C.M. Chadwick and D.R. Garrod, Eds.
   b. Receptors in Tumour Biology, C.M. Chadwick, Ed.
   c. Receptors and Ligands in Neurology, A.K. Sen and T.

Lee, Eds.

d. Receptors and Ligands in Psychiatry, A.K. Sen and T. Lee, Eds.

e. Intracellular Trafficking of Proteins, C.J. Steer and J. A. Hanover, Eds.

f. Vitamins as Ligands in Cell Communication—Metabolic Initiators, K. Dakshinamurti, Ed.

55. **Cinader, B.,** Contemporary Indian Art: the trail from the past to the future, exhibition catalogue, Mackenzie Gallery & Native Studies Program, Trent University, Peterborough, Ontario, 1977.

56. **Cinader, B., Daphne Odjig,** in *"100 Years of Native American Painting"*, The Oklahoma Museum of Art, Oklahoma City, 1978.

57. **Cinader, B.,** Manitoulin Island - The Third Layer, Thunder Bay Art Gallery (Thunder Bay National Exhibition Centre and Centre for Indian Art), 1987.

58. **Cinader, B., Carl Beam,** Art Post, Vol. 39, Winter 1990-91, pp. 20.

59. **Cinader, B., and Longboat, D.,** The Native Role of our Culture and of Canadian Education, Crucible; The Science Teachers Association of Ontario, 20(4), 6, 1989.

Chapter 6

WHAT HAPPENED TO TOLERANCE?

Erwin Diener

The basic tenet underlying our concept of adaptive immunity is the immune system's ability to distinguish between self and nonself. The formulation of hypotheses on mechanisms by which self-nonself discrimination is achieved has preoccupied immunologists for decades. In the past, many of us have based such formulations on experimental models where unresponsiveness is induced by a very select group of nonself antigens, thereby condescending to Hume's definition of scientific thought which is to assume that "instances of which we have no experience will conform to those of which we have experience." At present, we are faced with a body of data on tolerance to nonself, little of which has a high probability to be representative of tolerance to self.

Any theory concerned with self tolerance must acknowledge the fact that at the level of nominal epitope recognition *per se*, a T or B lymphocyte cannot tell whether it sees self or nonself. Constraints that would translate recognition into either immunity to nonself or tolerance to self must, thus, be postulated to operate either through a specified, temporally limited metabolic state during a lymphocyte's ontogenic development or thorough external regulatory influences. The first category of constraints is called for by the Clonal Abortion hypothesis.[1,2] In its original formulation, the hypothesis postulates that during ontogenic maturation, a potentially autoreactive lymphocyte passes through a transitional metabolic state during which antigen recognition results in paralysis and, thus, clonal abortion. Numerous sophisticated experimental models predominantly addressing B cell tolerance have lent support to this theory. However, one must not overlook the fact that most of the research data have been obtained from experiments that depended on two kinds of selected antigens: hapten derivatives of immunoglobulins—notably, human gamma globulin (HGG)—and, in some cases, polymeric proteins. Because the potential of immunoglobulins to induce tolerance is predominantly carrier related,[3] one must question interpretations of data from experiments concerned with Ig-mediated paralysis of immature B lymphocytes as being representative of clonal abortion to self. Furthermore, the well known observation that immunoglobulins are also tolerogenic for fully mature B cells, albeit at higher concentrations than for immature B cells, does not fully satisfy the basic assumption that only immature B cells perceive antigen recognition as a paralytic signal. The second category of antigens selected for tolerogenic potency are polymeric structures and their hapten-conjugates. It is important to recall that these antigens have been selected for their ability to induce unresponsiveness in fully mature immunocompetent B lymphocytes. From our own work with these antigens, we considered antigen-receptor crosslinking beyond a critical threshold as the condition for a paralytic signal to be induced.[4] The observation that induction of paralysis in immature B cells by antigens other than immunoglobulins also appears to depend on extensive receptor crosslinking by repeating epitopes,[5,6] constitutes yet another problem for defendants of clonal abortion, as it is unlikely that many self antigens present repetitive epitopes to potentially autoreactive lymphocytes. In the early days of cellular immunolo-

0-8493-4722-X/94/$0.00 + $.50

gy, most investigators believed that tolerance, particularly tolerance to self, meant the physical elimination of immunocompetent lymphocytes following antigen recognition under appropriate conditions. Not until the concept of immunoregulation by cell interaction circuits appeared on the scene, did investigators register the physical existence of self-antigen binding B lymphocytes in animals including man.[7] Along with this observation went the demonstration *in vivo* of what was coined "receptor blockade",[8] a state characterized by an apparent lack of receptor modulation by B lymphocytes following antigen binding. We interpreted receptor blockade to reflect a condition at which excessive degrees of receptor crosslinking would "freeze" the cell's mechanisms in control of surface structure modulation.[9] Similar effects which extend to surface structures that do not themselves function as antigen receptors may be observed. For example, following exposure of B lymphocytes to concanavalin A, surface Ig receptor modulation in response to antigen binding is inhibited. This, however, does not affect the cell's immunocompetence.[10,11] The phenomenon was shown to be due to the failure of polymerized microtubular protein to dissociate. When the cells so affected were exposed to colchicine, ligand-induced receptor modulation was restored.[12] Interestingly, inhibition of receptor modulation under conditions at which unresponsiveness is also induced was shown not to be related to the unresponsive state of the B cells concerned. Thus, tolerant B cells whose mechanism of receptor modulation was inhibited by antigen-mediated receptor blockade, when treated with colchicine underwent receptor redistribution and endocytosis or shedding, yet remained refractory to an immunogenic challenge even though they had a new set of antigen receptors expressed.9 We concluded that receptor blockade by antigen is likely to be independent of the tolerant state of the cell concerned, hence, the occurrence of receptor-bearing, yet tolerant, B cells *in vivo*. When the same phenomenon was also discovered in animals that had ben rendered tolerant as neonates, i.e., at an ontogenic state at which most B lymphocytes are considered immature, the term "clonal abortion" was replaced by the term "clonal anergy".[13] This further blunted the abortion hypothesis as a mechanism of tolerance to self as originally conceived.

Another theory which attempts to explain tolerance with persuasive intellectual elegance is the Two-Signal hypothesis of Bretscher and Cohn.[14] Based on the phenomenon of T-B cell cooperation, it defines a sequence of intracellular signals triggered by linked-associative recognition of hapten and carrier determinants involving hapten-specific B cells and carrier-specific helper T cells. In this model, two signals are required for immune triggering to occur: signal 1, derived from hapten recognition by B cell surface receptors, must coincide or be followed by an additional signal, 2, derived from the carrier-primed helper T cell. From the point of view of self tolerance, the most crucial constraint imposed by the theory is that signal 1 alone leads to paralysis. Given the assumption that T helper cells specific for self are absent from the environment in which potentially autoreactive B lymphocytes undergo ontogenic development, they will receive signal 1 only through recognition of self and, thereby, be clonally deleted. Like the Clonal Abortion theory, the Clonal Deletion hypothesis also hinges on the *ad hoc* assumption that potentially nonself reactive B lymphocytes emerging from bone marrow stem cells be protected from extrinsic antigens in order not to be deleted. There is no evidence, however, that the bone marrow is, in this sense, an immunologically privileged site.

The most effective method by which to assess a theory is to ask whether it is falsifiable by testing its own predictions. Given the molecular heterogeneity of self antigens, both the Clonal Abortion and Deletion hypotheses predict that the generation of a tolerogenic signal depends entirely on the binding affinity between the antigenic epitope and the receptor antigen combining site, regardless of the chemical structure presenting the epitope. Extensive studies from this laboratory led to the conclusion that B cell paralysis to nonself, regardless of the ontogenic state of the immune system, depends to a large extent on the molecular nature of the carrier that presents the B cell-specific epitopes (reviewed in Reference[15]).   Furthermore, antigens selected for lack of tolerogenicity to the adult immune system, regardless of the dose employed, also failed to tolerize the immature immune system, even when administered to the fetus *via* the placenta.[16]   Finally, hapten conjugates with different carriers but the same epitope at similar density, were found to induce unresponsiveness in the immature immune system either by what appeared to be clonal deletion or by accessory cell-mediated suppression, depending on the type of carrier used.[17]   These findings are incompatible with the predictions stated above and, hence, in disagreement with the Clonal Abortion/Deletion hypotheses.

The phenomenon of clonal anergy is of particular significance in view of the presence of B cells in normal animals, including man, that bind self antigens, for example myelin basic protein.[7]   Furthermore, it has been reported that in normal mice, B lymphocytes specific for thyroglobulin[18] are in a cycling state, and that B cells specific for autologous myosin and for albumin may be activated to generate autoantibodies *in vitro*.[19]   In all likelihood, self antigen-binding B cells could be triggered to yield an autoimmune response *in vivo* if given the proper circumstances.   One is reminded of the suggestion first proposed by Allison, that humoral unresponsiveness to self may be controlled by helper T cells rather than by deletion of B cells.[20]   Thus, potentially autoreactive B cells in the absence of functional autoreactive helper T cells could only be stimulated through linked recognition with helper T cells specific for a nonself antigenic determinant from, say, a virus or a drug, in association with self.   To postulate clonal deletion of potentially self-reactive T cells by direct contact with self is, however, controversial in view of new insights into the mechanisms by which T cells recognize antigens.   It is now clear that foreign proteins are internalized by antigen-presenting cells, broken down into peptide fragments, which are then exposed on the cell surface in association with self antigens encoded by the major histocompatibility (MHC) locus;[21] review.[22]   Recognition by a single-receptor combining site on T lymphocytes[23] of MHC-associated peptides becomes, thus, MHC restricted.   It follows that not only immune triggering but also clonal deletion of T cells would operationally appear MHC restricted. Experimental evidence, indeed, suggests this to be the case.[24,25,26,27,28] The likelihood that cells of the reticuloendothelial system not only process foreign proteins and present MHC-associated peptide fragments to the immune system, but that perhaps most cells of the body do the same with endogenous self proteins has been discussed.[22]   In the assumption that self tolerance results from clonal deletion of T cells,[21,29] the MHC-associated expression of self peptides would likely result in a state of immunologic incompetence of the animal to foreign antigens, as the probability for cross recognition with respect to self and nonself peptides is expected to be high, particularly so if the epitopes that are being recognized comprise a few amino acids only.   In recognition of this problem, the "Peptidic self model" of Claverie and Kourilsky[30] which, in its basic assumptions is corroborated by interpretations of recent experimental data, postulates the distinction between the "somatic self" and the "immunologic self," the two of which do not overlap.   The antigenic diversity of the somatic self is considered different from foreign proteins and peptides as the number of immunodominant amino acid sequences in a given protein is lower than expected and, hence, degrees of antigenic overlap between "self" and "foreign" may, in fact, be quite low. Tolerance to somatic self is thus considered unlikely to cause "holes" in the antigen recognition repertoire to a life-threatening extent.   In contrast to the "somatic self," the "immunologic self" is postulated by the authors to be displayed and recognized by immunocytes as part of the immunoregulatory machinery.   Clearly, the constraints imposed on mechanisms of tolerance to self call for a distinction to be made between recognition of "immunologic self" and "somatic self."   Such a distinction is difficult to reconcile with the simple notion of clonal deletion upon receptor-epitope recognition alone.

   To date, research on the fate of T cells directly affected by a tolerance-inducing mechanism has yielded relatively little information from which to deduce a generally applicable mechanism in control of tolerance to self. However, recently developed *in vitro* models have yielded the kind of data that point in a potentially fruitful direction.   T cell lines have been shown to assume a state of unresponsiveness akin to clonal anergy upon exposure to either high concentrations of free antigen in the absence of macrophages,[31] or to antigen bound to antigen-presenting cells (APC) by a coupling agent such as carbodiimide.[32]   As expected, paralysis induced by APC was shown to be I region restricted, in contrast to the presumably rare case where sufficiently high concentrations of free antigen can directly bind to T cells to bring about tolerance.   Treatment of APC with carbodiimide appears to be crucial to the abolishment of an as yet unidentified costimulant believed to be emitted by untreated APC to immunostimulate T cells.   In sympathy with the two signal hypothesis of Bretscher and Cohn, the authors suggest that in the absence of the costimulant (signal 2) from APC, antigen recognition (signal 1) by T cells leads to paralysis.   In this respect, the model bears similarity to that of Rheinherz,[33] concerning the functional relationship between the T3-Ti antigen/MHC-restricted antigen receptor complex and T11 surface molecules.   T3-T1 was shown to inhibit the alternative stimulatory pathway via T11, whose physiologic ligand has recently been identified as LFA-3.   In the model of Reinherz, T11, whose activation pathway is independent of macrophages and IL-1, is postulated to mediate expansion of thymocyte populations prior to T3-Ti receptor expression.   In the assumption that IL-1 is unavailable within the thymic cortex, intrathymic recognition of self by thymocytes emerging with T3-Ti receptors of appropriate specificity, would be incapable of undergoing expansion by either the IL-2 mediated or, the alternative, T11-dependent pathway.   In agreement with the two-signal hypothesis, the T3-Ti-mediated signal in the absence of IL-1, could be considered a paralytic signal.   Reinherz's model concerning intrathymic tolerance disagrees with that of Jenkins *et al.*,[32] insofar as T cell tolerance induced by carbodiimide treated APC's cannot be prevented by IL-1. Whether or not the two modes of antigen presentation lead to tolerance via similar mechanisms, remains unanswered.   Although, MHC-restricted T cell tolerance has been reported to occur *in vivo*, it remains to be investigated whether the phenomenon is due to the same mechanisms as tolerance *in vitro* cited above.

In vivo data on T cell tolerance are marred by a multitude of phenomena, apparently pointing at more than one mechanisms by which tolerance to self may be controlled. Intrathymically established tolerance in thymocytes appears to coexist with prethymically induced tolerance said to affect receptor-bearing thymocyte precursors.[34] The controversy as to T cell unresponsiveness being controlled by either clonal deletion/anergy or active suppression or by both these mechanisms, adds further to the complexity of issue. In view of the scarcity of *in vivo* data on self tolerance, the elegant experimental model of Borel and colleagues, concerning tolerance mechanisms to the complement component C5, is noteworthy.[35] By means of lymphocyte transfer studies between C5-sufficient and C5-deficient mice, the investigators were able to demonstrate the presence of C5-specific suppressor T cells in C5-sufficient and, hence, C5-tolerant mice. Not surprisingly, C5-specific B lymphocytes in C5-sufficient mice were fully immunocompetent but lacked the collaboration from helper T cells, which were found to be functionally deleted. Whether such deletion is causally related to the presence of suppressor T cells, is still an open question. Clearly, an experimental model such as this has the potential to further advance our knowledge about mechanisms of self tolerance, particularly if extended *in vitro* at the clonal level.

At the Symposium on Mechanisms on Immunological Tolerance held at Prague in 1961, the discussion chairman, Sir Peter Medawar, asked the participants to suggest, at the end of the sessions, the most likely course of therapy in case they suffered from fatal bilateral kidney disease. The answers were predictably varied; in essence, they centered around the homotransplantation of kidneys from closely matched donors combined with an attempt to induce tolerance to donor antigens by various means. If the same question were asked from a similar audience today, it is unlikely that anyone would seriously consider conditioning the recipient of the graft by a protocol that aims at tolerance induction to the donor's antigens. During the 26 years since the Prague conference, we have learned enough about tolerance to know that for us to apply it to clinical transplantation, we must know a lot more.

REFERENCES

1. Burnet, F.M., in *The Clonal Selection Theory of Acquired Immunity*, Cambridge University Press, New York, 1959.

2. Lederberg, J., Genes and antibodies: Do antigens bear instructions for antibody specificity or do they select cell lines that arise by mutation? *Science*, 129, 1649, 1959.

3. Waldschmidt, T.J., Borel, Y., and Vitetta, E.S., The use of haptenated immunoglobulins to induce B cell tolerance *in vitro*, The role of hapten density and the Fc portion of the immunoglobulin carrier, *J. Immunol.*, 131, 2204, 1983.

4. Diener, E. and Feldmann, M., Relationship between antigen and antibody induced suppression of immunity, *Transplant Rev.*, 8, 76, 1972.

5. Metcalf, E.S. and Klinman, N.R., *In vitro* tolerance induction of neonatal murine B cells, *J. Exp. Med.*, 143, 1327, 1976.

6. Pike, B.L., Battye, F.L., and Nossal, G.J.V., Effect of hapten valency and carrier composition on the tolerogenic potential of hapten-carrier conjugates, *J. Immunol.*, 126, 89, 1981.

7.   Yung, L.L.L., Diener, E., McPherson, T.A., Barton, M.A. and Hyde, H.A., Antigen binding lymphocytes in normal man and guinea pig to human encephalitogenic protein, *J. Immunol.*, 110, 1383, 1973.

8.   Borel, Y. and Aldo-Benson, M., Receptor blockade by tolerogen: One explanation of tolerance, in *Immunological Tolerance*, D.H. Katz and B. Benacerraf, Eds., Academic Press, New York, 1974, p. 333.

9.   Diener, E., Kraft, N., Lee, K.-C., and Shiozawa, C., Antigen recognition. IV. Discrimination by antigen-binding immunocompetent B cells between immunity and tolerance is determined by adherent cells, *J. Exp. Med.* 143, 805, 1976.

10. Diener, E. and Paetkau, V.H., Antigen recognition, II. Early surface receptor phenomena induced by binding of tritium-labeled antigen, *Proc. Natl. Acad. Sci. U.S.A.*, 69, 2364, 1972.

11. Lee, K.-C., Langman, R.E., Paetkau, V.H., and Diener, E., Antigen recognition, III. Effect of phytomitogens on antigen-receptor capping and the immune response, *Eur. J. Immunol.*, 3, 306, 1973.

12. Edelman, G.M., Yahara, I. and Wang, J.L., Receptor mobility and receptor cytoplasmic interactions in lymphocytes, *Proc. Natl. Acad. Sci. USA*, 70, 1441, 1973.

13. Nossal, G.J.V. and Pike, B.L., Clonal anergy: Persistence in tolerant mice of antigen-binding B lymphocytes incapable of responding to antigen as mitogen, *Proc. Natl. Acad. Sci. USA*, 77, 1602, 1980.

14. Bretscher, P.A. and Cohn, M.A., A theory of self-nonself discrimination, *Science*, 169, 1042, 1970.

15. Diener, E and Waters, C.A., Immunological quiescence toward self: Rethinking the paradigm of clonal abortion, in *Paradoxes in Immunology*, G.W. Hoffman, J.G. Levy, and G.T. Nepom, Eds., CRC Press, Inc., Boca Raton, 1986.

16. Diener, E., Waters, C.A., and Singh, B., Restraints on current concepts of self-tolerance, in *T and B Lymphocytes: Recognition and Function*, F.H. Bach, B. Bonavida, E.S. Vitetta, and C.F. Fox, Eds., Academic Press, New York, 1979, p. 209.

17. Waters, C.A. and Diener, E., Tolerance induction during ontogeny, II. Distinct unresponsive states in immature mice question the generality of clonal abortion, *Eur. J. Immunol.*, 13, 928, 1983.

18. Portnoi, D., Freitas, A. Holmberg, D., Bandeira, A., and Coutinho, A., Immuno-competent autoreactive B lymphocytes are activated cycling cells in normal mice, *J. Exp. Med.*, 164, 25, 1986.

19. Karray, S., Lymberi, P., Avrameas, S., and Coutinho, A., Quantitative evidence against inactivation of self-reactive B cell clones, *Scand. J. Immunol.*, 23, 475, 1986.

20. Allison, A.C., Denman, A.M., and Barnes, R.D., Cooperating and controlling functions of thymus-derived lymphocytes in relation to autoimmunity, *Lancet*, 2, 135, 1971.

21. Guillet, J.G., Lai, M.Z., Briner, T. J., Buus, S., Sette, A., Grey, H.M., Smith, J.A., and Gefter, M.L., Immunological self, nonself discrimination, *Science*, 235, 865, 1987.

22. Germain, R.N., The ins and outs of antigen processing and presentation, *Nature*, 322, 687, 1986.

23. Dembric, Z., Haas, W., Weiss, S., McCubrey, J., Kiefer, H., von Boehmer, H., and Steinmetz, M., Transfer of specificity by murine α and β T cell receptor genes, *Nature*, 320, 232, 1986.

24. Dos Reis, G.A. and Shevach, E.M., Antigen presenting cells from unresponsive strain 2 guinea pigs are fully competent to responder strain 13 T cells, *J. Exp. Med.*, 157, 1287, 1983.

25. Rammensee, H.G. and Bevan, M.J., Evidence from *in vitro* studies that tolerance to self antigens is MHC-restricted, *Nature*, 308, 741, 1984.

26. Groves, E.S. and Singer, A., Role of the H-2 complex in the induction of T cell tolerance to self minor histocompatibility antigens, *J. Exp. Med.*, 158, 1483, 1983.

27. Matzinger, P., Zamoyska, R., and Waldmann, H., Self tolerance is H-2 restricted, *Nature*, 308, 738, 1984.

28. Lowy, A., Drebin, J.A., Monroe, J.G., Granstein, R.D., and Green, M.I., Genetically restricted antigen presentation for immunological tolerance and suppression, *Nature*, 308, 373, 1984.

29. Kappler, J.W., Roehm, N., and Marrack, P., T cell tolerance by clonal elimination in the thymus, *Cell*, 49, 273, 1987.

30. **Kourilsky, P. and Claverie, J.M.,** The peptidic self model: A hypothesis on the molecular nature of the immunological self, *Ann. Inst. Pasteur*, 137D, 3, 1986.
31. **Zanders, E.D., Lamb, J.R., Feldmann, M., Green, N., and Beverley, P.C.L.,** Tolerance of T cell clones is associated with membrane antigen changes, *Nature*, 303, 625, 1983.
32. **Jenkins, M.K., Pardoll, D.M., Mizuguchi, J., Quill, H., and Schwartz, R.H.,** T cell unresponsiveness *in vivo* and *in vitro*: Fine specificity of induction and molecular characterization of the unresponsive state, *Immunol. Rev.*, 95, 113, 1987.
33. **Reinherz, E.L.,** A molecular basis for thymic selection: Regulation of T induced thymocyte expansion by the T3-Ti antigen/MHC receptor pathway, *Immunol. Today*, 6, 75, 1985.
34. **Bradley, S.M., Morrissey, P.J., Sharrow, S.O., and Singer, A.,** Tolerance of thymocytes to allogeneic I region determinants encountered prethymically, *J. Exp. Med.*, 155, 1638, 1982.
35. **Cairns, L., Rosen, F.S., and Borel., Y.,** Mice naturally tolerant to CS have T cells that suppress the response to this antigen, *Eur. J. Immunol.*, 16, 1277, 1986.

Chapter 7

ONE CELL - ONE ANTIBODY: IMPACT ON IMMUNOLOGICAL THEORY AND PRACTICE

G.J.V. Nossal

Now that international congresses of immunology attract 8,000 people, and that the immunological literature constitutes perhaps 15% of biomedical science, it is difficult to cast one's mind back to the middle 1950s, a period when a serious scholar in immunology still had a reasonable chance of finding out about, and understanding, every major discovery in the field. The "club" was small, and few people in Australia were members. I got my formal training in immunology, such as it was, in 1951 as a fourth year medical student, and from what little I learned from H.K. Ward about vaccines (Is it safe? Is it effective? Is it worthwhile?), I have been forgiven for concluding that the field was pretty sleepy. In fact, I interrupted my course for a year in 1951 to pursue laboratory studies in virology, in Ward's department, under P.M. de Burgh. During this period the ambition to work under F.M. Burnet in Melbourne first flowered. Viruses, the smallest forms of life, promised to reveal so much of the secrets of the life process! I finished my medical course in 1954 and my residency training in 1956 and plucked up enough courage to write to Burnet. Imagine my dismay when the great man wrote back saying he could be pleased to have me, provided he could rake up the necessary £700 per year, but I would have to work in immunology, as this was the coming new field! Such was the faith of the young in their mentors in those bygone days that I complied with hardly a demur. In 1957, I embarked on a Ph.D. degree within The Walter and Eliza Hall Institute of Medical Research in Melbourne.

BACKGROUND TO THE CLONAL SELECTION THEORY

Unbeknown to me, Burnet (experimentally a virologist) had been interested in immunological theory for at least 15 years.[1] He was deeply convinced that the direct template theory of antibody formation was incorrect, as it failed to explain, or indeed even address, some of the key observations of immunology, such as the exponential rise of antibody levels early after immunization; immunological memory and the booster effect; or affinity maturation of antibodies. Most important of all, the direct template theory had nothing to say on the subject of self-recognition, which Burnet considered critical to any understanding of immunity. He had predicted the discovery of immunological tolerance[2] on theoretical grounds, and constructed the "self-marker" theory[3] to explain it. Although at the time the self-marker theory lead nowhere, it gains renewed interest in the light of our present understanding of the processing and presentation of intracellular peptides in association with Class I molecules at the cell surface, and of clonal abortion within the thymus of at lest some anti-self T cells. The failure to find a truly satisfying cellular explanation for immunity and tolerance irked Burnet greatly, in particular as his book, *Enzyme, Antigen and Virus*[4] which attempted to construct a suitable framework, had received a very critical press.

The next major step forward was the articulation by Jerne of the natural selection theory of antibody formation.[5] This postulated that antibodies of every conceivable specificity were made randomly and entered the blood

0-8493-4722-X/94/$0.00 + $.50

plasma. An antigen had only to combine with the natural antibody specific for it to trigger excess production of that antibody, a thought which echoed Ehrlich's[6] side chain theory.   Even though the mechanism suggested (selective replication of the particular antibody of interest inside the macrophage which took up the antigen-antibody complex) contravened what later came to be known as the Crick dogma, Jerne's hypothesis intrigued and puzzled Burnet. He asked me what I thought of it. "Pretty crazy," came my conventional reply, chiefly because I simply could not conceive that the unimmunized immune system could create such a huge repertoire of pre-formed antibodies. Later that same year, Talmage[7] made the link between Jerne's proposal and Ehrlich's theory, and suggested that cells bearing natural antibodies with which the antigen could unite would be selected for multiplication. Talmage also noted the homogeneity of myeloma proteins, indicating that the clone of malignant cells was making just one antibody. Talmage's own perspective on this story is given elsewhere in this volume, but from my point of view he really deserves enormous credit for enunciating the central tenets of the clonal selection theory before Burnet, who actually cites Talmage in his first paper.[8]

Having been thinking along rather similar lines, but having been bruised by previous unsuccessful attempts to crack the problem of antibody formation, Burnet found that Talmage's article gave him the courage to publish his own version of the clonal selection theory.[8] Burnet placed great emphasis on the lymphocyte having just *one* kind of natural antibody as a receptor. Differences between different lymphocytes were attributed to somatic mutation. Tolerance was ascribed to contact with antigen when the cell was immature, leading to clonal deletion rather than activation. Autoimmunity was thought of as "forbidden clones," or some form of breakdown of the tolerance mechanism. As Jerne concluded in 1979: "I hit the nail, but Burnet hit the nail on its head"[9] Two experimental findings impressed Burnet. The first was growth of "pocks" on the chorio-allantoic membranes of chick embryos induced by lymphoid cells from another chicken, the numbers of which were related to the input number of lymphocytes. These were seen as localized graft-vs-host immune responses, with only a minority of donor cells capable of responding. The second was the observation that certain patients with macroglobulinemia, a monoclonal gammopathy, had high titers of autoantibodies in their serum, as if to suggest a "forbidden clone" had gone out of control and turned malignant. These experiments lent credence to multiplying unispecific cells as the central element of the immune response.

ANTIBODY FORMATION BY SINGLE CELLS

Six months into my Ph.D. course, I still harbored a fondness for viruses. In fact, the first project I tried was to induce immunological tolerance to influenza virus in embryonic mice, a project which failed rapidly and completely! I was still reading the virus literature with interest, including work on virus replication in mammalian cells. My earliest work as a medical student had been an attempt to generate one-step growth curves of ectromelia virus in mouse liver cells. I was therefore especially interested to see that it was now possible to grow viruses in single tissue-cultured cells grown in capillary tubes. One Monday morning, in about August 1957, Burnet came into the laboratory with a draft of his clonal selection paper.[8] Still not too impressed, but certainly more interested than before, I soon thought of a way of *disproving* the theory. If I could immunize an animal with two different antigens, and show that one single cell could make antibody against both of them, then the theory would be untenable. But how to do the experiment? I had no expertise in tissue culture, no idea how to get cells into or out of capillary tubes. Then fate took a hand. The whole laboratory was excited about a brief, three-month visit by the 32 year old genius who had founded the science of bacterial genetics, Joshua Lederberg, as a Fulbright Visiting Professor. Lederberg had in fact come to Melbourne to sort out influenza virus genetics, as Burnet's last major contribution to virology had been the demonstration of recombinational events between influenza virus strains. He had no prior interest in immunology. However, he had considerable experience in working with tiny droplets containing single bacteria which adhered to coverslips and were prevented from evaporating by a surrounding layer of paraffin oil. This seemed a promising way of culturing single lymphoid cells, and Lederberg generously offered to teach me the technique and to collaborate in the early experiments.

Next came a search for an antibody titration method that was sufficiently sensitive to detect the small amount of antibody secreted by a single cell. We chose to look at two possibilities. The first was the immobilization of motile bacteria by anti-flagellar antibody. A great deal was known about the so-called H antigens of *Salmonella* bacteria, which displayed remarkable diversity, frequently with no cross-reactivity. The second was the lysis of sheep erythrocytes by antibody plus complement. This second technique was frustrated by a very simple observation. The lymphoid cells from immunized mice were incubated in their little microdroplets, while handing from an inverted coverslip, sitting at a water:paraffin interface. They seemed perfectly happy there, but erythrocytes simply "popped" when they hit that interface. We had no anti-sheep erythrocyte assay, as the erythrocytes lysed, antibody or no antibody. One angle of this research is worth reporting, however. On his return to the United States, Lederberg wanted to try a version of this assay as a plaque technique in agar. He had a graduate student, Becca Patras, try to develop a hemolytic plaque assay using sheep erythrocytes, lymphoid cells and complement in agar. Neither Lederberg nor Patras knew that agar was strongly anti-complementary. Had they used agarose, or added DEAE-dextran, the hemolytic plaque technique would have been discovered five years earlier than it was!

The flagellar immobilization technique seemed to have the characteristics we were seeking. Luckily, the Bacteriology Department of the University had an old de Fonbrune micromanipulatory they were willing to lend us. There was only one major problem: we needed a microscope! The only proper binocular microscope in the Hall Institute was in Burnet's private office and obviously sacrosanct. So we got hold of a venerable old Bausch and Lomb microscope, without inclined oculars, and without phase or dark field optics. In those days, Australian pennies were very large, about 4 cm in diameter. We worked out that if we placed a penny in a judicious position just under the condenser of the microscope, and a bit off center, we could create a fair imitation of a dark-field effect and so see our motile bacteria! When Lederberg had taught me the delicate task of pulling micropipettes (by hand or by the de Fonbrune microforge), it was time for him to leave, before results came through. But fortunately, single cells incubated in droplets of 10^{-7} to 10^{-6} ml did secrete enough antibody to halt a little "cloud" of motile bacteria instilled into positive droplets by micromanipulation, and I soon showed that one lymph node cell from doubly-immunized rats could always form only one antibody specificity, not two.[10,11] Shortly thereafter, the same conclusion was reached by White on the basis of immunofluorescence studies.[12] Lederberg quickly concluded that Talmage and Burnet were on the right track, and became an ardent supporter of clonal selection.[13]

The first and most obvious contribution of the "one cell - one antibody" finding was that it was consistent with the clonal selection theory, although, from a formal point of view, it said nothing about the potential of the lymphocyte which generated the clone of antibody-forming plasma cells. The finding, and the technique which made it possible, had other consequences as well. It added credibility to the use of myeloma proteins as model immunoglobulins for the study of antibody structure; if single cells made a homogenous product, then the homogeneous proteins made by myeloma tumors might resemble true antibodies. It permitted a detailed study of the histology of antibody-forming cells[14] and of the cellular kinetics of antibody production. It also allowed the question to be posed as to whether cells could switch from IgM production to IgG without a change in specificity.[15] This switch was, in fact, noted in a small percentage of cells at critically chosen times of the immune response, when some cells produced both IgM an IgG of the same specificity. This work preceded the discovery of VDJ translocation as the basis of isotype switching. Single cell methods also proved of value in providing formal proof that, following T cell-B cell collaboration, it was the B cell that actually made the antibody.[16] But these later findings came after an interesting and difficult part of the story.

THE PROBLEM OF MEL COHN AND ED LENNOX

Unbeknown to me, a powerful group at Washington University had become interested in antibody formation by single cells.[17] Headed by M. Cohn and E.S. Lennox, this group immunized rabbits with unrelated phage strains, prepared single cell microdrops, and measured antibody formation by phage neutralization. They found that 15-22% of cells were double-producers! Burnet brought this news back to Australia from one of his trips; Mel Cohn was a protégé of Jacques Monod, who had even indulged in a little speculation of his own on the basis of the findings. You can imagine my dismay, as an essentially self-trained Ph.D. student (Burnet taught me some virological techniques but had never worked in cellular immunology himself), when I found such distinguished and established investigators in the opposite camp. Yet I was utterly confident of my findings, and in fact I thought I knew the explanation for the discrepancy. In my earliest studies, and in those of Attardi et al.,[17] lymphoid cells from immunized animals were dispensed as microdrops from a dense cell suspension. In those days, we had no metrizamide gradients, dead cell removal buffers, etc., and, no matter how hard you washed the cells, droplets thus dispensed contained traces of preformed antibody, perhaps leaching from cell debris, etc. I soon learned that the only way to avoid this background totally was to *wash each cell separately*, under the microscope, by micromanipulation. This was not too difficult once one had mastered the technique, and it made all the difference. Obviously droplets from doubly-immunized rats that contained preformed antibody would score as doubly-positive. Whether that was the *real* answer to the discrepancy will probably never be known. However, some years later, Mäkelä[18] repeated the phage-neutralization experiments almost exactly, *but* with the critical cell wash as an intermediate step, and he found no double producers.

In the meantime, the scientific controversy with Cohn and Lennox took a piquant human turn. Lederberg, having moved from Madison to Stanford to head up a new Department of Genetics, asked me to come there as a post-doctoral fellow (and later Assistant Professor). One of the chief attractions to Lederberg in coming to Stanford was that Arthur Kornberg was to occupy the laboratories literally next door to Genetics. Kornberg was bringing his whole team from Washington University, with Mel Cohn as a leading member! I do not mind admitting that my first meeting with Cohn in August 1959 was a little awkward. Happily, we eventually became the best of friends, and have had many (for me) constructive arguments about the immune system ever since. I met Ed Lennox in 1960 at an Antibody Workshop, and found him a charming and delightful person. Soon after Lennox and Cohn went to the Salk Institute in San Diego, I was invited to lecture there, and the early difficulties never impeded the development of our relationship as colleagues.

MÄKELÄ'S WORK ON HETEROCLITICITY

At Stanford, Lederberg asked a gifted Finnish post-doctoral fellow, Dr. Olavi Mäkelä, to work in close collaboration with me. It took him no time to learn all the micromanipulation techniques and we became firm colleagues and friends. We were soon joined by Avrion Mitchison, who came for a year as a Visiting Professor, and when we heard how sympathetically both he and another Visiting Professor, George Klein, looked on clonal selection, we were all riding high. This is not to say that the immunological establishment in the United States took us to their bosoms. In fact, most immunologists remained skeptical until the overwhelming evidence, by about the time of the 1967 Cold Spring Harbor Symposium, finally changed the climate of opinion.

Mäkelä did some beautiful work shortly after his return to Finland.[19] He took the phage neutralization single cell system invented by Attardi et al.[17] and used it to study antibody cross-reactivities. It was well known that antibody prepared against one phage could also neutralize another, cross-reactive phage, though to a lesser degree. Let us suppose phage 1, the immunogen, cross-reacted with phage 2 to the extent that neutralization of 1 was 5 times more than phage 2 at a particular dilution of serum. What Mäkelä showed was that this cross-reactivity was an *average* result based on the sum of the activities of many cells. When single cells were examined, each had its own unique fingerprint of cross-reactivity. While most cells neutralized phage 1 to a greater degree than phage 2, the ratios of neutralization varied widely, and some individual cells actually neutralized phage 2 to a greater degree than phage 1. Mäkelä termed this form of antibody *heteroclitic*. Not only did this study fit in beautifully with the idea of a random generation of diversity, as hypothesized in clonal selection, but it also showed what a precise and unique product, with its own particular properties, each cell made. It could thus fairly be argued that the study of antibody formation by single cells anticipated the qualities which monoclonal antibodies made by hybridoma technology would possess.[20]

For five or six years, with the exception of the Cohn-Lennox group (which effectively disbanded in 1959) the only people working on antibody formation by single cells were ourselves and the people we trained. Frank Fitch came to us at Stanford; as an experienced pathologist he picked up all the microscopic techniques with a speed that mortified us! I spent a happy month at New York University demonstrating the methods to Jonathan Uhr and his staff. On the whole, though, even our own students were reluctant to commit the time and effort into the tedious micromanipulations required for single cell work. I remember complaining to Burnet: "Why am I frequently cited, but rarely confirmed?"

All of this changed drastically one fine day in 1963. Jerne and his colleagues announced the discovery of the hemolytic plaque technique[21] and all of a sudden anyone with a Petri dish, some agarose, and some red cells, could play at antibody formation by single cells! I will not say that the vastly simpler method put us out of business, because there were still important things that one could find out only if one had access to the cell of interest (e.g. 15), but it certainly meant that now there was a whole army of new workers playing on our patch! It was satisfying to note that all our key findings were now rapidly confirmed, and of course the very handy, quantitative technique opened up a whole new chapter in cellular immunology, particularly for antibody production *in vitro* and for adoptive transfer studies. Furthermore, the plaque technique played a crucial role in the screening process for the first monoclonal antibody-producing hybridomas.

FORMAL PROOF OF CLONAL SELECTION

Quite early in the piece, Gordon Ada and I convinced ourselves that the direct template hypothesis could not possibly be correct, on the basis of the absence of antigen or antigen fragments in the cytoplasm of antibody-forming cells under circumstances where as few as 4 molecules of (radioactively labeled) antigen would have been detected.[22] During the earliest stages of antibody production, plasmablasts did show one or more patches of antigen at the cell surface[23] but although I commented on this location, I did not realize its crucial significance. It was Naor and Sulitzeanu[24] who first made a frontal attack on the question of antigen-specific receptors at the lymphocyte surface, finding that only a tiny minority of lymphocytes from an unimmunized animal could bind a particular labeled antigen to their surface. Moreover, the proportion rose after immunization and fell after the induction of a state of tolerance to the antigen concerned.[25] These findings certainly represented a big step forward for the clonal selection theory. However, it still remained to show conclusively that the antigen-binding cells were actually the direct precursors of the antibody-forming clone. Ada and Byrt[26] showed that attaching a sufficient quantity of high specific activity ^{125}I-antigen onto cells for 24 hr caused the lymphoid population to lose the potential to form the corresponding antibody. This important "hot antigen suicide" experiment did not formally eliminate the possibility that the antigen-binding cells had other potentials as well. Soon after Raff's work showing surface Ig as a convenient marker for B cells,[27] an ingenious co-capping experiment[28] made the monospecificity of B cells very likely. When a multivalent antigen attached to a small minority of B cells at saturating concentration, it capped essentially all the membrane Ig of that cell, so receptors of a different specificity were not present.

Enrichment of virgin antigen-specific B cells proved more difficult to achieve than depletion, although several successful attempts were reported in the early 1970s.[29,30,31,32] Using a technique dependent on the adhesion of hapten-specific cells to a thin layer of hapten-gelatin, followed by collagenase digestion of adherent antigen, we were finally able to provide formal proof of clonal selection for the B cell.[33] The requisite single cell cloning methods have been progressively improved and refined over the years,[34] so that now they constitute a useful tool for the study of B cell activation mechanisms. It is somewhat amusing to note that the formal proof some 18 years after we produced the first evidence for clonal selection occasioned little comment, because by then it was essentially what everyone had come to expect.

Looking back to the late 1960s I recall that there were two important questioners of clonal selection, each for a different reason. Morten Simonsen was perplexed by the high proportion of T lymphocytes with reactivity against a particular allogeneic MHC gene combination. This figure, which is around 5% is not really against one antigen, but probably against a large number of different self peptides fitting into the groove of the allogeneic MHC class I or class II molecules concerned. Alain Bussard was struck by the large proportion of murine peritoneal B cells which could apparently respond to a given antigen, sheep red blood cells. We now know that these were Ly-1 B cells making highly cross-reactive antibodies of a restricted range of specificities.[35] So these exceptional cases were not, in the last analysis, able to shake the clonal selection paradigm.

THE ROLE OF SOMATIC MUTATION

Curiously, Burnet was not particularly interested in the details of the mechanisms which set up the diversified repertoires of B and T lymphocytes. He used the term somatic mutation rather loosely. He meant thereby any somatic genetic process which ended up with the lymphocytes (a) having unique receptors and (b) being different from one another. Having retired in 1965, he did not follow the arguments about multiple germ line genes, versus somatic mutation in a single gene, versus somatic recombination among tandemly repeated genes. In the event, the construction of the primary repertoire depends on somatic translocations of chosen elements of sets of minigenes; and somatic hypermutation only occurs in B cells *after* antigen has acted to create post-antigenic B cell subsets. The elegant way in which nature arranged affinity maturation would surely have pleased Burnet, had he lived to experience our present level of knowledge revealed over the last few years.

A continuing question is why somatic mutation of T cell receptor V genes does not seem to occur in prolonged or repeated T cell responses. The conventional answer given is that, as the T cell receptor "sees" self-MHC plus foreign peptide, a mutation could risk creating regulatory cells of higher anti-self reactivity. However, this is a somewhat weak explanation, as mutations toward anti-self could also occur in B cells, and there appear to be mechanisms for controlling the effects.[36] As T cell responses to antigens clearly involve a range of cells of highly variable affinities, there are opportunities for affinity maturation, even without V gene mutation, through selective proliferation of the higher affinity T cell clones with declining antigen levels.

WIDER BIOLOGICAL SIGNIFICANCE OF
"ONE CELL - ONE ANTIBODY"

There is no doubt that the solution of the antibody puzzle which the last 35 years of research in cellular and molecular biology has given us represents one of the most elegant streams of twentieth century biomedical research, fully meriting the eleven Nobel Prizes which have resulted so far. The genesis of an amazing diversity of protein molecules using only a modest complement of genetic information through somatic genetic events naturally raises the questions of whether this is only one example of a mechanism which evolution has fashioned, and which it can use to address other complex tasks as well. For example, the question is frequently asked how the development of the brain with its immense number of synapses can be coded by genes which represent only a subset out of a total of 10^5 genes. Facile comparisons are sometimes made about memory in the brain and memory in the immune system. Speculation about a more general significance of the strategy on which the immune repertoire is based is fuelled by the extraordinary number of new members of the immunoglobulin supergene family generated each year as more sequence information becomes available. Yet, at the moment, no truly comparable division of labor between cells has been found in any other system. It may well be that we shall have to wait until the human genome project is well down the track until we find out whether a recognizably homologous genetic situation exists elsewhere in mammalian biology.

SUMMARY AND CONCLUSIONS

Many of the aspects of the "one cell - one antibody" story illustrate the chancy nature of much of scientific research. Had Talmage and Burnet not put a credible face on Jerne's theory; had Lederberg not been visiting the Hall Institute in 1957; had I not been interested in one-step growth curves of viruses; my scientific life might have been quite different. However, and even despite the early phage neutralization results, the true cellular basis of antibody formation would have been revealed soon enough. Apart from the immunofluorescence studies and the strong hint coming from the nature of myeloma proteins, the stream of work coming from the analysis of antibody structure and later from immunoglobulin gene structure and organization would have lead inexorably to an analysis of the unipotentiality of antibody-forming cells and their precursors.

It is difficult to escape the conclusion that my first decade in immunology (1957-1967) was a very exciting period, embracing, as it did, the flowering of cellular immunology as an independent discipline and the discovery of the structure of the antibody molecule. But each subsequent decade has had its triumphs as well, and immunology as a whole remains more promising than ever. Those of us who have been privileged to work in the field over these 30-odd years have truly been eyewitnesses to history in the making. This volume, therefore, tells a story of very significant dimensions.

ACKNOWLEDGMENTS

This work was supported by the National Health and Medical Research Council, Canberra, Australia; by Grant AI-03958 from the National Institute of Allergy and Infectious Diseases, United States Public Health Service; and by the generosity of a number of private donors to The Walter and Eliza Hall Institute.

REFERENCES

1.   Ada, G. L. and Nossal, G. J. V., *Sci. Am.*, 257, 62, 1987.
2.   Billingham, R.E., Brent, L. and Medawar, P.B., *Nature*, 172, 603, 1953.

3. **Burnet, F. M. and Fenner, F.**, *The Production of Antibodies*, 2nd edition, Macmillan, London, 1949.
4. **Burnet, F.M.**, *Enzyme, Antigen and Virus*, Cambridge University Press, Cambridge, 1956.
5. **Jerne, N.K.**, *Proc. Natl. Acad. Sci. USA*, 41, 849, 1955.
6. **Ehrlich, P.**, *Proc. Roy. Soc. Lond. B.*, 66, 424, 1900.
7. **Talmage, D. W.**, *Ann. Rev. Med.*, 8, 239, 1957.
8. **Burnet, F. M.**, *Austral. J. Sci.*, 20: 67, 1957.
9. **Jerne, N. K.**, *Ann. Rev. Walter and Eliza Hall Institute*, 1978-79, 34, 1979.
10. **Nossal, G. J. V. and Lederberg, J.**, *Nature*, 181, 1419, 1958.
11. **Nossal, G. J. V.**, *Brit. J. Exp. Path.*, 41, 89, 1960.
12. **White, R.G.**, *Nature*, 182: 1383, 1958.
13. **Lederberg, J.**, *Science*, 129, 1649, 1959.
14. **Nossal, G. J. V.**, *Brit. J. Exp. Path.*, 40, 301, 1959.
15. **Nossal, G. J. V., Szenberg, A., Ada, G. L. and Austin, C. M.**, *J. Exp. Med.*, 119, 485, 1964.
16. **Nossal, G. J. V., Cunningham, A., Mitchell, G. F., and Miller, J. F. A. P.**, *J. Exp. Med.*, 128, 839, 1968.
17. **Attardi, G., Cohn, M., Horibata, K. and Lennox, E. S.**, *Bacteriol. Rev.*, 23: 213, 1959.
18. **Mäkelä, O.**, *Cold Spring Harbor Symp. Quant. Biol.*, 32, 423, 1967.
19. **Mäkelä, O.**, *J. Immunol.*, 87, 447, 1965.
20. **Köhler, G. and Milstein, C.**, *Nature*, 256, 495, 1975.
21. **Jerne, N. K. and Nordin A. A.**, *Science*, 146, 405, 1963.
22. **Nossal, G. J. V., Ada. G. L. and Austin, C. M.**, *J. Exp. Med.*, 121, 945, 1965.
23. **Nossal, G. J. V.**, in *In Vitro*, Volume 2, M. N. Goldstein, Ed., Williams and Wilkins, Baltimore, MD, 1967, pp. 1-7.
24. **Naor, D. and Sulitzeanu, D.**, *Nature*, 214, 687, 1967.
25. **Naor, D. and Sulitzeanu, D.**, *Int. Arch. Allergy*, 36, 112, 1969.
26. **Ada, G. L. and Byrt, P.**, *Nature*, 222, 1291, 1969.
27. **Raff, M. C.**, *Immunol.*, 19, 637, 1970.
28. **Raff, M. C., Feldman, M. and de Petris, S.**, *J. Exp. Med.*, 137, 1024, 1973.
29. **Julius, M. H., Masuda, T. and Herzenberg, L. A.**, *Proc. Natl. Acad. Sci. USA*, 69, 1934, 1972.
30. **Henry, C., Kimura, J. and Wofsy, L.**, *Proc. Natl. Acad. Sci. USA*, 69, 34, 1972.
31. **Rutishauser, U., D'Eustachio, P. and Edelman, G. M.**, *Proc. Natl. Acad. Sci. USA*, 70, 3894, 1973.
32. **Haas, W. and Layton, J. E.**, *J. Exp. Med.*, 141, 1004, 1975.
33. **Nossal, G. J. V. and Pike, B. L.**, *Immunol.*, 30, 189, 1976.
34. **Pike, B. L., Alderson, M. R. and Nossal, G. J. V.**, *Immunol. Rev.*, 99, 119, 1987.
35. **Herzenberg, L. A., Stall, A. M., Lalor, P. A., Sidman, C., Moore, W. A., Park, D. R., and Herzenberg, L. A.**, *Immunol. Rev.*, 93, 81, 1986.
36. **Nossal, G. J. V., Karvelas, M. and Lalor, P. A.**, *Cold Spring Harbor Symp. Quant. Biol.*, 1987.

Chapter 8

REFLECTIONS ON THE LYMPHOMYELOID COMPLEX

Joseph M. Yoffey

INTRODUCTION

The lymphomyeloid complex[1] provides the effector apparatus for immune reactions in mammals. It has six constituents: bone marrow, thymus, spleen, lymph nodes, lymphoepithelial tissue, and connective tissue. The term "connective tissue" includes not only the connective tissue as usually understood, but also the blood, lymph, and serous fluids. Though the widely scattered constituents of the LMC are quite discrete, they are functionally integrated by streams of migrating cells passing in and out of the component parts of the complex, and migrating through blood, lymph, serous fluids and other connective tissues. Some aspects of these cellular migration streams have recently been reviewed.[2] The cellular migration streams consist largely of lymphocytes, though not exclusively, for they also contain a variety of cell types, among which are macrophages and other antigen-presenting cells, plasma cell precursors and plasma cells, primitive stem cells, and NK cells. Figure 1 is a schematic diagram of the lymphomyeloid complex.

The work which ultimately led to the formation of the concept of the lymphomyeloid complex started a long time ago, in a study of haemopoiesis in fish.[3] A key part of this study was performed on the spleen of the dogfish, a cartilaginous Elasmobranch in which there are neither bone marrow nor lymph nodes. A dogfish spleen consisted of masses of lymphoid tissue, surrounded by areas of erythropoiesis mainly, but also some granulopoiesis. At the edge of the lymphoid masses there was an ill-defined boundary zone in which one could see intermediate stages between the lymphocytes and the developing blood cells. Lymphocytes were then—and for many years after—identified solely as morphological entities, and were classed as small, intermediate, and large. The lymphoid masses never contained germinal centers, a finding confirmed later by Good and Finstadt.[4]

In the 1920's—and indeed for many years later—very little was known about lymphocytes, but that little was enough to make them the subject of acute controversy. Much of the work giving rise to this controversy was performed in mammals, in which, as compared with Elasmobranchs, two new tissues called for consideration, namely bone marrow and lymph nodes. In studying this more complex mammalian situation I did not quite know where to begin, so I decided to try to learn something about the magnitude of the problem, by quantitating both lymphocyte production and cell production in the bone marrow. The quantitative study of lymphocyte production was undertaken first, before the quantitative study of bone marrow, which was begun more than a decade later.

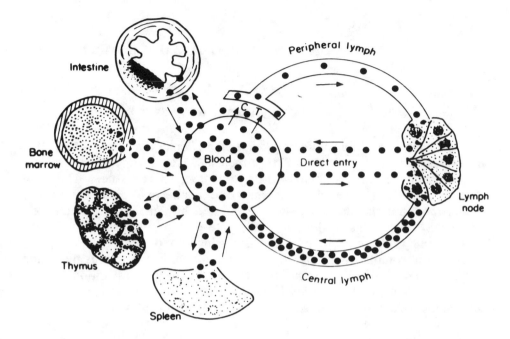

Figure 1.   Scheme to illustrate the main constituents of the lymphomyeloid complex and its cellular migration streams. Most of the migrating cells are lymphocytes, but macrophages and several other cell types are also involved, though in much smaller numbers. Cells can leave or enter the blood stream either by directly traversing the walls of the blood vessels ("direct entry") or by first obtaining access to the lymph stream, in which they then enter the blood ("indirect entry"). From Yoffey and Courtice 1970.[1]

THE QUANTITATIVE STUDY OF LYMPHOCYTE PRODUCTION

The early studies of lymphocyte production were based on several mistaken working hypotheses, so that though the reported data were correct, their interpretation was not. It was thought that lymphocytes were formed mainly in lymph nodes, where one could readily see the dividing cells in the germinal centers, one of the first mammalian tissues in which mitoses were observed.[5] In the light of later knowledge this was obviously not an auspicious start. But it is important to bear in mind the peculiar climate of opinion surrounding at the time almost all aspects of the lymphocyte problem. There were, for example, many who doubted that thymocytes could be regarded as lymphocytes. This, of course, sounds very odd at the present time, but no more odd than many other then prevailing misconceptions, such as that the small lymphocyte was a "mature" cell incapable of growth or differentiation or that the marrow tissue proper did not contain any lymphocytes. Lymphocytes present in marrow preparations were termed "extraparenchymatous".[6]

In the first quantitative studies, it was thought that after lymphocytes had been formed in lymph nodes, they all entered the blood indirectly, leaving the node in the efferent lymph, and finally reaching the blood via the thoracic and right lymph ducts, mainly the former. These cells were termed "indirect entry" lymphocytes as opposed to "direct entry" lymphocytes which in other situations entered the blood from their formative tissue by passing directly through the walls of the blood vessels. Little was known then about the large numbers of the direct entry lymphocytes, so in these early studies, counting the lymphocytes in thoracic duct lymph was thought to give a measure of lymphocyte production. The first such studies were performed in dogs[7] where it was observed that enough lymphocytes were daily entering the blood via the thoracic duct to replace those in the blood stream about 2½ x daily, and as later work showed, even more frequently in smaller laboratory animals.[1] But despite the large numbers of lymphocytes daily entering the blood, the level of the blood lymphocytes remained fairly constant. So it was concluded that they must constantly be leaving the blood. Where? Influenced by the dogfish studies, I speculated that they must be leaving the blood to enter the bone marrow where they could function as hemopoietic stem cells.

This working hypothesis had to be abandoned when it was shown not only that the bone marrow itself was the site of production of very large numbers of lymphocytes,[8] but also that thoracic duct lymphocytes were in the main recirculating.[9] We[10] had previously concluded that a small number of lymphocytes recirculated via peripheral lymph, but not on the massive scale on which lymphocyte recirculation was later shown to occur. However, the mistaken working hypothesis had one fruitful result. It led at an early stage to the concept of cellular migration streams which later underwent considerable development.

THE QUANTITATIVE STUDY OF BONE MARROW

The quantitative data on thoracic duct lymphocytes suggested the need for comparable data on bone marrow, and to this end we developed a quantitative technique for the study of bone marrow and some of the cellular changes occurring in it. These studies have been fully reported elsewhere.[11,12,13] Observations were made on the different cell groups under varying experimental conditions. Absolute counts per unit volume of marrow (Table 1), together with data on marrow volume[14] made it possible to estimate the total marrow population of the different cell groups, and compare them with cell populations in blood, thoracic duct lymph, and other parts of the lymphomyeloid complex (Table 2). The most extensive studies were performed in a standard experimental animal, a 400 g male guinea pig of the Dunklin-Hartley strain. But for some specific points they were supplemented by work on rats and mice.[15,16,17]

THE TRANSITIONAL (STEM) CELL COMPARTMENT

As will be seen in Table 1, the red marrow of the young adult guinea pig contains about 2,000,000 nucleated cells per mm³. The majority of these cells fall into three groups, myeloid, erythroid and lymphoid. There is also a small but fundamentally important group of cells which were termed "transitional," since I mistakenly thought that they were stages in development of small lymphocytes to become hemopoietic blast cells. But the name was retained since it turned out to be very apt in another sense. The compartment contains numerous transitions between cells of different sizes. The transition-

Table 1.
Absolute Counts (thousands/mm³) of Main Cell Groups in
Guinea Pig Marrow

	Mean ± SD
Early neutrophils	49 ± 21
Late neutrophils	405 ± 120
Total eosinophils	73 ± 22
Total basophils	17 ± 9
Myeloblasts	25 ± 13
Proerythroblasts	18 ± 9
Basophilic erythroblasts	358 ± 128
Polychromatic erythroblasts	53 ± 31
Orthochromatic erythroblasts	53 ± 31
Reticulocytes	197 ± 58
Lymphocytes	502 ± 114
Transitional cells	48 ± 16

al cell (TC) compartment proved to be eminently worthy of careful study, since it appears to be the cellular powerhouse not only of the bone marrow, but also of the entire lymphomyeloid complex.

It seems strange at first sight that this small group of transitional cells should make such a major contribution to maintaining the integrity both of the bone marrow, and of the entire lymphomyeloid complex, but as already noted[2] three important features must be taken into account: 1) even in the normal steady state the TC compartment is proliferating very actively; 2) the proliferation rate can become even higher when increased numbers of stem cells are required, as for example during the stimulation of erythropoiesis;[17] 3) especially important is the fact that once differentiation begins, powerful amplifying mechanisms are introduced, both intramyeloid and extramyeloid.

Table 2.

Comparative data on lymphocytes in bone marrow, blood and thoracic duct lymph (400 g guinea pig)	
Thoracic duct lymphocyte output in 24 hr	373 x 10⁶
Total blood lymphocytes	131 x 10⁶
Total marrow lymphocytes	2670 10⁶

Extramyeloid amplification is especially conspicuous in the case of lymphocytes, whether B or T. Antigenically stimulated B lymphocytes, for example, undergo marked clonal expansion.[18,19] In the case of T cells, thymocyte precursors migrating to the thymus have been thought to undergo as many as eight mitoses before the mature T lymphocyte stage is reached.[1] On this basis, one prothymocyte would give rise to over 200 T cells (see Reference).[20] In the case of erythropoiesis and granulocytopoiesis, the final amplification stage appears to be intramyeloid.

A full account of the TC compartment has been given elsewhere,[12] including a discussion of the very confused terminology, which appears to have been an important contributory factor in obscuring the true role of the compartment. No other cells in the bone marrow have been given so many different names. Throughout nearly a century transitional cells have repeatedly been rediscovered, redescribed, reillustrated, and renamed. One of the earliest examples was the "micromyeloblast" of Naegeli,[21] a typical small transitional cell as shown by later illustrations in color.[6] In recent years immunologists viewing TC from an immunological standpoint have contributed their own quota of additional names, with important functional connotations. The "pre-B" cells, "progenitor B cells," "B-lymphocyte precursors," T-cell precursors," or "prothymocytes" are all transitional cells in morphology. Of the many different names given to transitional cells, "lymphoid" and "lymphocyte-like" now appear to be those most commonly employed. But these terms cover such a wide range of cells that it would seem preferable to use a more distinctive name for the outstandingly important group of cells which constitute the TC compartment.

The TC compartment consists of a spectrum of cells, with a high N:C ratio, of different sizes and varying degrees of basophilia. The TC nucleus is predominantly leptochromatic, the leptochromasia being more marked in the larger than in the smaller cells. The TC compartment proliferates very actively. In the normal steady state the guinea pig transitionals have a thymidine labeling index of around 35% while in the rat the index is close to 50%. The compartment exhibits a typical proliferation gradient, the labeling index being low in the small cells, and becoming progressively higher the larger the cells.[12,13,22] The index is lower in the pale than in the basophilic transitionals. The large basophilic cells have an index of 70%.

It would appear from the proliferation gradient that one way of increasing stem cell production would be to stimulate more of the small cells to enlarge and enter the larger end of the compartment containing the more rapidly proliferating cells. An analysis of the available experimental data indicates that this change has repeatedly been found to occur.[23]

In postnatal life the bone marrow appears to be the primary habitat of TC, though some scattered stem cells are always to be found throughout the LMC. In the fetus, once the bone marrow has attained its full development, it contains a higher percentage of TC than at any other time of life, while a considerable number may also be found in the circulation and throughout the LMC, very notable in the thymus.[24,25,26,27] The role of pluripotential stem cells in situations such as the peritoneum and connective tissues is unknown, though in the rapidly growing fetal thymus they could conceivably be functioning as T cell precursors. However, since in this situation relatively few T cell precursors are required,[20] it is conceivable that at this stage of development the thymus also can be a temporary site for stem cell proliferation.

From an extensive series of experiments it seems clear that there are two basic processes in the TC compartment. On the one hand there is self-maintenance, which by itself would merely increase the size of the compartment. On the other hand there is differentiation, in which the pluripotential TC can undergo commitment and differentiate along a variety of pathways, lymphocytic or otherwise, and leave the compartment. Differentiation starting from a common stem cell pool opens up the possibility of stem cell competition, involving lymphocytes as well as the other cell groups. The TC compartment contains both the committed and the uncommitted stem cells.

We owe to the pioneer studies of Osmond and Everett[8] the demonstration that lymphocytes in the bone marrow are formed from transitional cells. They studied inter alia the sequence of labeling changes in TC and lymphocytes following a single pulse of tritiated thymidine. From an analysis of the labeling curves and grain counts, they concluded not only that it is transitional cells which give rise to small lymphocytes, but also that the normal population of marrow lymphocytes in the guinea pig is maintained in a dynamic steady state, with an average turnover time of 3 days or less.

It is pertinent at this point to emphasize that the CFU-S and other colony-forming cells all appear to have transitional cell morphology. Moore, Williams and Metcalf[28] were the first to emphasize this in the case of the CFU-GM, the granulocyte macrophage precursors.

DISTINCTIVE FEATURES OF MARROW LYMPHOCYTE PRODUCTION

The fact that there is a size spectrum in the TC compartment can readily be seen even at a cursory inspection of a bone marrow smear. More careful analysis of the size spectrum brings out the basic fact that there are three size groups in the compartment.[29] Several of the colony-forming units have also been shown to exist in three sizes which is what one might expect from the morphological identity of colony-forming units and transitional cells. Furthermore, it is interesting to note that the three sizes are present in both the uncommitted stem cells, the CFU-S, and in the committed erythropoietic and granulopoietic progenitor cells. In all these instances, these size differences are associated with the same relationship between cell size and the percentage of cells in DNA synthesis[23] as already established for the TC compartment.

On immunological grounds it has been suggested that B lymphocyte production starts from a pool of large actively synthesizing cells with cIgM+, i.e., presumably the large basophilic transitionals.[19,30,31] If this is the case it would appear that at the most there can only be three mitoses in the course of lymphocyte production in the bone marrow to which we therefore refer as the Short Lymphocyte Production Pathway, as compared to the Long Lymphocyte Production Pathway of six to eight mitoses in thymus and lymph nodes.[1] The occurrence of only three mitoses should result in less dilution of label, and therefore heavier labeling in radioautographs of marrow small lymphocytes as compared with thymocytes. Everett and Caffrey[32] observed that this was actually the case, and for this reason they considered it unlikely that there was extensive migration of thymocytes to the marrow. However, some migration of thymocytes to the marrow is thought to occur.[33,34] In addition to the part they may play in immunological reactions, these myelopetal thymocytes may have other important functions, such as augmenting marrow growth as a whole[35] and stimulating erythropoiesis.[36] It has recently been suggested that the control of erythropoiesis may require both helper and suppressor T cells.[37]

MARROW LYMPHOCYTES WITH DIFFERENT TURNOVER TIMES

Though the majority of marrow lymphocytes are being rapidly renewed, this does not apply to them all. In the case of the guinea pig, Rosse[38] had adduced evidence to indicate that while 86% of marrow lymphocytes turn over rapidly, with only a short stay in the marrow, 14% turn over more slowly and about half of these may have a life span exceeding four weeks. The same general conclusion was reached by Haas *et al.*[39] in whose studies the labelling of the fetal tissues with ^{3}H-thymidine was actually begun via the pregnant mother[40] and then continued for 26 days after birth. Four weeks after discontinuing the thymidine, a small number of marrow lymphocytes are still labeled. In all these long-term labelling experiments there is of course the possibility that some of the labelled lymphocytes in the marrow may belong to the recirculating pool which have entered the marrow from outside. That this is a possibility is clear from the parabiosis experiments of Rosse (33).

COMPARATIVE DATA ON LYMPHOCYTE PRODUCTION

The scale of lymphocyte production in the marrow is readily appreciated if a comparison is made with the thoracic duct lymphocytes and the number of lymphocytes in the circulation. Table 2 presents these data for the standard guinea pig. For every lymphocyte present in the blood, three are daily entering the blood stream via the thoracic duct and about 20 are present in the marrow where they can readily be seen both in smears and in sections.[41,42] Allowances must be made for species differences, which have been fully discussed elsewhere.[1] Since the data of Osmond and Everett[8] indicate a turnover time for marrow lymphocytes of about three days, it would appear that the daily lymphocyte production by the marrow is around five to six times the normal blood lymphocyte population. There is no evidence of lymphocyte destruction in the marrow to any marked extend, so it follows that large numbers must be constantly discharged as "direct entry" lymphocytes into the blood stream, in which they must spend a relatively short time.

HISTOLOGICAL OBSERVATIONS ON MARROW LYMPHOCYTES

Histological study of marrow lymphocytes presents several features of interest. In both light and electronmicroscope studies[41,42] lymphocytes may be seen: 1) scattered irregularly throughout the marrow parenchyma; 2) lined up against the sinusoidal endothelium presumably on the point of leaving the marrow; 3) transversing the sinusoidal endothelium, when the characteristic motion pattern of the small lymphocyte indicates the direction of movement;[42,43] 4) in the lumen of marrow sinusoids, often in considerable numbers. The accumulation of small lymphocytes in the lumen of the sinusoids was termed "lymphocyte loading".[44] Osmond and Batten[45] have recently suggested that the cells involved in lymphocyte loading are nearly all sIgM+ B small lymphocytes.

The occurrence of lymphocyte loading has been explained on the basis of the peculiar circulatory conditions in bone marrow, giving rise to stagnant sinusoids containing a disproportionately large amount of plasma with hardly any red cells.[44] It is presumably in such stagnant sinusoids that an occasional lymphocyte may be seen adhering to the sinusoidal endothelium. This adherence could well be the first stage in the entry of lymphocytes into the marrow from the blood stream. However, this is an infrequent appearance, suggesting that the uptake of lymphocytes by the marrow occurs on a much smaller scale than lymphocyte discharge. Everett *et al.*[46] were among the first to show the uptake of lymphocytes by normal, as opposed to irradiated, marrow. They performed exchange transfusions in rats between pairs of littermates, one of which had received tritiated thymidine 24 hr previously. Some labeled lymphocytes were subsequently found in the marrow of the animal which had not received thymidine, but no quantitative data were obtained. Rosse,[33] working with parabiotic guinea pigs, concluded that an appreciable number of labeled long-lived lymphocytes entered the marrow from the blood, which they subsequently re-entered. Ropke *et al.*[34] found long-lived T and B lymphocytes in the marrow.

Factors Influencing Lymphocyte Production

In view of the fundamental importance of lymphocyte production by the bone marrow, it is obviously desirable to know how this production is controlled. Though we are not yet in a position to speak with any certainty about control mechanisms, it seems reasonable to suppose that stimuli which give rise to immunological reactions should also stimulate marrow lymphocyte production. There is some recent evidence that this may actually be the case. Fulop *et al.*[47] reported increased B lymphocyte production following multiple intraperitoneal injections of sheep red blood cells.

It is interesting to note, however, that one of the best ways of increasing lymphocyte production by the marrow is not associated with any obvious immunological stimulation, but with the kinetic changes following the stimulation of erythropoiesis in a decompression chamber, and the sequence of changes which subsequently occur when the animal is returned to ambient air, the phase known as "rebound".[48] During the hypoxic phase erythropoiesis is stimulated and the animal becomes polycythemic, but in rebound, erythropoiesis in the polycythemic animals is greatly depressed and almost ceases. During hypoxia the marrow lymphocytes fall sharply, at first possibly because they are discharged from the marrow to make way presumably for the rapidly expanding erythropoiesis but subsequently because the actively proliferating transitional cells are nearly all differentiating along the erythropoietic pathway, so that very few are available for either lymphocyte or granulocyte production. In consequence, both lymphocytes and granulocytes fall markedly. In rebound, when in the polycythemic animal in ambient air erythropoiesis almost ceases, the increased transitional cell proliferation seems unable to cease immediately, but continues for a few days during which these cells reach an unusually high level. However, as the erythropoietic stimulus has now almost ceased, TC are now able to resume differentiation into both lymphocytes and granulocytes, so these latter rebound in the marrow to their normal level, and then in the case of the lymphocytes they rise to well above this level. It was for this reason that the post-hypoxic phase was termed "rebound." In fact, during rebound there is a phase when the marrow lymphocytes form 70% of the total nucleated cells, giving the marrow a leukemic appearance.[49]

Rosse[50] administered ³H-thymidine to guinea pigs at the beginning of rebound, and then observed that in a day or so labeled small lymphocytes began to appear. But he then noted that if at the beginning of rebound erythropoiesis was suddenly stimulated by blood withdrawal, it was labeled erythroid cells which appeared in the marrow rather than labeled small lymphocytes. Presumably the TC proliferation occurring in rebound was a proliferation of non-committed cells, which if stimulated by bleeding became committed to erythropoiesis, but if not so stimulated followed the lymphocyto-poietic pathway. These results tempt one to speculate that the *in vivo* proliferating stem cells compartment gives rise primarily to lymphocytes unless specific stimuli induce differentiation in other directions. This is obviously a speculation which requires further investigation. If one could devise a technique by which granulopoiesis could be greatly reduced in the same way as erythropoiesis is reduced in rebound, and if granulopoiesis and erythropoie-sis could be depressed simultaneously, it should be possible to put this speculation to a more convincing test.

FOETAL OBSERVATIONS

The lymphomyeloid complex in the fetus presents several features of interest. These are in part associated with the enormous stem cell demands of the fetus, necessitated by the very rapid growth of both the immunological and the hemopoietic components of the LMC. The postulated early origin of stem cells from the yolk sac[51] may be followed by the liver as a source of these cells for a time,[52] then finally by the bone marrow and its transitional cell population as the definitive permanent source of stem cells.[12] Once the fetal marrow has developed fully, it contains a higher percentage of TC than at any other time of life.[53] Furthermore, the cells are constantly migrating through the blood stream, in which they are present in appreciably larger numbers than in postnatal life. Whereas in adult blood only an occasional transitional cell may be seen, in the blood of the neonate, they form around 3-4% of the lymphoid cells. Winter *et al.*[54] found that in neonatal blood about 2% of the lymphoid cells are transitional cells in DNA synthesis (see Reference)[55] In fetal blood TC are even more numerous.[24]

In view of the greater numbers of transitional cells, it is not surprising that there are appreciably more colony-forming units in fetal and neonatal than in adult blood. Barnes *et al.*,[56] working with mice, found about 100 times as many CFUs in fetal as in adult blood. Since then, many observations have been made in man on *in vitro* colony-forming cells. A few CFU-GEMM are already present in fetal marrow blood at 13 wks.[57] High levels of CFU-CM and BFU-E are found in fetal blood but fall rapidly after birth.[58,59]

The many different varieties of stem or progenitor cells in fetal blood may either be proliferating in the blood stream, or may be presumed in the main to be migrating to the rapidly growing members of the LMC. The human fetal thymus, for example, appears to contain large numbers of transitional cells,[27] "prothymocytes".[60] Since relatively small numbers of prothymocytes seem to be required for the production of T cells in the fetal thymus (20), it is difficult to understand why so many stem cells are present in this situation. One possibility is that the stem cell requirement in the fetus is so great that they are forming multifocally for a time.

REACTIVITY OF FETAL AND NEONATAL LYMPHOCYTES

A striking feature of the circulating fetal and neonatal lymphocytes is that they react more vigorously to mitogenic stimulation than adult lymphocytes. Papiernik[61] noted this in the case of fetal blood while Yoffey *et al.*[62] reported similar results for the response of neonatal cord blood lymphocytes to PHA and Con A. The neonatal lymphocytes responded more rapidly, and in larger numbers than adult ones. In some cultures of cord blood there was an appreciable increase in the number of labeled cells at 24 hrs, whereas in the adult hardly any were labeled at this stage. In the PHA culture, 43.96% of cells in cord blood were labeled at 48 hrs, as compared with 20.3% of adult cells. A similar difference was found in the Con A cultures at 48 hrs—42.9% DNA-synthesizing cells in cord blood, as compared with 14.3% in the adult cells.

MORPHOLOGY OF CORD BLOOD AND FETAL LYMPHOCYTES

A TEM study of cord blood demonstrated the characteristic structure of the transitionals.[55] It also brought out the fact that many of the lymphocytes in cord blood had a higher N:C ratio, and were somewhat larger and more leptochromatic than the typical pachychromatic small lymphocytes. In fact they were intermediate in size and structure between the pachychromatic small lymphocyte and the transitional cell. It is possible that these are the cells which respond to mitogens in larger numbers and more rapidly than the pachychromatic small lymphocyte of the adult.

CONCLUDING REMARKS

The explosive growth of immunology has opened up so many new avenues that there is no difficulty in selecting fruitful areas for research. One of the most exciting is the bone marrow, described in a recent review as the "dynamo of the lymphomyeloid complex".[2] The bone marrow is directly responsible for the production of the antibody-forming B cells,[63] and indirectly for the production of T cells via the prothymocytes migrating to the thymus.[64] Furthermore, it gives rise to many of the antigen-presenting cells, such as macrophages, Langerhans cells, and dendritic cells.[65] When one adds to all these the different varieties of granulocytes and the NK cells, it becomes evident that about two-thirds of the total bone marrow cells are concerned with one aspect or another of the body's immune reactions.

The fundamental role of the bone marrow in all these areas calls for further clarification. How the production of B lymphocytes is controlled, what factors influence prothymocyte development, to what extent do recirculating lymphocytes which enter the marrow influence its activity, all these and many other questions call for further elucidation. Perhaps most fundamental of all is the way in which the uncommitted stem cells become finally and irreversibly committed. As Nossal[18] has emphasized, the intermediate steps between the pluripotential stem cell and the committed small lymphocyte progenitors are still obscure. Similarly, there is uncertainty with regard to the changes involved in the formation of T cell subsets from prothymocytes.

ACKNOWLEDGMENTS

This paper has been written during the tenure of a grant from the Joint Research Fund of the Hebrew University and Hadassah.

REFERENCES

1. **Yoffey, J. M. and Courtice, F. C.,** *Lymphomyeloid Complex*, Academic Press, New York, 1970.
2. **Yoffey, J. M.,** Cellular migration streams. The integration of the lymphomyeloid complex, *Lymphology,* 18, 5, 1985.
3. **Yoffey, J. M.,** A contribution to the study of the comparative histology and physiology of the spleen, with reference chiefly to its cellular constituents, I. In fishes, *J. Anat. (London),* 63, 314, 1929.
4. **Good, R.A. and Finstad, J.,** The phylogenetic development of immune responses and the germinal center system, in *Germinal Centers in Immune Responses,* H. Cottier, N. Odartchenko, R. Schindler and C.C. Congdon, Eds., Springer-Verlag, New York, 1967, pp. 4-27.
5. **Flemming, W.,** Studien uber Regeneration der Gewebe, *Arch. Mikr. Anat. Entw. Mech.*, 24, 50, 1885.
6. **Naegeli, O.,** *Blutkrankheiten und Blutdiagnostik,* Julius Springer, Berlin, 1931.
7. **Yoffey, J.M.,** The quantitative study of lymphocyte production, *J. Anat.*, 67, 250, 1933.
8. **Osmond, D.G. and Everett, N.B.,** Radioautographic studies of bone marrow lymphocytes *in vivo* and in diffusion chamber cultures, *Blood,* 23, 1, 1964.
9. **Gowans, J.L.,** The recirculation of lymphocytes from blood to lymph in the rat, *J. Physiol.*, 146, 54, 1959.
10. **Yoffey, J.M. and Drinker, C.K.,** The cell content of peripheral lymph and its bearing on the problem of circulation of the lymphocyte, *Anat. Rec.*, 73, 417, 1939.
11. **Yoffey, J.M.,** *Bone Marrow Reactions,* Edward Arnold, London, 1966.
12. **Yoffey, J.M.,** Transitional cells of hemopoietic tissues: origin, structure and development potential, *Int. Rev. Cytol.*, 62, 311, 1980.
13. **Tavassoli, M. and Yoffey, J.M.,** *Bone Marrow. Structure and Function,* Alan R. Liss, New York, 1983.
14. **Hudson, G.,** Bone marrow volume in guinea pigs, *J. Ana.*, 92, 150, 1958.
15. **Ramsell, T.G. and Yoffey, J.M.,** The bone marrow of the adult male rat, *Acta Anat.*, 47, 55, 1961.
16. **Turner, M.S., Hurst, J.M. and Yoffey, J.M.,** Studies on hypoxia VIII, Effect of hypoxia and post-hypoxic polycythaemia (rebound) on mouse marrow and spleen, *Brit. J. Haemat.*, 13, 942, 1967.
17. **Yoffey, J.M. and Yaffe, P.,** Studies on transitional cells, I. Kinetic changes in rat bone marrow in hypoxia and rebound, *J. Anat.*, 130, 333, 1980.
18. **Nossal, G.J.V.,** The double cascade of lymphocyte proliferation: current challenges and problem areas, *Am. J. Anat.*, 170, 253, 1984.
19. **Osmond, D.G. ,** The ontogeny and organization of the lymphoid system, *J. Invest. Dermatol.*, 85, 23, 1985.
20. **Owen, J.J.T. and Jankinson, E.J.,** Early events in T lymphocyte genesis in the fetal thymus, *Am. J. Anat.*, 170, 301, 1984.
21. **Naegeli, O.,** Ueber rothes Knochenmark und Myeloblasten, *Deutsch. Med. Wschr.*, 26, 287, 1900.

22. **Moffatt, D.J., Rosse, C. and Yoffey, J.M.,** Identity of haemopoietic stem cell, *Lancet*, ii, 547, 1967.

23. **Yoffey, J.M.,** Stem cell kinetics, Correlation of *in vivo* and *in vitro* data, *Experimental Hematology*, 15, 110, 1987.

24. **Yoffey, J.M.,** The stem cell problem in the fetus, *Israel J. Med. Sci.*, 7, 825, 1971.

25. **Yoffey, J.M.,** Fetal Immunohemopoietic stem cells, in *The Intrauterine Life. Management and Therapy*, J.G. Schenkar and D. Weinstein, Eds., Elsevier Science Publications, 1986, pp. 445-449.

26. **Barg, M., Mandel, T.E. and Johnson, G.R.,** Haemopoietic stem cells in the foetal thymus, *Aust. J. Biol. Med. Sci.*, 56, 195, 1978.

27. **Kelemen, E., Calvo, W. and Fliedner, T.M.,** *Atlas of Human Hematopoietic Development*, Springer-Verlag, Berlin and New York, 1979.

28. **Moore, M.A.S., Williams, N. and Metcalf, D.,** Purification and characterization of the in vitro colony-forming cell in monkey hemopoietic tissue, *J. Cell Physiol.*, 179, 283, 1972.

29. **Patinkin, D., Grover, N.B and Yoffey, J.M.,** The lymphocyte production pathway in bone marrow: possible significance of the size spectrum of lymphocytes and their precursors, *Brit. J. Haematol.*, 41, 309, 1979.

30. **Owen, J.J.T., Wright, D.E., Haba, S., Raff, M.C. and Cooper, M.D.,** Studies on the generation of B lymphocytes in fetal liver and bone marrow, *J. Immunol.*, 118, 2067, 1977.

31. **Osmond, D.G.,** The contribution of bone marrow to the economy of the lymphoid system, *Monographs Allergy*, 16, 157, 1980.

32. **Everett, N.B. and Caffrey, R.W.,** Radioautographic studies of bone marrow small lymphocytes, in *The Lymphocyte in Immunology and Haemopoiesis*, J.M. Yoffey, Ed., Edward Arnold, London, 1967, pp. 108-119.

33. **Rosse, C.,** Migration of long-lived lymphocytes to the bone marrow and to other lymphomyeloid tissues in normal and parabiotic guinea pigs, *Blood*, 40, 90, 1972.

34. **Ropke, C., Hougen, H.P. and Everett, N.B.,** Long-lived T and B lymphocytes in the bone marrow and thoracic duct lymph of the mouse, *Cell Immunol.*, 15, 82, 1975.

35. **Pritchard, L.L., Shinpock, S.G. and Goodman, J.W.,** Augmentation of marrow growth by thymocytes separated by discontinuous albumin density-gradient centrifugation, *Exp. Hematol.*, 3, 94, 1975.

36. **Nathan, D.G., Chess, L., Hillman, D.G., Clark, B., Beard, J., Merler, E. and Houseman, D.E.,** Human erythroid burst-forming units: T cell requirement for proliferation *in vitro*, *J. Exp. Med.*, 14, 124, 1978.

37. **Sharkis, S.J., Cremo, C., Collector, M.I., Noga, S.J. and Donnenberg, A.D.,** Thymic regulation of hematopoiesis. III. Isolation of helper and suppressor populations using counterflow centrifugal elutriation, *Blood*, 68, 787, 1986.

38. **Rosse, C.,** Lymphocyte production and life span in the bone marrow of the guinea pig, *Blood*, 38, 372, 1971.

39. **Haas, R.J., Bohne, F., Fliedner, T.M.,** Cytokinetic analysis of slowly proliferating bone marrow cells during recovery from radiation injury, *Cell Tiss. Kinet.*, 4, 31, 1971.

40. Fliedner, T.M., Haas, R.J., Stehle, H. and Adams, A., Complete labeling of all cell nuclei in rats with ^{3}H-thymidine, *Lab. Invest.*, 18, 249, 1968.

41. Yoffey, J.M., Hudson, G. and Osmond, D.G., The lymphocyte in guinea pig bone marrow, *J. Anat.*, 99, 841, 1985.

42. Hudson, G. and Yoffey, J.M., The passage of lymphocytes through the sinusoidal endothelium of guinea pig bone marrow, *Proc. Roy. Soc. (London)*, 165, 486, 1966.

43. deBruyn, P.P.H., Michelson, S. and Thomas, T.B., The migration of blood cells of the bone marrow through the sinusoidal wall, *J. Morph.*, 133, 417, 1971.

44. Yoffey, J.M., Lymphocyte loading of bone marrow sinusoids. A microcirculatory puzzle, *Adv. Microcirculation*, 7, 49, 1975.

45. Osmond, D.G. and Batten, S.J., Genesis of lymphocytes in the bone marrow: extravascular and intravascular localization of surface IgM-bearing cells in mouse bone marrow detected by electron microscope radioautography after *in vivo* perfusion of ^{125}I anti-IgM antibody, *Am. J. Anat.*, 170, 349, 1984.

46. Everett, N.B., Rieke, W.O., Reinhardt, W.O. and Yoffey, J.M., Radioisotopes in the study of blood cell formation with special reference to lymphocytopoiesis, in *Ciba Foundation Symposium on Haemopoiesis, Cell Production and Its Regulation*, G.E.W. Wolstenholme and M. O'Connor, Eds., Churchill, London, 1960, pp. 43-66.

47. Fulop, G.M., Pietrangeli, C.E. and Osmond, D.G., Regulation of marrow lymphocyte production, IV. Altered kinetic steady state of lymphocyte production after chronic changes in exogenous stimuli, *Exp. Hematol.*, 14, 27, 1986.

48. Yoffey, J.M., Jeffreys, R.V., Osmond, D.G., Turner, M.S., Tabsin, S.C. and Niven, P.A.R., Studies on hypoxia. VI. Changes in lymphocytes and transitional cells in the marrow during the intensification of primary hypoxia and rebound, *Ann. N.Y. Acad. Sci.*, 149, 179.

49. Jones, H.B., Jones, J.J. and Yoffey, J.M., Studies in hypoxia. VII. Changes in lymphocytes and transitional cells in the bone marrow during prolonged rebound, *Brit. J. Haemat.*, 13, 934, 1967.

50. Rosse, C., Precursor cells to erythroblasts and to small lymphocytes of the bone marrow, in *Haemopoietic Stem Cells*, G.E.W. Wolstenholm and M. O'Connor, Eds., Ciba Foundation Symposium 13, Associated Scientific Publishers, 1973, pp. 105-126.

51. Moore, M.A.S. and Metcalf, D., Ontogeny of the haemopoietic system. Yolk sac origin of *in vivo* and *in vitro* colony-forming cells in the developing mouse embryo, *Brit. J. Haemat.*, 18, 279, 1970.

52. Bodger, M.P., Janossy, G., Bollum, F.J., Burford, G.D. and Hoffbrand, A.V., The ontogeny of terminal doxynucleotidyl transferase positive cells in the human fetus, *Blood*, 61, 1125, 1983.

53. Yoffey, J.M., Thomas, D.B., Moffatt, D.J., Sutherland, I.H. and Rosse, C., Non-immunological functions of the lymphocyte, in *Biological Activity of the Leucocyte*, G.E.W. Wolstenholme and M. O'Connor, Eds., Ciba Foundation Study Group No. 10, J. and A. Churchill, London, 1961, pp. 45-54.

54. Winter, G.C.B., Byles, A.B. and Yoffey, J.M., Blood lymphocytes in newborn and adult, *Lancet*, ii, 932, 1965.

55.   **Faulk, W.P., Goodman, J.R., Maloney, M.A., Fudenberg, H.H. and Yoffey, J.M.,** Morphology and nucleoside incorporation of human neonatal lymphocytes, *Cellular Immunol.*, 8, 166, 1973.

56.   **Barnes, D.W.H., Ford, C.E. and Loutit, J.F.,** Haemopoietic stem cells, *Lancet*, i, 1395, 1964.

57.   **Hann, J.M., Bodger, M.P. and Hoffbrand, A.V.,** Development of pluripotent hematopoietic progenitor cells in the human fetus, *Blood*, 62, 118, 1983.

58.   **Knott, L.J., Rodeck, C.H. and Huehns, E.R.,** Studies of circulating hemopoietic progenitor cells in human fetal blood, *Blood*, 59, 976, 1982.

59.   **Prindull, G., Prindull, B. and Meulen, N.,** Hematopoietic stem cells in human cord blood, *Acta Paediat. Scand.*, 67, 413, 1978.

60.   **Galili, U., Polliack, A., Okon, E., Leizerovitz, R., Gamliel, H., Korkesh, A., Schenkar, J.G and Izak, G.,** Human prothymocytes. Membrane properties, differentiation patterns, glucocorticoid sensitivity and ultrastructural features, *J. Exp. Med.*, 152, 796, 1980.

61.   **Papiernik, M.,** Comparison of human foetal with child blood lymphocyte kinetics, *Biol. Neonate*, 19, 165, 1971.

62.   **Yoffey, J.M., Ron, A., Prindull, G. and Yaffe, P.,** Earlier onset of DNA synthesis in mitogen-stimulated lymphocytes of cord blood than in lymphocytes of adult blood, *Clin. Immunol. Immunopathol.*, 9, 491, 1978.

63.   **Osmond, D.G.,** Population dynamics of bone marrow B lymphocytes, *Immunological Rev.*, 93, 103, 1986.

64.   **Yoffey, J.M.,** Stem cells and the thymus with special reference to cellular migration streams, in *The Thymus Gland*, M. Kendall, Ed., Academic Press, New York, 1981, pp. 185-202.

65.   **Tew, J.G., Thorbecke, G.J. and Steinman, R.M.,** Dendritic cells in the immune response: characteristics and recommended nomenclature, *J. Reticuloendoth. Soc.*, 31, 371, 1982.

Chapter 9

THE MINNESOTA SCENE: A CRUCIAL PORTAL OF ENTRY TO MODERN CELLULAR IMMUNOLOGY

Robert A. Good

Many have suggested that I attempt to describe interactions of people and the intellectual scene at the University of Minnesota which permitted and fostered generation of many new concepts and insights into the bodily defense, cellular immunology, and the nature and treatment of immunological diseases during that highly productive score of years during the 1950's and 1960's. I will attempt, in a somewhat self-focused analysis, to try to capture the Minnesota scene and hopefully to shed light on what may have been a special moment in a special place in biomedical and immunological history.

Of greatest importance was the foment that existed in the Medical School at the University of Minnesota for several decades during and following the tenure of Elias Potter Lyon.[1] Especially within the basic science faculty, outstanding scholars and teachers were abundant. Free and generous interaction of basic scientists with one another and with clinical faculty characterized the University of Minnesota Medical School during the 1940s, 1950s and 1960s. This foment was rooted in true scholarship and in deep respect, real appreciation, yes, almost a worship, of creative scientific contributions in both basic and clinical medical sciences. A faculty spirit existed that was generated and nurtured by a great dean, Elias Potter Lyon.[2] Lyon had brought together an almost unbelievable basic scientific faculty with immense strengths in most of the sciences basic to medicine. A dozen world-renowned scholars and scientists led that faculty. These included C.M. Jackson and E.A. Boyden in anatomy, Richard Scammon in embryology, A.T. Rassmussen in neuroanatomy, H. Downey in microscopic anatomy and hematology, A.R. Henrici in soil microbiology, R. Green and C. Evans in virology, H.O. Halvorson in microbial physiology and what later came to be called molecular biology when it focussed on nuclear control of physiological events, M.B. Visscher, E. Gellhorn and J. Bittner in physiology, E.T. Bell and B. Clawson in pathology, A.D. Hirschfelder in pharmacology, G. Burr, Leo Samuels, C. Barnum, Jr., Harlan Wood and W. Armstrong in biochemistry, and G.W. Anderson, J.A. Meyers and later Emerson, L. Schuman and A. Treloar in preventative medicine and public health. All were intellectual giants devoted to both the highest standards of science and to true scholarship. They fostered creative expression as well as productivity in basic research. Each was in vigorous interaction with one another and most impressively also each was involved in genuine ongoing interactions with a somewhat home-grown but brilliant and creative group of clinical scientists. The latter group was led by Wangensteen, a man of many roles and incredible creativity, Richard Varco, C.W. Lillehei and J. Lewis, the leaders who pioneered open heart surgery and who also were teachers at the highest level. Watson and Spink were the leaders in medicine, Irvine McQuarrie and John Adams in pediatrics, J.C. Litzenberg, J.L. McKelvey and R.O. Meyer in obstetrics and gynecology, S. Hathaway and Hastings in psychology and psychiatry. G.T. Evans launched the discipline of laboratory medicine at Minnesota. Later, Kottke and Kubechek became pioneers in rehabilitative medicine, Benson developed laboratory medicine, and Lewis Thomas for

0-8493-4722-X/94/$0.00 + $.50

several years led the way in pediatrics and medicine. May in pediatrics was a most skillful teacher and investigator, and Lewis Wannamaker, W. Krivit, R. L. Vernier, Ulstrom and Michael and J. White in pediatrics and Holtz in dermatology joined or succeeded this impressive group.

Each of these clinicians could be identified with a very leading edge of investigations in either or both clinical and basic sciences, and each seemed determined to outdo all of the others in nurturing and developing what became significant schools of productive young scholars, scientists and clinicians. Each of these giants engaged in constantly shifting active collaborations and competitions, both with each other and with the continuous flood of young aspiring scientists who appeared in their laboratories in the basic sciences and in the clinics from all parts of the world. Thus, young and scientifically vigorous academicians were constantly being generated at all levels in the Minnesota medical school. As the young scientists matured, they were in turn dispatched as academic disciples to populate new departments in the rapidly expanding medical school faculties all over the United States. Many of these young scholar-scientists became important academic leaders in either or both basic and clinical sciences throughout the nation and, indeed, throughout the world.

An impressive graduate school developed at the University of Minnesota which became a real complement to the development of the medical school. The graduate school, while setting high standards of research and education, became a most important component in the creation of a unique scientific force in medical science at Minnesota. Rather uniquely, graduate education encompassed both the sciences basic to medicine and also the applied clinical scientific disciplines. It was thus commonplace for the young surgeons, internists, pediatricians, yes, occasionally even extraordinary dermatologists, orthopedists, obstetricians-gynecologists or neurosurgeons, to take sufficient training and education in one of the basic sciences and occasionally even in one of the enabling sciences of chemistry, physics, mathematics or applied sciences like engineering to qualify, with an appropriate thesis, based on original research, for a Ph.D. degree. Thus, for an aspiring youngster such as myself who was dedicated to a career in academic medicine, this was an exciting and challenging environment in which to develop as a clinical investigator.[1]

Another influence that contributed greatly to the development of cellular immunology at Minnesota was Dr. Irvine McQuarrie's conviction that the history of medicine may be incisively viewed as a succession of critical investigations of Experiments of Nature. McQuarrie considered the interaction of young clinical investigators with Experiments of Nature—by studying rare diseases after being steeped at once in science and in clinical medical knowledge, to be a most powerful means for generating new medical knowledge and fundamental new insights into normal physiology. In his ward rounds, formal lectures and skilled written exposition,[3,4,5,6] McQuarrie presented untiringly and reviewed repeatedly his views that analysis of Experiments of Nature represented a major scientific vehicle to generate the most relevant basic information. McQuarrie taught with great enthusiasm, employing as illustrations his own experiences interspersed with elaborate accounts from the literature describing how Experiments of Nature had led to much new understanding and new perspectives in shaping medical history. McQuarrie traced the concept that understanding of the great power of nature's experiments could often be achieved by study of rarer forms of disease, first to William Harvey,[7] in turn to William Osler, culminating in Archibald Garrod's clear expression of this perspective in his description of inborn errors of metabolism.[8]

McQuarrie's concepts concerning the importance of Experiments of Nature shaped all of my research in immunology. To capture this philosophy so enthusiastically espoused by McQuarrie, it seems appropriate to quote from William Harvey's beautiful letter to Jan Vlakfeld—who he addressed as the distinguished and accomplished Physician at Harlem. This letter was written just six weeks before Harvey died:

> "It is even so. Nature is nowhere accustomed more openly to display her secret mysteries than in cases where she shows traces of her workings apart from the beaten path; nor is there any better way to advance the proper practice of medicine than to give our minds to the discovery of the usual law of nature, by the careful investigation of cases of rarer forms of disease. For it has been found in almost all things, that what they contain of useful or of applicable, is hardly perceived unless we are deprived of them, or they become deranged in some way. The case of the plasterer to which you refer is indeed a curious one, and might supply a text for a lengthened commentary by way of illustration. But it is in vain that you apply the spur to urge me, at my present age, not mature merely but declining, to gird myself for any new investigation. For I now consider myself entitled to my discharge from duty. It will, however, always be a pleasant sight for me to see distinguished men like yourself engaged in this honorable arena. Farewell, most learned sir, and whatever you do, still love."[7]

Besides being a student of, seeker for, and interpreter of Nature's experiments in clinical medicine, McQuarrie was a people watcher. As later became apparent, in the course of his people-watching he somehow selected me for special attention, wooed me into the pediatric field, nurtured me and challenged me to become a serious academician. McQuarrie provided opportunity at every turn for me to realize my full academic and scientific potential. With long and determined discussions, spurred, I believe, by my first mentor Berry Campbell, Dr. McQuarrie convinced me early in my medical school days that if I wished to have a truly productive career, I must devote my entire scientific life to interpreting Experiments of Nature in the pediatric perspective.

It is difficult to conceive today, but at the time my work in immunology began in 1944 we knew nothing of the cells, nothing, really, of the molecules, and very little about the function of the major organs now known to be crucial to immunological development. For example, at that time almost everyone believed that macrophages were the cells that make antibody because this had been the erroneous conclusion drawn by the famous Florence Sabin from her research at the Rockefeller Institute.[9] A few were beginning to be attracted to new conclusions put forth by White and Dougherty at Yale who argued that antibodies are generated by lysis of lymphocytes effected by the influence of adrenal cortical hormones.[10,11] Little or nothing was known in those days of the crucial immunologic functions of the thymus, lymph nodes, spleen, fetal liver, Peyer's patches or appendix. Nothing really was known or established concerning the functions and interactions of lymphocytes and the role played by plasma cells as immunoglobulin secreting, antibody producing cells. I have had the privilege to live and work at a time when I could contribute to development of the burgeoning knowledge in each of these fields of immunology.

I actually began research in Berry Campbell's neurophysiology laboratory. I was studying, at first, the physiology and pathologic physiology of the two neuron-two axon reflex. As a poorly paid technician I was also generating data to facilitate my mentor Berry Campbell's analysis of electroarchetectonics, which he was attempting to relate to the cytoarchitectonics of the spinal cord. I got involved in this line of investigation because, paralyzed from the knees down from what in retrospect seems to have been a severe attack of Guillain-Barré syndrome, I was left without knee jerks. In my research, I was attempting to alter the tempo of electrical transmission over the two neuron-two axon reflex by producing chromatolytic changes in the anterior horn cells of the spinal cord. I was manipulating the two neuron-two axon reflex by initiating retrograde degeneration using nerve section or, alternatively, by producing a virus infection within these beautiful neural elements—the anterior horn cells of the spinal cord.

My studies of lymphocytes, plasma cells and stem cells (called reticulum cells by H. Downey) began while I was working in the neurophysiology laboratory in 1944 with Campbell. Campbell was a Ph.D. from Hopkins who, at that time, was a somewhat renegade associate professor at the University of Minnesota. He seemed most important to me because he had spent time as a fellow at the Rockefeller Institute for Medical Research where he had worked in Gasser's department. Campbell introduced me to a rather outlandish but most attractive personality—a surgical resident named Fred Kolouch.[1] Kolouch, at that time, was scheduled to be Wangensteen's succeeding chief resident and so like each of Wangensteen's chief resident trainees he had to spend time hard at work in Wangensteen's experimental surgery laboratory, called the "dog laboratory," in the physiology department. Wagensteen insisted this long period of scientific preparation, usually one year, was essential to succession to the chief residency in his Department of Surgery.

Kolouch took notice of my industry in the laboratory and enticed me to help him with some experiments on inflammation in rabbits. In turn, he taught me hematologic morphology in the Downey tradition[12]. After several weeks of working together, Kolouch came to my laboratory late one night in 1944 and in all seriousness said, "Why don't you cut out all this foolish research on the knee jerks and help me with my really important unfinished research to define the antibody-producing cell—namely, the plasma cell." Kolouch was so enthusiastic and spoke so convincingly from intimate knowledge of the literature and his own personal experience that I paid close attention to him. Because of his enthusiasm I became enamored with the line of reasoning he was pursuing and with the clinical Experiments of Nature and laboratory studies by which he linked plasma cells to that crucial still unfathomed component of the bodily defense—antibody production.

Kolouch's interest in plasma cells had been ignited by a conjunction of three separate Experiments of Nature. While studying the role of lymphocytes, monocytes and PMNs in acute inflammation, Kolouch came across a paper written in 1937 by the Danish investigators Bing and Plum.[13] In their report these scientists described three among 14 patients with agranulocytosis who, at the same time, exhibited both striking bone marrow plasmacytosis and rather marked hyperglobulinemia. From their clinical-pathological-biochemical analyses of these patients, Bing and Plum raised a question: "could it be that plasma cells were the cells that were producing the globulin that accumulated in the serum of these special patients among those with agranulocytosis?"

As fortune would have it, Kolouch, in his studies as a pathology student with Clawson, the professor of pathology, had examined under Downey's guidance slides from the tissues and particularly smears from the bone marrow from a patient who suffered from subacute bacterial endocarditis. These slides impressed Kolouch enormously. The patient's bone marrow was, in Kolouch's terms, "chock-a-block" full of plasma cells. In another investigation with Downey, Kolouch also had been studying blood and bone marrow from a patient who suffered from serum sickness, produced by treatment with horse serum as a prophylactic passive immunization against tetanus. This patient with serum sickness also showed impressive plasmacytosis of the bone marrow and furthermore exhibited a flood of plasma cells which even came out into the peripheral blood.[14]

Kolouch inquired of Downey, the hematologist, whether the latter knew the function of plasma cells. Downey, a consummate morphologist, said he had concluded from morphological analyses that plasma cells must have some sort of secretory function because their morphological features seemed very similar to those of known secretory cells, e.g., salivary gland or pancreatic acinar epithelial cells. Kolouch inquired of Clawson, the pathologist, "what do plasma cells do?" Clawson responded that although he didn't actually know the physiologic function of plasma cells, he regularly observed these cells to accumulate in chronic inflammatory exudates, such as those of chronic infections or granulomatous diseases like tuberculosis or syphilis, and also in bronchiectatic lesions or in other chronic inflammations. Clawson also pointed out to Kolouch that plasma cells were present in large numbers in spleen and marrow when in his experiments he produced rheumatic fever-like valvular and myocardial lesions in rats by repeated injections or infections with *Streptococcus viridans*.[15] Clawson believed the rheumatic-fever like lesions that he had produced in both heart and joints were generated by antibodies formed against the *S. viridans* he had injected, so Clawson associated the plasma cells with antibodies.

Challenged by these three Experiments of Nature, the plasma cell accumulation in SBE, serum sickness and tuberculosis, Kolouch immunized rabbits repeatedly with a *S. viridans* vaccine prepared by Clawson until the rabbits regularly developed anaphylactic shock following injections of the vaccine. After such provocative injections of the *S. viridans* vaccine, Kolouch studied serial imprints and sections from bone marrow and spleen and also studied smears of the blood. The rabbits that exhibited anaphylaxis regularly showed a burst of plasma cells in the bone marrow and, when looked for, also in the spleen. In his experiments, Kolouch almost never saw plasma cells coming into the blood as had occurred in his patient with serum sickness, but the bone marrow especially and also, in some experiments, spleen promptly developed impressive and, indeed, what Kolouch called a "beautiful" plasmacytosis following each injection of vaccine in the previously immunized rabbits.[12,16] Because of the limitations of morphology alone, Kolouch had confused osteoblasts with the earliest plasma cell precursors, but the association of bone marrow plasmacytosis with anaphylaxis was both real and highly reproducible.

These findings led Kolouch to conclude that the vaccine he had given generated the plasmacytosis and that the associated anaphylactic shock could perhaps have been a stimulus to production of impressive plasma cell accumulation within the hematopoietic tissues. Kolouch's experiments, performed in 1937, were published as a small paper in the Proceedings of the Society of Experimental Biology and Medicine the following year.[16] Kolouch did further experiments attempting to link plasma cells to anaphylaxis and antibody production, and his impressive results became the subject of a Master's degree thesis at the University of Minnesota graduate school.[12] From his interpretation of the three Experiments of Nature and as a consequence of the derivative laboratory experimentation, Kolouch became convinced that the plasma cell, indeed, was an antibody-producing cell and probably **the** antibody-producing cell. As part of his thesis, Kolouch summarized a rather lengthy literature extending like a loose thread through the years from 1890, when the plasma cell was first described by Cajal[17] as a morphological entity, to 1938 which linked plasma cells to both globulin and antibody production.[12]

In 1944, Kolouch turned over all his evidence and even some recent papers by Bjoerneboe and Gormsen[18,19] as his legacy to me. He literally gave me the plasma cell and the lymphocyte, as subjects for my life's work, and he did so with much enthusiasm because he knew I would work hard to elucidate the challenge of the plasma cell he had given me. I knew, even as a student, that additional experiments would be needed to help sort out what were the true relationships of plasma cells and the other lymphoid cells, but I was flattered by being given Kolouch's challenge. I thought for example that it might be conceivable that plasma cells are generated by the physiological events associated with anaphylaxis which regularly occurred in Kolouch's experiments or, alternatively, that the plasmacytosis might have occurred in the *S. viridans* vaccine-injected rabbits in association with a vigorous **secondary antibody response** that had been generated by the **repeated** stimulation with antigen which had also, but incidentally, been responsible for the anaphylactic shock.

Thus, after further discussions with Kolouch, I carried out in 1944 and 1945 my initial immunological experimentation and in these investigations compared in quantitative detail plasma cell development in bone marrow after anaphylaxis that had been generated by secondary injection of antigen (active anaphylaxis) to anaphylaxis generated by a primary injection of antigen (passive anaphylaxis). Both procedures could be counted on to produce anaphylactic shock and regularly did, but I postulated that if plasma cells were associated with antibody production that only active sensitization would be accompanied by an extensive plasmacytosis as a consequence of the secondary immune response with its known accompanying burst of antibody production. If active but not passive anaphylaxis generated the plasmacytosis, I could conclude that it was the secondary immune response that had generated the plasmacytosis in my experiments[21] and that was associated with anaphylactic shock in Kolouch's earlier studies and not the anaphylactic shock per se.

The results of my experiments came out clear and decisive. When anaphylactic shock was produced by a primary injection of antigen, an increase in plasma cell numbers was not detectable in the marrow of my rabbits. By contrast, anaphylaxis which was consequent to active immunization via a secondary injection of antigen, regularly induced impressive and quantifiable plasmacytosis.[20,21] Thus I concluded that plasma cells are, indeed, a regular morphological signal of stimulation of lymphoid cells and bone marrow cells to enter antibody production.[14,20,21] In many different experiments using a variety of different antigens and injections into numerous different bodily sites I showed that plasmacytosis was regularly associated, in many organs and tissues, with preceding antigenic stimulation and with either measured or presumed vigorous antibody responses. This line of research became the basis of my Ph.D. thesis, which I completed as part of what I believe was the very first conjoined Ph.D.-M.D. educational program to be pursued at the University of Minnesota.[20,21,22]

After finishing medical school and receiving both the Ph.D. and M.D. degrees in the same ceremony in 1947, just four years after I had entered medical school, I began studies of Pediatrics at the University of Minnesota. This seemingly rather impossible achievement was actually made possible by a wartime medical curriculum that shortened the period in medical classes and clerkships to three short years. During an internship and residency in pediatrics at the University of Minnesota, I continued to hunt plasma cells and I launched numerous clinical-pathological investigations. Each of these investigations seemed to me to strengthen the link I was forging between plasma cells, which appeared to be the derivatives of morphologically transformed lymphocytes or, alternatively, to be antibody producing cells which were derived from larger, so-called "reticular" or (blastic) lymphoid cells,[20,21,22] and the immune response and antibody production.

As part of a clinical investigation carried out during my pediatric residency in 1947-1949, I showed, for example, that in patients with rheumatic fever the slope of the curve of rapid accumulation of gammaglobulin in the serum which I had learned to quantify precisely could be beautifully correlated to the absolute numbers of plasma cells in the marrow.[23] I developed methods for most accurately quantifying the Ig levels in serum and for quantifying the absolute numbers of plasma cells in the marrow.[23] The method for quantification of the plasma cells I used was based on 5,000 cell counts to enumerate plasma cells (or other infrequent elements) in a tiny smear of marrow collected in a precise and measured way.[20,23] This and several other methods which I used to quantify plasma cells in tissues became invaluable tools for recognizing and quantifying the relationships of plasma cells to the antibodies and immunoglobulins that I had begun to analyze.

Kolouch completed a Ph.D. degree in surgery and physiology but he did not delve further into hematological issues and never returned to work on the plasma cells. He felt he knew enough already about these magnificent cells. He developed himself as a brilliant experimental and clinical surgeon. He cultivated an interest in hypnosis and employed hypnosis to facilitate preoperative and postoperative care of surgical patients. He introduced the second look procedure in surgery and spoke always as a proper surgeon of doing his post mortem examinations antemortem. I remember being most impressed in 1948 or 1949 when Kolouch's research with hypnosis as an approach to pre- and post-operative care was featured in the news magazine, *Time*. This research became increasingly important when Kolouch later left surgical practice after sustaining loss of an eye in a skiing accident. He became, in turn, a skilled neuropsychiatrist and a splendid professor of psychiatry at the University of Utah School of Medicine. I believe it was his work with hypnosis in surgery that inspired me some years later to study the effect of hypnosis on expression of immunity in PK reaction.

I feel certain that as Kolouch repeatedly later reviewed my research with the lymphocytes and plasma cells he always considered me to be a particularly competent, high-quality technician.[24] With me in the picture, however, I believe Kolouch felt quite relaxed about turning his attention away from his beloved lymphocytes and plasma cells and felt confident that these, to him, vitally important cellular elements were in what he considered to be "Good" hands.

Kolouch believed in all sincerity that he had rescued the plasma cells from an obscurity to which they had been assigned by the pathologists. In those days pathologists spoke of lymphocytes and plasma cells as being similar to medical students—always there, never doing very much, but standing around looking on when important things were going on in medicine. Kolouch repeatedly said that plasma cells reminded him of the appearance of someone looking out of the corner of his eye, anticipating something unexpected to happen.

After completing medical school, obtaining both Ph.D. and M.D. degrees and taking house staff training in pediatrics with McQuarrie, I accepted a Helen Hay Whitney Fellowship. This fellowship was presented to me by T. Duckett Jones and was given with the express requirement that after a year as Helen Hay Whitney Fellow at Minnesota I must leave the University of Minnesota for at least one year. So off I went for a year to the Rockefeller Institute, where I was scheduled to work and study in the laboratory of Maclyn McCarty.   I realized McCarty was already a great and famous scientist and that it was because of Mac's outstanding reputation that McQuarrie had arranged for me to study with McCarty. It was McCarty, along with O.T. Avery and C. McLeod, who had carried out the investigations many have called the experiments of the century.[25]   I was immensely impressed when I learned that these investigators worked nearly 10 years between publications, but when they finally did publish their important research it was to show that DNA was **the** molecule responsible for introduction of the inheritable information in Griffiths' bacterial transformation of pneumococci.[26] It must have been Avery's untimely, relatively early death which robbed these three scientists of the Nobel Prize. I say this because no research could have been more important to the ultimate development of biology and medicine and especially to modern molecular biology than their very first identification of DNA as the molecule responsible for inherited characteristics.

I came to the Rockefeller Institute directly from Minnesota. This was my first true move outside my beloved home state. Oh, yes, I had spent one summer during childhood working on a farm in Illinois and had made a brief three-day trip to Colorado where I had competed for a Markle Scholarship and had come home with the Helen Hay Whitney Fellowship instead. On arriving at the Rockefeller I first continued with research on bone marrow plasma cells, gammaglobulins and antibodies in patients with rheumatic fever. That seemed fine, because I was working in McCarty's rheumatic fever laboratory with McCarty, Stuart Elliot, Rebecca Lancefield, Chandler (Al) Stetson and Harrison Wood. Rheumatic fever patients were easy to obtain for my studies and I still had a bit more to do to clean up the analyses I had undertaken. The situation, however, was not satisfactory to me because I could have done the same work I was doing while at home.

Soon after arriving at the Rockefeller I met and was greatly influenced by Chandler (Al) Stetson. Through Stetson I met many people, both within and outside the Rockefeller Institute. These people included among others, the dynamic and creative Lewis Thomas who frequently came up first from Hopkins and then from New Orleans where he had gone to work as a young professor, and the dogged and highly critical and creative Henry Kunkel. Through Stetson I met or made friends with George Cotzias, Lew Dahl, Peyton Rous, Rene Dubos, David Karnofsky, Gregory Shwartzman, Merril Chase and many others. I later did exciting collaborative research with Al Stetson on the Shwartzman phenomenon.[27] However, while I was at the Rockefeller, encounters with two new Experiments of Nature exerted an impressive influence on my research and scientific career.

When I met Kunkel he was a young man with a fire in his belly. He wanted to use his newly acquired skills in immunochemistry to analyze myeloma proteins and to compare individual myeloma proteins both to other myeloma proteins and also to the normal gammaglobulins. His only problem was that he was having difficulty obtaining myeloma serums from which to prepare the purified paraproteins for his immunochemical analyses. Because of my prior research on plasma cells at Minnesota, I was recognized in certain quarters of New York as a "plasma cell hunter". Mary Peterman at the Sloan-Kettering Institute, a friend of my chemistry teacher, David Glick[28] and David Barr, Chairman of Medicine at Cornell and himself a plasma cell hunter, befriended me. Barr had given me an opportunity to teach my perspective on plasma cells both formally and informally in departments of medicine at Cornell Medical College and Mary Peterman did the same at the nearby cancer center—the Sloan-Kettering Institute for Cancer Research and Memorial Hospital.

Kunkel proposed that if I would help him collect myeloma serums he would teach me modern serology and immunochemistry. Consequently, with the help of my plasma cell hunting friends, I found seven different untreated myeloma patients who provided their beautiful plasmas for our research. These serums proved to be exactly what Kunkel needed for his initial immunochemical analyses of myeloma proteins. In return, Kunkel taught me quantitative immunochemistry and together, we carried out a series of studies that showed clearly that each myeloma protein was immunochemically similar to all the others, each was immunochemically distinct from the others, and each was also immunochemically similar to normal gammaglobulins.[29] I enjoyed this collaboration and learned a great deal from Kunkel.

But what fascinated me even more than the data generated by my research were revelations which stemmed from my talking at length to the myeloma patients from whom I obtained the blood for my collaborative studies. Gregarious as I was, I befriended each of the myeloma patients and sat sometimes for hours taking with them when I went to draw the rather large samples of their blood we needed for our studies. Each patient gave me a history of almost incredible susceptibility to infections. Each had repeatedly suffered from pneumonias, skin infections and septicemias. Each told me in turn how antibiotic treatment, usually with penicillin, had proved to be his or her lifesaver. Study of these patients' hospital records regularly revealed that they had been repeatedly infected by the organisms which René Dubos had been teaching me to consider the high-grade extracellular bacterial pathogens: *Streptococcus pneumoniae, Streptococcus pyogenes, Hemophilus influenza* and occasionally even *Pseudomonas aeruginosa*. I realized that each of these high-grade pathogens could be characterized as being encapsulated by a rather large capsule in the pathogenic state. It became clear to me, as my own research and that of others would later show, that the multiple myeloma patients each exhibited a profound deficiency of normal bodily defenses, particularly they were deficient in ability to produce antibody. But their immunodeficiency seemed to make them vulnerable to infections and reinfections primarily by an impressive but almost monotonous set of high-grade encapsulated bacterial pathogens. They did not have nearly so much trouble with infections by the lower grade pathogens, or what have become known today as opportunistic pathogens, e.g., facultative intracellular bacteria, fungi or certain viruses. I began to wonder why the myeloma patients exhibited this selective susceptibility to this particular set of organisms.

Soon after this experience and while I was digesting the provocative insight provided by the myeloma patients, I also began a study of patients with Hodgkin's disease. These patients exhibited a more or less counterpoint clinical-microbiological-immunological relationship to the myeloma patients. I did not set out to investigate the immunity systems of patient's with Hodgkin's disease. Indeed, my work with these patients began in quite a different way (see below). However, they too exhibited increased susceptibility to infections, but their susceptibility was to a completely different set of pathogens from those that plagued my myeloma patients—and I knew and realized this profound difference.

As stated, I had come to the Rockefeller Institute to work with Maclyn McCarty. McCarty didn't believe in assigning fellows or visiting investigators to any specific tasks. He wanted each to generate his own research project. I learned this valuable approach to fellows from Mac and have always tried to follow this lead in working with younger associates. It sometimes seems all too easy to make research assignments, and I learned that that temptation must be religiously avoided. There are now more than 200 of my former students, each of whom spent at least one year in my laboratory, who are now professors and another 200 who are rising through the academic ranks—100 are associate professors. I sincerely believe that controlling my enthusiasm and thus withholding direct assignments from them has been one of the most important contributions I made to the development of each of these incipient scholars. I learned that from Maclyn McCarty.

At that time, however, I was feeling an internally generated pressure to identify a line of research which might interest my new boss. While McCarty was on summer vacation I even got a bit depressed. I felt I wasn't doing much that I couldn't have done back in Minnesota, or even that I couldn't have done in any garage for that matter, and here I was at the Rockefeller Institute, where the greatest scientific minds and the best equipment for research were available to me. Yet I was still working on plasma cells and their relationship to antibody and immunoglobulin production, and for that reason I was unhappy.

One morning, Al Stetson bounced into my office-laboratory and, noticing my rather "brown study," said, "When I need occupational therapy for my depressions I crystallize proteins." I asked, "You do what?" Stetson bounced out and returned immediately with part of Northrup's still unpublished monograph on crystallizing proteins. He suggested I start with egg albumin. I was off like a shot. I bought three dozen eggs from the delicatessen across the street and started the indicated protein fractionation according to a protocol provided by Stetson. It was fun to be doing something different, and by the following day I had a preparation of concentrated purified egg albumin and was ready to try my hand at crystallization. In retrospect I know that the crystallization progressed far too easily and I am quite sure that Al Stetson dropped a few egg albumin crystals which he had prepared some months earlier into my concentrated protein solution to make my needed occupational therapy proceed rapidly. The results were fantastic. Crystals were all over the place! And my depression was gone! Al then said, why not crystallize C reactive protein—Mac would like that. Thus my problems seemed quickly to end. With Stetson's help I had picked a question that would permit me to learn from Mac, which I also thought might please Mac, that would be fun and that could be important.

Mac had told me earlier that the key to his original and I believe unpublished success in crystallizing C reactive protein (CRP) was to get the proper starting material which contained CRP in high concentration and was relatively free of lipid. In McCarty's earlier work this resource had been the clear chest effusion fluids obtained from patients suffering from streptococcal empyema. Because CRP is an acute phase reactant, it had captured my imagination. However, when I tried to find patients with streptococcal empyema I was completely frustrated. None were to be found in the hospitals anywhere in New York. Streptococcal empyemas had been dried up almost entirely because of the effective treatment of streptococcal pneumonias with penicillin. However, David Karnofsky at the then new Sloan-Kettering Institute, who was helping Stetson and me launch investigations of the role of leukocytes and platelets in the Shwartzman reaction, suggested that I might try to get the effusions I needed from the chests or abdominal cavities of patients with Hodgkin's disease. Hodgkin's disease patients often had massive pleural or peritoneal effusions and also frequently were quite ill with fevers, sweats and other indications of acute disease—even life-threatening infections. When I tested their blood for CRP, the levels were regularly very high: recorded by me as 6+ (a Rockefeller standard I learned from Harrison Wood). With the help of Karnofsky I began to collect effusion fluids from patients with Hodgkin's disease. In certain of the effusions, especially pleural effusions, CRP was present in the especially useful form since it was not obviously bound to lipid.

After much hard work I obtained a small amount of crystalline CRP from this source. That minor victory was not of much scientific moment. However, as I worked with my Hodgkin's disease patients to withdraw quarts and occasionally even gallons of fluid from their pleural and peritoneal effusions, I became friends with each of them and spent long hours talking with them about the awful diseases from which they suffered. I thus learned a great deal about the life-threatening infectious illnesses which they often experienced and feared. Some of them were looking forward to chemical treatment of their cancer, which was just beginning at the Sloan-Kettering Institute following the lead of Farber in Boston.

This research all took place long before serious cancer chemotherapy had become available. These patients were regularly dying of their neoplastic disease, and they knew it. To make matters worse, one after another of these Hodgkin's patients told me that their greatest dread was the infections that plagued the lives of fellow patients with this disease. Indeed, life for these patients, just as was life for patients with multiple myeloma, seemed to be one life-threatening infection after another. But the infections in the two groups of patients were very different. Instead of the *pneumococcus, streptococcus, Hemophilus influenza* and *P. aeruginosa* that caused the greatest trouble for the myeloma patients, patients with Hodgkin's disease repeatedly were under attack by viruses, e.g. Herpes simplex, fungi such as *Candida albicans*, and sometimes the cryptococcus (torula) or alternatively one or another low-grade or opportunistic bacterial infection. Tuberculosis and occasionally atypical acid-fast organisms also caused frequent and sometimes fatal infections in patients with Hodgkin's disease and generated much suffering. I remember attending several post-mortem examinations on my patients and observing that often it was these particular infections which they could not resist normally that led to their demise. By contrast it seemed that the patients with Hodgkin's disease, unlike the myeloma patients, rarely suffered from infections with the high-grade encapsulated extracellular bacterial pathogens.

I began to think that perhaps there might exist two separate universes of microorganisms—one that plagued and destroyed myeloma patients, and a very different set of infectious organisms that plagued patients with Hodgkin's disease. Many of the infections in the myeloma patients could be treated effectively with antibiotics and/or sulfa drugs, but the infections in Hodgkin's patients were more indolent, more difficult to treat, more persistent and more often lethal, even when sulfas and antibiotics were used. I discussed these strange relationships with Kunkel, Karnofsky, Peterman, Mrs. Lancefield, Al Stetson, Rene Dubos, Stan Rogers, David Barr and McCarty—anyone who would listen. None of these people of great mind could give me a clue as to why this striking difference in apparent microbial universes existed, but all agreed that these differences in microbial populations fit with their experience or knowledge and were indeed very likely real differences. Perhaps I should investigate that!

At about this time I became aware of and was impressed by the work Merrill Chase had been doing at the Rockefeller Institute. Merrill was quite austere, at least toward me. First with Landsteiner[30] and then independent-ly,[31] Chase had done most impressive work on two separate kinds of immunities. In Landsteiner's last research, he and Chase realized that tuberculin type reactions in guinea pigs and later tuberculin-like reactions to chemicals in guinea pigs could be **specifically** transferred from sensitized animal to nonsensitized animal with lymphoid cells, especially with peritoneal lymphoid cells. Such transfers were not possible with serum. Similarly, other delayed allergic or tuberculin type reactions, could be specifically transferred with cells, whereas immediate skin sensitivity of several types, as in Prausnitz and Kustner's classical experiments,[32] could be transferred only by serum, as could Arthus reactions. Both of the latter were, of course, attributable to antibodies. Chase's studies implicated the small lymphocytes in the transfer of the delayed allergic reactions and serum, with its antibodies, as the basis for transferring immediate, or so-called "early" allergies.[31]

While I was at the Rockefeller Institute, a sometimes visitor to Peyton Rous's laboratory was Peter Medawar, who Stetson told me was a truly brilliant British scientist from the University of London. In 1949 or 1950, Medawar gave a dynamic Friday conference on skin graft rejection in which he described research with cattle, guinea pigs, mice and rabbits which he interpreted to indicate that rejection of skin grafts was due to immunity, was not transferrable by serum but could be transferred by cells. I was impressed by Medawar and took the lessons he taught quite seriously. He was tall, handsome, filled with great animal vigor and exhibited immense confidence. He also had a marvelous sense of humor. His findings concerning homograft rejections indicated that a kind of immunity was involved in homograft rejection, but his work seemed to implicate cells and not the usual antibodies in the rejection process.[33,34,35] Stanfield Rogers, who also worked with Dr. Rous, was, like Kunkel, a bridge buddy of Al Stetson. He was investigating immunity to certain mouse tumors, which he said sometimes but not always involved antibodies transferrable with sera and sometimes seemed to involve an immunity attributable to cells. I remember being impressed by the way in which Rogers set up his experiments. He had numerous experiments going at any one time, so that even though experiments might take a full year from start to finish, he was busy harvesting experimental results nearly every week. I wondered if I could ever learn to be as orderly as Rogers so that I could do experiments that took a full year to complete and yet start and conclude them on such a regular schedule. I doubted my capacity to do this and was thus impressed by Rogers and admired very much his mentor Peyton Rous.

While at the Rockefeller I launched and completed several experiments, but none challenged my imagination as much as my observations concerning the different natures of the frequent infections in patients with Hodgkin's disease on the one hand and multiple myeloma on the other. Kunkel and I completed a first phase of the myeloma protein immunochemistry project. Odds and ends had to be completed before a publication would result and these were left behind to be completed by R. Slater, who had joined Kunkel's lab in 1950. Later, Slater and Kunkel did far more extensive analyses of the immunochemistry of the myeloma proteins and still later the chemist Edelman came into Kunkel's laboratory and used multiple myeloma and myeloma proteins as the Experiment of Nature to permit him to get a sufficient amount of the homogenous IgG myeloma protein so that he could achieve full chemical definition of IgG, including the amino acid sequencing, of the IgG immunoglobulin molecule.

Stetson and I did quite serious research on the pathogenesis of the Shwartzman reaction which led to an important publication in the Journal of Experimental Medicine. This research was basic to several investigations that I carried out later in collaboration with Lewis Thomas after I returned to Minnesota.[27,36,37,38,39] As a byproduct of my research with Stetson, Dr. Rous taught me how to write a *Journal of Experimental Medicine* (JEM) paper. He literally crossed out with red ink and rewrote every word I had written in a jointly authored manuscript with Stetson. I also began research with Kunkel on a group of young girls who suffered from a form of chronic active hepatitis and who had massive hypergammaglobulinemia. In this research I showed that these girls who had a considerable plasmacytosis of bone marrow regularly had an almost unbelievably extensive plasmacytosis in their hepatic tissue exudates. I later dubbed this disease "plasma cell hepatitis".[40,41,335,336] Kunkel and I submitted a description of the disease and its impressive cellular pathology focussed on the plasma cell to the Johns Hopkins Bulletin because Kunkel had come from Hopkins and wanted to publish there. My data on the association of these extreme forms of hypergammaglobulinemia with very extensive liver plasmacytosis did not impress Arnold Rich, who reviewed the paper, and so our paper was rejected by the Johns Hopkins Hospital Bulletin. Nonetheless, a few years after returning to Minnesota I finally published on this disease in which I was able to emphasize the plasma cell-gammaglobulin associations in this disease that was featured by massive hypergammaglobulin-emia.[40,41] Bearn, Kunkel and Slater had also published on different aspects of the disease some years earlier even though Bearn came to Kunkel's lab after I had left.[42] Before it could be an appropriate time for me to publish on this new disease or old disease in a new perspective, I had to convince the hypercritical Cecil Watson, the liver expert at Minnesota, that I was studying and treating patients with what really was a special form of liver disease in which plasma cells and gammaglobulin levels were both massively increased and intimately linked, and which I could often cure or place into dramatic remission by adrenal steroid treatment. Watson wanted to think of plasma cell hepatitis as just another form of early cirrhosis. My approach, using for that time rather high-dose adrenal steroid treatment, dramatically eliminated both the liver plasmacytosis and the massive hypergammaglobulinemia as well as all manifestations of disease in these patients. Such treatment was rather ineffective in patients with chronic active hepatitis attributable to chronic infection with the hepatitis B virus. The results of my treatment were so much bettern than we obtained with adrenal steroid treatment in other forms of early cirrhosis that I finally convinced Watson that I, indeed, was on to something new, and so I finally published a proper reviewed report linking plasma cells and gammaglobulins together in that form of chronic active hepatitis. In subsequent research Page and I also showed that the immuno-suppressive drug we had found to be an antiinflammatory agent as well, amethopterin, was also effective in treating this severe and otherwise rapidly progressive disease.[40,335,336]

After spending only one year at the Rockefeller Institute I returned to Minnesota. However, I was still fired up about the apparent bisection of immunity and bisection of the different classes of microorganisms implicit in my studies of the two diseases in which deficient resistances to different microorganisms seemed characteristic—Hodgkin's disease and myeloma. Study of these patients made it clear to me that there must be two distinct microbial universes as revealed by the different infectious problems which plagued these two sets of patients.

After I came home to Minnesota McQuarrie gave me a small office and an adjacent small laboratory. I completed my residency requirement by helping McQuarrie as chief resident while carrying the title of instructor on the pediatric service. I also had sufficient time to begin conducting research on pediatric patients as Experiments of Nature. McQuarrie had been so successful in placing his trainees as department heads around the United States and around the world that the pediatric department had been grossly depleted and could use much attention from a quite junior staff. This greatly improved the opportunity for and fostered the rapid development of men and women in the junior ranks such as myself. I did research on the Shwartzman reaction, the Arthus reaction and other kinds of allergic necrotizing inflamma-tory reactions and was seeking common denominators for these skin reactions that were each produced in very different ways. I also continued studies of acute phase reactions, especially C-reactive protein,[43] and set up systems to evaluate the cellular and humoral aspects of immunity.

When in 1950 I was asked to visit St. Louis to consider a junior pediatric position under Hartman at the Children's Hospital at Washington University, I remember spending a full hour arguing, inconclusively, with the microbiolo-gist Bronfenbrenner about whether or not tuberculin reactions, delayed allergies and Arthus reactions and also the different means of resistance to different infections were intimately related and specialized parts of each other or could, indeed, be considered to be fundamentally different immunity processes. Bronfenbrenner, who had studied at the Rockefeller, took the view that all immunities were basically the same and all were based on antibodies. He said, "there can only be one basis of specificity," and that is represented by immunity based on antibodies. I tried in vain to convince Bronfenbrenner, who represented one established view, that there were at least two different and separate forms of immunity which were fundamentally and distinctly different from each other. This I felt was revealed by the different susceptibilities to different microorganisms I had observed in my myeloma and Hodgkin's disease patients and that also was clearly reflected in Chase's experiments. I felt the two were represented by lymphocytes on the one hand and plasma cells on the other. I could not convince Bronfenbrenner that anything more than antibodies were needed. I was disgusted with myself when I left Bronfenbrenner's office because I felt the experiments to convince a skeptic remained far too incomplete.

During the early 1950's I also cared for the children with leukemias for Dr. McQuarrie's department. We provided the entire diagnostis, treatment and management of approximately 30-35 new leukemia patients each year. At the time we were just beginning to see responses to aminopterin, and so these patients were at long last of some interest and not just terribly depressing experiences in which the children died usually within weeks or months. I set up rheumatic fever and rheumatoid arthritis clinics and saw rheumatology patients, patients with acute and chronic liver disease, patients with mesenchymal and collagen diseases, and patients with acute and chronic kidney disease. I began to conceive of and design for myself a clinical subspecialty in pediatrics that had immunology as its focus. Indeed, by my actions I had become a clinical immunologist and had created my own new subspecialty.

Then one morning in 1952 I opened my green pediatric journal, and there was an article by Colonel Ogden Bruton entitled, "Agammaglobulinemia".[44] In that paper, Bruton described a single patient for whom (like the myeloma patients I had been studying) life was just one severe life-threatening bacterial infection (most often attributable to the pneumococcus) after another. That patient could not produce antibodies and lacked gammaglobulin in the blood—he was agammaglobulinemic. I literally trembled as I read the article and feared that this disease might be so rare that I would never have the chance to study such a patient and thus might never be able to test in such a challenging Experiment of Nature whether my plasma cells might be present or absent in patients who could produce neither antibody or gammaglobulin. I predicted, of course, from my prior research that plasma cells could not be formed by such a patient.

At the time Bruton's paper appeared in Pediatrics, and as luck would have it, I was responsible for the care and diagnosis of three similar patients who had presented diagnostic problems on the wards at the University of Minnesota Hospital. Armed with Bruton's description and my big old Klett electropoiesis apparatus, which yielded Schlieren patterns of the plasma proteins and which I was skilled at using, it was possible for me to make the diagnosis of agammaglobulinemia in each of these three children. What luck. Two of the initial three of these patients were brothers, and the family history, which included other male infant deaths in the mother's family, suggested that an X-linked recessive inheritance might be involved. All three patients had been diagnostic problems. Life for these children was one threatening episode of pneumonia, meningitis, septicemia, cellulitis, sinusitis or severe bronchitis after another. The two brothers also had exhibited intermittent episodes of neutropenia. When I did bone marrow biopsies on each of these three boys, no leukemia was present and I found the bone marrow of each to be completely lacking in plasma cells—I mean completely.[4,45,46,47,48,49] However, lymphocyte counts in blood and bone marrow were not decreased. The children each had very small tonsils, and their lymph nodes and spleen were small and the lymph nodes seemed poorly developed when I performed biopsies and studied them histologically after stimulating them with diphtheria, pertussis and tetanus vaccines. I studied primary, secondary and tertiary antibody responses in these patients after antigenic stimulation with diptheria, tetanus and pertussis vaccines. I also compared responses of the lymph nodes of these patients to those of normal children and adults following antigenic stimulation. I discovered that germinal centers usually present in what I called the secondary lymphoid follicles were completely lacking. Lymphocyte development was also deficient in lymph nodes of these children. In the deep cortical regions of the nodes the lymphocyte population was quite abundant. By contrast, at the periphery of the nodes, which I called the far cortical areas, a marked deficiency of lymphoid cells was evident and the humps on the lymph node surface were lacking. The medullary cords of the lymph nodes were devoid of plasma cells, even after the children had been stimulated with secondary or tertiary injections of antigen. This was quite a different picture from the striking development of secondary follicles, germinal centers and plasma cells that could be found in the nodes of healthy adults and children that had also been repeatedly stimulated with the same antigen or antigens.[4,46,47,50]

During the next year I discovered on the medical services of the University Hospital and the pediatric and medical services of the large county hospital, the Hennipen County General Hospital. The private children's hospital in St. Paul and the Anker Municipal Hospital in St. Paul had a relatively large number of patients (8 or 9, as I remember) who suffered from different forms of agammaglobulinemia or hypogammaglobulinemia. Many clinicians helped me to identify and study these patients.[4,45,46,48,49,50] Even the pediatric staff at the Mayo Clinic sent patients to me for diagnosis and analysis. To some degree the patients were heterogeneous; some seemed to have an acquired disease which began later in life, and some were boys with a familial, apparently X-linked, inherited disease. Delayed allergic reactions were often quite normal but these, too, were deficient in certain of the patients with hypogammaglobulinemia. One of my patients kept a skin engraftment in place without rejection for more than one year. Other hypogammaglobulinemic patients, especially those with apparent XLA, rejected skin grafts with impressive vigor.[48,49] In the children with hypogammaglobulinemia, especially those with what appeared to be an X-linked form of agammaglobulinemia (XLA), vigorous delayed allergic reactions, e.g. poison ivy, could be developed and expressed normally in these children. In spite of the agammaglobulinemia, these delayed allergic responses could sometimes be specifically transferred from such patients to normal, nonsensitized recipients by injecting, into the subcutaneous tissues, muscle or preferably into the skin of nonsensitized normal persons, peripheral blood lymphocytes of specifically sensitized agammaglobulinemic patients.[4] Antibody responses in each of the agammaglobulinemic and most of the hypogammaglobulinemic patients were almost always absent or, when present in the adults or children with hypogammaglobulinemia, the antibody responses were always exceedingly feeble. The tonsils of the boys with XLA were very small and lacked the characteristic huge germinal center development and the lymphoid follicular structure which is so characteristic of tonsils in immunologically normal children.[4]

It thus became clear from my early analysis of immunity in these agammaglobulinemic and hypogammaglobulinemic patients that they were always markedly immunodeficient. Often, however, they were not deficient in all of the different immune responses. The patients with very early clinical onset of X-linked agammaglobulinemia, XLA, usually developed disease during the second half of the first year. These XLA patients were regularly the most deficient of all patients with respect to antibody production, but at the same time many of them truly displayed the most vigorous cell-mediated immunities observed in any of the agammaglobulinemic patients. These responses were often unusually vigorous even when compared to those of normal persons. Sometimes the agammaglobulinemic patients, had brothers with the disease or brothers or male cousins or uncles who had died of infections in infancy.[4,45,46,48,51] They usually had vigorous and quite normal delayed allergic skin reactions, and could reject skin grafts. They were prone to suffer many infections with high-grade encapsulated bacteria, especially streptococci, pneumococci, *Hemophilus influenzae, Neisseria meningitides*, or *P. aeruginosa*. They also were susceptible to staphylococcus infection but did not appear to be as susceptible to these organisms as to pneumococci. They had normal lymphocyte counts in blood but did not have plasma cells in bone marrow, and they lacked plasma cells and secondary follicles (germinal centers) in their lymph nodes after repeated antigenic stimulation.[4,45,46,48,49] In contrast to their susceptibility to bacterial infection, which I determined by cultures as well as by susceptibility to antibiotic treatment they expressed normally, recovered from and seemed to develop immunity to several of the usual childhood exanthems—rubella, measles, chicken pox or mumps—even though they did not produce demonstrable antibody to these pathogens".[4,45,46,48,49] One of the boys who had an extremely deficient or non-existent antibody response had been given BCG during infancy in a refugee rehabilitation camp in Europe before being permitted to come to America. He had developed the usual localized skin infection that resulted in a vigorous tuberculin reaction. I could passively transfer this delayed allergic reaction to non-sensitized normal persons with viable lymphocytes from the agamma-globulinemic child's blood.[4] These boys with the apparent X-linked disease did not appear to be unusually susceptible to fungus infections and they showed normal resistance to infections by certain viruses even though they could not make demonstrable antibodies to these viruses.[4,45,46]

It became clear as we studied further the patients with XLA that these patients like my Hodgkin's disease patients and myeloma patients appeared to be bisecting at one time several very different universes. They were clearly bisecting the lymphoid cell universe into plasma cells and the special lymphocytes of the germinal centers which they lacked, and lymphocytes, phagocytes and inflammatory cells responsible for certain cell-mediated immunities which were present and seemed to be quite intact in these patients.[45,46,47] These patients developed delayed and contact allergies (poison ivy, for example) quite normally, reacted normally to gram-negative endo-toxins and even developed increased ability to tolerate endotoxins after repeated injection, yet they produced no demonstrable antibodies even when extremely sensitive measures such as immunization with E. coli (bactericidal antibody formation) were employed to search for antibodies which they might have produced.[4,50] Thus these agammaglobulinemic children were bisecting the immunological universes into antibodies and ability to produce antibodies which they lacked on the one hand and cell-mediated immunities (delayed allergic and contact allergies) which they possessed in quantitatively normal amount on the other.[4,40,50,52]

And these patients were also clearly bisecting the microbial universe. Infections with *pneumococci, Hemophilus influenzae, P. aeruginosa, meningococci, Streptococcus pyogenes* and to some extent also *staphylococci*—the high-grade encapsulated bacterial pathogens—caused great trouble and were always life-threatening to these children. By contrast, these patients handled tuberculosis well and resisted with normal vigor infections by atypical acid-fast bacilli, fungi and numerous viruses even though no antibodies to any of these organisms could be found in their blood. We looked very hard in their serums and responses for such antibodies.[4,47,48,49]

Certain viruses unlike others did, however, cause these patients to have unusually severe clinical disease. Hepatitis B infection occurred in three of our patients through the years and in each of them progressed fatally,[41] as did non A, non B hepatitis later in another. The agammaglobulinemic boys seemed especially prone to develop paralytic disease as a consequence of poliomyelitis. A dermatomyositis-like clinical disease occurred in several such patients whom others and we discovered later to be due to echovirus infection.[53] Mycoplasma and uroplasma infections, the former involving the respiratory apparatus, and the latter involving sometimes the respiratory apparatus but especially involving joints, have also been a special problem in some of these agammaglobulinemic patients especially but not exclusively those with X-linked disease, as we later showed.

We were almost forced from study of these patients to reason that they lacked capacity to produce gammaglobulins and antibodies in association with an inability to generate plasma cells, but the that their ability to develop certain cell-mediated immunities was intact as was ability to produce certain classes of lymphocytes.[4,40,47] Thus these patients, as Experiments of Nature, at once bisected the microbial universe and the immunologic universe just as they had bisected the lymphoid cell universe. In our earliest descriptions of the lymph nodes of these patients, not only did we find plasma cells to be absent, for example, but expected follicles containing germinal centers (so-called secondary follicles) could not be located in the lymph node cortex. The bisection of the microbial universe by these X-linked infantile agammaglobulinemic patients was very similar to the dissection which had been exhibited by the two groups of patients we were also studying with hematologic malignancies, namely, those with Hodgkin's disease on the one hand and those with multiple myeloma on the other.[40,54,55,56,57,58]

It is especially important to reflect on the lessons, taught with incredible clarity by these agammaglobulinemic patients, which were compatible with certain propositions developing from other directions of immunologic inquiry. The findings in the XLA patients were incompatible with the point of view expressed by Bronfenbrenner (see above) that all immune responses are based on the same mechanism and are only somewhat different expressions of this single immune mechanism—antibody production. Our plasma cell theory, although supported by several lines of telling evidence, had not yet been generally accepted up to the time of our study of agammaglobulinemia (XLA) in late 1953. Support for Kolouch's plasma cell theory had come from several quarters, but that plasma-cellular-antibody linkage was clearly and definitively established by the studies of patients with X-linked agammaglobulinemia. Among the most telling supports for the plasma cell theory had been the brilliant and quite definitive studies analyzing antibody production in tissue fragments carried out by Astrid Fagraeus that had been set in motion in response to her encounters with multiple myeloma as an Experiment of Nature.[59] Also, the immunohistochemical analyses using fluorescent microscopy carried out by Coons and his collaborators[60,61,62,63] had indicated that plasma cells and not lymphocytes or other cells contained and probably produced gammaglobulins and antibodies. Ehrlich switched his allegiance from lymphocyte to plasma cell after he carried out detailed collaborative observations with his brilliant research fellow Carolyn Forman.[64] Each of these investigations seemed to us to be important. Some of these observations we already considered crucial supports for the concept that the plasma cell was *the* antibody producing cell. However, our studies of the agammaglobulinemic (XLA) children who could produce *no* antibodies and also very little or *no* gammaglobulin represented an opportunity for immediate disproof of our plasma cell hypothesis. Instead of disproving the hypothesis that the plasma cells were the antibody-producing cell, the agammaglobulinemic patients, of course, represented another strong support for the theory that it is actually the plasma cells which produce antibodies.[4,45,46,47]

I named the infantile X-linked recessive agammaglobulinemia Bruton's agammaglobulinemia to recognize the unique contributions made by Colonel Ogden Bruton, who was a pediatrician and had been the first to recognize and describe such a patient.[44] In a bit of irony, it turned out that, much later, when I studied Bruton's original case in detail after his patient had reached adulthood, I found the patient not to have the lymphoid cell characteristics of X-linked agammaglobulinemia (XLA) at all.[40,45,46,47] Indeed, we showed that Bruton's original case had suffered from the form of immunodeficiency we, with Seligmann and Fudenberg, had later named the common variable form of hypogammaglobulinemia.[65]

Following Bruton's discovery of agammaglobulinemia and our detailed analysis of X-linked agammaglobulinemic patients, we also had the opportunity to study and define patients with several different kinds of primary and secondary immunodeficiencies. Many patients with different primary immunodeficiency diseases have represented revealing Experiments of Nature. The X-linked agammaglobulinemic patient, it seems to me, as an Experiment of Nature, has provided in immunology an additional major support for Karl Popper's argument[66] that a scientific hypothesis has true power in direct proportion to its refutability. These patients also supported William Harvey's teaching that much can be learned of the useful and applicable functions in normals from studying patients with rarer forms of disease in which an important component of the bodily functions has been left out or has become deranged in some way.[7] The possibility of immediate refutation of the plasma cell theory of antibody production in the X-linked agammaglobulinemic patients who could produce no gammaglobulins, immunoglobulins or antibodies clearly reflected the scientific importance and power of our plasma cell postulate. These findings, together with our own basic experimental findings and those of the others that linked plasma cells to antibody synthesis and dissociated the latter from the cell-mediated immunities, impelled further studies both by us and by many clinical investigators of the immunological concomitants of the patients with X-linked agammaglobulinemia and other primary and secondary immunodeficiency diseases.

But what of Hodgkin's disease and multiple myeloma, the clinical studies of which had launched our inquiries? Schier used skin tests[67] to show that patients with Hodgkin's disease are often anergic when tested with a readily available battery of six skin test antigens, namely tuberculin, trichophyton, candidin, streptococcal antigens, mumps and diptheria toxoid. These in the aggregate produce delayed skin reactions in a very high proportion of normal persons. We confirmed and extended Shier's findings of anergy in Hodgkin's disease[40,50,52,55,56] and showed that patients with Hodgkin's disease failed also to respond not only to this battery of skin tests but also failed to develop contact allergy to 2,4-dinitrofluorobenzene or 2,4-dinitrochlorobenzene. By contrast, patients with X-linked agammaglobulinemia developed vigorous delayed and contact allergies. We also showed that Hodgkin's patients, unlike the X-linked agammaglobulinemic patients, were grossly deficient in skin allograft rejection.[56] They exhibited all of the usual immunoglobulins in at least normal amounts and sometimes made quite normal antibody responses. Thus these patients presented a fascinating counterpoint to patients with X-linked agammaglobulinemia who made no antibodies but who possessed vigorous cell-mediated immunities. By contrast, Horace Zinneman and Wendall Hall[57,58] at the University of Minnesota as well as I myself,[40] showed that patients with multiple myeloma rejected skin grafts vigorously, developed second-set skin graft rejections and showed vigorous cell-mediated immunities to the batteries of antigens we used for testing delayed type allergy to which most immunologically normal persons regularly reacted. They were also readily sensitized to 2-4 dinitrochloro or 2-4 dinitrofluorobenzene. The untreated patients with Hodgkin's disease were usually quite effective as antibody producers, but the multiple myeloma patients, like the agammaglobulinemic patients, did not produce antibodies well in response to antigenic challenges. Since we had already reasoned that the set of microorganisms to which Hodgkin's disease patients were susceptible was very different from the set of microbial pathogens that plagued myeloma patients and the agammaglobulinemic patients, it seemed that these two malignant diseases, which clearly involved different sets of lymphoid cells, were teaching the same basic lessons about the different forms of immunity that were being taught by the children with X-linked agammaglobulinemia. In light of the immunological findings in these groups of patients, it became eminently clear that the microbial, lymphoid and immunological universes comprised two separate and distinct complexes clearly distinguishable by these incisive Experiments of Nature. These clinical analyses that sorted out and definitively revealed two universes within the major specific defenses of the body now seemed to confirm and greatly extend the evidence for this same dissection that had been achieved by Chase and Landsteiner ten years earlier.[30,31]

During this same period we were analyzing all of these relationships I was asked to see another patient who proved ultimately to be a most telling Experiment of Nature. In 1952 a farmer from Moorehead, Minnesota, came to Dr. Richard Varco's chest disease clinic and was ultimately admitted to Varco's surgical service.[4,45,46,68] Fortunately, Varco and his staff had been working in collaboration with us doing all of the surgical biopsies that were needed to help in the essential analyses of agammaglobulinemic and hypogammaglobulinemic patients and the liver biopsies on my hypergammaglobulinemic girls. Although I was a pediatrician, I was asked to see this immunodeficient adult patient. The patient, F.H., confided to me that one of his chief concerns was that perhaps he had become addicted to a new antibiotic called terramycin. This antibiotic was the first of the tetracyclines and one which now is used entirely in animal feeding. This 54 year old had been very well up to 46 years of age. Life had then changed for him and he had suffered 16 episodes of pneumonia over an eight-year period. His susceptibility to infection had occurred in temporal association with appearance of a huge mediastinal mass that, when extirpated by Dr. Varco, proved to be a 540 gram benign stromal epithelial *thymoma*. This tumor was associated with profound hypogammaglobulinemia, and the patient also was shown to have a broadly based immunodeficiency. In association with his immunodeficiency disease, this patient was grossly lacking in all immunoglobulins and had a profound deficiency of antibody production, and was also impressively deficient in all cell-mediated immunities. The latter was reflected by an anergy toward all of the delayed allergic responses after administration of the battery of antigens similar to that which we had used to evaluate immunodeficiency in patients with Hodgkin's disease and the other agammaglobulinemic patients. Plasma cells were deficient in this patient, but unlike in the patients with XLA, plasma cells were not completely absent. Furthermore, the patient had relatively low lymphocyte numbers and showed defective allograft (homograft) immunity as revealed by a markedly slow and ultimately delayed rejection of skin allografts. Removal of the thymus mass did not correct the patient's immunodeficiency disease.[4,45,46,48,49,68]

The association of this peculiar stromal epithelial thymus tumor with the broadly based immunodeficiency in our patient provoked us to begin to question what role is played by the thymus in immunity. Up to that moment the thymus had been considered to be a "vestigial" organ. Robert Hebbel, a very skillful professor of surgical pathology warned me not to make too big a deal of the thymus and its possible immunity functions as I had been doing from the findings in my patient. He considered the thymus to be of no importance because it was what he called a "vestigial organ." Furthermore, pathologists disdained the thymus because of errors generated by the erroneous concept that of status thymicolymphaticus was associated with sudden death in children. One of Varco's fellows, MacLean, and my medical student associate Sol Zak and I, inspired by this patient, nonetheless set out to remove the thymus early in life in young rabbits to try to determine what the thymus might be doing in the development and establishment of immune reactions. Zak and MacLean, under my direction, extirpated the thymus in as small rabbits, as young as 4-5 wks of age—as yong as we then thought possible. To say the least, we were all disappointed when these rather extensive investigations involving complete extirpation of the thymus did not reveal, in relatively short-term experiments that the thymus exerted any measurable influence on immunity functions. In 1956 and 1957 we reported both the studies of our thymoma patient and our thus-far negative experiments with thymic function in rabbits.[68,69] However, in the discussion portion of our scientific report which contained the description of the clinical association of thymoma and immunodeficiency we clearly stated that although our initial experimental results with rabbits had not been revealing, we considered our Experiment of Nature as represented by our patient with thymoma and immunodeficiency to suggest that the thymus does, indeed, play a crucial role in immunity functions. Because of Boyd and Scammon's influence[70,71,72,73] at the University of Minnesota we knew that the thymus was of relatively maximal size and presumably thus is exerting its maximal influence very early in life. It was for this reason that the initial experiments were done in very young rabbits. We later learned that even in choosing to thymectomize very young (4-wk-old rabbits) in these first experiments, the rabbits we had chosen were not young enough so that thymic extirpation might reflect in short term experiments the crucial function of the thymus in immunological development which we later discovered.

Another chance event—a different kind of Experiment of Nature—then influenced the direction of our research. Bruce Glick was a graduate student at Ohio State University. He had been told by his mentor Professor Knauff that if he wanted to become a famous scientist he would carry out investigations that would elucidate the function of the bursa of Fabricius in chickens. Glick, being an enthusiastic graduate student, jumped into this endeavor with exemplary vigor. He extirpated the bursa of Fabricius at different ages, from early to old age, even removing it from newly hatched chickens. He then attempted to relate the bursa of Fabricius to many different components of chicken physiology. All to no avail. As is often the case with graduate students, he and a fellow graduate student, Timothy Chang, had another assignment. That task was to prepare a class demonstration of an immunologic agglutination reaction for a short course in immunology. Glick had carried out this simple assignment in a prior year and had chosen immunization with *Salmonella pullorum* and the bacterial agglutination as the basis for a most reliable class demonstration. Because he had done the demonstration before, he sloughed off the immunization of the chickens for the class demonstration to Chang. Unbeknownst to Glick, Chang chose for the class demonstration to immunize chickens which Glick had earlier bursectomized in the newly hatched period. The class demonstration failed: no antibody response could be revealed by the agglutination reaction. Glick and Chang, after discussion, recognized that the class demonstration failure was almost certainly attributable to the fact that the chickens which had been immunized were, indeed, chickens that had been bursectomized very early in life—before the tenth day after hatching.

These graduate students had made a major discovery. Chickens, bursectomized in the newly hatched period, failed to make antibodies!! The faulted short-course demonstration had revealed fortuitously a crucial role for the bursa of Fabricius in immunologic development. After subsequent confirmatory experiments, the investigators prepared with Jaap a brief but quite definitive paper to announce their discovery. They submitted this paper to one of America's most prestigious scientific journals, *Science*. The paper was reviewed, and the editorial opinion drawn that although the science involved seemed adequate to the task, the reviewers could not convince themselves that the research had the broad general significance essential for a paper to be published in the prestigious journal *Science*. Thus the editor could not recommend that Glick's crucial paper be published in *Science*.

Not to be daunted, the three[74] published what has been a watershed paper describing the bursa of Fabricius as an organ crucial to immunologic development in the journal *Poultry Science* in 1956. This paper showed that the Bursa of Fabricius is essential if chickens are to develop ability to produce antibody. Being published in *Poultry Science*, the paper escaped attention of almost all immunologists. Perhaps all except one, Harold Wolfe Professor of Immunology at the University of Wisconsin. A major part of Wolfe's life's work had been a most impressive series of 21 elegant papers published in *The Journal of Immunology*; each of these was published with one of Wolfe's graduate students as first coauthor. These papers, in each instance based on elegant methodologies, were entitled "Precipitin production in chickens: papers 1-21." Paper 21 in this series[75] was a clear confirmation and extension of the research done by Glick and colleagues. Instead of bacterial agglutination, the elegant immunochemical analytic methods introduced by Heidelberg had been used. Harold Wolfe was a good friend of mine at a neighboring academic institution, namely the University of Wisconsin. Thus, at the FASEB meetings in the Spring of 1959, after I had given a report on immunodeficiency diseases to the experimental pathologists, Harold Wolfe sought me out and told me of his convincing confirmation of the experiments of Glick et al which were being done in his laboratory by his student Mueller and associate Meyer.[75]

Armed with this exciting new information about the role of the bursa in developmental immunology I felt I knew exactly what to do with our thymus experiments. It was clear what had been wrong with our experiments to this point. We had been taking the thymus out too late in life. As a student of Hal Downey, who more than anything else was a comparative morphological hematologist, I had been taught that Jolly, early in the century,[76,77] had become interested in the morphology, development and involution of the bursa of Fabricius and had recognized similarities between thymus in mammals and bursa in fowl. Jolly, citing the common lymphoepithelial nature of both organs, the regular involution of both organs following sexual maturation, and the fact that the two organs were morphologically similar in that they had lobular and follicular structures with distinct and prominent cortical and medullary regions, referred to the bursa of Fabricius as the "Cloacal Thymus."

Thus in 1959 and continuing through 1960, several of my young associates and my trusted colleague Martinez and I performed a major series of experiments in which we once again turned to extirpating the thymus. Now, however, instead of working with 4-6 week-old rabbits, we studied baby immediately newborn rabbits (hot little newborns, as I called them),[78,79] infant mice.[80,81,82,83,84,85,86] Later we also extirpated the thymus in neonatal hamsters,[87] all with similar results. The thymectomies instead of in 4 week old rabbits were now performed in the immediate neonatal period—in those hot little newborns of each of the species. The results we obtained, of course, in this second go-round were very different from those with rabbits we had reported earlier.[68,69] In rodents, rabbits, chickens and hamsters, neonatal thymic extirpation or prevention of normal development of thymus and/or bursa interfered with ability to make antibodies,[78,79,86,88] ability to reject homografts (now allografts) of skin,[80] develop tumor immunity[81] or develop capacity of the animals' lymphoid cells to induce GVHR.[82] Our extensive experiments showed that cell-mediated as well as the humoral immunities were all inhibited from developing normally by neonatal thymectomy or by inhibition of thymic development using 19-nor-testosterone treatment given early in embryonic life.

The very first announcement of our discovery that the thymus could be shown to play a crucial role in the development of immunity came in an abstract which we submitted for publication and scientific presentation in December 1960—the deadline for submission of abstracts for the FASEB meeting. This scientific presentation of our findings was made by my master's degree fellow, Olga Archer, who had come from Sydney, Australia with her husband who was a young faculty member at University of South Wales and had come to Minneapolis as a senior fellow in aeronautical engineering in the Institute of Technology. O. Archer, my student, had been educated as a serologist in Australia. She was aided in both execution of the thymectomies in newborn rabbits and in the experimental analyses by Dr. Richard Varco's highly competent junior surgical fellow, James Pierce. Our abstract describing this crucial research was submitted for presentation at the American Association of Immunologists meeting in December 1960.[78]   By April 1961, when the immunology meeting was held, Carlos Martinez, John Kersey, Gus Dalmasso, Papermaster and I already had obtained much evidence from studies in mice as well as rabbits and chickens which showed clearly that thymectomy or prevention of thymus development very early in life prevented the normal development of both humoral and cell-mediated immunities, prevented homograft or allograft rejection of normal tissues and even prevented rejection of both allogeneic and syngeneic tumors. Neonatal thymectomy or hormonal thymectomy during development also had inhibited the cellular development necessary for generation of cells that could initiate a graft-vs-host reactions.[83,85,89]

In the discussion period that followed Archer's presentation at the April 1961 meeting of the American Association of Immunologists,[78] I summarized all these collective data which had been generated in my laboratory and which we, of course, considered to established once and for all time that the thymus does, indeed, play a crucial role in development of immunity. In my usual rather audacious way I announced that at long last we now had established the essential function of the thymus. That function, I stated, was to make possible the normal development of **both** cellular and humoral immunities. (Unpublished discussion, Robert A. Good et al, annual meeting of the American Association of Immunologists, Atlantic City, New Jersey, April 1961).

Our definitive papers were prepared with great care. We didn't hurry because we did not realize that a horse race might be on. The plan was that on one of these first papers I would be the first author and that this paper would be presented in the *Journal of Experimental Medicine*.[83]   On another paper which was to emphasize the presentation of data on allograft immunity, Carlos Martinez, originally an embryologist trained by the Nobel Laureate Houssay of Argentina, would be first author.[80] This paper was to be published in the *Proceedings of the Society for Experimental Biology and Medicine*. In a third paper our student Olga Archer would be first author and that paper should be published in *Nature*[79] and in still other papers my graduate student, Papermaster, would be first author[85,86,88] or Martinez's new fellow, Dalmasso, would be first author.[81,82] Further, our *Proc. Soc. Exp. Biol. Med.* report on the influence of thymectomy on skin graft rejection was unusually long in press, unusual especially for a Proc. Soc. paper, because of a printers' strike that delayed publication of the Proc. Soc. for approximately two months. J.F.A.P. Miller's announcement[90] of his initial but also quite definitive experiments that established a role for the thymus in developmental immunology appeared in the *Lancet*. We published our most detailed results in the *Journal of Experimental Medicine*.[83] Basically, the two sets of investigations—Miller's and mine— were most complementary to each other. From our point of view, because of the initial abstract from our laboratory which preceded all the other publications, including Miller's *Lancet* paper. We felt the events clearly established our priority in the discovery of the thymus function.

There has been much dispute about whether I should be credited with the discovery of the biologic function of the thymus or whether that credit should go rather to J.F.A.P. Miller, then of London's Chester Beatty Research Institute.[90] I sincerely believe that each of us independently made the discoveries which have established the biologic function of the thymus. The experimental work, extensive from each group, surely had to be have been simultaneous and independent. Miller was working in a cancer research facility — the Chester Beatty Research Institute—and so it was quite natural that he, or if not he, someone else should pursue the lead generated by the earlier research of Jacob Furth.[91,92] The latter had discovered that leukemia in AKR mice (Jacob Furth's strain) is prevented by thymectomy if this operation is performed in the neonatal period. Miller, studying this issue further, had exhibited the ingenuity to test also immunological functions of his neonatally thymectomized mice.[90,93,94,95,96] Miller did not know at all the line of reasoning that led to our research on the thymus which had been provoked by the developmental, morphologic and involutional similarities of this organ to the bursa of Fabricius. Nor did he know of Glick's investigations of the function of the bursa of Fabricius—morphologically similar to the thymus— which was established both by early extirpation or removal or selective hormonally-based prevention of development of the bursa early in life. I am sure Miller was certain that he had discovered independently the function of the thymus,[96] and from his perspective that was the case. We were equally certain the contribution had been mine. By the time we submitted our abstract with its definitive data in December 1960, there was no way that we could have known of Miller's research. He had not made a single utterance of any kind about the thymus in immunology prior to our first submission and the presentation of the observations from our laboratory.

Further, in a presentation at the discussions of Archer's paper at the immunology meeting, I summarized our extensive research on skin graft rejection across multi-minor and major histocompatibility barriers and inhibition of development of tumor immunity in neonatally thymectomized mice and prevention of development of capacity to induce graft vs. host reactions.[80,81,82,83,84] This session of the American Association of Immunologists which I chaired and at which approximately 100 leading American immunologists were in attendance. Thus, we all would certainly have had to be clairvoyant to have been led by or in any way to have copied Miller's research.[78,79,80,81,82,83,84]

Indeed, the very first I heard of Miller's work was when his paper had appeared in *Lancet*[90] after a very short prepublication period (three weeks, I am told). I heard of Miller's report while attending a meeting on immunologic progress held at Brook Lodge in Michigan in November 1961. Byron Waksman announced Miller's findings reported in the Lancet to this assemblage and also described some recent studies he himself was conducting with Arnason and Jankovic.[97] I must reiterate that one of our definitive papers on the crucial role of the thymus in developmental biology by that time had already been submitted and was in press in the *Proceedings of the Society for Experimental Biology and Medicine*.[80] That paper was submitted in August or early September 1961. Thus, even this *Proc. Soc.* paper was submitted prior to submission of Miller's *Lancet* paper. At the Brook Lodge meeting, Waksman also announced that he and Jankovic had also been extirpating thymuses in neonatal rats and that such extirpation inhibited only the development of cell-mediated immunities and didn't alter capacity for antibody production.[98,99]   I disagreed with Waksman and my position subsequently was proved to be correct, because we already had presented clear evidence of an influence also on the influence of thymus on development of capacity for antibody production.[78,79,84]   Later I learned that Parrott[100,101,102] working in the laboratory of the impeccable John Humphrey, had also been independently studying thymic function and had generated impressive data in mice that linked the thymus to development of both humoral and cell-mediated immunities. Parrott et al also emphasized that neonatally thymectomized mice developed an early wasting syndrome later recognized to be a most characteristic finding in neonatally thymectomized mice which were raised in conventional and not in specific pathogen-free environments.[102]

Because of all this excitement concerning the thymus and the obvious importance and significance of the research as well as the intense struggle for the credit for the thymus discovery, I decided to convene an international conference on the thymus that would bring together everyone with a real interest in the thymus and the bursa of Fabricius. The conference was held in Minneapolis in November 1962.[103]

Not one speaker whom we invited to this conference on this rather narrow subject in immunologic development turned down the invitation. The proceedings of that conference contain nearly all of the crucial data, later published in many different locations, and taken all together these establish the several important, yes crucial, influences that the thymus exerts in developmental immunology.[97,102,103,104,105,106,107,108,109,110]   Thus, from the data presented from a half dozen laboratories, action of the thymus to foster development of both immunological systems and lymphoid development,[79,101,102] development of all forms of cell-mediated immunities[89,90,108] ability to develop tumor immunities[82] and ability to produce antibodies[79,86,88,101,102,109] could all be attributed to an influence exerted by the thymus early in life. Yes, even in some strains or species increasing susceptibility to development of autoimmunities was one consequence of neonatal thymectomy which our group first recognized in rabbits.[111] We studied this evidence of immunologic disorganization attributable to early thymectomy in several strains of mice extensively with Yunis a bit later.[112]

The influences of the bursa of Fabricius on antibody-producing capacity was described at this conference by both Glick and the now very strong Wisconsin group led by Wolfe and also the developmental biologist Auerbach[113,114,115,116] and by Papermaster et al., from my laboratory.[84,86] Metcalf of Australia at the thymus conference once again emphasized a theme he had been pursuing for several years[117,118,119,120,121] that from his perspective the thymus had long been known to be important for generating small lymphocytes and for producing humoral factors that influenced growth of lymphoid cells.

At the same thymus conference, Fichtelius, too, thanked all the scrambling and intensive new thymecologists for leaving the thymus to him for so long.[122,123,124,125,126,127]

I insisted that plasma cell development could either be well preserved after neonatal thymectomy or could be significantly depressed when thymectomized animals were challenged with a "thymus-dependent antigen," e.g., in a secondary response, a response in which antibody production was clearly depressed for certain antigens by thymectomy.

Then Noel Warner spoke at the conference. Warner was a young graduate fellow working at the Eliza Hall Institute. When he got up to speak he seemed to me to be so very young. I remember thinking that this young man probably hadn't even started to shave. Warner electrified the entire international gathering of about 100 scientists as he presented his research done with the more seasoned Szenberg.[110] From this research, Warner concluded that the thymus and bursa do not subserve the same function. Far from it. Prevention of development of either the thymus or bursa using different timing of administration of steroid hormones, a method, of hormonal inhibition of development of the thymus or bursa or both thymus and bursa, which he had adapted from Glick's[113] and Wolfe's research[114,116] inhibited quite differently the different immunological developments. Warner asserted that the inhibition of bursa development alone inhibited antibody production and also prevented development of delayed allergies. Inhibition of development of only the thymus controlled allograft rejection. He interpreted his findings to indicate that initiation of graft-vs-host reactions depended on cells that were not under the direct influence of either the thymus or the bursa. These were the organs that by then I was already calling central as opposed to peripheral lymphoid organs.[83,105]

Warner's presentation at the 1962 conference[110] generated much discussion. He had clearly proposed a division of labor within the lymphoid cell system that seemed attributable to divisions of developmental influence of two different lymphoid developmental functions of the thymus on the one hand or bursa on the other. However, the division of labor he proposed was very different from the division of labor into two separate systems the lymphoid structure and immunological functions we had been proposing that was derived from much data and analysis we believed to be correct. The division of labor within the lymphoid system that had been proposed in Minneapolis was derived in Minneapolis from studying patients with both primary and secondary immunodeficiency diseases and analyzing effects of neonatal thymectomy in rabbit and mouse and from Papermaster's now rather extensive experiments using hormonal suppression of the central lymphoid organs, thymus or bursa, in the chicken. For us, just too much of Warner's interpretation didn't fit our scheme of separation of labor within the lymphoid system which we had been developing from study of patients with congenital agammaglobulinemia, patients with Hodgkin's disease and patients with multiple myeloma. Further, our experiments showing suppression of antibody production by thymectomy and inhibitory action of thymectomy on both GVHD and graft rejection in neonatally thymectomized mice, rats, rabbits and even hamsters[87] did not agree with the conclusions Warner and Szenberg had reached from study of hormonal thymectomy and bursectomy or both which required precise timing and influences exclusively of the hormones on the central lymphoid organs and their function which was difficult for us to accept.

For us the thymus could be assigned responsibility for development of all the cell-mediated immunities, namely allograft rejections, all delayed allergies and ability to initiate graft-vs-host reaction. The plasma cell lineage which we deemed responsible for antibody production surely represented a completely separate development from this thymus-dependent, cell-mediated set of immunities, as revealed by agammaglobulinemic and myeloma patients. But the thymus also had to be cross-linking, because its function was essential for development of antibody production as well. We realized and presented much data to support the view that early thymectomy inhibited antibody responses to what we called thymus-dependent antigens. The Warner-Szenberg proposal that the bursa controlled development of the antibody-producing cells was attractive to us but seemed to need further study in a simple system in which all components could be under precise control rather than relying on potentially complex manipulations involving prevention of development as had been achieved by hormonal thymectomy, hormonal bursectomy or both hormonal thymectomy and bursectomy. Warner, Szenberg and Burnet had linked development of graft rejection to the thymus all right, but they interpreted their experiments to show that delayed allergy was under the control of bursa, and graft-vs-host reactions were not influenced by either hormonal bursectomy or thymectomy, a conclusion unacceptable to the information we had generated.

We left the 1962 thymus conference resolved to reinvestigate the influences of thymus and bursa as central lymphoid organs with respect to development of different populations of lymphoid cells and the several distinct immunologic functions. We planned to use appropriate extirpation of the central lymphoid organs appropriately in the chicken to properly dissect the division of labor of the central lymphoid organs in development of the lymphoid systems.

By then Raymond D.A. Peterson had come to my laboratory, He was a rather senior and mature research fellow. While on active duty in the armed services as a pediatrician, Peterson had already been trained in pediatrics as well as in allergy and also in dermatology. Peterson by this time had already focussed his laboratory approach on using our new perspective on the role of thymus and bursa in developmental immunology to take another look at Jacob Furth's discovery that leukemia could be prevented by thymectomy.[91] Ray Peterson especially wanted to know whether the bursa of Fabricius as a central lymphoid organ might, like the thymus, be a site for development of leukemias and lymphomas. Quite on his own he took the initiative to generate a collaboration with Ben Burmeister and Burmeister's young associate, Purchase, who worked at the East Lansing poultry laboratory where many investigations of the virology and pathogenesis of the leukemia-lymphoma complex known as the avian leukosis system was already well underway. Ray set up crucial and highly productive collaborative arrangements with Burmeister and his group to investigate the role of thymus or bursa or thymus plus bursa in development of leukemia-lymphoma complex.[128,129] As part of this development, Peterson worked out magnificent techniques for extirpating thymus and bursa in chickens.

I was anxious to have one of my junior fellows work with Peterson to reinvestigate in parallel, in this ideal situation, the role of the thymus and bursa in the development of lymphoid cell populations and different components of the immunological functions. Ray agreed to help and also to participate in all phases of the immunological studies as well. He agreed that we might best be able to achieve our mutually desired goals if I would find just the right fellow from my laboratory to assist in the effort.

Henry Hilgard, then a fellow in the laboratory who had begun to work with my collaborator Martinez,[130] demurred because he considered our goal to be too competitive with the efforts of his close friends at the Eliza Hall Institute in Australia. Hilgard had worked earlier as a student with the group at Eliza Hall Institute, and he considered that our competition with that group had become much too intense. However, a clinical research fellow who was new to our laboratory was a young pediatrician from Tulane who also had trained earlier as an allergist in California. His name was Max Cooper. At his own volition, Max took an interest in collaborating with Peterson and me on this project. Ray Peterson took Max Cooper under his wing and the two, along with Ray's technician Ronnie Henderson, began to make regularly scheduled trips to East Lansing, Michigan, to carry out investigations of the roles of the two central lymphoid organs in genesis of both the viral induced leukemia-lymphoma complex in chicken and also to reinvestigate the roles of the bursa and thymus in the immunological and lymphoid tissue development of the chicken using the techniques of surgical extirpation of thymus and bursa.

Ray taught Max the tricks of bursectomy and thymectomy and, together with Ray's close friend and associate Burmeister they hit on a critical experiment which was to resolve cleanly and correctly the issue of how the functions of the thymus and bursa of Fabricius as central lymphoid organs, were divided in the process of controlling the development of the lymphoid systems in chickens. They gave near lethal total body irradiation (600R) to the newly hatched chickens and then extirpated either the bursa or thymus or both the bursa and thymus together. Removal of each and every one of the thymus lobes in newly hatched chickens took considerable skill and determination because the several thymus lobes often extended very far posteriorly, and sometimes the removal of the most posterior thymus lobe led to inadvertent penetration of the pleural space with fatal consequences. In short, this rather arduous but definitive set of experiments showed that when the thymus had been removed following sublethal total body irradiation in newly hatched chickens, thymus-dependent aggregates of lymphoid cells in the spleen and in the small lymph nodes (which were present, contrary to popular view, and could be located along blood vessels in chickens), failed to develop. The circulating lymphocyte count was depressed, and all cell-mediated immune functions, i.e., allograft immunity, ability to develop delayed allergies and ability to initiate graft-vs-host reactions, were suppressed or absent altogether. By contrast, selective and complete removal of the bursa of Fabricius in irradiated newly hatched chicks prevented the development of the very distinct bursa-dependent *germinal* centers in spleen and lymph nodes and prevented as well the development of all the plasma cells in the body.[131,132,133] The latter was most readily seen in the splenic red pulp but also could be recognized in the bone marrow and gut. This maneuver of early bursectomy after total body irradiation prevented antibody production but did not prevent at all the development of any of the cell-mediated immunologic functions. In the wake of the thymus conference and all of its discussions, Warner and Szenberg, with Burnet, drew similar conclusions from further manipulations using hormones to depress thymus or bursal development or both together.[134,337] Their approach was, after all, quite different, yet turned out to be an approach also quite complementary to the one we were taking.

With all of our experimental work now in such substantial agreement both with our earlier extrapolations from long and extensive clinical investigations and also with experimental investigations in mice, we could speak with much greater confidence about the existence of two separate and distinct immunity systems.[131,132,133,135,136,137,138,139] We called the two systems the thymus-dependent and thymus-independent cellular immunological systems, and we identified morphologically the regions in chickens where the lymphoid cells of the distinct and different cellular systems were prone to aggregate within the major lymphoid organs. The latter we called the thymus-dependent lymphoid areas and the alternative system we called the bursal-dependent or bursa-equivalent-dependent lymphoid regions.[131,132,133,136,137,139,140,141]

Max Cooper insisted, against my advice, on giving the first public presentation of what I called the new view of the lymphoid systems, based on these critical experimental data generated with Ray Peterson and me, at the American Pediatric Society meetings in 1965.[132] I would rather have had him make this presentation at the immunology meetings in the spring of 1965. However, Cooper argued because he was a pediatrician, he should first present these exciting new findings about the lymphoid system development to the pediatricians rather than to my beloved immunologists. Ray Peterson and I finally agreed to this proposal.

It is well Cooper presented this perspective to the pediatricians. Cooper finished his presentation. The initial discussion was by Fireman (then of Boston). He said he thought it best to keep an open mind on this new perspective. This didn't bother us, because we were quite accustomed by this time to opposition from members of the school of pediatrics at the Children's Hospital in Boston, led by Gitlin. Then Angelo DiGeorge, an endocrinologist from St. Christopher's Hospital in Philadelphia, ran for the microphone shouting, "That's it, that's it! That explains what we have been seeing in Philadelphia!"[142] DiGeorge proceeded to describe children born without a thymus and without parathyroid glands. These children generally presented with neonatal tetany and/or disease based on congenital outflow tract abnormalities of the heart. However, these children often died of infections caused by viruses, fungi, or atypical acid-fast bacteria.[142,143] These patients could produce apparently sufficient amounts of immunoglobulins but did not make antibodies well. They failed to develop cell-mediated immunities normally and lacked the lymphoid cell population in the deep cortical regions of the lymph nodes. Nonetheless, they had quite well developed accumulations of cells in the periphery of the cortical regions of the lymph nodes in the areas I was then calling the far cortical regions. I immediately named that disease the DiGeorge syndrome, although had I known better I would have called the disease the Harrington-DiGeorge syndrome,[144] and linked it to failure to differentiate the epithelial derivatives of the third and fourth pharyngeal pouches, including the thymus, as DiGeorge did a bit later.[143]

At that time Pierson van Alten, an experimental embryologist, came into our lab on a sabbatical leave from the University of Illinois. He found he could operate quite well right within the egg on late chicken embryos (18-21 days of embryonation), and with him leading the way we found it possible to produce the same clear-cut assortment of lymphoid cell populations and functions as Cooper, Peterson and I had done in the X-irradiated newly hatched chickens subjected to thymectomy or bursectomy or both thymectomy and bursectomy.[145] This was an important step because it eliminated the need for the initially clarifying but later possibly confounding X irradiation needed for the Cooper-Peterson experiments. The observations clearly supported a true two-component concept of the specific immunoreactive cells in the form we had initially constructed.[136,145,146,147,148]

With all these data in hand, under Peterson's leadership[136] we felt able to write definitively to establish in cellular terms the pathogenesis of the primary human immunodeficiency diseases we had been studying through the years.[4,47,105,136,147,148] The X-linked agammaglobulinemia patients lacked plasma cells and did not develop germinal centers. Their lymph nodes lacked all lymphocytes in the far cortical regions—the thymus-independent regions. These patients were represented experimentally by the irradiated-bursectomized chickens.[136] The patients with the Harrington-DiGeorge syndrome, who had a broadly based immunodeficiency, lacked lymphoid cells in the spongy deep cortical areas of the nodes but possessed lymphocytes predominantly in the far cortical areas of the lymph nodes.[135,136,139,148,149,150,151] These children developed germinal centers poorly. They seemed to be the equivalent of the neonatally thymectomized mice and the chickens that had been thymectomized in ovo or those given total body irradiation plus thymectomy in the newly hatched period.

I had earlier been impressed with a form of primary immunodeficiency disease I regularly referred to as Swiss-type agammaglobulinemia, as I had encountered it on my first visits to Switzerland in 1957 and 1959. These patients—first described as lymphocytothesis by Glanzmann and Riniker[152]—were often virtually devoid of all lymphoid cells. This disorder had been studied by Tobler and Cottier[153] in Bern and by Hitzig and Willi in Zurich.[154] We likened these patients to the chickens that had been irradiated and subjected to bursectomy plus thymectomy after sublethal total body irradiation in our experiments in the newly hatched period or bursectomy plus thymectomy in ovo.[131,133,135,136,138,145] With passage of time and certainly after additional experimentation, Warner also had also linked endocrinological manipulation (testosterone or 19-nor-testosterone administration) that prevented bursal development to selective inhibition of plasma cell development.[110,134] Maria de Sousa joined Parrott and East at Mill Hill and together they studied the lymphoid tissues of thymectomized mice. Parrott and De Sousa came forward with a similar and, in some regards, somewhat more detailed definition of the locations in lymph nodes and spleen of the thymus-dependent and thymus-independent regions of the lymphoid tissues in the mouse.[155] All of the experimental research as well as all the clinical investigation over a period of at least two decades fell clearly and agreeable into dramatic alignment. The scientific meetings at which these findings were presented and discussed were filled with joy, excitement and anticipation of the incredible future which we visualized as lying ahead in cellular immunology.[135,138,141,146,147,149,150,156]

As was by now a characteristic methodology, I organized and held a fourth small international conference. This one was to be concerned with consideration of immunodeficiency diseases of man as they could be viewed in light of our new view of the lymphoid systems that had been as clarified through the perspectives derived from the research on chickens and mice.[158] This conference was the third in a series of four I had organized with my former fellow Richard Smith and Peter Miescher of New York University[151,158] and so with the thymus conference in 1962 was the 4th conference in this series.

The latter group of conferences were held on Sanibel Island in Florida. It was especially exciting to anticipate the Sanibel Conference on Immunodeficiencies because we now thought we knew enough not only to define the separate immunity systems but also perhaps might know enough to begin to plan further how to identify, diagnose, analyze, and even correct (possibly cure) the abnormalities present in still to be encountered patients with several different primary immunodeficiency diseases of man.[158] We would be able to draw on knowledge of development of the two separate immunological systems as revealed by the research in chickens and mice which had in turn been guided through the years by our clinical investigations. We also had new knowledge from Moore and Owen's finding[159] that cells travel from bone marrow to thymus or bursa via the blood circulation.

Several puzzling aspects of the new view of the lymphoid systems and of the immunologic functions then began to be clarified. Claman had discovered rather by chance that it does, indeed, take two to tango, as Henry Azar had proposed at the thymus conference and then again at one of these Sanibel conferences[160]. Miller was also now describing essential interactions of the thymus-dependent and thymus-independent cells of the lymphoid systems[161,162] to achieve antibody production to thymus dependent antigens. Indeed, Miller even wrote of a **new** "golden era" of thymus research, focused on working out the nature of the cell-cell interactions of the two separate populations of cells within the lymphoid systems.[109]

This 1967 conference was the first major conference on the pathogenesis of the immunodeficiency diseases and was held under the auspices of the March of Dimes National Foundation. The latter a lay group which had supported much of my research through the years. It was also the organization that had supported much of the research which had led to the development of both the Salk and Sabin polio vaccines. All of the new findings in experimental systems and the related findings and interpretation of the new findings for human immunodeficiency diseases were presented and analyzed at this conference.[158] We felt that at long last we could understand the major immunodeficiency diseases in terms of which of the cell systems were involved in each and what approaches might be offered to provide potential treatments that might cure some of the patients who, as critical Experiments of Nature, along with our laboratory mice and chickens had been *the* great teachers of modern immunology.[135,136,147,148,158] Study of these patients had been guiding us step-by-step in our analysis of the cellular basis of immunologic function. They had represented for immunology the essential Experiments of Nature.

Further, by this time we were also beginning to be increasingly skillful in recognizing and defining patients who suffered from selective deficiency of phagocytic effector cells. We separated out from among children with increased susceptibility to infection a group which had what I called "fatal granulomatous disease of childhood" which we later named the chronic granulomatous disease.[147,163,164,165,166,167,168,169,170,171] We were beginning to carry out definitive investigations of patients with increased susceptibility to infection who exhibited also autoimmune disease in high frequency and in which both sets of diseases could be attributed to deficiencies of one or another of the complement components.[172,173,174] We also had defined and analyzed, as had Lars Å Hanson in Sweden,[175] patients who lacked only IgA or IgG and IgA.[176,177] Like the other immunodeficiency patients before them, each of these new groups of patients seemed to be dissecting further and further both the microbial universes and the several distinct components of the immunological universe, its amplification mechanisms and fundamental effector processes.

A very good example of the numerous discoveries we made in my laboratory during this exciting period was one reflected in our definition and analysis of patients with chronic granulomatous disease of childhood. These patients surely contributed an additional rather neat bisection of the microbial universe. They divided microbes into two distinct new subpopulations. The organisms that caused disease in these patients were organisms that possessed catalase enzyme(s) and thus were catalase positive. Those organisms which, by contrast, did not produce infections in these children, were the catalase negative bacteria.[178] The organisms to which the chronic granulomatous disease patients were susceptible, we recognized included *Staphylococcus aureus*, a variety of *Coliform bacilli*, *Serratia marcescens*, and numerous fungi. *Aspergillus fumigatus* was an especially difficult problem clinically in such patients. These patients were found also to be susceptible to other catalase-positive organisms and to have life-threatening infections caused by these microbes. In collaboration with a young associate professor, Paul Quie, my former student Arthur Page and my young graduate student Beulah Holmes who had come to pursue a Ph.D. degree with me, we discovered that these patients, whom we had recognized and defined earlier as a clinical entity[163,164] and who usually presented evidence of an X-linked inheritance, exhibited a metabolic abnormality of their phagocytic cells.[166] Their neutrophils and monocytes failed to kill catalase-positive organisms, including catalase-positive microorganisms even though the phagocytic cells of these patients ingested all organisms quite well. Also, the neutrophils of these patients could not be induced by a phagocytic process to express the hexose monophosphate shunt metabolic pathway or generate H_2O_2 after they phagocytosed catalase-positive microorganisms, catalase-negative organisms or even latex particles. Obligate carriers of this disease and the patients themselves who had an X-linked form of chronic granulomatous disease could be readily distinguished from normal persons and from each other because in the patients none of the leukocytes reduced the nitroblue tetrazolium dye to the formasan pigment and in the obligate carriers of the gene some of the phagocytic cells (about half) could reduce the tetrazolium dye to the purple-staining formasan pigment.[170] By contrast, all or nearly all of the phagocytic cells of normal persons could reduce the nitroblue tetrazolium dye after phagocytosis. Thus carrier detection became quite possible.[170]

With this group of patients we had seized the opportunity to separate a distinct group of patients from among several groups which comprised the complex population of patients which exhibited impressive hypergammaglobulinemia but still were inordinately susceptible to infections.[163] We identified these patients clinically as having a previously unrecognized new disease,[164] and discovered that their disease was based on an X-linked inheritance associated with a defect of phagocytic function;[163,164,170,178] we identified a basic killing defect of the phagocytic neutrophils and monocytes;[178] and we defined quite precisely the basic chemical nature of the failure to kill ingested organisms that was potentially the pathogenic defect.[166] We showed the intracellular killing defect involved only catalase positive microorganisms and did not hold for catalase negative microorganisms.[167,168] We were also able to identify the carriers of the common form of the disease.[170] In collaboration with Quie and White we showed there were forms of the disease transmitted genetically as an autosomal recessive trait as well.[147,169]. Later we showed with others that this disease could be cured by bone marrow transplantation using the technique for marrow transplantation from an MHC-matched sibling donor which I introduced to clinical medicine in 1967 and 1968.[179,180,181] Subsequently patients with this disease have been found to have a defective membrane oxidase system associated with deficiency of a peculiar cytochrome b enzyme[182,183] which was worked out independently by spectroscopic analyses of the patient's membranes that revealed deficiency of a heme-containing component[182] and by a new approach to genetic analysis which might be referred to as reverse genetic analysis.[184,185]

When Henry Gewurz joined our laboratory and clinics directly from the student body at Johns Hopkins, I repeatedly urged him to focus his attention on the complement system. In this one instance I deviated a bit from my usual approach to new fellows. I actually urged him to become an expert in complement biology and chemistry. I did this because with the progress that I recognized had already been made by Manfred Mayer[186,187] and his group and independently by Robert Nelson[188,189] and his colleagues studying guinea pigs, and Hans Müller-Eberhard,[190] I recognized that what may have appeared to be the impossibly complex complement system was approaching full molecular definition. I was absolutely certain that such a complex system of interacting precursors, biologically active molecules and stabilizing molecules which functioned as a tightly knit cascade would have to be of major survival advantage to have been kept essentially intact throughout vertebrate evolution.[191] Thus the importance of components of this system might be quite dissectable by studying patients who suffered from immunodeficiency diseases involving the C system. This of course had been our approach that served so well to provide the essential underpinnings of our contributions to understanding the specific immunologic systems and in turn the analysis and definition of the primary or secondary specific immunodeficiency diseases themselves.

By the time we entered the field with the contributions of Henry Gewurz, Richard Pickering and N.K. Day,[172,173,192,193,194,195,196,197,198,199,200,201] a patient with profound complement deficiency was known to be a healthy immunologist who had no disease. In spite of his good health this patient exhibited a gross or complete deficiency of the second complement component.[202] However, our earliest studies had used both phylogenetic and ontogenetic approaches and had shown that the C system was indeed most venerable and thus must be of great importance in the body economy.[173,195] Investigations from Boston Children's Hospital[203,204] described a physician's family members in whom C2 deficiencies were frequent but who apparently were without disease had concluded again that C2 deficiency might not be disease producing. They argued that these findings strengthened the interpretation that a virtual absence of the functional complement system is well tolerated clinically. Our findings in C deficient patients suggested just the opposite. We found that despite the C2 deficiency, the famous C2-deficient immunologist's plasma exhibited vigorous bactericidal activity and immune adherence even in the absence of C2. But in our patients we also associated C2 deficiency with recurrent pneumonias, recurrent respiratory disease as well as lupus erythematosus.[192,194,200] Then Alper et al., in Boston[205,206,207] described a defect of the third complement component that was consequent to absence of a stabilizer of C3. That patient had a greatly increased susceptibility to infection which was comparable to the susceptibility observed in patients with XLA. Alper and Rosen[208] also described a patient who failed to produce C3 and that patient also was very susceptible to infections. Michael E. Miller and his colleagues described a family in which defective functioning of C5 was associated with Leiner's disease who also exhibited marked susceptibility to infection.[209,210] The involved children in this family could be treated effectively by plasma replacement therapy. Pickering et al discovered a patient who lacked C2 who also had severe progressive renal disease.[197] We also studied patients with C2, C1 esterase inhibitor or C1r deficiencies[196] each of whom suffered from autoimmune or mesenchymal disease and also had frequent infections.[197] Day associated a number of complement deficiencies with susceptibility to kidney and other mesenchymal and autoimmune diseases and infections.[176,198,199,200,201,211,212] Independently[213,214] came to the same conclusions that patients with complement deficiency often develop lupus, lupus-like or other connective tissue disease, and so complement deficiencies were associated with autoimmune disease, mesenchymal and renal disease in also with far too high frequency to be explained by chance.

Now that sufficient time has elapsed to have permitted many patients with complement deficiency to be identified from clinics from all around the world, it has become clear that deficiency of each of the complement components involving either the primary activation pathway, the alternative activation pathway, or the components of the attack pathway of the complement system, are most susceptible to infection. These findings have established that the C system is crucial to defense against infection.[215] Each of the C systems also appear to be crucial to defense against systemic autoimmune diseases, lupus, lupus-like diseases or other mesenchymal disease.[198,199,200,201,202,212,214] Particularly, isolated C component deficiencies that involve the components of the attack sequences open the door to the occurrence of infections with Neisserial pathogens[215] as well as to mesenchymal diseases.[201] It is also clear that deficiency or abnormality of properdin, a stabilizer of the alternative activation pathway, leads to serious disease in high frequency.[216,217] Thus, patients with immunodeficiency diseases involving the C system have also helped greatly to dissect the microbial universe into those pathogens that particularly are defended by the complement systems and those where defense by the complement system may be less important. Also, once again, they have helped sort out the role of proper integration of the components of the immunological systems for prevention of immunologically based diseases. These patients also have revealed that protection against development of systemic autoimmunities, protection against immune complex-based diseases and protection against mesenchymal diseases also involves the complement system.

Study of each of the specific forms or groups of immunodeficient patients have repeatedly revealed that patients with primary, generally genetically determined immunodeficiencies do, indeed, represent most revealing Experiments of Nature. These Experiments of Nature have continued to guide the bisections and dissections of the microbial universes. They have helped define the separate immunological mechanisms that are essential to maintenance of the physical integrity of the body. These immunodeficient patients have, without question, assisted more than any other means the definition and dissections of the lymphoid systems, the most important biologic amplification systems and basic effector processes involved in the bodily defenses.

At approximately this same time, all of this insight was developing, we reasoned from experimental investigations which showed that thymus transplants could correct deficits due to neonatal thymectomy in the mouse[84,96,101,102,218] that the DiGeorge syndrome attributable to failure of thymic development which resulted in selective T cell immunodeficiency leads to an immunological abnormality that might be correctable by thymus transplantation.[82,112,131,133,136,140] We then surmised that a thymus transplantation should be attempted to correct the failure of thymus development in man. According to our reasoning, this approach was tried and treatment of the DiGeorge athymic syndrome was attempted (see below).[219,220,221]

We reasoned further that the lethal Swiss type agammaglobulinemia (a name I had given to the Glanzmann-Riniker syndrome) which is now called severe combined immunodeficiency disease (SCID) should be curable by bone marrow or fetal liver transplantation.[222] We reasoned this way since we could show that both of the two major specific cellular components of immunity were absent or very much underdeveloped in these patients and both of these cell systems were known or could be presumed to descend from bone marrow derived lymphoid stem cells.   Thus we concluded that restoration by transplantation of normal stem cells from marrow might correct this genetically determined defect.[222]

We already knew that patients with X-linked agammaglobulinemia, associated with a deficiency of plasma cell development, could benefit greatly by treatment with the missing antibodies (derived from plasma cells) passively delivered as gammaglobulin injections. I.M. injection of gammaglobulin was a treatment established as an effective therapy in Bruton's first case of agammaglobulinemia. It was also shown to be effective in the Boston series of agammaglobulinemia cases, and in our own patients with X-linked, acquired and common variable immunodeficiency. Unfortunately, in those early days we could give gammaglobulin injections only by the intramuscular route and this procedure was of relatively less value than it might have been because it was so painful and only a limited dosage of gammaglobulin could be delivered intramuscularly.   Because of Barandun's investigations,[223,224,225] things have become far better for these agammaglobulinemic and hypogammaglobulinemic patients because this series of investigations provided approaches to preparing gammaglobulins so they can be now given safely by the intravenous route.   We now know that treatment with intravenous immunoglobulin is now both safe and much more effective than when gammaglobulin administration is limited to the IM route.[223,224,225,226,227,228]

The proposal to treat immunodeficiency in the DiGeorge syndrome by thymus transplantation was brought to fruition by Cleveland et al.,[219] using thymus from an aborted fetus of approximately 14 weeks embryonation. With our reasoning and essentially our blueprint before him, Cleveland, who was not an immunologist but an endocrinologist, corrected for the first time the immunodeficiency associated with DiGeorge syndrome.[219] Shortly thereafter, and published at the same time, thymus transplantation was also applied by August et al of the Boston group[220] to correct the immunodeficiency of DiGeorge syndrome.   These results were somewhat difficult to ascertain because DiGeorge syndrome is often incomplete and some degree of improvement can occur with time as a result of the contributions by a small, underdeveloped thymus.

At this same time, as a consequence of our concerted analyses, we concluded it should also be possible to treat severe combined immunodeficiency (SCID) from this new cellular perspective. I proposed that SCID could be corrected by transplantation of normal lymphoid stem cells obtained from either fetal liver or bone marrow. We reasoned that because the patients were immunodeficient and both T-cells and B-cells were grossly deficient immunosuppression or myeloablation might not be necessary. Our first effort employed fetal liver cells. Richard Hong and several of my younger associates and I carried out this transplant with fetal liver provided by Humphrey Kay in England. The transplant appeared to correct the cellular immunodeficiency which characterized that initial patient, N.F., who suffered from autosomal recessive SCID.[229] However, as the patient's immunologic reconstruction was being established, a transfusion was given by the house staff at the University of Minnesota Hospitals in an effort to raise the patient's low Hb level. This transfusion, given without irradiation of the blood to be transfused, led to a fulminating and fatal graft-vs-host reaction—a devastating complication of the hospital management of this child with SCID. For this reason, and directed by extensive laboratory research,[222,230] we established a rule that no blood transfusions should ever be given to severely immunodeficient children without first irradiating the blood to render all lymphocytes post-mitotic.[222,229,230]

We then began to reflect on what we knew at the time about the major histocompatibility system from lessons learned from mice that has been provided by Gorer and later, Gorer with Snell and Snell and his coworkers.[231,-232,233,234,235] With Martinez and a rather large group of students and fellows in the basic sciences with whom we had been working since the mid-'50s, we had used tissue-typing and matching of strains of mice to facilitate tolerance production and skin and organ allotransplantation even during adult life.[112,236,237,238,239,240,241,242,243,244,245,246] We also had used tissue-typing as a means to diminish susceptibility to graft-vs-host disease.[247,248] Thus by 1968 we felt we had learned enough about tissue typing and matching to employ tissue typing as an approach to facilitate organ transplantation in animals. Further, tissue typing for humans had become progressively sophisticated through investigations of Daussett, Van Rood, Amos and Terasaki.[249,250,251,252,253,254,255,256] Thus we felt we could predict from simple Mendelian principals that an MHC-matched sibling might represent a suitable donor of bone marrow cells to permit treatment of a recipient suffering from SCID. We had good reason from our experiments with mice to believe that such transplantation might not initiate severe or lethal graft-vs-host disease. With Richard Hong and Richard Gatti we wrote a theoretical paper proposing that a cure of SCID might be possible if we transplanted bone marrow cells from an MHC-matched sibling donor.[222] We reasoned that stem cells as precursors for both the thymus-dependent (T cells now) and thymus-independent (B cells now) systems must both be lacking or underdeveloped in these patients with SCID.[136,137,257,258,259] Precursors of thymus and precursors of bursal cells were known to be present in both bone marrow and fetal liver and to have passed through the blood on the way to each of the central lymphoid organs—the thymus or bone marrow in mammals and man and thymus or bursa in chickens. To our new view of lymphoid development, the cells common to the two-cell systems resided in the bone marrow and were represented by the cells we referred to as lymphoid stem cells. After these cells had been exposed to educational events in the central lymphoid sites—the thymus or the bursa—(bursal equivalent in man) the cells might be expected to differentiate to cells that distinguish self from non-self and thereafter be exported to the periphery.[180] From the central lymphoid organs, the now well differentiated lymphoid cells would be expected to be expanded, at first independent of antigenic influence and after differentiation as cells capable of recognizing antigen and cell populations also being further expandable as specific populations following contact with antigen after distribution to the peripheral lymphoid sites. It would be in the peripheral sites that the definitive immunologic functions (cell-mediated immunities or antibody production) would be performed. Either fetal liver or bone marrow should be quite satisfactory as a source of lymphoid stem cells. We further concluded that these common lymphoid precursors (stem cells) must represent the cells that are basically abnormal in SCID since the SCID patients could be shown sometimes at least, to be deficient in functions of *both* the thymus-dependent (T lymphocytes) and the thymus-independent system of cells (B lymphocytes). It was already clear at that time and it has now been very well established that the immunoglobulin-producing plasma cells were the cells that actually secreted definitive antibodies.[20,21,22,59]

I discussed the theoretical possibility of curing SCID by bone marrow transplantation in many national and international forums and also widely in the medical and scientific community. Consequently, a pediatrician who had heard me speak, Dr. Jerome L'Heureux of Meriden, Connecticut, contacted me regarding a patient and the patient's family he was following. This family was one in which SCID of the X-linked type had already been the cause of death of 11 male children over four generations in the family of the mother of the sick baby. The propositus which Dr. L'Heureux was caring for was a 4-month-old baby with apparent SCID who had four female siblings. He had already suffered from several bouts of pneumonia and his life and been saved each time by antibiotic treatment. We had reasoned that transplantation of bone marrow from an MHC-matched sibling donor should permit us to cure the SCID[222] if a matched sibling donor were available and was the only treatment which could be used. We also reasoned that the chance of having a perfectly matched sibling donor should be approximately 1 in 4.

With this reasoning as background Dr. L'Heureux sent the entire family to Minneapolis in hope of finding a miracle cure for this baby in our clinics and laboratories. The family was comprised of a mother and father, the sick baby and 4 healthy female siblings. Dr. Richard Gatti had just joined our group as a beginning research fellow. Hilaire Meuwissen, a more senior fellow, was also interested in carrying out transplants of stem cells from marrow to treat SCID, and Richard Hong was the associate professor who was helping me train the research and clinical fellows in basic immunochemistry and who was taking much of the responsibility for analysis, care and treatment of the immunodeficient patients. Hong was an independent, well-trained scientist who had been engaged in analyzing, defining and managing clinically many of the children who came to my clinics with primary or secondary immunodeficiency diseases. Edmund Yunis, had become director of the University of Minnesota blood bank. He was also working hard to develop a tissue typing laboratory and in those days worked in close collaboration with Bernard Amos. Thus his presence and ongoing investigations brought us to the very forefront of research on the complexity of the genetic loci that determined the major histocompatibility system in man and that would be involved in the essential tissue typing for our undertaking. Consequently we were able to use state of the art methods to type the patient with severe combined immunodeficiency. After the tissue typing had been accomplished we carried out reciprocal unidirectional mixed leukocyte typing on the patient using Bach's[260,261,262] adaptation to unidirectional matching with Bain's mixed leukocyte culture technique.[263,264] Further, Edmund Yunis had also been doing collaborative research on lymphoid and hematopoietic transplants in experimental animals with Carlos Martinez and me. In a beautiful set of experiments which we published in 1965 in the *Journal of Experimental Medicine*, Edmund Yunis and we showed that in neonatally thymectomized mice, by employing transplants of lymphoid tissues from MHC-matched but not from MHC-mismatched donors, we could achieve by lymphoid cell transplants long-term correction of the immunodeficiencies otherwise produced by neonatal thymectomy[112,246] (see reference 265 for review) without inducing lethal GVHD.

The tissue matching for this first successful bone marrow transplant was achieved with some difficulty. This was due to the fact that the baby had a very low number of lymphoid cells. However, from the family study and the tissue typing results we were able to conclude that the patient's eight-year-old female sibling, Doreen, although not an absolutely perfect match with little David, was probably a good enough match to permit us to attempt a bone marrow transplantation that might cure the otherwise lethal SCID from which this child suffered. We later showed that this sister donor and the recipient SCID child represented a single antigen mismatch attributable to differences between the two at the A locus, a difference due in turn to a genetic cross-over event which had occurred in the patient. However, although the A locus was mismatched the C, B and D loci of the patient and sister were perfectly matched and the mixed leukocyte culture (MLC) showed little or no reaction. Since the MLC response was low we decided, after talking with Bach and consulting with Yunis, to attempt to correct the SCID by a bone marrow transplantation from the 8-yr-old sister to this child with SCID. The excitement was at a very high level because this was to be the first serious effort to cure by allogeneic bone marrow transplantation an otherwise hereditary and lethal disease. Richard Gatti, my new research fellow supervised by Meuwissen and Hong, actually carried out this first bone marrow transplantation. Gatti was assisted by the clinical resident on the case, Hugh Allen. We actually administered this first successful marrow graft by the intraperitoneal route in an unnecessary effort to avoid any untoward events that might occur in the circulation from the clinical administering the grafted cells intravascularly.

Sure enough, without using any myeloablative preparative treatment or any other manipulation of the marrow except gauze filtration to remove bony spicules and without using immunosuppression we performed the transplant of marrow cells and waited. Fortunately a dramatically successful transplantation of bone marrow occurred that was followed rather shortly by clear evidence of immunologic reconstitution.

Reconstitution of both *thymus-dependent* immunities and *plasma cell-associated* (or bursal dependent) immunities were actually well underway in our patient within 30 days.[179]

However, we did not get off with this first successful marrow transplantation scot-free of trouble. A graft-vs-host reaction that led to aplastic anemia ensued.[257,266] This reaction, in retrospect, almost certainly was due to the histoincompatibility at what is now known to be the A locus. Indeed, as part of this GVHR the child developed profound aplasia of the cells of all of the bone marrow lineages. Lymphocytes and plasma cells were present and continued to be attributable to the donor. Most of the clinicians in the University of Minnesota pediatric department who were observing my efforts and naturally kibitzing on the undertaking, and even the members of my own clinical research team who carried out the transplantation, tried to persuade me to destroy the graft that was both apparently reconstituting immunologic function in the patient but also had produced a serious, immunologically based, graft-vs-host reaction that had culminated in the development of a severe aplastic anemia. I recognized that the reaction which had occurred and the complicating immunologically based aplastic anemia was similar to the consequences of graft-vs-host reactions that had been described by Simonsen in his earlier studies of graft-vs-host reactions in chickens.[267,268,269] Consequently, to the entreaties that I destroy my graft I responded "No!,"

I could not permit destruction of the graft. I reasoned that even if an effort to destroy the graft were to be successful, this success would result only in bringing us back to the starting gate. The patient would still have the surely fatal SCID we were attempting to correct by marrow transplantation. I proposed that instead of destroying the original graft, since the child was suffering from life-threatening aplastic anemia we should perform a second bone marrow transplantation in an effort to cure the patient of his complicating aplastic anemia. This transplant we then reasoned should be given from the marrow of the same sister donor that had provided cells for the initial immunoreconstitution. We realized that this second effort represented both a first effort to treat this different, complicating and probably also fatal disease, aplastic anemia, by a bone marrow transplantation[180,181,266] but also might facilitate further the immunologic reconstitution of the SCID. My colleagues and the now well-informed family agreed that the approach to be taken should be a second bone marrow transplant. Thus we carried out a second transplant using the same well-matched sister as the best possible donor.

This second marrow transplant achieved magnificent engraftment and with it we cured the life-threatening aplastic anemia completely. The patient's bone marrow began to produce not only lymphoid cells but also blood cells of all kinds. Mature red blood cells, white blood cells and platelets promptly appeared in the circulating blood. The patient's red blood cell type switched over entirely from cells of the patient's genetic A type to production of red cells from the marrow that were now entirely of donor origin—blood group O cells. Progressively, the child also recovered full immunological capacity following this second bone marrow transplant.[180,181,257,266,270] Further, all of the patient's proliferating red blood cell precursors, leukocyte precursors and, indeed, all the proliferating and all the developing hematopoietic cells that could be made to divide or were dividing, exhibited the female karyotype and thus could be established as having been derived from precursors of the sister who was the bone marrow donor. The patient's lymphocytes began to form plasma cells in abundance, and the blood levels of immunoglobulin began to increase rapidly from the agammaglobulinemic state into the normal range. Indeed, the patient, after exhibiting several monoclonal gammaglobulin spikes and some degree of B cell overshoot since the controlling T cell system had not fully matured, gradually developed a perfectly normal and well balanced immunoglobulin profile. All cellular and humoral immunological functions became normal. This new, impressively fully balanced, immune system had replaced the lymphopenic T and B cell deficient agammaglobulinemic pattern with which the child had been sent to us prior to our attempt to cure his disease that was based on our new view of the immunity systems. I recall that the B-cell overshoot was of greatest concern to us because the IgG and IgM circulating immunoglobulins temporarily reached levels that were significantly greater than normal. Indeed, we feared at first that the patient might be developing a lymphoma or myeloma involving B lymphocytes or plasma cells. But the patient did not develop any malignant disease. All cells in the bone marrow which were dividing and all the peripheral blood lymphocytes which could be made to divide by mitogenic stimuli continued to be cells with a female karyotype, the immunoglobulin levels settled down and the spiking gammaglobulin pattern smoothed out into a normal pattern.

We have now followed this patient intermittently for more than 22 years. He has remained immunologically normal in every way. He still has normal numbers of both T and B lymphocytes. He forms beautiful plasma cells normally and has entirely normal blood-forming tissue, including bone marrow, lymph nodes and peripheral blood cells. All of his cell lineages continue after 22 years to be in magnificent balance. All of this young man's blood cells can be shown to have been derived from precursors that are descended from the bone marrow precursors present in his female sibling's marrow. Throughout his normal childhood he has grown normally, resisted infections normally, developed normally sexually and matured without any apparent abnormalities. He has now grown up fully and is a healthy man. He is already happily married, gainfully employed and well-adjusted in every way.

This first successful allogeneic bone marrow transplant thus cured for the very first time a surely fatal primary immunodeficiency disease with which the patient was born: His disease was SCID of the relatively common X-linked recessive type. The marrow transplant in this patient also cured for the very first time a second complicating, probably also lethal disorder, the immunologically based aplastic anemia that was consequent to his graft-vs-host reaction.

The findings in this patient showed in a dramatic way that bone marrow transplantation would surely become adaptable, with appropriate tissue typing and matching, to the treatment and cure of many otherwise lethal diseases that are attributable to abnormalities located in or arising in stem cells present in the marrow.

In the intervening years, of course, bone marrow transplantation has become a well developed clinical discipline and we are using marrow transplantation as a treatment for many lethal diseases. Sometimes, as an alternative, transplantation of stem cells from fetal liver can also be used as a viable approach to curing a multiplicity of otherwise lethal diseases. This approach has been especially well developed, after first trials in our laboratory,[176,222,229] and subsequent extensive independent development by my former fellow J.L. Touraine[271] and R. O'Reilly.[272]

Our successes with this initial patient's treatment showed that bone marrow transplantation could be used to reconstruct completely and dramatically an hereditarily defective immunological apparatus. The observations also showed that bone marrow transplantation could be used to correct profound deficiencies both of structure and function of the entire hematopoietic system attributable to an acquired disease. It is no wonder that because of its wide applicability to reconstruct deficient immunologic and hematological functions I dubbed this approach to correction of immunodeficiency "cellular engineering" when as a newly elected Regents Professor at the University of Minnesota I was called upon to address the faculty of the Institute of Technology at my home university.[180,273]

Soon after we performed this first successful bone marrow transplantation to two distinct but otherwise fatal diseases, Bach, Bortin and their colleagues at the University of Wisconsin applied massive doses of cyclophosphamide as both myeloablatant and immunosuppressant followed by bone marrow transplantation to achieve partial correction of the complex hematological-immunological disease known as Wiskott-Aldrich Syndrome using bone marrow transplantation.[262] A few months later de Koning et al in Holland successfully treated an apparent autosomal recessive case of SCID by bone marrow transplantation as well.[274]

In the years immediately following our initial successes in treating both SCID and aplastic anemia in the same patient, we also treated and cured for the first time a patient with SCID attributable to lack of the enzyme adenosine deaminase. Now 20 years later I still follow this patient who is quite normal immunologically, but exhibits marrow and blood which reveal a balanced stable mixed chimeric status. Her red blood cells lack the enzyme adenosine deaminase as do most lineages of her white blood cells. However, all of her lymphocytes contain adenosine deaminase and are certainly derived from lymphoid cells which came from her MHC-matched sibling donor. In addition, we treated successfully four additional children with SCID and this for the first time launched the development of a bone marrow transplantation unit. This unit was conceived as a clinical unit to be devoted solely to bone marrow transplantation. We established such a unit for the first time at the University of Minnesota. It was our plan that this unit should be dedicated to application of marrow transplantation in efforts to cure a wide variety of malignant, hematopoietic, metabolic or aplastic disorders as well as the immunodeficiency disorders with which we had begun the enterprise. With Meuwissen, we also began efforts to treat otherwise high-risk leukemias, advanced lymphomas and patients with advanced (e.g., Stage IV) Hodgkin's disease.[270]

After I left Minnesota to go the Sloan-Kettering Institute in New York, my bone marrow transplantation unit at Minnesota was taken over and was regenerated and redeveloped by John Kersey, one of my former students. It was John Kersey who as a sophomore medical student had performed the initial experiments on neonatal thymectomy in mice in collaboration with Carlos Martinez, Papermaster and me.[80] It was necessary for John Kersey to redevelop this unit because when I moved to New York, much but not all of my Minnesota team moved to the Sloan-Kettering Institute in New York with me where we set up another bone marrow transplantation unit. Others of this group have gone on to other training or definitive academic posts elsewhere.

Donnell Thomas and his group, with most impressive and commendable persistence and tenacity, achieved with great difficulty a low frequency of bone marrow transplant successes when they applied bone marrow transplantation to the treatment advanced end-stage leukemias.[275] This tiny glimmer of success, achieving only 11 percent long-term survivals in the otherwise uniformly fatal acute myeloid leukemia, however, was the achievement that opened the door to application of bone marrow transplantation, when properly used, as a relatively early treatment for high-risk leukemias which could not be treated successfully in any other way. This approach also became the treatment of choice through extensive application of bone marrow transplantation in Seattle, Minneapolis and at the Sloan-Kettering Institute in New York to treat many different forms of immunodeficiency, a wide variety of different types of aplastic anemias, numerous high risk leukemias, lymphomas and other kinds of malignancies. Now even advanced breast cancer is being treated with aid of this methodology. In addition, several genetic abnormalities of red blood cell and leukocyte development, and now also successful treatment of a variety of metabolic diseases have been accomplished by bone marrow transplantation.[276,277,278,279,280,281] I now count more than 60 otherwise lethal diseases (see Table 1) which can and are quite frequently cured by allogeneic bone marrow transplantation which I first accomplished with my clinical team in 1968. To date, more than 25,000 bone marrow transplants have been done. And I am sure that we are only at the beginning of the application of both allogeneic and autologous marrow transplants as the means of treatming many more otherwise lethal or highly morbid diseases.

Table 1
Diseases Now Curable by Bone Marrow Transplantation,
as Grouped by Major Category

1. Hematological abnormalities and genetic defects of RBC, platelets and leukocytes.
2. Primary immunodeficiency diseases - genetically determined.
3. Acquired severe immunodeficiency disease.
4. High risk acute and chronic leukemias, lymphomas.
5. Metabolic diseases—inborn errors of metabolism, e.g., mucopolysaccharidoses, mucolipidoses.
6. Numeorus forms of aplastic anemias, including constitutional aplastic anemias.
7. Other disseminated cancers and either autologous or allogeneic bone marrow transplantation may be used - neuroblastomas, breast cancers, and other disseminated cancers.

After I moved to the Sloan-Kettering Institute in New York, working with Betty Smithwick, Richard O'Reilly, Rajendra Pahwa, John Hansen, Caspar Jersild and Bo Dupont, I was able to set up and launch a second bone marrow transplantation unit at the Memorial Hospital. A young assistant professor, John Hansen, was the leader of this bone marrow transplant unit and Joao Ascensao, Richard O'Reilly, Neena Kapoor and Rajendra Pahwa, Elliot Grossbard and Thomas Garrett were the first six fellows who helped me launch that unit. Now four of them head independent and important bone marrow transplant program at their own respective medical centers. Two hematology-oncology fellows, Elliot Grossbard and Tom Garrett did well too, but the latter two fellows turned in other directions and didn't continue to develop bone marrow transplantation as a life's work.

These and many other former fellows and trainees from our program who work with bone marrow transplantation, much more than our own currently small bone marrow transplant program at the All Children's Hospital in St. Petersburg, are continuing to contribute to the burgeoning application of this still demanding clinical discipline. Bo Dupont joined us in New York and became a true immunogeneticist in residence and with Casper Jersild and John Hansen developed the essential expertise in tissue typing and immunogenetics that is now a major cornerstone to modern clinical bone marrow and organ transplantation. John Hansen, from our program, later served the same function for the Seattle bone marrow transplantation unit. Recently John has succeeded Donnell Thomas as head of research at the Hutchison Cancer Center in Seattle.

While I was at the Memorial Hospital as head of research, my young associates and I launched investigations and analyses which led to several additional exciting developments in cellular engineering. We showed for the first time that one can use not only matched sibling donors but also occasionally can find a suitable donor among non-sibling members of an extended family.[282,283,284] Additionally, we showed for the first time that one may be able sometimes to locate a suitable donor among members of the general population[285] and we performed the very first although only partially successful bone marrow transplantation to correct SCID[285] from a donor we had located in the general population. That patient developed chronic graft-vs-host disease and ultimately what turned out to be a lethal squamous cell carcinoma on one of his hands that had been severely affected by the GVHD. Nonetheless, I am sure our struggles to find a bone marrow donor for this child with SCID, which was led by Bo Dupont and John Hansen, gave these scientists and me as well the resolution to help Robert Graves and Admiral Zumwalt and some of their other friends and associates launch a National Bone Marrow Donor Program in the United States to facilitate volunteer bone marrow donations after appropriate MHC typing and matching. These volunteer donors make curative allogeneic bone marrow transplantation a reality in high frequency when the immediate or extended family lacks a suitable MHC-matched sibling donor. Such registries of MHC-matched volunteers are well developed and functioning now in several countries, inlcuding Canada, England, France, Holland and Germany. To my knowledge, these registries were first proposed and developed in England at the behest of John Hobbs at Westminster.

Yair Reisner joined us in New York. In parallel, he had experienced success using mismatched experimental bone marrow transplantation in mice that was based on removal of T-cells—purging the marrow of all T cells and all committed T cell precursors.[286,287,288] Because of our interest, Reisner came to my laboratory in the Sloan-Kettering Institute at my invitation to help develop bone marrow transplantation for patients who did not have an MHC-matched sibling whose mismatched parents or siblings might be used as donors. HE had developed a lectin separation technique that worked well in mice based on lectin fractionation. He had developed a lectin separation technique that worked well in mice based on lectin fractionation. We also had developed a T-cell purging technique in mice based on antibody removal of T cells.[288,289] When Reisner's lectin separation method did not work to remove T cells completely in humans, Reisner had developed for mice did not work for humans, Reisner conducted subsequent critical research in my laboratory[290,291] which led to the first clinical adaptation of the T-cell purging technique for human donor marrow. This method permitted us, with Richard O'Reilly, then head of our bone marrow transplant unit at Memorial Hospital, to develop the parental or sibling (haploidentical) donor transplantation which has been adapted as a method suitable to permit cure of children with SCID when no matched sibling donor is available.[292,293] Later, Rebecca Buckley, working with SCID, and also Richard O'Reilly, both for SCID and also for other diseases, have successfully applied our technique of purged haploidentical parental marrow transplants to large numbers of children.[294] Modifications of this method which will ultimately permit treatment of many lethal diseases other than SCID when no matched marrow donor can be found.

In the laboratory, we had been spurred by the contributions of Tyan[295] and of von Boehmer and colleagues,[296,297] to purge bone marrow of T cells to make bone marrow transplantation in mice possible and successful where it otherwise could not work. These investigators showed that T-cell purging made parental—>F_1 transplants across major histocompatibility barriers possible without GVHD. With Onoé and Fernandes[288,289,298] we employed experimentally a combination of T cell and T cell precursor purging using in vitro treatment of prospective donor marrow by anti Thy-1 polyclonal or monoclonal antibodies to prepare bone marrow of mice so that we might transplant the marrow across major histocompatibility barriers without inducing graft-vs-host reactions. In collaboration with Onoé and his group,[298,299,300,301,302,303,304,305,306,307] as well as later with Ikehara[308,309] and in collaboration with Ikehara and his associates[310,311,312,313,314,315] and his group, we have used purging bone marrow of T cells and have been analyzing the effectiveness of bone marrow transplantation in mice both within and across MHC barriers as an approach to treatment of many classes of disease which continue to represent unsolved problems when they occur in humans. For example, we have treated with impressive success advanced renal disease,[314] treated and prevented organ-specific autoimmune diseases such as diabetes and treated cell-specific or systemic autoimmune diseases successfully in experimental animals by bone marrow transplantation. Our collective investigations show that bone marrow transplantation can be used experimentally to cure, in mice and rat models of many diseases that are very similar to certain human diseases in which current treatment leaves much to be desired. These diseases include insulin-dependent juvenile diabetes mellitus,[309,310,311] systemic lupus erythematosus,[314] autoimmune thrombocytopenic purpura,[313] coronary cardiovascular disease[316] and even advanced renal diseases. This T-cell purging approach and MHC matched marrow transplantation has also been used in our laboratory as a means to introduce resistance genes that are effective in preventing retrovirus-induced cancers.[317,318,319]

Consequently it has beome clear that as bone marrow transplantation becomes safer and safer and thus more generally available, it will become a method that certainly will be able to be used as a dominant approach for treatment of many more lethal diseases and, in addition, numerous highly morbid diseases which cannot yet be treated by bone marrow transplantation. Already we have seen that it is possible to greatly shorten the recovery period following bone marrow transplantation. This approach involves the use of cytokines or growth factors that stimulate and/or expand populations of hematopoietic cells. I can now visualize a time in the not too distant future when cellular engineering through allogeneic bone marrow, stem cell or stem cell plus stromal cell transplants or even transplantation of genetically modified stem cell transplants will be able to be employed even as outpatient procedures to provide long-term correction or cure of a great many more human diseases—some of which are now only ineffectively treated or cannot be treated effectively. Listed on Table 2 are diseases we cannot treat effectively now in which marrow transplantation or stem cell transplantation have already been used as effective treatment in animals. (See Table 2).

Already, by transplanting into fatally irradiated recipients isolated populations representing only a very small proportion of the bone marrow cells which in turn contain a high concentration of stem cells, we have been able to cure and, in reciprocal experiments, to cause systemic autoimmune diseases as well as organ-specific autoimmunities, cell-specific autoimmunities and systemic autoimmunities.[314,315] We are sure these experimental successes utilize approaches which can and will be applied clinically in the years ahead. Great strides are surely in the offing for cellular engineering as we learn better to define and isolate stem cells, treat these cells as transplants to treat and cure otherwise poorly responsive diseases.

Further, it seems certain that such stem cell preparations will surely soon begin to use somatic cell genetics—by altering genetically a patient's own stem cell populations—to correct inborn errors of metabolism. Already many of the emotional, legal and ethical hurdles for approval of the very first undertakings in gene therapy have been overcome by Blaese, Anderson, Rosenberg and

Table 2
Diseases of Experimental Animals Preventable or
Treatable by bone marrow Transplantation

1. Juvenile form of diabetes in NOD mice.
2. Juvenile form of diabetes in BB rats.
3. Lupus-like autoimmune disease, including renal disease in B/W mice.
4. Lupus-like renal disease and autoimmunity in NZB mice.
5. Coronary vascular disease in BXSB mice.
6. Idiopathic autoimmune thrombocytopenia in BXSB mice.
7. Systemic autoimmune disease and lymphoproliferative disease in MRL/lpr lpr mice. Stromal cell + stem cell, or bone marrow transplant.
8. Progressive globoid degeneration in Twitcher mice.
9. Others.

their colleagues at the National Institutes of Health (See New York Times, Wednesday, August 1, 1990, page 1).

We can now be certain that bone marrow transplantation, and its ultimate derivative, stem cell transplantation[314,315,319,320,321] as approaches to cellular engineering are still at only a beginning stage. I am certain that we will soon realize the fullest potentials of this kind of cellular engineering, and we can now be certain that this development will occur. The stem cell transplants may become even more useful as bone marrow stromal cells are identified, cultured and utilized along with the stem cells.

It now is possible to see that the enthusiastic predictions I made in those early days following our first successes in curing by cellular engineering two highly lethal diseases using bone marrow transplantation have been gross underestimates.[323,324,325] Nonetheless, in spite of underestimating the potential of our approach, I called correction of disease by BMT cellular engineering. It is now certain to become applicable for many more diseases. Indeed, it appears certain that the true somatic cell genetic treatment of lethal disease will often use the host's own stem cell transplants after genetic manipulation of these precursor cells. This form of genetic engineering will surely borrow greatly from the methods we and others have employed as we have introduced bone marrow transplantation into the clinical arena. I feel certain that cellular engineering using modified stem cells will be one of the major platforms from which somatic cell genetic engineering to the cure human disease will be launched.[277,278,279] (See New York Times, Wednesday, August 1, 1990, page 1.)

There is one final area of promising research inquiry that my colleagues and I initiated and which I directed at the University of Minnesota that I feel has great potential, but has not yet reached full fruition. When I began at the behest of my friend Harold Wolfe to take Bruce Glick's research on the bursa of Fabricius seriously and thus to realign my thymus research, I noticed a striking morphologic and histologic similarity between the structure of the Bursa of Fabricius in the rabbit and the Peyer's patch type of tissue in the rabbit. The latter tissue is especially well developed in the Sacculus rotundas appendix and Peyer's patches of the rabbit. It is also well developed in the Peyer's patches of bovine and ovine species and in Peyer's patches of some other animals. In collaborative studies of the lymphoid tissue of many of what we found with Fichtelius and Finstad, numerous tissues with similar morphology, that are bursal equivalents of vertebrates, we found very similar tissues in many vertebrates.[326]

We did rather extensive initial experiments with Kellum[111] and Archer and Sutherland[327,328] to try experimentally to link these tissues to bursal-type functions. These efforts were of interest in that they did suggest that profound influences on immunologic development could be produced by early removal of sacculus rotundas, appendix and Peyer's patches in the rabbit.

Then a young pediatric surgeon, Daniel Perey, joined my laboratory group as a fellow. We were determined to continue research in this direction and to try to ascertain whether removal of all or as much as possible of this type of bursa-like tissue in neonatal rabbits might interfere with plasma cell development, antibody production, and development of immunoglobulin levels as does removal of the bursa of Fabricius in irradiated chickens. The short of this story was that we made numerous investigations to follow up our earlier leads that had been obtained with my student colleagues Archer, Sutherland and Kellum. Perey extirpated the appendix, Sacculus rotundas and Peyer's patches of rabbits. This manipulation, indeed, greatly decreased immunologic development in the rabbits. The appendectomized plus saculectomized plus Peyer's patch-ectomized rabbits developed autoimmunities regularly and also developed profound amyloidosis and increased susceptibility to infection. They also had significant deficiencies of the antibody producing systems. With Cooper, Perey later extended these experiments impressively. The investigations showed that reduced survival as well as antibody deficiency was produced by this type of neonatal surgery in these rabbits.[135,146,329] Max Cooper was the senior fellow who had introduced Dan Perey to our line of thinking and working, just as Peterson had introduced Cooper to our approach to ontogenetic, phylogenetic and clinical laboratory investigations. However, unlike Peterson, who was very permissive and generous with Cooper, Max Cooper insisted on being first author on all the papers that were, indeed, features by Perey's very skillful application of his rather unique pediatric surgical skills. Max's insistence on being first author on what Perey considered to be his quite independent surgical-immunologic research initiated a quarrel between these two young scientists. I am quite certain the two never spoke to one another again after their quarrel. Perey died of coronary artery disease as a relatively young man and took his anger about the first author scientific credit for his work to his grave. He felt he should have been first author on each of these scientific papers, but Max would not permit that.

I tell this story because we felt at that time from my morphological studies, and I feel still today that the Peyer's patch type tissue, the sacculus rotundas and the Peyer's patches themselves, do indeed, possess incredibly similar morphological features to those that characterize the bursa of Fabricius. These similarities which I noted are so striking that I am certain there must be an important relationship in the function of these tissues and organs. I continue to believe these morphological similarities that I emphasized more than a quarter of a century ago now have been shown by the research of several of my fellows to have crucial functional concomitants. However, I still believe, in spite of John Cebra and Lars Å. Hanson's important investigations of the role for these tissues in generating cells which have undergone isotype switching to become the cells that produce dimeric IgA[330,331] that the full, developmental function of these special follicular lymphoid components of the local immune system remains to be fully elucidated.   After he left my laboratory Cooper maintained an interest in the morphology of the Peyer's patch type of tissue.   With outhers, he elucidated further the morphology of the dome epithelium M cells (microfold) especially at the ultrastructural level.

Cooper and his British colleagues Moore and Raff later showed in studies that seem at this time to be quite convincing that pre-B cells which possess cytoplasmic Ig develop early in life in the mammalian fetal liver.   These investigators will probably turn out to be correct in their conclusion that the fetal liver subserves some of the same functions for most vertebrates that is subserved, for a time at least during development, by the bursa of all orders of birds.   However, there is no similarity in structure between the bursa and the fetal liver lymphoid tissue.   Thus, I continue to believe the last chapter has not been written about the bursal equivalents of the bursaless vertebrates. To be written definitively this chapter needs much further effort, especially using techniques and analyses of the events involved in their development, including the methods of generation of diversity—G.O.D.   It must be determined whether the specialized forms of gene rearrangement that occur within the bursa, e.g., insertional mutagenesis that involve insulin-producing genes, are also occurring at these specialized lymphoid tissue sites.   The critical experiments, I believe, remain still to be done.

The influence of those incredible Minnesota days as a portal of entry to modern lymphoid cell biology has been incredible. We have gone a long way toward understanding in impressive detail the ontogeny, phylogeny, development and interactions of the immunologically competent cells, the biologic amplification systems of immunity and the nature of the effector processes. The contributions from the Minnesota years have been legion. In all of this Minnesota-based elucidation from the very earliest days critical experiments of nature and a view from both ontogenetic and phylogenetic developmental perspectives have been the crucial features.

Because of these efforts we have gained impressive knowledge and understanding of how it is possible for humans and other vertebrates to maintain their individuality even while living in a veritable sea of bacteria, viruses, fungi, protozoa and potentially invasive Helminths. Our increasing understanding, although surely still barely at a beginning, has permitted over and over again not only impressive bisections and dissections of the microbial universe, and bisections and dissections of the immunological and lymphoid universe, but also has permitted development of new treatments applicable to the curing many otherwise fatal diseases.   We feel certain that these investigations hold today important keys to the launching of genetic engineering as an approach to medical treatment of many otherwise fatal human diseases.

As we speed down the modern immunologic highways paved with modern cell biology and molecular biology we must realize and appreciate that we owe a great debt to our fine teachers of modern immunology. These teachers have repeatedly been our sometimes rare or unusual patients whose diseases and clinical problems with infections and whose disturbed immune functions we have encountered and analyzed in our clinics, at the bedside and in the laboratories.   The study of these patients, as I have repeatedly pointed out,[5,241,332] has taken us often to the laboratory or laboratory bench with critical questions. In the laboratory we have been able to seek answers which have often returned to the bedside with useful new approaches to diagnosis, clinical treatment or penetrating analyses of human disease.   Thus, our patients as Experiments of Nature have raised crucial questions or have pointed in revealing investigative directions. THey have shed light into many dark corners of biology, genetics, immunology and even biochemistry. Today such patients still provide leads to important new issues even in molecular biology.[333,334]

Such patients provide not only directions to follow for immunologic progress, but also represent often superb opportunities to test the applicability of new knowledge as it is generated and while understanding of complex human systems continues to evolve. Attempts to treat these sometimes rare patients who often have had otherwise lethal diseases have also provided critical testing grounds for our developing knowledge. These patients have been great teachers of clinical hematology and immunology and now they are or will become crucial teachers of molecular biology. They represent Experiments of Nature which have been most effective for immunology when analyzed in close interaction with those three other great teachers of immunology: the exalted inbred laboratory mouse, the instructive little bunny rabbits, and even the lowly chicken.

REFERENCES

1. **Good, R.A.,** Following the Lyon's Trail, in *Elias Potter Lyon: Minnesota's Leader in Medical Education*, Warren H. Green, St. Louis, MO, 1981, p. 81.
2. **Wangensteen, O.H.,** Ed., *Elias Potter Lyon: Minnesota's Leader in Medical Education*, Warren H. Green, St. Louis, MO, 1981, p. 3.
3. **Good, R.A., and Platou, E.S.,** Eds., in *Essays on Pediatrics*, In Honor of Irvine McQuarrie, *Lancet Publications*, Minneapolis, MN, 1955.
4. **Good, R.A., and Zak, S.J.,** Disturbances in gamma globulin synthesis as "experiments of nature", *Pediatrics*, 18, 109, 1956.
5. **Good, R.A.,** Presidential address: The whetstones, *J. Lab. Clin. Med.*, 69, 6, 1967b.
6. **Good, R.A.,** Experiments of nature in immunobiology, *N. Eng. J. Med.*, 279, 1344, 1968a.
7. **Harvey, W.,** To the Distinguished and Elegant Gentleman and Experienced Physician, Jan Vlackveld, of Haarlem (1657), in *The Circulation of the Blood*, Harvey, W., Everyman's Library 262, J.M. Dent & Sons, London, 1966.
8. **Garrod, A.E.,** The debt of science to medicine. The Harveian oration. *Brit. Med. J.*, Oct. 24, 1924.
9. **Sabin, F.,** Cellular reactions to a dye-protein with a concept of the mechanism of antibody formation, *J. Exp. Med.*, 70, 67, 1939.
10. **White, A. and Dougherty, T.F.,** Effect of prolonged stimulation of the adrena cortex and adrenalectomy on the numbers of circulating erythrocytes and lymphocytes, *Endocrinology*, 36, 16, 1945a.
11. **White, A. and Dougherty, T.F.,** The pituitary adrenotropic hormone control of the rate of release of serum globulins from lymphoid tissue, *Endocrinology*, 36, 207, 1945b.
12. **Kolouch, F.,** The Bone Marrow Plasma Cell, A Thesis, University of Minnesota, 1938b.
13. **Bing, J. and Plum, P.,** Serum proteins in leucopenia: contribution on the question about place of formation of serum proteins, *Acta. Med. Scandinav.*, 92, 415, 1937.
14. **Kolouch, F. Good, R.A. & Campbell, B.,** The reticulo-endothelial origin of the bone marrow plasma cells in hypersensitive states, *J. Lab. Clin. Med.*, 32, 749, 1947.
15. **Clawson, E.J.,** Experimental streptococcic inflammation in normal immune and hypersensitive animals, *Arch. Pathology*, 9, 1141, 1930.
16. **Kolouch, F.,** Origin of bone marrow plasma cell associated with allergic and immune states of rabbits, *Proc. Soc. Exp. Biol. Med.*, 39, 147, 1938a.
17. **Cajal, S.R.,** *Manual de Anatomia Patologico General*, Ed. 1, Barcelona, Spain, 1890.
18. **Bjoerneboe, M. and Gormsen, H.,** Preliminary report on investigations on occurrence of plasma cells in experimental hyperglobulinemia in rabbits, *Nordisk. Medicin*

Hospitalstid., 9, 891, 1941.

19. **Bjoerneboe, M. and Gormsen, H.,** Experimental studies on the role of plasma cells as antibody producers, *Acta path. et microbiol. Scandinav.*, 20, 649, 1943.

20. **Good, R.A.,** The morphologic mechanisms of hyperergic inflammation in the brain; with special reference to the significance of local plasma cell formation, Doctoral Dissertation, University of Minnesota, 1947.

21. **Good, R.A.,** Effect of passive sensitization and anaphylactic shock on rabbit bone marrow (Introduced by B. Campbell), *Proc. Soc. Exp. Biol. Med.*, 67, 203, 1948.

22. **Good, R.A.,** Experimental allergic brain inflammation, a morphological study, *J. Neuropathol. Exp. Neurol.*, 9, 78, 1950.

23. **Good, R.A., and Campbell, B.,** Relationship of bone marrow plasmacytosis to the changes in serum gamma globulin rheumatic fever, *Am. J. Med.* IX, 330, 342, 1950.

24. **Good, R.A.,** Runestones in immunology: inscriptions to journeys of discovery and analysis, *J. Immunol.*, 117, 1413, 1976.

25. **Avery, O.T., MacLeod, C.M. and McCarty, M.,** *J. Exp. Med.*, 79, 137, 1944.

26. **Griffiths, F.,** The significance of pneumococcal types, *J. Hyg.*, 27, 113, 1928.

27. **Stetson, A. & Good, R.A.,** Studies on the mechanism of the Shwartzman phenomenon: evidence for the participation of polymorphonuclear leucocytes in the phenomenon, *J. Exp. Med.*, 93, 49, 1951.

28. **Good, R.A., and Glick, D.,** Mucolytic enzyme systems. XVI. Factors influencing hyaluronidase inhibitor levels in serum, role of adrenal cortex, *Am. J. Physiol.*, 166, 555, 1951.

29. **Kunkel, H.G., Slater, R.J. & Good, R.A.,** Relationship between certain myeloma proteins and normal gamma globulin, *Proc. Soc. Exp. Biol. Med.*, 76, 190d, 1951.

30. **Landsteiner, K. & Chase, M.W.,** Experiments on transfer of cutaneous sensitivity to simple compounds, *Proc. Soc. Exper. Biol. Med.*, 67, 225, 1942.

31. **Chase, M.W.** Production of local skin reactivity by passive transfer of antiprotein sera, *Proc. Soc. Exp. Biol. Med.*, 52, 238, 1943.

32. **Prausnitz, C., and Kustner, H.,** Studien uber die Ueberempfindlichkeit, *Zentralbl. Bakteriol.*, 86, 160. *J. Bact.*, 86, 160, 1921.

33. **Medawar, P.B.,** The behaviour and fate of skin autografts and skin homografts in rabbits, *J. Anat.*, 78, 176, 1944.

34. **Medawar, P.B.,** A second study of the behaviour and fate of skin homografts in rabbits, *J. Anat.*, 79, 157, 1945.

35. **Medawar, P.B.,** Relationship between the antigens of blood and skin, *Nature* (London), 157, 161, 1946.

36. **Thomas, L. and Good, R.A.,** Studies on the generalized Shwartzman reaction. I. General observations concerning the phenomenon, *J. Exp. Med.*, 96, 605, 1952a.

37. **Thomas, L. and Good, R.A.),** The effect of cortisone on the Shwartzman reaction: the production of lesions resembling the dermal and generalized Shwartzman reactions by a single injection of bacterial toxin in cortisione-treted rabbits, *J. Exp. Med.*, 95, 409, 1952b.

38. **Good, R.A., and Thomas, L.,** Studies on the generalized Shwartzman reaction. II. The production of bilateral cortical necrosis of the kidneys by a single injection of bacterial toxin in rabbits previously treated with thorotrast or trypan blue, *J. Exp. Med.*, 96, 624, 1952.

39. **Good, R.A., and Thomas, L.,** Studies on the generalized Shwartzman reaction. IV. Prevention of the local and generalized Shwartzman reactions with heparin, *J. Exp. Med.*, 97, 871, 1953.

40. **Good, R.A.,** Morphological basis of the immune response and hypersensitivity, in *Host-Parasite Relationships in Living Cells*, Felton, H.M. et al., Eds., Charles C. Thomas, Springfield, IL, 1957, p. 78.

41. **Good, R.A., and Page, A.R.,** Fatal complications of virus hepatitis in two patients with agammaglobulinemia, *Am. J. Med.*, 29, 804, 1960.

42. **Bearn, A., Kunkel, H.G. and Slater, R.J.,** The problem of liver disease in young women, *Am. J. Med.*, 21, 3, 1956.

43. **Good, R.A.,** Acute-phase reactions in rheumatic fever, in *Symposium on Rheumatic Fever*, Univ. of Minnesota Press, Minneapolis, MN, 1952, p. 115.

44. **Bruton, O.C.,** Agammaglobulinemia, *Pediatrics*, 9, 722, 1952.

45. **Good, R.A.,** Agammaglobulinemia—a provocative experiment of nature, *Bull. Univ.*

Minn. Hosp. Minn. Med. Found. 26, 1, 1954a.

46. **Good, R.A.,** Absence of plasma cells from bone marrow and lymph nodes following antigenic stimulation in patients with agammaglobulinemia, *Revue d'Hematol.*, 9, 502, 1954b.

47. **Good, R.A.,** Studies on agammaglobulinemia. II. Failure of plasma cell formation in the bone marrow and lymph nodes of patients with agammaglobulinemia, *J. Lab. Clin. Med.*, 46, 167, 1955b.

48. **Good, R.A., and Varco, R.L.,** A clinical and experimental study of agammaglobulinemia, *J. Lancet*, 75, 245, 1955a.

49. **Good, R.A., and Varco, R.L.,** Successful homograft of skin in a child with agammaglobulinemia: studies on agammaglobulinemia, *J. Am. Med. Assoc.*, 147, 713, 1955b.

50. **Mazzitello, W.F. & Good, R.A.,** The clinical problem of agammaglobulinemia, *Postgrad. Med.*, 20, 95, 1956.

51. **Porter, H.M.,** Congenital agammaglobulinemia: A sex-linked genetic train and demonstration of delayed skin sensitivity, *Am. J. Dis. Child*, 90, 617, 1955.

52. **Kelly, W.D., Good, R.A., Varco, R. and Levitt, M.,** The altered response to skin homografts and to delayed allergens in Hodgkin's disease, *Surg. Forum*, 9, 785, 1959.

53. **Page, A.R., Hansen, A.E. and Good, R.A.,** Occurrence of leukemia and lymphoma in patients with agammaglobulinemia, *Blood*, 21, 197, 1963.

54. **Good, R.A., and Kelley, V.C.,** Adrenal cortical function in patients with agammaglobulinemia, *Proc. Soc. Exp. Biol. Med.*, 88, 99, 1955.

55. **Kelly, W.D., Good, R.A. and Varco, R.L.,** Anergy and skin homograft survival in Hodgkin's disease, *Surg. Gynecol. Obstet.*, 107, 565, 1958.

56. **Lamb, Pilney, F., Kelly, W.D. and Good, R.A.,** A comparative study of the incidence of anergy in patients with carcinoma, leukemia, Hodgkin's disease and other lymphomas, *J. Immunol.*, 89, 555, 1962.

57. **Zinneman, H.H. and Hall, W.H.,** Steatorrhea and probable tuberculosis with acquired hypogammaglobulinemia, *Am. Rev. Tuberc.*, 74, 773, 1956.

58. **Zinneman, H.H., Hall, W.H. and Heller, B.I.,** Recurrent pneumonia in multiple myeloma and some observations on immunological response, *Ann. Int. Med.*, 41, 1152, 1954.

59. **Fagraeus, A.,** Antibody production in relation to the development of plasma cells: *In vivo* and *in vitro* experiments, *Esselte Aktiebolag*, Stockholm, 1948.

60. **Coons, A.H., Leduc, E.H. and Connolly, J.M.,** Studies on antibody production. I. A method for the histochemical demonstration of specific antibody and its application to a study of the hyperimmune rabbit, *J. Exp. Med.*, 102, 49, 1955a.

61. **Coons, A.H., Leduc, E.H. and Connolly,** Studies on antibody production. II. The primary and secondary responses in the popliteal lymph node of the rabbit, *J. Exp. Med.*, 102, 61, 1955b.

62. **White, R.G., Coons, A.H. & Connolly, J.M.,** Studies on antibody production. III. The alum granuloma, *J. Exp. Med.*, 102, 1955a.

63. **White, R.G., Coons, A.H. & Connolly, J.M.,** Studies on antibody production. IV. The role of the wax fraction of mycobacterium tuberculosis in adjuvant emulsions on the production of antibody to egg albumin, *J. Exp. Med.*, 102, 83, 1955b.

64. **Ehrlich, W.E., Drabkin, D.L. and Forman C.,** Nucleic acids and the production of antibody by plasma cells, *J. Exp. Med.*, 90, 157, 1949.

65. **Seligmann M., Fudenberg, H., Good, R.A.,** A proposed classification of primary immunologic deficiencies, *Am. J. Med.*, 45, 817, 1968.

66. **Popper, K.R.,** *Conjectures and Refutations*, Routledge and Kegan Paul, London, 1963.

67. **Schier, W.W.,** Cutaneous anergy and Hodgkin's disease, *New Engl. J. Med.*, 250, 353, 1954.

68. **MacLean, L.D., Zak, S.J., Varco, R.L. and Good, R.A.,** Thymic tumor and acquired agammaglobulinemia: a clinical and experimental study of the immune response, *Surgery*, 40, 1010, 1956.

69. **MacLean, L.D., Zak, S.J., Varco, R.L. and Good, R.A.,** The role of the thymus in antibody production: an experimental study of the immune response in thymectomized rabbits, *Transplant. Bull.*, 4, 21, 1957.

70. **Boyd, E.,** Growth of the thymus: Its relation to status thymicolymphaticus and thymic symptoms., A.M.A., *Am. J. Dis. Child.*, 33, 867, 1927.

71. **Boyd, E.** The weight of the thymus gland in health and disease, A.M.A., *Am. J. Dis.*

Child., 43, 1162, 1932.

72. **Scammon, R.E.**, The prenatal growth of the human thymus, *Proc. Soc. Exper. Biol. & Med.*, 24, 906, 1927.

73. **Scammon, R.E.**, Developmental anatomy, in *Morris' Human Anatomy*, Ed., 11, Schaeffer, J.P., Ed., McGraw-Hill, New York, 1953, p. 1.

74. **Glick, B., Chang, T.S. and Jaap, R.G.**, The bursa of Fabricius and antibody production, *Poultry Sci.*, 35, 224, 1956.

75. **Mueller, A.P., Wolfe, H.R. and Meyer, R.K.**, Precipitin production in chickens. XXI. Antibody production in bursectomized chickens and in chickens injected with 19-nortestosterone on the fifth day of incubation, *Journal of Immunology*, 85, 172, 1960.

76. **Jolly J.**, Sur la function hematopoiettique de la bourse de Fabricius, *Comp. Rend. Soc. Biol.*, 70, 498, 1911.

77. **Jolly J.**, La bourse de Fabricius et les organes lymphoepithaliaux, *Arch. Anat. Microbiol.*, 16, 363, 1914.

78. **Archer, O.K. and Pierce, J.C.**, Role of the thymus in development of the immune response, *Fed. Proc.*, 20, 26, 1961.

79. **Archer, O.K., Pierce, J.C., Papermaster, B.W. and Good, R.A.**, Reduced antibody response in thymectomized rabbits, *Nature*, 191, 191, 1962.

80. **Martinez, C., Kersey, J., Papermaster, B.W. and Good, R.A.**, Skin homograft survival in thymectomized mice, *Proc. Soc. Exp. Biol. Med.*, 109, 193, 1962.

81. **Dalmasso, A.P., Martinez, C. and Good, R.A.**, Failure of spleen cells from thymectomized mice to induce graft-vs-host reactions, *Proc. Soc. Exp. Biol. Med.*, 110, 205, 1962a.

82. **Dalmasso, A.P., Martinez, C. and Good, R.A.**, Further studies of suppression of the homograft reaction by thymectomy in the mouse, *Proc. Soc. Exp. Biol. Med.*, 111, 143, 1962b.

83. **Good, R.A., Dalmasso, A.P., Martinez, C., Archer, O.K., Pierce, J.C. and Papermaster, B.W.**, The role of the thymus in the development of immunologic capacity in rabbits and mice, *J. Exp. Med.*, 116, 773, 1962.

84. **Papermaster, B.W., Bradley, S.G., Watson, D.W. and Good R.A.**, Antibody-producing capacity of adult chicken spleen cells in newly hatched chicks: A study of sources of variation in a homologous cell transfer system, *J. Exp. Med.*, 115, 1191, 1962.

85. **Papermaster, B.W., Friedman, D.I. and Good, R.A.**, Relationship of the bursa of Fabricius to immunologic responsiveness and homograft immunity in the chicken, *Proc. Soc. Exp. Biol. Med.*, 110, 62, 1962.

86. **Papermaster, B.W. and Good, R.A.**, Relative contributions of the thymus and the bursa of Fabricius to the maturation of the lymphoreticular system and immunological potential in the chicken, *Nature*, 196, 836, 1962.

87. **Hard, R.C., Martinez, C. and Good, R.A.**, Intenstinal crypt lesions in neonatally thymectomized hamsters, *Nature*, 204, 455, 1964.

88. **Papermaster, B.W., Dalmasso, A.P., Martinez, C. and Good, R.A.**, Suppression of antibody forming capacity with thymectomy in the mouse, *Proc. Soc. Exp. Biol. Med.*, 111, 41, 1962.

89. **Martinez, C., Dalmasso, A. and Good, R.A.**, Acceptance of tumor homografts by thymectomized mice, *Nature*, 194, 1289, 1962.

90. **Miller, J.F.A.P.**, Immunological function of the thymus, *Lancet 2*, 748, 1961a.

91. **McEndy, D.P., Boon, M.C., Furth, J.**, On the role of thymus, spleen and goands in the development of leukemia in a high leukemia stock of mice, *Cancer Res.*, 4, 377, 1944.

92. **Furth, J.**, Prolongation of life with prevention of leukemia by thymectomy in mice, *J. Gerontol.*, 1, 46, 1946.

93. **Miller, J.F.A.P.**, Studies on mouse leukaemia. The role of thymus in leukaemogenesis by cell-free leukaemic filtrates, *Brit. J. Cancer*, 14, 93, 1960.

94. **Miller, J.F.A.P.**, Analysis of the thymus influence in leukaemogenesis, *Nature*, 191, 248, 1961b.

95. **Miller, J.F.A.P.**, Etiology and pathogenesis of mouse leukemia, *Advances in Cancer Research*, 6, 291, 1961c.

96. **Miller, J.F.A.P.**, Role of the thymus in transplantation immunity, *Ann. New York Acad. Sci.*, 99, 340, 1962.

97. **Arnason, B.G., Jankovic, B.D. and Waksman, B.H.,** The role of the thymus in immune reactions in rats, in *The Thymus in Immunobiology*, Good, R.A. and Gabrielsen, A.E., op. cit., 1964, p. 492.

98. **Waksman, B.H., Arnason, B.G. and Jankovic, B.D.,** Role of the thymus in immune reacitons in rats. III. Changes in the lymphoid organs of thymectomized rats, *J. Exp. Med.*, 116, 187, 1962.

99. **Arnason, B.G., Jankovic, B.D., Waksman, B.H. and Wennersten, C.,** Role of the thymus in immune reactions in rats. II. Suppressive effect of thymectomy at birth on reactions of delayed (cellular) hypersensitivity and the circulating small lymphocyte, *J. Exp. Med.*, 116, 177, 1962.

100. **Parrott, D.M.V.,** Strain variation in mortality and runt disease in mice thymectomized at birth, *Transpl. Bull.*, 29, 102, 1962.

101. **Parrott, D.M.V. and East, J.,** The role of the thymus in neonatal life, *Nature*. 195, 347, 1962.

102. **Parrott, D.M.V. and East, J.,** Studies on a fatal wasting syndrome of mice thymectomized at birth, in *The Thymus in Immunobiology*, Good, R.A. and Gabrielsen, A.E., Eds., op. cit., 1964, p. 523.

103. **Good, R.A., and Gabrielsen, A.E.,** Eds., *The Thymus in Immunobiology*, Harper & Row, New York: Hoeber Medical, 1964, p. v - 778.

104. **Good, R.A., and Gabrielsen, A.E.,** Preface, in *The Thymus in Immunobiology*, op. cit., 1964, p. xv.

105. **Good, R.A., Martinez, C. and Gabrielsen, A.,** Clinical considerations of the thymus in immunobiology, in *The Thymus in Immunobiology*, Good, R.A. and Gabrielsen, A.E., op. cit., 1964, p. 3.

106. **Archer, O.K., Papermaster, B.W. and Good, R.A.,** Thymectomy in rabbit and mouse: consideration of time and lymphoid peripheralization, in *The Thymus in Immunbiology*, Good, R.A. and Gabrielsen, A.E., Eds., Hoeber Medical, Harper & Row, New York, 1964, p. 414.

107. **Dalmasso, A.P., Martinez, C. and Good, R.A.,** Studies of immunologic characteristics of lymphoid cells from thymectomized mice, in *The Thymus in Immunobiology*, op. cit., 1964, p. 489.

108. **Martinez, C., Dalmasso, A.P. and Good, R.A.,** Effect of thymectomy on development of immunological competence in mice, *Ann. N.Y. Acad. Sci.*, 113, 933, 1964.

109. **Miller, J.F.A.P.,** The thymus and the development of immunologic responsiveness. The thymus directs the maturation of immunologic capabilities by means of a humoral mechanism, *Science*, 144, 1544, 1964b.

110. **Warner, N.L. and Szenberg, A.,** Immunologic studies on hormonally bursectomized and surgically thymectomized chickens: Dissociation of immunologic responsiveness, in *The Thymus in Immunobiology*, op. cit., p. 395, 1964.

111. **Kellum, M.J., Sutherland, D.E.R., Eckert, E., Peterson, R.D.A. and Good, R.A.,** Wasting disease, Coombs-positivity, and amyloidosis in rabbits subjected to central lymphoid tissue extirpation and irradiation, *Intl. Arch. Allergy Appl. Immunol.*, 27, 6, 1965.

112. **Yunis, E.J., Hilgard, H.R., Martinez, C. and Good, R.A.,** Studies on immunologic reconstitution of thymectomized mice, *J. Exp. Med.*, 121, 607, 1965.

113. **Glick, B.,** The bursa of Fabricius and the development of immunologic competence, in *The Thymus in Immunobiology*, Good, R.A. and Gabrielsen, A.E., op. cit., 1964, p. 343.

114. **Mueller, A.P., Wolfe, H.R. and Cote, W.P.,** Antibody studies in hormonally and surgically bursectomized chickens, in *The Thymus in Immunobiology*, Good R.A. and Gabrielsen, A.E., Eds., op. cit., 1964, p. 359.

115. **Auerbach, R.,** Experimental analysis of mouse thymus and spleen morphogenesis, in *The Thymus in Immunobiology*, Good, R.A. and Gabrielsen, A.E., op. cit., 1964, p. 95.

116. **Aspinall, R.L. and Meyer, R.K.,** Effect of steroidal and surgical bursectomy and surgical thymectomy on the skin homograft reaction in chickens, in *The Thymus in Immunobiology*, Good, R.A. and Gabrielsen, A.E., op. cit., 1964, p. 376.

117. **Metcalf, D.,** The thymic origin of the plasma lymphocytosis stimulating factor, *Brit. J. Cancer*, 10, 442, 1956.

118. **Metcalf, D.,** The effect of thymectomy on the lymphoid tissues of the mouse, *Brit. J. Haematol.*, 6, 324, 1960.

119. **Metcalf, D.,** Lymphocyte production and differentiation in the preleukaemic mouse thymus, in *Morphologic Precursors of Cancer*, Severi, L., Ed., Perugia University Press, Perugia, 1962, p. 269.

120. **Metcalf, D.,** A thymus responsive phase in leukaemogenesis in AKR mice, *Nature*, 195, 88, 1962.

121. **Metcalf, D.,** The thymus and lymphopoiesis, in *The Thymus in Immunobiology*, Good, R.A. and Gabrielsen, A.E., op. cit, p. 150, 1964.

122. **Fichtelius, K.E.,** Further studies on the difference between lymphocytes of lymph nodes and thymus, *Acta Haemat.*, 19, 187, 1958.

123. **Fichtelius, K.E.,** On the destination of thymus lymphocytes, in *CIBA Foundation Symposium on Haemopoiesis*, Wolstenholme, G.E.W. and O'Connor, M., Eds., Little, Boston, 1960, p. 204.

124. **Fichtelius, K.E. and Diderholm, H.,** (1959) Transfusion of labelled thymus lymphocytes in rats under secondary resonse to S. thyphi H. antigen. Acta path. et microbiol. scandinav. 47, 304.

125. **Fichtelius, K.E., Diderholm, H. and Stillstrom, J.,** The importance of different lymph nodes in lymphocyte recirculation, *Acta Anat.*, 44, 177, 1961.

126. **Fichtelius, K.E., Laurell, G. and Philipsson, L.,** The influence of thymectomy on antibody formation, *Acta path. et microbiol. Scandinav.*, 51, 81, 1961.

127. **Fichtelius, K.E. and Bryant, B.J.,** On the fate of thymocytes, in *The Thymus in Immunobiology*, Good, R.A. and Gabrielsen, A.E., op. cit., 1964, p. 274.

128. **Peterson, R.D.A., Burmester, B.R., Fredrickson, T.N., Purchase, H.G. and Good, R.A.,** The effect of bursectomy and thymectomy on the development of visceral lymphomatosis in the chicken, *J. Nat. Cancer Inst.*, 32, 1343, 1964.

129. **Peterson, R.D.A., Purchase, H.G., Burmester, B.R., Cooper, M.D. and Good, R.A.,** Relationships among visceral lymphomatosis, the bursa of Fabricius and the bursa-dependent lymphoid tissue of the chicken, *J. Nat. Cancer Inst.*, 36, 585, 1966.

130. **Hilgard, H.R., Sosin, H., Martinez, C. and Good, R.A.,** Specifically increased graft-vs-host reactivity of thymus cells from immunized mice, *Nature*, 207, 208, 1965.

131. **Cooper, M.D., Peterson, R.D.A. and Good, R.A.,** Delineation of the thymic and bursal lymphoid systems in the chicken, *Nature*, 205, 143, 1965.

132. **Cooper, M.D., Peterson, R.D.A. and Good, R.A.,** A new concept of the cellular basis of immunity, *J. Ped.*, 67, 907, 1965b.

133. **Cooper, M.D., Peterson, R.D.A., South, M.A. and Good, R.A.,** The functions of the thymus system and the bursa system in the chicken, *J. Exp. Med.*, 123, 75, 1966.

134. **Warner, N.L., Szenberg, A. and Burnet, F.M.,** The immunological role of different lymphoid organs in the chicken. I. Dissociation of immunological responsiveness, *Australian J. Exper. Biol. & M. Sc.*, 40, 373, 1962.

135. **Cooper, M.D., Perey, D.Y., Peterson, R.D.A., Gabrielsen, A.E. and Good, R.A.,** The two-component concept of the lymphoid system, in *Immunologic Deficiency Diseases in Man*, Bergsma, D. and Good, R.A., op. cit., 1968, p. 7.

136. **Peterson, R.D.A., Cooper and Good, R.A.,** The pathogenesis of immunologic deficiency diseases, *Am. J. Med.*, 38, 579, 1965.

137. **Good, R.A., Peterson, R.D.A., Finstad, J. and Gabrielsen, A.E.,** Morphologic studies of the development of the lymphoid tissues, *Sem. Haematol.*, 8, 1, 1965.

138. **Good, R.A., Gabrielsen, A.E., Finstad, J. and Cooper, M.D.,** Ontogenetic and phylogenetic development of the lymphoid system and relation to immunologic deficiency states, in *Lymph and the Lymphatic Systems: Proceedings*, Charles C. Thomas, Springfield, IL, 1968, p. 130.

139. **Good, R.A.,** Disorders of the immune system, *Hosp. Pract.*, 2, 38, 1967a.

140. **Cooper, M.D., Gabrielsen, A.E. and Good, R.A.,** Role of the thymus and other central lymphoid tissues in immunological disease, *Ann. Rev. Med.*, 18, 113, 1967.

141. **Good, R.A., Gabrielsen, A.E., Cooper, M.D. and Peterson, R.D.A.,** The role of the thymus and bursa of Fabricius in the development of effector mechanisms, *Ann. N.Y. Acad. Sci.*, 129, 130, 1966.

142. **DiGeorge, A.M.,** Discussion (following presentation by M.D. Cooper). Perlman and Good, *J. Ped.*, 67, 908, 1965.

143. **DiGeorge, A.M.,** Congenital absence of the thymus and its immunologic consequences: Concurrence with congenital hypoparathyroidism, in *Immunologic Deficiency Diseases in Man*, Bergsma, D. and Good, R.A., op. cit., 1968, p. 116.

144. Harrington I.H., Absence of thymus gland, *London Med. Gaz.*, (3)314, 1828, 1829.

145. van Alten, P.J., Cain, W.A., Good, R.A. and Cooper, M.D., Gamma globulin production and antibody synthesis in chickens bursectomized as embryos, *Nature*, 217, 358, 1968.

146. Cooper, M.D., Perey, D.Y., Gabrielsen, A.E., Sutherland, D.E.R., McKneally, M.F. and Good, R.A., Production of an antibody deficiency syndrome in rabbits by neonatal removal of organized intestinal lymphoid tissues, *Int. Arch. Allergy*, 33, 65, 1968.

147. Good, R.A., Peterson, R.D.A., Perey, D.Y., Finstad, J. and Cooper, M.D., The immunological deficiency diseaes of man: consideration of some questions asked by these patients with an attempt at classification, in Bergsma, D. and Good, R.A., Eds., op. cit., 1968, p. 17.

148. Hoyer, R., Cooper, M.D., Gabrielsen, A.E. and Good, R.A., Lymphopenic forms of congenital immunologic deficiency: Clinical and pathologic patterns, in *Immunologic Deficiency Diseases in Man*, Bergsma D. and Good, R.A., Eds., op. cit. 1968, p. 91.

149. Good, R.A., and Gabrielsen, A.E., The thymus and other lymphoid organs in the development of the immune system, in *Human Transplantation*, Rapaport, F., Dausset, J., Eds., Grune & Stratton, New York, 1968, p. 526.

150. Good, R.A., Gabrielsen, A.E., Peterson, R.D.A., Finstad, J., and Cooper, M.D., The development of the central and peripheral lymphoid tissue: ontogenetic and phylogenetic considerations, in *The Thymus: Experimental and Clinical Studies; Ciba Foundation Symposium*, Wolstenholme, G.E.W. and Poeter, R., Eds., Little, Brown & Co., Boston, MA, 1966, p. 181.

151. Good, R.A., Miescher, P.A. and Smith, R.T., Nomenclature, therapy and the ethics of investigation: a general discussion and concluding remarks, in *Immunologic Deficiency Diseases in Man*, Bergsma, D. and Good, R.A., op. cit., 1968, p. 459.

152. Glanzmann, E. and Riniker, P., Essentielle lymphozytophthise, *Wien. Med Wochschr.*, 100, 35, 1950.

153. Tobler, R. and Cottier, H., Familiare lymphopenie mit agammaglobulinamie und schwerer moniliasis, *Helvet. Pediatr. Acta*, 13, 313, 1958.

154. Hitzig, W.H. and Willi, H., Hereditare lymphoplasmocytare dysgenesie ("Alymphocytose mit Agammaglobulinamie"), *Schweiz Med Wochschr.*, 91, 1625, 1961.

155. Parrott, D.V.M., De Sousa, M. and East, J., Thymus-dependent areas in the lymphoid organs of neonatally thymectomized mice, *J. Exp. Med.*, 123, 191, 1966.

156. Good, R.A., and Finstad, J., The Gordon Wilson Lecture: The development and involution of the lymphoid system and immunologic capacity, *Trans. Am. Clin. Climatol. Assoc.*, 79, 69, 1967.

157. Good, R.A., and Finstad, J., Relation between structure and function of the lymphoid system. A developmental perspective, in *International Convocation on Immunology: Proceedings*, S. Karger, Buffalo, NY, 1969, p. 52.

158. Bergsma, D. and Good, R.A., Eds. *Immunologic Deficiency Diseases in Man*, in *Birth Defects Original Article Series*, Vol. 4, National Foundation Press, New York, 1968.

159. Moore, M.A.S. and Owen, J.T., Chromosome marker studies on the development of the hematopoietic system in the chick embryo, *Nature*, 208, 956, 1965.

160. Claman, M.N., Chaperon, E.A. and Triplett, R.F., Thymus marrow cell combination; synergism in antibody production, *Proc. Soc. Exp. Biol. Med.*, 122, 1167, 1964.

161. Miller, J.F.A.P. and Mitchell, G.F., Influence of the thymus on antigen-reactive cells and their precursors, in *Advance in Transplantation*, in *Proceedings of the first international congress of the transplantation society*, Dausset, J., Hamburger, J., Mathé, G., Eds., The Williams and Wilkins Company, Baltimore, MD, 1967.

162. Miller, J.F.A.P., Mitchell, G.F. and Weiss, N., Cellular basis of the immunological defects in thymectomized mice, *Nature*, 214, 992, 1967.

163. Berendes, H., Bridges, R.A. and Good, R.A., A fatal granulomatosus of childhood: the clinical study of a new syndrome, *Minn. Med.*, 40, 309, 1957.

164. Bridges, R.A., Berendes, H. and Good, R.A., A fatal granulomatous disease of childhood: the clinical, pathological, and laboratory features of a new syndrome, *A.M.A., J. Dis. Child.*, 97, 387, 1959.

165. Holmes, B., Quie, P.G., Windhorst, D.B. and Good, R.A., Fatal granulomatous disease of childhood: an inborn abnormality of phagocytic function, *Lancet*, 1, 1225, 1966.

166. Holmes, B., Page, A.R. and Good, R.A., Studies of the metabolic activity of leukocytes from patients with a genetic abnormality of phagocytic function, *J. Clin. Invest.*, 47,

1422, 1967.

167. Holmes, B., Page, A.R., Windhorst, D.B., Quie, P.G., White, J.G. and Good, R.A., The metabolic pattern and phagocytic function of leukocytes from children with chronic granulomatous diseases, *Ann. N.Y. Acad. Sci.*, 155, 888, 1968a.

168. Holmes, B., Page, A.R., Windhorst, D.B., Quie, P.G., White, J.G. and Good, R.A., Fatal granulomatous disease: a genetic defect of phagocytic function, in *Immunologic Deficiency Diseases in Man*, Bergsma, D. and Good, R.A., Eds., op. cit., 1968b, p. 433.

169. Quie, P.G., White, J.G., Holmes, B. and Good, R.A., *In vitro* bactericidal capacity of human polymorphonuclear leukocytes: diminished acitvity in chronic granulomatous disease of childhood, *J. Clin. Invest.*, 46, 668, 1967.

170. Windhorst, D.B., Page, A.R., Holmes, B., Quie, P.G. and Good, R.A., The pattern of genetic transmission of the leukocyte defect in fatal granulomatous disease of childhood, *J. Clin. Invest.*, 47, 1026, 1968.

171. Windhorst, D.B., White, J.G., Dent, P.B., Decker, J. and Good, R.A., Defective defense associated with genetic disease of subcellular organelles, in *Immunologic Deficiency Diseases in Man*, Bergsma, D. and Good, R.A., Eds., op. cit., 1968, p. 424.

172. Gewurz, H., Pickering, R.J., Clark, D.S., Page, A.R., Finstad, J. and Good, R.A., The complement system in the prevention, mediation and diagnosis of disease and its usefulness in the determination of immunopathogenetic mechanisms, in *Immunologic Deficiency Diseases in Man*, Bergsma, D. and Good, R.A., Eds., op. cit., 1968a, p. 396.

173. Day, N.K.B., Pickering, R.J., Gewurz, H. and Good, R.A., Ontogenetic development of the complement system, *Immunology*, 16, 319, 1969.

174. Day, N.K., and Good, R.A., Deficiencies of the complement system in man, in *Immunodeficiency in Man and Animals*, Good, R.A., Finstad, J. and Paul, N.W., Eds., in *Birth Defects: Orginal Article Ser.* XI (1), 306, Sinauer Associates, Sunderland, MA, 1975.

175. Hanson, L.A., Aspects of the absence of the IgA system, in *Immunodefiency Diseases in Man*, Bergsma, D. and Good, R.A., op. cit., 1968, p. 298.

176. Hong, R., Pickering, R.J. and Good, R.A., Immunochemical studies in hypogammaglobulinemia, in *Immunologic Deficiency Diseases in Man*, Bergsma, D. and Good, R.A., Eds., op. cit., 1968c, p. 212.

177. South, M.A., Cooper, M.D., Wollheim, F.A. and Good, R.A., The IgA system. II. The clinical significance of IgA deficiency: studies in patients with agammaglobulinemia and ataxia-telangiectasia, *Am. J. Med.*, 44, 168, February, 1968.

178. Holmes, B., Quie, P.G., Windhorst, D.B., Pollara, B. and Good, R.A., Protection of phagocytized bacteria from the killing action of antibiotics, *Nature*, 210, 1131, 1966.

179. Gatti, R.A., Meuwissen, H.J., Allen, H.D., Hong, R. and Good, R.A., Immunolgical reconstitution of sex-linked lymphopenic immunological deficiency, *Lancet*, 2, 1366, 1968.

180. Good, R.A., Immunologic reconstitution: the achievement and its meaning, *Hosp. Practice*, 4, 41, 1969.

181. Meuwissen, H.J., Gatti, R.A., Terasaki, P.I., Hong, R. and Good, R.A., Treatment of lymphopenic hypogammaglobulinemia and bone marrow aplasia by transplantation of allogeneic marrow, *N. Engl. J. Med.*, 382, 691, 1969.

182. Segal, A.W., Cross, A.R., Garcia, R.C., et al., Absence of cytochrome b-245 in chronic granulomatous disease: a multicenter European evaluation of its incidence and relevance, *New Eng. J. Med.*, 308, 245, 1983.

183. Segal, A.W., Absence of both cytochrome b-245 subunits in x-linked chronic granulomatous disease, *Nature* (London), 326, 88, 1987.

184. Dinauer, M.C., Orkin, S.H., Brown, R., et al., The glycoprotein encoded by the X-linked chronic granulomatous disease locus is a component of the neutrophil cytochrome b complex, *Nature* (London), 327, 717, 1987.

185. Dinauer, M.C. and Orkin, S.H., Molecular genetics of chronic granulomatous disease, *Immunodeficiency Reviews* 1, 55, 1988.

186. Mayer, M.M., Complement and complement fixation, in *Experimental Immunochemistry*, Kabat, E.A., Ed., Charles C. Thomas, Springfield, IL, 1961, p. 113.

187. Mayer, M.M., Mechanism of haemolysis by complement, in *Complement*, Ciba Foundation Symposium, 1964, p. 4.

188. **Nelson, R.A., Jr.,** The role of complement in immune phenomena, in *The Inflammatory Process*, Zweifach, B.W., Grant, L., McCluskey, R.T., Eds., Academic Press, New York, 1965.

189. **Nelson, R.A., Jr., Jensen, J., Gigli, I. and Tamura, N.,** Methods for the separation purification and measurement of nine components of hemolytic complement in guinea pig serum, *Immunochemistry*, 3, 111, 1966.

190. **Müller-Eberhard, H.J., Nilsson, U.R., Dalmasso, A.P., Polley, M.J. and Calcott, M.A.,** A molecular concept of immune cytolysis, *Arch. Path.*, 82, 217, 1966.

191. **Gewurz, H., Finstad, J., Muschel, L.H. and Good R.A.,** Phylogenetic inquiry into the origins of the complement system, in *Phylogeny of Immunity*, Smith, R.T., Miescher, P.A. and Good, R.A., Eds., University of Florida Press, Gainesville, FL, 1966, p. 105.

192. **Gewurz, H., Pickering, R.J., Muschel, L.H., Mergenhagen, S.E. and Good, R.A.,** Complement-dependent biological functions in complement deficiency in man, *Lancet*, ii, 356, 1966.

193. **Gewurz, H., Pickering, R.J., Christian, C.L., Snyderman, R., Mergenhagen, S.E. and Good, R.A.,** Decreased C'1, protein concentration and agglutinating activity in agammaglobulinaemia syndromes: an inborn error reflected in the complement system, *Clin. Exp. Immunol.*, 3, 437, 1968b.

194. **Gewurz, H., Pickering, R.J. and Good, R.A.,** Complement and complement component activities in diseases associated with repeated infections and malignancy, *Int. Arch. Allergy*, 33, 368, 1968c.

195. **Gewurz, H., Shin, H.S., Pickering, R.J., Snyderman, R., Lichtenstein, L.M., Good, R.A. and Mergenhagen, S.E.,** Interactions of the complement system with endotoxic lipopolysaccharides: complement-membrane interactions and endotoxic-induced inflammation, in *Cellular Recognition*, Smith, R.T. and Good, R.A., Eds., Appleton-Century-Crofts, New York, 1969, p. 305.

196. **Pickering, R.J., Naff, G.B., Stroud, R.M., Good, R.A. and Gewurz, H.,** Deficiency of C1r in human serum: effects on the structure and function of macromolecular C1, *J. Exp. Med.*, 141, 803, 1970.

197. **Pickering, R.J., Michael, A.F., Jr., Herdman, R.C., Good, R.A. and Gewurz, H.,** The complement system in chronic glomerulonephritis: three newly associated aberrations, *J. Pediatr.*, 78, 30, 1971.

198. **Day, N.K., Geiger, H., Stroud, R., deBracco, M.M.E., Moncada, B., Windhorst, D., and Good, R.A.,** C1r deficiency. An inborn error associated with cutaneous and renal disease, *J. Clin. Invest.*, 51, 1102, 1972.

199. **Day, N.K., Geiger, H., McLean, R., Michael, A. and Good, R.A.,** C2 deficiency: development of lupus erythematosus, *J. Clin. Invest.*, 52, 1601, 1973.

200. **Day, N.K., Geiger, H., McLean, R., Resnick, J., Michael, A. and Good, R.A.,** The association of respiratory infection, recurrent hematuria, and focal glomerulonephritis with activation of the complement system in the cold, *J. Clin. Invest.*, 52, 1698, 1973.

201. **Day, N.K., Moncada, B. and Good, R.A.,** Inherited deficiencies of the complement system, in *Biological Amplification Systems in Immunology*, Day, N.K. and Good, R.A., Eds., Vol. 2, Comprehensive Immunology Series, Plenum Press, New York, 1977, p. 229.

202. **Silverstein, A.M.,** Essential hypocomplementemia: report of a case, *Blood*, 16, 1338, 1960.

203. **Klemperer, M.R., Woodworth, H.C., Rosen, F.S. and Austen, K.F.,** Hereditary deficiency of the second component of human complement: Transmission as an autosomal codominant trait, *J. Lab. Clin. Med.*, 66, 886, 1965.

204. **Klemperer, M.R., Woodworth, H.C., Rosen, F.S. and Austen, K.F.,** Hereditary deficiency of the second component of complement (C'2) in man, *J. Clin. Invest.*, 45, 880, 1966.

205. **Alper, C.A., Abramson, N., Johnston, R.B., Jr., Jandl, J.H., and Rosen, F.S.,** Increased susceptibility to infection associated with abnormalities of complement-mediated functions and of the third component of complement (C3), *N. Engl. J. Med.*, 282, 349, 1970.

206. **Alper, C.A., Colten, H.R., Rosen, F.S., Rabson, A.R., Macnab, G.M., and Gear, J.S.S.,** Homozygous deficiency of the third component of complement (C3) in a patient with repeated infections, *Lancet*, 2, 1179, 1972.

207. **Alper, C.A., Colten, H.R., Gear, J.S.S., Rabson, A.R., and Rosen, F.S.,** Homozygous

C3 deficiency. The role of C3 in antibody production, C1s-induced vasopermeability, and cobra venom reduced passive hemolysis, *J. Clin. Invest.*, 57, 222, 1976.

208.   **Alper, C.A., Rosen, F.S.**, Studies of the *in vivo* behavior of human C3 in normal subjects and patients, *J. Clin. Invest.*, 46, 2021, 1967.

209.   **Miller, M.E., Seals, J., Kaje, R., and Levitsky, L.C.**, A familial plasma-associated defect of phagocytosis. A new cause of recurrent bacterial infections, *Lancet* 2, 60, July, 1968.

210.   **Miller, M.E. and Nilsson, U.R.**, A familial deficiency of the phagocytosing enhancing activity of serum related to a C5 dysfunction of the fifth component of complement (C5), *N. Engl. J. Med.*, 282, 354, 1970.

211.   **Day, N.K., L'Esperance, P., Good, R.A., Michael, A.F., Hansen, J.A., Dupont, B., and Jersild, C.**, Hereditary C2 deficiency: Genetic studies and association with the HL-A system, *J. Exp. Med.*, 141, 1464, 1975b.

212.   **Good, R.A.**, Immunodeficiency in developmental perspective, *Harvey Lect.*, 67, 1, 1973.

213.   **Agnello, V., de Bracco, M.M.E., and Kunkel, H.G.**, Hereditary C2 deficiency with some manifestations of systemic *lupus erythematosus*, *J. Immunol.*, 108, 837, 1972.

214.   **Agnello, V., Ruddy, S., Winchester, R.J., Christian, C.L. and Kunkel, H.G.**, Hereditary C2 deficiency in systemic *lupus erythematosus* and acquired complement abnormalities in an unusual SLE-related syndrome, in *Immunodeficiency in Man and Animals*, Good, R.A., Finstad, J. and Paul, N.W., Eds., in *Birth Defects: Original Article Ser.*, XI(1), 312, Sinauer Associates, Sunderland, MA, 1975.

215.   **Ross, S.C. and Densen, P.**, Complement deficiency states and infection: Epidemiology, pathogenesis and consequences of Neisserial and other infections in an immune deficiency, *Medicine*, 63, 243, 1984.

216.   **Sjöholm, A.G., Braconier, J.H. and Söderström, C.**, Properdin deficiency in a family with fulminant meningococcal infections, *Clin. Exp. Immunol.*, 50, 291, 1982.

217.   **Densen, P., Weiler, J., Griffis, M., and Hoffmann, L.G.**, Familial proferdin deficiency and fatal meningococcemia, *N. Eng. J. Med.*, 316, 922, 1987.

218.   **Miller, J.F.A.P.**, Effect of thymic ablation and replacement, in *The Thymus in Immunobiology*, Good, R.A. and Gabrielsen, A.E., Eds., op. cit., 1964a, p. 436.

219.   **Cleveland, W.W., Fogel, B.J., Brown, W.T. and Kay, H.E.**, Foetal thymic transplant in a case of DiGeorge's syndrome, *Lancet*, 2, 1211, 1968.

220.   **August, C.S., Rosen, F.S., Filler, R.M. et al.**, Implantation of a foetal thymus restoring imunological competence in a patient with thymic aplasia (DiGeorge's syndrome), *Lancet*, 2, 1210, 1968.

221.   **Biggar, W.D., Good, R.A. and Park, B.H.**, Immunologic reconstitution of a patient with combined immunodeficiency disease, *J. Pediatr.*, 81, 301, 1972.

222.   **Hong, R., Gatti, R.A. and Good, R.A.**, Hazards and potential benefits of blood transfusion in immunological deficiency, *Lancet*, 2, 388, 1968a.

223.   **Barandun, S., Huser, H.J. and Hassig, A.**, Klinishce erscheinungsformen des antikorpermangelsyndroms, *Schweiz. med. Wschr.*, 88, 78, 1958.

224.   **Barandun, S., Kistler, P., Jeunet, F., Isliker, H.**, Intravenous administration of human gamma globulin, *Vox Sang.*, 7, 157, 1962.

225.   **Barandun, S.**, Die gammaglobulintherapie, *Bibl. haemat. fasc.*, 17, Basel, S. Karger, 1964.

226.   **Barandun, S., Cottier, H., Hassig, A. and Riva, G.**, *Das Antikorpermangelsyndrom*, Basel/Stuttgart, Benno Schwabe & Co., 1959.

227.   **Barandun, S., Riva, G. and Spengler, G.A.**, Immunologic deficiency diagnosis, forms and current treatment, in *Immunologic Deficiency Diseases in Man*, Bergsma, D. and Good, R.A., op. cit., 1968, p. 40.

228.   **Cunningham-Rundles, C., Siegal, F.P., Smithwick, E.M., Lion-Boulé, A., Cunningham-Rundles, S., O'Malley, J., Barandun, S. and Good, R.A.**, Efficacy of intravenous immunoglobulin in primary humoral immunodeficiency disease, *Ann. Intern. Med.*, 101(4), 435, 1984.

229.   **Hong, R., Kay, H.E.M., Cooper, M.D., Meuwissen, H., Allan, M.J.G. and Good, R.A.**, Immunologic restitution in lymphopenic immunologic deficiency syndrome, *Lancet*, 1, 503, 1968b.

230.   **Coifman, R.E., Good, R.A. and Meuwissen, H.J.**, The function of irradiated blood elements. I. Limitations on the response to phytohemagglutinin as an indicator of immunocompetence in irradiated lymphocytes, *Proc. Soc. Exp. Biol. Med.*, 137,

155, 1971.

231. Gorer, P.A., The genetic and antigenic basis of tumour transplantation, *J. Path. Bact.*, 44, 691, 1937.

232. Gorer, P.A., The antigenic basis of tumour transplantation, *J. Path. Bact.*, 47, 231, 1938.

233. Gorer, P.A., Lyman, S., and Snell, G.D., Studies on the genetic and antigenic basis of tumour transplantation. *Proc. Roy. Soc. London*, (B)135, 499, 1948.

234. Snell, G.E., Russell, E., Fekete, E. and Smith P.,, Resistance of various inbred strains of mice to tumor homotransplants and its relation to the H-2 locus which each carries, *J. Natl. Cancer. Inst.*, 14, 485, 1953.

235. Snell, G.D. and Stimpfling, J.H., Genetics of tissue transplantation, in *Biology of the Laboratory Mouse*, Green, E.L., Ed., McGraw-Hill, New York, 1966.

236. Aust, J.B., Martinez, C., Bittner, J.J. and Good, R.A., Tolerance in pure strain newborn mice to tumor homograts, *Proc. Soc. Exp. Biol. Med.*, 92, 27, 1956.

237. Aust, J.B., Martinez, C., Bittner, J.J. and Good, R.A., Tumor homotransplantation in inbred mice during the newborn period, Vol. III, *Surgical Forum*, 478, 1957.

238. Shapiro, F., Martinez, C., Smith, J.M. and Good, R.A., Homologous skin transplantation from F1 hybrid mice to parent strains, *Proc. Soc. Exp. Biol. Med.*, 101, 94, 1959.

239. Shapiro, F., Martinez, C., Smith, J.M. and Good, R.A., Tolerance of skin homografts induced in adult mice by multiple injections of homologous spleen cells, *Proc. Soc. Exp. Biol. Med.*, 106, 742, 1961.

240. Mariani, T., Martinez, C., Smith, J.M. and Good, R.A., Induction of immunological tolerance to male skin isografts in female mice subsequent to the neonatal period, *Proc. Soc. Exp. Biol. Med.*, 101, 596, 1959.

241. Martinez, C., Aust, J.B. and Good, R.A., Acquired tolerance to ovarian homografts in castrated mice, *Transplant Bull.*, 3, 128, 1956.

242. Martinez, C., Smith, J.M. and Good, R.A., Acquired tolerance to homologous transplantation of endocrine glands in inbred strains of mice, *Br. J. Exp. Pathol.*, 39, 574, 1958.

243. Martinez, C., Smith, J.M., Shapiro, F. and Good, R.A., Transfer of acquired immunologic tolerance of skin homografts in mice joined in parabiosis, *Proc. Soc. Exp. Biol. Med.*, 102, 413, 1959.

244. Martinez, C., Shapiro, F. and Good, R.A., Essential duration of parabiosis and development of tolerance to skin homografts in man, *Proc. Soc. Exp. Biol. Med.*, 104, 256, 1960.

245. Martinez, C., Shapiro, F., Kelman, H., Onstad, T. and Good, R.A., Tolerance of F1 hybrid skin homografts in the parent strain induced by parabiosis, *Proc. Soc. Exp. Biol. Med.*, 103, 266, 1960.

246. Yunis, E.J., Martinez, C. and Good, R.A., Studies on immunologic reconstitution of thymectomized mice, *Proc. Soc. Exp. Biol. Med.*, 121, 607, 1967.

247. Stutman, O., Yunis, E.J., Martinez, C. and Good, R.A., Reversal of post-thymectomy wasting disease in mice by multiple thymus grafts, *J. Immunol.*, 98, 79, 1967.

248. Stutman, O., Yunis, E.J. and Good, R.A., Reversal of post-thymectomy wasting in mice with immunocompetent cells: influence of histocompatibility differences, *J. Immunol.*, 102, 87, 1969.

249. Terasaki, P.I., Marchioro, T.L. and Starzl, T.E., Serotyping of human lymphocyte antigens. II. Preliminary trials on long term kidney homograft survivors, in *Histocompatibility Testing*, Nat. Acad. Sci., 1965.

250. Terasaki, P.I., Vredevoe, D.L., Porter, K.A., Mickey, M.R., Marchioro, T.L., Faris, T.D., Herrmann, T.J. and Starzl, T.E., Serotyping for homotransplantation. V. Evaluation of a matching scheme, *Transplantation*, 4, 688, 1966.

251. Dausset, J., Leuko-agglutinin IV leukoagglutinins and blood transfusion, *Vox Sang.*, 4, 190, 1954.

252. Dausset, J., Iso-leuko anticorps, *Acta haemat.*, 20, 156, 1958.

253. van Rood, J.J., van Leeuwen, A., Schippers, M.J., Vooys, W.H., Fredericks, E., Balner, H. and Eernisse, J.G., Leukocyte groups, the normal lymphocyte transfer test and homograft sensitivity, in *Histocompatibility Testing*, p. 37. Series *Haematologica* 11, Munksgaard, Copenhagen, 1965.

254. van Rood, J.J., Leucocyte groups and histocompatibility, *Vox Sang* 11, 276, 1966.

255. Amos, D.B., Hutchin, P., Hattler, B.G., McCloskey, R., and Zmijewski, C.M., Skin donor selectin by leukocyte typing, *Lancet*, 1, 300, 1966.

256.   **Amos, D.B., Hattler, B.G., MacQueen, J.M., Cohen, I., and Seigler, H.F.,** An interpretation and application of cytotoxicity typing, in *Advance in Transplantation*, Proceedings of the First International Congress of the Transplantation Society, Dausset, J., Hamburger, J., Mathé, G., Eds., The Williams and Wilkins Company, Baltimore, MD, 1967.

257.   **Good, R.A., Gatti, R.A., Hong, R. and Meuwissen, H.J.,** Successful marrow transplantation for correction of immunological deficit in lymphopenic agammaglobulinemia and treatment of immunologically induced pancytopenia, *Exp. Hematol.*, 19, 4, 1969b.

258.   **Good, R.A., Gatti, R.A., Meuwissen, H.J., and Stutman, O.,** Treatment and analysis of the DiGeorge syndrome, *Lancet*, 1, 946, May 3, 1969, (Letters to the Editor).

259.   **Good, R.A., Meuwissen, H.J., Hong, R., and Gatti, R.A.,** Bone marrow transplantation: correction of immune deficit in lymphopenic immunologic deficiency and correction of an immunologically induced pancytopenia, *Trans. Assoc. Am. Physicians*, 82, 278, 1969.

260.   **Bach, F.H. and Hirschhorn, K.,** Lymphocyte interaction: a potential histocompatibility test *in vitro*, *Science*, 143, 813, 1964.

261.   **Bach, F.H. and Voynow, N.K.,** One way stimulation in mixed leukocyte reaction, *Science*, 153, 545, 1966.

262.   **Bach, F.H., Albertini, R.J., Joo, P., Anderson, J.L.X., and Bortin, M.M.,** Bone marrow transplantation in a patient with Wiskott-Aldrich syndrome, *Lancet*, 2, 1364, 1968.

263.   **Bain, B., Vas, M.R. and Lowenstein, L.,** The development of large immature mononuclear cells in mixed leukocyte culture, *Blood*, 23, 108, 1964.

264.   **Bain, B. and Lowenstein, L.,** Genetic studies on mixed leukocyte reaction, *Science*, 156, 1506, 1967.

265.   **Yunis, E.J., Fernandes, G., Smith, J. and Good, R.A.,** Long survival and immunologic reconstitution following transplantation with syngeneic or allogeneic fetal liver and neonatal spleen cells, in *Immunobiology of Bone Marrow Transplantation*, Dupont, B. and Good, R.A., Eds., Grune & Stratton, New York, 1976, p. 173.

266.   **Good, R.A., Gatti, R.A., Hong, R. and Meuwissen, H.J.,** Graft treatment of immunological deficiency, *Lancet*, 1, 1162, June 7, 1969a, (Letters to the Editor).

267.   **Simonsen, M,** The impact on the developing embryo and newborn animal of adult homologous cells, *Acta. Path. Microbiol. Scand.*, 40, 480, 1957.

268.   **Simonsen, M., Engelbreth-Holm, J., Jensen, E. and Poulsen, H.,** A study of the graft-vs-host reaction in transplantation to embryos, F1 hybrids and irradiated animals, in *Annals of the New York Academy of Sciences*, Whitelock, O., Furness, F. and Sturgeon, P., Eds., Vol. 73, Art 3, 1958, p. 834.

269.   **Simonsen, M.,** Graft vs. host reactions. Their natural history and applicability as tools of research, *Prog. Allergy*, 6, 349, 1962.

270.   **Meuwissen, H.J., Rodey, G., McArthur, J., Pabst, H., Gatti, R., Chilgren, R., Hong, R., Frommel, D., Coifman, R. and Good, RA.,** Bone marrow transplantation. Therapeutic usefulness and complications, *Am. J. Med.*, 51, 513, 1971.

271.   **Touraine, J.L., Griscelli, C., Vossen, J., Hitzig, W.H., Hobbs, J.R., Hugh-Jones, K., Stoop, J.W., Zegers, B.J.M. and Fasth, A.,** Fetal tissue transplnatation for severe combined immunodeficiency; European experience, *Transplant Proc.*, 15, 1427, 1983.

272.   **O'Reilly, R.J., Kirkpatrick, D., Kapoor, N., Collins, N., Brochstein, J., Kernan, N., Flomenberg, N., Pollack, M., Dupont, B., Lopez, C. and Reisner, Y.,** A comparative review of the results of transplants of fully allogeneic fetal liver and HLA-haplotype mismatched, T cell depleted marrow in the treatment of severe combined immunodeficiency, in *Fetal Liver Transplantation*, Gale, R.P., Touraine, J.L., and Lucarelli, G., Eds., Alan R. Liss, Inc., New York, 1985, p. 327.

273.   **Good, R.A., O'Reilly, R.J. and West, A.,** Cellular engineering in immunodeficiency diseases, in *Thymus, Thymic Hormones and T Lymphocytes: Proceedings of the Seronon Symposia*, Vol. 38, Aiuti, A. and Wigzell, H., Eds., Academic Press, New York, 1980, p. 339.

274.   **deKoning, J., Dooren, L.J., van Bekkum, D.W. et al.,** Transplantation of bone marrow cells and fetal thymus in an infant with lymphopenic immunological deficiency, *Lancet*, 1, 1232, 1969.

275.   **Thomas, E.D., Bryant, J.I., Buckner, E.D., Cleft, R.A., Fefer, A., Johnson, F.L., Numan, P., Kamberg, R.E. and Storb, R.,** Leukaemic transformation of engraften human marrow cells *in vivo*, *Lancet*, 1, 1310, 1972.

276. **Good, R.A.,** Toward safer marrow transplantation, *J. Clin. Immunol.*, 2(2) Suppl., 5S, April, 1982.

277. **Good, R.A.,** Progress in bone marrow transplantation, in *Genetic Disease: Diagnosis and Treatment*, in *Proceedings of the Fifth A.O. Beckman Conference in Clinical Chemistry*, Dietz, A.A., Ed., American Association for Clinical Chemistry, Washington, D.C., 1983a, p. 263.

278. **Good, R.A.,** Immunologic reconstitution: Achievements and potentials, in *The Biology of Immunologic Diseases*, Dixon, F. and Fisher, D., Eds., Sinauer, Sunderland, MA, 1983b, p. 359.

279. **Good, R.A., Kapoor, N. and Reisner, Y.,** Bone marrow transplantation—An expanding approach to treatment of many diseases, *Cell. Immunol.*, 82, 36, 1983.

280. **Kapoor, N., Good, R.A.,** Bone marrow transplantation in 1985, in *Recent Advances in Primary and Acquired Immunodeficiencies*, Aiuti, F., Rosen, F. and Cooper, M.D., Eds., Raven Press, New York, 1986, p. 327.

281. **Krivit, W., Whitley, C.B., Chang, P.N., Shapiro, E., Belani, K., Snover, D., Summers, C.G. and Blazar, B.,** Lysosomal storage diseases treated by bone marrow transplantation: Review of 21 patients, in *Bone Marrow Transplantation in Children*, Johnson, F.L. and Pochedly, C., Eds., Raven Press, New York, 1990, p. 261.

282. **Koch, C., Herriksen, K., Juhl, F., Wiik, A., Faber, V., Andersen, V., Dupont, B., Hansen, G.S., Svejgaard, A., Thomsen, M., Ernst, P., Killmann, S.A., Good, R.A., Jensen, K. and Müller-Berat, N.,** (Copenhagen Study Group of Immunodeficiencies): Bone-marrow transplantation from an HL-A non-identical but mixed-lymphocyte-culture identical donor, *Lancet*, 1, 1146, 1973.

283. **Hansen, J.A., O'Reilly, R.J., Good, R.A. and Dupont, B.,** Relevance of major human histocompatibility determinants in clinical bone marrow transplantation, *Transplant. Proc.*, 8, 581, December, 1976.

284. **Dupont, B., Andersen, V., Ernst, P., Faber, V., Good, R.A. et al.,** Immunologic reconstitution in severe combined immunodeficiency with HLA-incompatible bone marrow graft. Donor selection by mixed lymphocyte culture, *Transplant. Proc.*, 5, 905, 1973.

285. **O'Reilly, R.J., Dupont, B., Pahwa, S. et al.,** Reconstitution in severe combined immunodeficiency by transplantation of marrow from an unrelated donor, *N. Engl. J. Med.*, 297, 1311, 1977.

286. **Reisner, Y., Itzicovitch, L., Meshorer, A. and Sharon, N.,** Hemopoietic stem cell transplantation using mouse bone marrow and spleen cells fractionated by lectins, *Proc. Natl. Acad. Sci. USA*, 75, 2933, 1978.

287. **Reisner, Y., and Sharon, N.,** Cell fractionation by lectins, *Trends Biochem. Sci.*, 5, 29, 1980.

288. **Onoé, K., Fernandes, G. and Good, R.A.,** Humoral and cell-mediated immune responses in fully allogeneic bone marrow chimera in mice, *J. Exp. Med.*, 151, 115, 1980.

289. **Krown, S.E., Coico, R., Scheid, M.P., Fernandes, G. and Good, R.A.,** Immune function in fully allogeneic mouse bone marrow chimeras, *Clin. Immunol. Immunopathol.*, 19, 268, 1981.

290. **Reisner, Y., O'Reilley, R.J., Kapoor, N., and Good, R.A.,** Allogeneic bone marrow transplantation using stem cells fractionated by lectins: VI, *in vitro* analysis of human and monkey bone marrow cells fractionated by sheep red blood cells and soybean agglutinin, *Lancet*, 2, 1320, 1980.

291. **Reisner, Y., Kapoor, N., Hodes, M.Z. et al.,** Enrichment for CFU-C from murine and human bone marrow using soybean agglutinin, *Blood*, 59, 360, 1982.

292. **Reisner, Y., Kapoor, N., Kirkpatrick, D. et al.,** Transplantation for acute leukemia with HLA-A and -B nonidentical parental marrow cells fractionated with soybean agglutinin and sheep red blood cells, *Lancet*, 2, 327, 1981.

293. **Reisner, Y., Kapoor, N., Kirkpatrick, D., Pollack, M.S., Cunningham-Rundles, S., Dupont, B., Hodes, M.S., Good, R.A. and O'Reilly, R.J.,** Transplantation for severe combined immunodeficiency with HLA A, B, D, Dr incompatible parental marrow cells fractionated by soybean agglutinin and sheep red blood cells, *Blood*, 61, 341, 1983.

294. **Buckley, R.H., Schiff, S.E., Sampson, H.A., Schiff, R.I., Markert, M.L., Knutsen, A.P., Hershfield, M.S., Huang, A.T., Mickey, G.H., and Ward, F.E.,** Development of immunity in human severe primary T-cell deficiency following haploidentical bone marrow stem cell transplantation, *J. Immunol.*, 136, 2398, 1986.

295. **Tyan, M.L.,** Modification of severe graft-vs-host-disease with antisera to the O antigen or to whole serum, *Transplantation*, 15, 601, 1973.

296. **Sprent, J., von Boehmer, H. and Nabholz, M.,** Association of immunity and tolerance to host H-2 determinants in irradiated F1 hybrid mice reconstituted with bone marrow cells from one parental strain, *J. Exp. Med.*, 141, 322, 1975.

297. **Von Boehmer, H., Sprent, J. and Nabholz,** Hematopoietic reconstitution obtained in F1 hybrids by grafting of parental marrow cells, in *Immunobiology of Bone Marrow Transplantation*, Dupont, B., Good, R.A. Eds., Grune & Stratton, New York, 1976, p. 29.

298. **Onoé, K., Yasumizu, R., Oh-ishi, T., Kakinuma, M., Good, R.A. and Morikawa, K.,** Restricted antibody formation to sheep erythrocytes of allogeneic bone marrow chimeras histoincompatible at the K end of the H-2 complex, *J. Exp. Med.*, 153, 1009. 1981.

299. **Onoé, K., Fernandes, G., Shen, F.W. and Good, R.A.,** Sequential changes of thymocyte surface antigens with presence or absence of graft-vs-host reaction following allogeneic bone marrow transplantation, *Cell. Immunol.*, 68, 207, 1982.

300. **Noguchi, M., Onoe, K., Ogasawara, M., Iwabuchi, K., Geng, L., Ogasawara, K., Good, R.A. and Morikawa, K.,** H-2 incompatible bone marrow chimeras produce donor-H-2 restricted Ly-2 suppressor T cell factor (s), *Proc. Natl. Acad. Sci.* USA, 82, 7063, 1985.

301. **Onoé, K., Yasumizu, R., Geng, L., Iwabuchi, K., Ogasawara, M., Kakinuma, M., Okuyama, H., Good, R.A. and Morikawa, K.,** Analyses of Ia restriciton specificity of helper T cells in H-2 subregion compatible bone marrow chimera in mice, *Immunobiology*, 169, 71, 1985.

302. **Onoé, K., Yasumizu, R., Noguchi, M., Noguchi, M., Iwabuchi, K., Ogasawara, M., Kakinuma, M., Okuyama, H., Good, R.A. and Morikawa, K.,** Analyses of H-2 restriction specificity of helper T cells in fully allogeneic bone marrow chimera in mice, *Immunobiology*, 169, 60, 1985.

303. **Onoé, K., Good, R.A. and Yamamoto, K.** (1985) Anti-bacterial immunity to Listeria monocytogenes in allogeneic bone marrow chimera in mice. J. Immunol. 136, 4264-4269.

304. **Iwabuchi, K., Ogasawara, K., Ogasawara, M., Yasumizu, R., Noguchi, M., Geng, L., Fujita, M., Good, R.A. and Onoé, K.,** A study on proliferative responses to host Ia antigens in allogeneic bone marrow chimera in mice: sequential analysis of the reactivity and characterization of the cells involved in the responses, *J. Immunol.*, 138, 18, 1987.

305. **Iwai, H., Yasumizu, R., Sugiura, K., Inaba, M., Kumazawa, T., Good, R.A. an dIkehara, S.,** Successful pancreatic allografts in combination with bone marrow transplantation in mice, *Immunology*, 62, 457, 1987.

306. **Ogasawara, M., Iwabuchi, K., Geng, L., Good, R.A. and Onoe, K.,** Bone marrow cells from allogeneic bone marrow chimeras inhibit the generation of cytotoxic lymphocyte responses against both donor and recipient cells, *J. Immunol.*, 141, 3306, 1988.

307. **Iwabuchi, K., Katsume, C., Arase, H., Hatakeyama, S., Ogasawara, K., Good, R.A. and Onoée, K.,** A T-cell subpopulation positively selected in the thymus where it develops, *Proc. Natl. Acad. Sci.* USA, 86, 5089, 1989.

308. **Nakamura, T., Good, R.A., Yasumizu, R., Inoe, S., Oo, M.M., Hamashima, Y. and Ikehara, S.,** Successful liver allografts in mice by combination with allogeneic bone marrow transplantation, *Proc. Natl. Acad. Sci.* USA, 83, 4529, 1986.

309. **Ikehara, S., Good, R.A., Nakamura, T., Sekita, K., Inoue, S., Oo, M.M., Muso, E., Ogawa, K. and Hamashima, Y.,** Rationale for bone marrow transplantation in the treatment of autoimmune diseases, *Proc. Natl. Acad. Sci.* USA, 82, 2483, 1985.

310. **Ikehara, S., Ohtsuki, H., Good, R.A., Asamoto, H., Nakamura, T., Sekita, K., Muso, E., Tochino, Y., Ida, T. and Kuzuya, H.,** Prevention of type I diabetes in non-obese diaetic mice by allogenic bone marrow transplantation, *Proc. Natl. Acad. Sci.* USA, 82, 7743, 1985.

311. **Yasumizu, R., Sugiura, K., Iwai, H., Inaba, M., Makino, S., Ida, T., Imura, H., Hamashima, Y., Good, R.A. and Ikehara, S.,** Treatment of type 1 diabetes mellitus in non-obese diabetic mice by transplantation of allogeneic bone marrow and pancreatic tissue, *Proc. Natl. Acad. Sci.* USA, 84, 6555, 1987.

312. **Yasumizu, R., Hiai, H., Sugiura, K., Oyaizu, N., Hongxue, F., Ohnishi, Y., Inaba, M., Kakinuma, M., Onoé, K., Good, R.A. and Ikehara, S.,** Development of donor-derived thymic lymphomas after allogeneic bone marrow transplantation in AKR/J mice, *J. Immunol.*, 141, 2181, 1988.

313. **Oyaizu, N., Yasumizu, R., Miyama-Inaba, M., Nomura, S., Yoshida, Y., Shigeki, M., Shibata, Y., Mitsuoka, M., Kojiro, Y., Morii, S., Good, R.A. and Ikehara, S.,** (NZW-BXSB)F1 mouse, a new model of idiopathic thrombocytopenic purpura, *J. Exp. Med.*, 167, 2017, 1988.

314. **Ikehara, S., Yasumizu, R., Inaba, M., Izui, S., Hayakawa, K., Sekita, K., Toki, J., Sugiura, K., Iwai, H., Nakamura, T., Muso, E., Hamashima, Y. and Good, R.A.,** Long-term observations of autoimmune-prone mice treated for autoimmune disease by allogeneic bone marrow transplantation, *Proc. Natl. Acad. Sci.* USA, 86, 3306, 1989.

315. **Ikehara, S., Kawamura, M., Takao, F., Inaba, M., Yasumizu, R., Than, S., Hisba, H., Koide, Y., Yoshida, T., Ida, T., Imura, H. and Good, R.A.,** Etiopathogenesis of organ-specific and systemic autoimmune diseases resides in abnormalities at stem cell level, In press, *Proc. Natl. Acad. Sci.* USA.

316. **Good, R.A. and de la Morena, D.,** unpublished data.

317. **Wustrow, T.P., Andreeff, M., Fernandes, G. and Good, R.A.,** DNA and RNA analysis by flow cytometry of the leukemia in AKR mice, *Leuk. Res.*, 9, 1283, 1985.

318. **Wustrow, T.P., Good, R.A.,** Expression of antigens coded in murine leukemia viruses on thymocytes of allogeneic donor origin in AKR mice following syngeneic or allogeneic bone marrow transplantation, *Cancer Res.*, 45, 6428, 1985.

319. **Wustrow, T.P., Katopodis, N., Stock, C.C. and Good, R.A.,** Prevention of leukemia and the increase of plasma levels of lipid-bound sialic acid by allogeneic bone marrow transplantation in mice, *Cancer Res.*, 45, 1097, 1985.

320. **Sardiña, E.E., Sugiura, K., Lay, S. and Good, R.A.,** Wheat germ agglutinin positive (WGA+), low density cells contain progrnitors capable of transferring or correcting autoimmune disease in lethally irradiated, histocompatible autoimmune disease in lethally irradiated, histocompatible mice (Selected for oral presentation), *FASEB J.* 4(4)A, 1133, 1990.

321. **Sardiña, E.E.,** Hematopoietic stem cell transfer in mice demonstrates the pivotal role of stem cells in the development of systemic autoimmune disease, Doctoral dissertation, University of South Florida, 1990.

322. **Sardiña, E.E., Good, R.A., Sugiura, K. and Ikehara, S.,** In press, *Proc. Natl. Acad. Sci.* USA, 1990.

323. **Good, R.A.,** Cellular engineering, in *Varieties of Academic Experience: A Series of Seminars*, Department of Chemical Engineering, University of Minnesota, Minneapolis, 1970a, p. 35.

324. **Good, R.A.,** Progress toward a cellular engineering (Lasker Award Lecture), *J. Am. Med. Assoc.*, 214, 1289, 1970b.

325. **Good, R.A., Finstad, J. and Gatti, R.A.,** Bulwarks of the bodily defense, in *Infectious Agents and Host Reactions*, Mudd, S., Ed., W.B. Saunders, Philadelphia, 1970, p. 76.

326. **Fichtelius, K.E., Finstad, J. and Good, R.A.,** Bursa equivalents of bursaless vertebrates, *Lab. Invest.*, 19, 339, 1968.

327. **Archer, O.K., Sutherland, D.E.R. and Good, R.A.,** Appendix of the rabbit: a homologue of the bursa in the chicken? *Nature*, 200, 337, 1963.

328. **Archer, O.K., Sutherland, D.E.R. and Good, R.A.,** The developmental biology of lymphoid tissue in the rabbit. Consideration of the role of thymus and appendix, *Lab. Invest.*, 13, 259, 1964.

329. **Cooper, M.D., Perey, D.Y., McKneally, M.F., Gabrielsen, A.E., Sutherland, D.E.R. and Good, R.A.,** A mammalian equivalent of the avian bursa of Fabricius, *Lancet*, 1, 1388, June 25, 1966.

330. **Cebra, J.J., Kamat, R., Gearhart, P., Robertson, S.M. and Tseng, J.,** The secretory IgA system of the gut, in *Immunology of the Gut*, Ciba Fed. Symp., 46, Amsterdam Alsever/Exerpta Medica North Holland, 1977, p. 5.

331. **Hanson, L.A. and Brandtzaeg, P.,** The mucosal defense system, in *Immunologic Disorders in Infants and Children*, Stiehm, R., Ed., W.B. Saunders, Philadelphia, 1989, p. 116.

332. **Good, R.A.,** Presidential address: keystones, *J. Clin. Invest.*, 47, 1466, 1968b.

333. **Weinberg, K. and Parkman, R.,** Severe combined immunodeficiency due to a specific defect in the production of interleukin-2, *N. Eng. J. Med.*, Vol. 322, No. 24, p. 1718, June 14, 1990.

334. **Gelfand, E.W.,** SCID continues to point the way, *N. Eng. J. Med.*, 322, 1741, 1990.

335. **Page, A.R. and Good, R.A.,** Plasma cell hepatitis, in *Current Pediatric Therapy* 4, Gellis, S.S., Kagan, B.M., Eds., W.B. Saunders, Philadelphia, 1962a, p. 363.

336. **Page, A.R. and Good, R.A.,** Plasma cell hepatitis, *Lab. Invest.*, 11, 351, 1962b.

337. **Warner, N.L. and Szenberg, A.,** Effect of neonatal thymectomy on the immune response in the chicken, *Nature*, 196, 784, 1962.

Chapter 10

IMMUNOLOGICAL FUNCTION OF THE THYMUS AND THYMUS-DERIVED CELLS

J. F. A. P. Miller

I have been asked by the editors of this book to write a "personal article" in an "autobiographical style" describing some of the "basic work" which has led to "important advances in immunology today." As I have been involved in the last 25 years with the immunological function of cells derived from the thymus, I will concentrate on the early work establishing this function. It was performed at a time when immunologists considered the thymus as a vestigial structure filled with incompetent cells. It is not the purpose of this chapter to give a detailed review of this work; extensive reviews have been published elsewhere.[1,2]

EARLY WORK ON THYMECTOMY

"The outstanding feature of the development of
immunology in the last 10 years has been the recognition
of the function of the lymphocyte and of the importance
of the thymus in the immune process".[3]

In 1958, when I enrolled for the degree of Ph.D. at the Chester Beatty Research Institute in London, the competence of the lymphocyte was being debated,[4] and many did not consider the thymus capable of taking part in immune processes: "We interpret these observations as evidence that the thymus gland does not participate in the control of the immune system".[5] The thymus was known to be involved in the development of lymphocytic leukemia in mice and its removal (thymectomy) at 6 to 8 wks of age prevented leukemogenesis in high leukemic strain mice as well as in low-leukemic strains giving ionizing irradiation or chemical carcinogens [for review see].[6] In 1951 Ludwik Gross discovered that injection of filtrated material extracted from leukemic tissues of mice with spontaneous leukemia would induce the disease in low leukemic strains, but only if given in the neonatal period.[7] The thymus was also involved in this case and I decided to find out whether thymectomy after weaning would prevent the disease. It did so.[8] Thymus implantation 6 months after thymectomy (which was performed at 1 month of age) restored the potential for leukemia development in mice inoculated at birth with cell-free filtrates (containing the Gross virus).[9] Clearly the virus must have remained latent and the next experiment was a logical follow-up: virus could be recovered from the non-leukemic tissues of thymectomized mice.[10] I asked the question whether virus could multiply *outside* thymus tissue (it was subsequently shown to do so). Since, however, the virus had to be given at birth in order for leukemia to develop, the question could be studied only by thymectomizing *before* the virus was inoculated, i.e., immediately after birth. At that time I had no idea that the thymus may have a role in establishing the development of the immune system. The experiment met with some difficulties: "Subsequent mortality was very high in mice that had been thymectomized at 1 day of age, more than 50 percent of these dying between 2 and 4 months (whether they had

0-8493-4722-X/94/$0.00 + $.50
© 1994 by CRC Press, Inc.

been inoculated with virus or not), suggesting that the thymus at birth may be essential to life".[11]   This was totally unlike the situation in adult thymectomized mice which had never shown untoward effects or curtailment of lifespan. It was clear that mice without a thymus from the time of birth were susceptible to infection because, when kept in "clean" conditions, the incidence of wasting and death was less.   Examination of their tissues revealed "atrophy" of the lymphoid system and blood counts showed a marked diminution in lymphocyte levels and reversal of the lymphocyte polymorph ratio.[12]

During the late 1950's, I had the opportunity to discuss aspects of lymphocyte function in normal animals with Jim Gowans in Oxford and in immunologically tolerant animals with Sir Peter Medawar and his group, then at University College, London. Gowans[13] had unequivocally established the small lymphocyte's long lifespan, its recirculating property and its immunological competence, e.g., its capacity to initiate graft-versus-host reactions in incompatible hosts.   The studies of Medawar's group in immunologically tolerant mice had fascinated me so much that, having learned various techniques from them, including skin grafting, I induced tolerance between high and low leukemic strains to determine whether the failure of the Gross virus to cause leukemia in adults could be ascribed to immunological incompatibility.[14]   Hence, when I found lymphoid atrophy in neonatally thymectomized mice, I could immediately test their immune functions by skin grafting.   All grafts survived, even those incompatible at the major histocompatibility complex (the H-2 locus), and even skin from other species such as rats. The grafts grew luxuriant tufts of hair easily distinguishable from host hair, usually by their color. These results were shown in various seminars and meetings in 1961 in London and Oxford, in two Ciba Foundation Symposia, one in Perugia in June 1961,[15] the other in London in November 1961[16] and in great detail at the February 1962 meeting of the New York Academy of Sciences.[17]   I concluded: "during embryogenesis the thymus would produce the originators of immunologically competent cells many of what would have migrated to other sites at about the time of birth. This would suggest that lymphocytes leaving the thymus are *specially selected* cells".[12]

These results, or their interpretation, were not universally accepted, probably because most considered the thymus as having no role to play in immune processes. In many experiments, thymus cells had failed to transfer immunity or break tolerance.[18] Medawar[19] suspected "that we shall come to regard the presence of lymphocytes in the thymus as an evolutionary accident of no very great significance." R.J.C. Harris, at the June 1961 Ciba Foundation Symposium stated: "Dr. Delphine Parrott in our laboratory has been thymectomizing day-old mice and there is at present no evidence that these animals are immunologically weaker than normal animals. They do not retain skin grafts, they are living and breeding quite normally. They do not die of laboratory infections".[15] Even Robert Good's group who, independently and for reasons entirely different from mine, neonatally thymectomized animals to study their immune functions, observed prolonged skin graft survival "only in strains of mice isogeneic at the H-2 histocompatibility locus but homologous with respect to other weaker histocompatibility genes".[20] Later Good offered an explanation for the discrepancy between our results: "Careful autopsies performed in the thymectomized animals often revealed minute amounts of residual thymic tissue in these animals. With perfection of our technique a large proportion of neonatally thymectomized mice accepted H-2 incompatible grafts in contrast to partially thymectomized mice".[21] In my experience, however, partial thymectomy was never associated with any immune defects, an observation in keeping with the clearly demonstrated fact that the thymus is composed of multiple autonomous subunits, each of which is independent of the other and not subject to external feedback mechanisms.[1]

The importance of the thymus in establishing immune competence was soon confirmed, notably by Waksman's group[22] and in experiments using the newly available athymic nu/nu mouse strain.[23]

TWO DISTINCT UNIVERSES OF LYMPHOCYTES

A separate line of investigation led Glick and co-workers[24] to conclude that the bursa of Fabricius, a lymphoid organ of birds somewhat analogous to the thymus, seemed essential in early life for normal antibody-forming capacity in chickens. Szenberg and Warner[25] were the first to show a division of labor among lymphocytes in this species: early thymectomy impaired cellular immunity and early bursectomy humoral immunity. This suggested that in birds, in contrast to other vertebrates which do not have a bursa, lymphoid differentiation occurred in two separate and distinct organs. Since, in the mouse, neonatal thymectomy not only impaired cellular immunity but also antibody production to some antigens,[26,27] the mammalian thymus was believed to fulfill the function of *both* the thymus and bursa of birds. Yet an explanation had to be found for the observation that neonatal thymectomy in mice was associated with a marked reduction of lymphocytes normally found in those areas of lymphoid tissues associated with cellular immunity (e.g., paracortical areas of lymph nodes and periarteriolar lymphocyte sheaths in spleen), and not so much in those areas where antibody formation normally took place (e.g., follicles and germinal centers).[28] How then should one account for defects in antibody formation to some antigens after neonatal thymectomy?

An important observation was made in 1966 by Henry Claman and his co-workers:[29] irradiated mice given mixtures of cells from marrow and thymus together with antigen produced far more antibody than when given either cell source alone. It was not possible, from the design of these experiments to define the precise role of the thymus and marrow cells. At that time I had moved from London to the Walter and Eliza Hall Institute of Medical Research in Melbourne where I began, with my Ph.D. student, Graham Mitchell, a systematic study of the role of various cell types in the reconstitution of immune functions in immunoincompetent animals. Marrow cells had no effects in either irradiated or thymectomized mice. To our surprise, thymus cells were as effective as recirculating lymphocytes (obtained by thoracic duct cannulation) in restoring antibody-forming capacity when given simultaneously with antigen, but only in neonatally thymectomized hosts, not in irradiated mice. The latter required marrow cells to be given as well, and responded better with thoracic duct cells than with thymus cells. If, however, the thymus cells had previously been exposed to antigen in a first irradiated host, their ability to restore responsiveness in a second irradiated host given marrow cells was considerably enhanced for that specific antigen. This introduced the novel concept of "thymus cell education" and implicated some interaction between educated thymus cells and marrow cells.[30,31] With genetically marked cells, susceptible to destruction by specific antisera, we "demonstrated that the precursors of the hemolysin-forming cells are derived not from either thymus or thoracic duct lymphocytes but from bone marrow".[30] This was the first unequivocal proof that thymus-derived cells did not become antibody formers but were required in many antibody responses to help potential antibody formers produce antibody. Our results were published in great detail in four successive papers in the *Journal of Experimental Medicine* in 1968 and reviewed extensively in the first issue of *Transplantation Reviews* (later renamed *Immunological Reviews*).[32] They were met with some skepticism when I presented them at the Brook Lodge Symposium on Immunological Tolerance in September 1968.[33] Gowans, who had clearly shown that the recirculating small lymphocyte could initiate both cell-mediated immunity and humoral antibody responses, admitted: "Had it not been for Dr. Miller's experiments I would have assumed that a single variety of small lymphocyte was involved in each of our experiments".[33] Good was "concerned at separating thymus derived from marrow derived cells" since the former "are, in fact, marrow derived cells"[33] (p. 136). A multipotential stem cell was known to exist in the marrow and to differentiate in different environments: in the thymus it would give rise to thymus cells of which some would migrate out to become thymus derived cells and thus be distinct from those which never passed through the thymus and which we, for the sake of brevity, named "marrow derived." We postulated that thymus-derived cells had first to react with antigen and could then "release some pharmacologically active agents which *nonspecifically* induce the recruitment of bone marrow derived cells into activity".[33] I offered this as one of several possible mechanisms of cell interaction.

The establishment of cell interaction in antibody responses provided a suitable explanation for the "carrier effect," viz., the fact that successful immunization to a hapten (a small chemically defined molecule, which by itself is not immunogenic) requires the hapten to be coupled to a carrier molecule. Proof was obtained by groups led by Mitchison and Rajewsky for the cooperation of two distinct and separate classes of lymphocytes, one recognizing the carrier and the other the hapten, cooperation between these involving a carrier-hapten "antigen bridge." It was soon shown that the carrier reactive cells were thymus derived and hapten sensitive cells marrow derived. The former were designated "helper" cells since they did not produce the antibody but enabled the latter to do so.[34] For simplicity, thymus derived cells were called T cells and bone marrow derived cells (or bursa derived cells) B cells.

The demonstration of lymphocyte cooperation in antibody responses led to a reappraisal of numerous immunological phenomena including tolerance, autoimmunity, genetically determined unresponsive states, "original antigenic sin," immunogenicity, etc. As I suggested in my 1971 Burnet Lecture of the Australian Academy of Science,[35] "it may turn out that tolerance to self-components is a property confined exclusively to the T cell population, tolerance in B cells being merely a laboratory artifice. Autoantibodies are not normally produced, though not because there are no B cells which can synthesize them, but because T cells with receptors specific for so-called 'carrier determinants' on these self-components have been rendered tolerant during development." It has now, however, been proven that tolerance can be induced in the B cell compartment under certain circumstances[36] although tolerance in helper T cells is probably the major component that accounts for self tolerance.

A PLETHORA OF LYMPHOCYTE SUBSETS AND THEIR PRODUCTS

By the late 1960s, both the immunological importance of the thymus and the existence of two major subsets of lymphocytes had clearly been established. T and B cells could not be easily distinguished by morphological criteria alone. A major step forward was made when various cell surface components became identifiable by the use of specific antisera. The existence of the Thy-1 antigen on T cells[37] and the high density of surface immunoglobulin on B cells[38] was a convenient way of distinguishing and separating T from B cells. It was soon found that T cells, themselves could be further subdivided according to function and cell-surface markers: cytotoxic T cells[39] and suppressor T cells[40,41] were generally Lyt-2^{+}[42] whereas helper cells were generally L3T4^{+}.[43] A plethora of other T cell subsets, such as various types of helper and suppressor cells, contra-suppressors and inducers have also been postulated and in some cases identified.

Suppressor T cells probably play a crucial role in regulating a great variety of immune responses, both cellular and humoral, in antigenic competition, in the induction and maintenance of some forms of immune tolerance and in the control of allergic and autoimmune reactions. They may also serve to control potential B cell autoreactivities. Unravelling the complex interactions occurring between various T cells, B cells and macrophages is a goal of cellular immunologists today. For it is clearly evident that the immune response does not unfold following a simple interaction of antigen and immunocompetent cells: it is the result of the activation of an elaborate network of interacting cells.[44] In addition, each response is a highly amplified reaction and, as is the case with other amplification systems, each step must be subjected to appropriate control mechanisms. Cells involved in this control must be identified if we are to learn how to manipulate the immune response to our advantage.

Largely as a result of the work of Mackaness[45] evidence accumulated for the release by sensitized T lymphocytes of factors which activated macrophages to kill some intracellular bacteria. Similar mechanisms are likely to be involved in resistance to a variety of pathogens and hence in protection. Among the factors produced by activated T cells are the lymphokines, gamma interferon, the interleukins [e.g., IL-2,[46] IL-3,[47] IL-4 and other B cell specific lymphokines (reviewed in reference)[48] and GM-CSF (reviewed in reference).[49] These lymphokines have a variety of target cells. They are produced for a short period of time after activation and there is evidence of coordinated regulation of their synthesis but much more work remains to be done to unravel the molecular events involved.

ANTIGEN RECOGNITION

Burnet's clonal selection theory[50] accounted for antigen recognition and the distinction between self and nonself. It predicted that only a minority of lymphocytes would bind a given antigenic determinant. This was clearly demonstrated for B cells, only a small proportion of which (< 0.1 percent) bound radiolabelled antigen specifically, the binding being inhibited by anti-immunoglobulin reagents.[51] Hence, the immunoglobulin detected on the B cell surface must have been specific receptors for antigen.

The situation with T lymphocytes is much more complex. Using the graft-versus-host reaction in chick embryos, Simonsen[52] had estimated the frequency of alloreactive lymphocytes (later shown to be T cells) to be some 100 to 1000 times as high as the frequency of cells reacting to other antigens.

A similar conclusion was reached by others using *in vitro* cytotoxic T cell assays.[53] To account for the high frequency of alloreactive T cells, Jerne[54] proposed that the repertoire of T cell reactivities depended on a set of germline v genes (those coding for the *variable* regions of T cell antigen receptors) which coded for structures essentially complementary to the major histocompatibility complex (MHC) alleles of the species (e.g., the H-2 in mice). After entering the thymus, potentially alloreactive T cells, which form a relatively large proportion of the T cell pool, would not be influenced. By contrast, T cells with anti-self H-2 reactivities would proliferate in response to H-2 structures present in the thymus. This must not be allowed to continue, for it was argued that such cells could kill self-H-2 bearing cells. Random somatic mutations in the genes coding for receptors to self-H-2 would accumulate and thus decrease the strength of anti-self-H-2 binding receptors (negative selection). Hence, only T cells without anti-self-H-2 reactivities would mature. These would have their receptors directed to non-H-2 antigens and each specific set would thus constitute a much smaller proportion of the total T cell pool than alloreactive T cells. Because of this particular way in which T cell reactivities are selected, virtually all T cells would retain some "memory" of their anti-self-H-2 past and would be directed to antigens which contained some measure of H-2ness.

Jerne's negative selection theory accounted for the high frequency of alloreactive T cells and actually predicted "MHC restriction," a phenomenon which may indeed be considered as the major discovery of the 70's. Early in the work on lymphocyte collaboration we had observed failure of cooperation between allogeneic cells. I stated at the 1968 Brooke Lodge Symposium on Immunological Tolerance: "Unfortunately no interaction took place between allogeneic cells".[33] Kindred and Shreffler[55] also noted this and documented it in detail. Katz and Benacerraf[56] soon showed the need for identity at the I-A region of the H-2 locus if T and B cells were to cooperate successfully in antibody responses. They interpreted their findings in terms of a requirement for matching of "cell interaction molecules" on T and B cells. Zinkernagel and Doherty[57] extended these observations, documenting a requirement for H-2 matching, this time between cytotoxic T cells and their targets. They termed the phenomenon "H-2 restriction" and mapped the genes imposing it in cytotoxic T cells in the K and D regions of H-2. In the case of delayed type hypersensitivity reactions to a variety of protein antigens, we mapped the restriction to the I region of H-2.[58] Further experiments by Zinkernagel and his colleagues,[59] using thymectomized and thymus-grafted radiation chimeric mice, gave data implying that H-2 restriction had been imposed at the level of differentiation of pre-T cells within the thymus, not as a result of priming. Once differentiated, emigrant T cells could then perceive antigen only if presented by antigen-presenting cells (APC) in association with the appropriate MHC gene product (called restriction element) identical to that present on thymus stromal cells; i.e., the T cells and the APC (or T cell target) need not have identical restriction elements. These results were therefore *not* consistent with a hypothesis which would explain H-2 restriction on the basis of a requirement for matching between *like* MHC-coded cell interaction molecules on activated T cells and their targets. On the contrary, they were consistent with a model proposing that T cells have either one receptor directed towards both antigen and the MHC component involved in restriction, or two distinct receptors, one for antigen, the other for the MHC component. Since the restriction is established within the thymus, the question arises as to whether incoming T cells are committed irreversibly towards differentiation to a particular subset, within a specific thymus microenvironment which uniquely expresses the MHC gene product involved in restriction of that subset. Thus, the Lyt-2$^+$ T cells are generally class I (i.e., H-2K or H-2D) restricted and L3T4$^+$ T cells class II (i.e., I region of H-2).[42,60] To scan the thymus environment (e.g., the epithelial or reticular framework) for heterogeneity, revealed by differential MHC gene expression and associated T cell subset differentiation, seems highly desirable.

The discovery of MHC restriction led to some modification of the original antigen-focusing hypothesis of T and B cell collaboration. This is because the same restriction imposed by the MHC on T cell activation by APC-associated antigen was also found to be imposed at the level of T and B cell cooperation.[61] Thus T cell recognition of MHC-associated antigen on APC and on specific B cells must be similar. As I suggested at that time, "T cells specific for Ia and 'processed' antigen would seek out those B cells displaying identical structures. Of course, only B cells with specific receptors for either hapten or carrier determinants should 'capture' sufficient hapten-carrier conjugates via their surface Ig receptors. Only these B cells should be able to 'process' carrier determinants and associate them with Ia determinants on their cell surface, thus displaying the correct structure for specific carrier reactive T_H cells".[62] I thus considered B cells as cells able to present antigen to T cells in an MHC-restricted fashion and this was in line with a suggestion I had made prior to the discovery of MHC restriction when our data made me conclude that "antigen bound to immunoglobulin determinants on B cells seems to be very effective in activating T cells".[63] In 1985, Lanzavecchia[64] published data which established B cells as capable of presenting antigen to T cells.

That MHC genes did indeed govern T cell antigen recognition had been apparent since the discovery of MHC-linked immune responsiveness (Ir) genes.[65,66] The immune response to a large number of antigens was found to be controlled by genes mapping in the I region of the H-2 complex. These genes governed the activities of T cells (e.g., delayed type hypersensitivity, *in vitro* induced antigen proliferation) or T cell-assisted functions like antibody production. After the discovery of MHC restriction, it was possible to envisage identity of Ir gene products and I region gene coded restriction elements. To be consistent with such a view, however, one would expect localization of the Ir genes controlling the activities of K and D restricted cytotoxic T cells in the K and D regions of the MHC. This was soon found to be the case in a variety of experimental systems.[58,67] In general, therefore, one could conclude that class II gene products govern the immune response of L3T4$^+$ T cells and class I products influence that of Lyt-2$^+$ T cells. The exact mechanism of this control is still controversial and opposing views have been formulated to explain nonresponsiveness. According to one, some form of association between antigenic determinants and MHC gene products is essential for T cell recognition.[68,69] T cells recognize the "associative" antigen and are thus MHC-restricted. A "nonpermissive" interaction between an antigenic determinant and a particular MHC component leads to nonresponsiveness. It remains a major challenge to molecular immunologists to determine the precise nature of this association in physicochemical terms [cf. the discussion of amphipathic structures by Berzofsky].[70] An alternative view seeks to explain nonresponsiveness in terms of a gap in the T cell repertoire.[71]

The major discovery of the 80's has been the elucidation of the nature of the T cell antigen recognition receptor (TcR) and identification of the genes which code for it. Use of monoclonal antibodies[72] and T cell clones[73] were instrumental in isolating the TcR.[74,75] It is a disulfide bonded heterodimeric glycoprotein composed of two chains termed α and ß. Its coding sequences were cloned independently in mouse[76] and man[77] by differential hybridization techniques followed by identification of rearranging genes. A third genetic locus coding for a gamma chain was identified[78] but the function of this chain has yet to be clarified. Evidence soon became available to show that the TcR α-ß heterodimer was entirely responsible for both antigen specificity and MHC restriction[75] thus vindicating the hypothesis of the one TcR model directed to both antigen and associated MHC component. There is, however, no correlation between α and ß v region gene usage and MHC or antigen specificity.[79] Hence the phenomenon of MHC restriction has yet to be clarified both at the molecular and genetic level.

THE FUTURE

I have alluded above to a number of areas in immunology which require further basic work. Although a great deal of knowledge has accumulated since the discovery of immunological tolerance in 1953, we still do not have a comprehensive view of the fundamental aspects of self-tolerance at the cellular and molecular levels, nor do we have a simple and practical means of inducing tolerance when it would be most useful clinically. Perhaps more work on T cell differentiation pre- and intra-thymically, on the molecular basis of MHC restriction, and on the factors which regulate repertoire selection, will eventually assist our understanding of how self-reactive cells are "censured."

In 1979, I wrote: "Although the feeling has been expressed that immunology was born from the demand for protection against infectious disease, and that essentially what was needed was provided, it may be worthwhile pointing out that a recent World Health Organization Survey (1974) estimated that approximately 200 million people are infected with schistosomes, 300 million with filariae and other helminths, 250 million with malaria, and 1000 million with a variety of intestinal parasites. Furthermore, of the immunological methods available, none can satisfactorily halt the spread of gonococcal and syphilitic infections".[80] Now, 8 years later, the situation has not improved, and to the list of infectious diseases we have to add AIDS, a disease clearly showing the importance of the T cell system in protective immunity. Here, again, in spite of the tremendous growth of immunological knowledge and the proliferation of immunologically oriented journals, we still lack the capacity to immunize against many infectious diseases, in particular parasitic infestations. We need reliable adjuvants safe for human use and we require more detailed knowledge of what constitutes good T and B cell epitopes for protective immunization and how these should be put together in an artificial vaccine.

This chapter was written in 1987 and therefore, much relevant recent work is not included. An update can be found in reference.[81]

REFERENCES

1. **Metcalf, D.,** *The Thymus*, Springer-Verlag, Berlin, 1966.
2. **Miller, J.F.A.P. and Osoba, D.,** Current concepts of the immunological function of the thymus, *Physiol. Rev.*, 47, 437, 1967.
3. **Burnet, F.M.,** , Chairman's opening remarks, in *The Thymus: Experimental and Clinical Studies*, G.E.W. Wolstenholm and R. Porter, Eds., CIBA Foundation Symposium, Churchill, London, 1966, pp. 1-2.
4. **Wolstenholme, G.E.W. and O'Connor, M.,** Eds., *Cellular Aspects of Immunity*, Ciba Foundation Symposium, Churchill, London, 1960.
5. **MacLean, L.D., Zak, S.J., Varco, R.L., and Good, R.A.,** The role of the thymus in antibody production: an experimental study of the immune response in thymectomized rabbits, *Transpl. Bull.*, 41, 21, 1957.
6. **Miller, J.F.A.P.,** Aetiology and pathogenesis of mouse leukaemia, *Adv. Cancer Res.*, 6, 291, 1961a.
7. **Gross, L.,** Pathogenic properties and "vertical" transmission of the mouse leukemia agent, *Proc. Soc. Exp. Biol. Med.*, 78, 342, 1951.
8. **Miller, J.F.A.P.,** Role of the thymus in murine leukaemia, *Nature*, 183, 1069, 1959a.
9. **Miller, J.F.A.P.,** Fate of subcutaneous thymus grafts in thymectomized mice inoculated with leukaemic filtrates, *Nature*, 184, 1809, 1959b.
10. **Miller, J.F.A.P.,** Recovery of leukaemogenic agent from non-leukaemic tissues of thymectomized mice, *Nature*, 187, 703, 1960a.
11. **Miller, J.F.A.P.,** Analysis of the thymus influence in leukaemogenesis, *Nature*, 191, 248, 1961b.
12. **Miller, J.F.A.P.,** Immunological function of the thymus, *Lancet*, 2, 748, 1961c.
13. **Gowans, J.L.,** The immunological activity of lymphocytes, in *Biological Activity of the Leucocyte*, G.E.W. Wolstenholme and M. O'Connor, Eds., Ciba Foundation Study Group, Churchill, London, 1961, pp. 32-44.
14. **Miller, J.F.A.P.,** Studies on mouse leukaemia, III. The fate of thymus homografts in immunologically tolerant mice, *Brit. J. Cancer*, 14, 244, 1960b.
15. **Miller, J.F.A.P.,** Role of the thymus in virus-induced leukaemia, in *Ciba Foundation Symposium, Tumour Viruses of Murine Origin*, G.E.W. Wolstenholme and M. O'Connor, Eds., Churchill, London, 1962a, pp. 262-288.
16. **Miller, J.F.A.P.,** Role of the thymus in transplantation tolerance and immunity, in *Ciba Foundation Symposium, Transplantation*, G.E.W., Wolstenholme and M.P. Cameron, Eds., Churchill, London, 1962b, pp. 383-403.
17. **Miller, J.F.A.P.,** Role of the thymus in transplantation immunity, *Ann. N.Y. Acad. Sci.* 99, 340, 1962c.
18. **Billingham, R.E. and Brent, L.,** Quantitative studies on tissue transplantation immunity. IV. Induction of tolerance in newborn mice and studies on the phenomenon of runt disease, *Phil. Trans. Roy. Soc. London*, 242B, 439, 1959.
19. **Medawar, P.B.,** Discussion of Miller, J.F.A.P. and Osoba, D. The role of the thymus in the origin of immunological competence, in *The Immunologically Competent Cell*, G.E.W. Wilstenholme and J. Knight, Eds., Ciba Foundation Study Group, Churchill, London, 1963, p. 70.
20. **Martinez, C., Kersey, J., Papermaster, B.W., and Good, R.A.,** Skin homograft survival in thymectomized mice, *Proc. Soc. Exp. Biol. Med.*, 109, 193, 1962.
21. **Martinez, C., Dalmasso, A.P., and Good, R.A.,** Homotransplantation of normal and neoplastic tissue in thymectomized mice, in *The Thymus in Immunobiology*, R.A. Good and A.E. Gabrielsen, Eds., Harper and Row, New York, 1964, pp. 465-477.
22. **Arrnason, B.G., Jankovic, B.D., and Waksman, B.H.,** Effect of thymectomy on "delayed" hypersensitive reactions, *Nature*, 194, 99, 1962.
23. **Rygaard, J.,** *Thymus and Self: Immunobiology of the Mouse Mutant Nude*, Wiley, London, 1973.
24. **Glick, B., Chang, T.S., and Japp, R.G.,** The bursa of Fabricius and antibody production, *Poultry Sci.*, 35, 224, 1956.
25. Szenberg, A. and Warner, N.L. Dissociation of immunological responsiveness in fowls with a hormonally arrested development of lymphoid tissue. Nature **194**: 146-147, 1962.

26. **Miller, J.F.A.P.,** Effect of neonatal thymectomy on the immunological responsiveness of the mouse, *Proc. Roy. Soc. London,* 156B, 410, 1962d.

27. **Miller, J.F.A.P.,** Tolerance in the thymectomized animal, in *La Tolérance Acquise et la Tolérance Naturelle à l'égard de Substances Antigéniques Définies,* C.N.R.S. Colloque, Paris, 1963, pp. 47-75.

28. **Parrott, D.M.W., de Sousa, M.A.B., and East, J.,** Thymus-dependent areas in the lymphoid organs of neonatally thymectomized mice, *J. Exp. Med.,* 123, 191, 1966.

29. **Claman, H.N., Chaperon, E.A., and Triplett, R.F.,** Thymus-marrow cell combinations - synergism in antibody production, *Proc. Soc. Exp. Biol. Med.,* 122, 1167, 1966.

30. **Miller, J.F.A.P., and Mitchell, G.F.,** The thymus and the precursors of antigen-reactive cells, *Nature,* 216, 659, 1967.

31. **Mitchell, G.F., and Miller, J.F.A.P.,** Immunological activity of thymus and thoracic duct lymphocytes, *Proc. Natl. Acad. Sci. USA,* 59, 296, 1968.

32. **Miller, J.F.A.P. and Mitchell, G.F.,** Thymus and antigen-reactive cells, *Transpl. Rev.,* 1, 3, 1969.

33. **Miller, J.F.A.P.,** Cell to cell interaction in the immune response of mice to sheep erythrocytes, in *Immunological Tolerance: A Reassessment of Mechanisms of the Immune Response,* Brook Lodge Symposium, M. Landy and W. Braun, Eds., Academic Press, New York, 1969, pp. 125-133.

34. **Miller, J.F.A.P.,** Lymphocyte interactions in antibody responses, *Intern. Rev. Cytol.,* 33, 77, 1972.

35. **Miller, J.F.A.P.,** The thymus in immunity, *Records of the Australian Academy of Science,* 2, 82, 1971.

36. **Goodnow, C. C., Adelstein, S., and Basten, A.,** The need for central and peripheral tolerance in the B cell reprtoire, *Science,* 248, 1373, 1990.

37. **Reif, A.E. and Allen, J.M.W.,** The AKR thymic antigen and its distribution in leukemias and nervous tissues, *J. Exp. Med.,* 120, 413, 1964.

38. **Raff, M.C.,** Surface antigenic markers for distinguishing T and B lymphocytes in mice, *Transpl. Rev.,* 6, 52, 1971.

39. **Cerottini, J.-C. and Brunner, K.T.,** Cell-mediated cytotoxicity, allograft rejection and tumor immunity, *Adv. Immunol.,* 18, 67, 1974.

40. **McCullagh, P.J.,** The abrogation of immunological tolerance by means of allogeneic confrontation, *Transpl. Rev.,* 12, 180, 1972.

41. **Gershon, R.K.,** T cell control of antibody production, *Contemp. Topics Immunobiol.,* 3, 1, 1974.

42. **Boyse, E. A. and Old, L.J.,** The immunogenetics of differentiation in the mouse, *Harvey Lect.,* 71, 23, 1975.

43. **Dialynas, D.P., Wilde, D.B., Marrack, P., Pierres, A., Wall, KA., Havran, W., Otten, G., Loken, M.R., Pierres, M., Kappler, J., and Fitch, F.W.,** Characterization of the murine antigenic determinant, designated L3T4a, recognized by monoclonal antibody GK1.5: expression of L3T4a by functional T cell clones appears to correlate primarily with class II MHC antigen-reactivity, *Immunol. Rev.,* 74, 29, 1983.

44. **Jerne, N.K.,** Towards a network theory of the immune system, *Ann. Immunol. Inst., Pasteur,* 125C, 373, 1974.

45. **Mackaness, G.B.,** Delayed hypersensitivity and the mechanism of cellular resistance to infection, *Prog. Immunol.,* 1, 413, 1971.

46. **Gillis, S., Ferm, M.M., Ou, W., and Smith, K.A.,** T cell growth factor: parameters of production and a quantitative microassay for activity, *J. Immunol.,* 120, 2027, 1978.

47. **Yung, Y.-P., Eger, R., Tertian, G., and Moore, M.A.S.,** Long-term *in vitro* culture of murine mast cells, II. Purification of a mast cell growth factor and its dissociation from TCGF, *J. Immunol.,* 127, 794, 1981.

48. **Klaus, G.G.B.,** Unravelling the control of B cells, *Nature,* 324, 16, 1986.

49. **Metcalf, D.,** The granulocyte-macrophage colony-stimulating factors, *Science,* 229, 16, 1985.

50. **Burnet, F.M.,** *The Clonal Selection Theory of Acquired Immunity,* Cambridge University Press, 1959.

51. **Ada, G.L.,** Antigen binding cells in tolerance and immunity, *Transpl. Rev.,* 5, 105, 1970.

52. **Simonsen, M.,** The clonal selection hypothesis evaluated by grafted cells reacting against their host, *Cold Spring Harbor Symp. Quant. Biol.,* 32, 517, 1967.

53. **Skinner, M.A. and Marbrook, J.,** An estimation of the frequency of precursor cells which generate cytotoxic lymphocytes, *J. Exp. Med.*, 143, 1562, 1976.

54. Jerne, N.K. The somatic generation of immune recognition. Eur. J. Immunol. 1: 1-9, 1971.

55. **Kindred, B. and Schreffler, D.C.,** H-2 dependence of cooperation between T and B cells *in vitro*, *J. Immunol.*, 109, 940, 1972.

56. **Katz, D.H. and Benacerraf, B.,** The function and interrelationship of T cell receptors, Ir genes and other histocompatibility gene products, *Transpl. Rev.*, 22, 175, 1975.

57. **Zinkernagel, R.M. and Doherty, D.C.,** Immunological surveillance against self components by sensitized T lymphocytes in lymphocytic chorio-meningitis, *Nature*, 251, 547, 1974.

58. **Miller, J.F.A.P., Vadas, M.A., Whitelaw, A., and Gamble, J.,** H-2 gene complex restricts transfer of delayed-type hypersensitivity in mice, *Proc. Natl. Acad. Sci. USA*, 72, 5095, 1975.

59. **Zinkernagel, R.M., Callahan, G.N., Althage, A., Cooper, S., Klein, P.A., and Klein, J.,** On the thymus in the differentiation of "H-2 self-recognition" by T cells: evidence for dual recognition? *J. Exp. Med.*, 147, 882, 1978.

60. **MacDonald, H.R., Glasebrook, A.L., Bron, C., Kelso, A., and Cerottini, J.-C.,** Clonal heterogeneity in the functional requirement for Lyt2/3 molecules on cytolytic T lymphocytes (CTL): possible implications for the affinity of CTL antigen receptors, *Immunol. Rev.*, 68, 89, 1982.

61. **Sprent, J.,** Restricted helper functions of F_1 hybrid T cells positively selected to heterologous erythrocytes in irradiated parental strain mice. II. Evidence for restrictions affecting helper cell induction and T-B collaboration, both mapping to the K-end of the H-2 complex, *J. Exp. Med.*, 147, 1159, 1978.

62. **Miller, J.F.A.P.,** Cellular interactions in immune responses, *Seminars Hematol.*, 16, 283, 1979a.

63. **Miller, J.F.A.P.,** Cellular cooperation in the immune response, in *Proceedings of the VIIIth Congress of the Internatl. Assoc. of Allergol.*, Tokyo, Exc. Medica, ICS, 323, 155, 1973.

64. **Lanzavecchia, A.,** Antigen-specific interaction between T and B cells, *Nature*, 314, 537, 1985.

65. **Benacerraf, B. and Katz, D.H.,** The histocompatibility-linked immune response genes, *Adv. Cancer Res.*, 21, 121, 1975.

66. **McDevitt, H.O., Delovitch, T.L., Press, J.L., and Murphy, D.B.,** Genetic and functional analysis of the Ia antigens: their possible role in regulating the immune response, *Transpl. Rev.*, 30, 197, 1976.

67. **Meruelo, D., Nimelstein, S.H., Jones, P.P., Lieberman, M., and McDevitt, H.O.,** Increased synthesis and expression of H-2 antigens on thymocytes as a result of radiation leukemia virus: a possible mechanism for H-2 linked control of virus-induced neoplasia, *J. Exp. Med.*, 147, 470, 1978.

68. **Benacerraf, B.,** A hypothesis to relate the specificity of T lymphocytes and the activity of I-region-specific Ir genes in macrophages and B lymphocytes, *J. Immunol.*, 120, 1809, 1978.

69. **Rosenthal, A.S.,** Determinant selection and macrophage function in genetic control of the immune response, *Immunol. Rev.*, 40, 136, 1978.

70. **Berzofsky, J.A., Cornette, J., Margalit, H., Berkower, I., Cease, K., and Delisi, C.,** Molecular features of class II MHC-restricted T cell recognition of protein and peptide antigens: the importance of amphipathic structures, *Current Topics Microbiol. Immunol.*, 130, 13, 1986.

71. **Nagy, Z.A. and Klein, J.,** Macrophage or T cell - that is the question, *Immunol. Today*, 2, 228, 1981.

72. **Milstein, C.,** Monoclonal antibodies, in *Accomplishments in Cancer Research*, Lippincot, Philadelphia, PA, 1981, pp. 86-94.

73. **Samelson, L.E. and Schwartz, R.H.,** The use of antisera and monoclonal antibodies to identify the antigen-specific T cell receptor from pigeon cytochrome c-specific T cell hybrids, *Immunol. Rev.*, 76, 59, 1983.

74. **Allison, J.P., McIntyre, B.W. and Block, D.,** Tumor-specific antigen of murine T lymphoma defined with monoclonal antibody, *J. Immunol.*, 129, 2293, 1982.

75.   **Haskins, K., Kubo, R., White, J., Pigeon, M., Kappler, J. and Marrack, P.,** The major histocompatibility complex restricted antigen receptor on T cells. I. Isolation with a monoclonal antibody, *J. Exp. Med.,* 157, 1149, 1983.

76.   **Hedrick, S.M., Cohen, D.I., Nielsen, E.A. and Davis, M.M.,** Isolation of cDNA clones encoding T cell-specific membrane-associated proteins, *Nature,* 308, 149, 1984.

77.   **Yanagi, Y., Yoshikai, Y., Leggett, K., Clark, S.P., Aleksander, I. and Mak, T.W.,** A human T cell-specific cDNA clone encodes a protein having extensive homology to immunoglobulin chains, *Nature,* 308, 145, 1984.

78.   **Saito, H., Kranz, D.M., Takagaki, Y., Hayday, A.C., Eisen, H.N. and Tonegawa, S.,** A third rearranged and expressed gene in a clone of cytotoxic T lymphocytes, *Nature,* 312, 36, 1984.

79.   **Goverman, J., Minard, K., Shastri, N., Hunkapiller, T., Hansburg, D., Sercarz, E., and Hood, L.,** Rearranged ß T cell receptor genes in a helper T cell clone specific for lysozyme: no correlation between Vß and MHC restriction, *Cell,* 40, 859, 1985.

80.   **Miller, J.F.A.P.,** Experimental thymology has come of age, *Thymus,* 1, 3, 1979b.

81.   **Miller, J. F. A. P.,** The Croonian Lecture, The key role of the thymus in the body's defence strategies, *Phil. Trans. Roy. Soc. London,* 337B, 105, 1992.

Chapter 11

T CELL-B CELL COLLABORATION

Henry N. Claman

I have been asked to describe the genesis of our experiments, published in 1966, showing that two cells, one from the thymus and one from the bone marrow, were needed to make antibody. Immunologically speaking, this is ancient history indeed, but this is how it went.

THE GENERAL IMMUNOLOGICAL SCENE

In the early 1960's, the accent was on antibody formation and immunoglobulin structure. However, the thymus came to prominence in 1961 with the startling experimental results of J.F.A.F. Miller and R.A. Good. Miller showed that neonatally thymectomized mice had deficient allograft rejection and antibody production.[1] Good showed that neonatally thymectomized rabbits had impaired antibody production.[2] These were astounding papers because they clearly put the thymus (hitherto a "mystery organ") at the center of the immune response. Cellular immunology was born.

THE SCENE IN DENVER

A less astounding event was my debut as a postdoctoral fellow in the laboratory of David W. Talmage, at the University of Colorado Medical School in Denver. Talmage was known as a brilliant immunologist who had a small but innovative group. (This group included one of the editors of this book, Dr. A. Szentivanyi). I was just starting my experimental career and worked on the effects of irradiation on antibody production and the mechanisms of tolerance in adult mice. Most of my experiments did not work, but I enjoyed myself greatly. I was lucky enough to go to the thymus conference convened by Good in Minneapolis in 1962.[3] Subsequently I met J.F.A.P. Miller who came to Denver for two summers to do thymectomies on newborn possums which were still in the pouch. As they were extremely immature, this presented Miller with a chance to remove the thymus extremely early in ontogeny, so that the effects of the thymectomy could be studied in adult life.

I do not remember exactly when I became interested in the thymus. In 1962-1963, Talmage and I did experiments showing that in tolerized mice thymectomy delayed the return of immunocompetence.[4] This was consistent with the notion that acquired immunological tolerance wanes when new untolerized cells are born in the thymus and seed the peripheral lymphoid tissues. However, it was not clear just what the thymus did. Thus, it was a "mystery organ" still, and this intrigued me.

THE ROLE OF THYMUS IN ANTIBODY FORMATION - EARLY 1960'S

Here was a dilemma. The thymus was needed for the development and maintenance of the lymphoid system. Yet, we knew very well that the thymus did not make antibodies in the primary immune response. (To be sure, germinal follicles could be seen in the thymus in such conditions as systemic lupus erythematosus, but this was a highly abnormal situation).

At this time there was a lot of interest in a putative blood-thymus barrier, a concept promulgated by Sam Clark (whom I knew from my internship at

0-8493-4722-X/94/$0.00 + $.50
© 1994 by CRC Press, Inc.

Washington University in St. Louis). Clark showed that radiolabeled antigen would get into the lymphoid areas of the spleen but in the thymus it seemed to stay in the stroma and not get to the thymocytes.[5] If this blood-thymus barrier was the physiological basis of the inability of the thymus to make antibody, perhaps isolated thymocytes would respond differently.

CELL TRANSFER EXPERIMENTS

Transfer of lymphoid cells to irradiated recipients was becoming popular at this time. We knew that spleen cell suspensions transferred to lethally irradiated recipients which were then injected with antigen would respond by making antibodies. The favored antigen was sheep erythrocytes (SRBC) which were highly immunogenic in mice. Furthermore, the antibody response could be quantitated at the cellular level using the newly-invented Jerne hemolytic plaque method published in 1963 in a paper one-half of a page long.[6] The results of spleen transfer experiments indicated that the spleen had all the machinery needed for antibody formation in an irradiated recipient.

OUR BASIC EXPERIMENT

We wished to know if thymus cells transferred to an irradiated recipient, in suspension, would be able to mount an antibody response if stimulated with SRBC. In this situation the blood-thymus barrier would presumably be broken by the making of the spleen cell suspension. For antibody detection, we used the method of Playfair, Papermaster and Cole.[7] Spleens from the recipient mice were cut into many fragments and plated out on a lawn of SRBC in agar in a petri dish in a kind of map where the disposition of the fragments reflected their position in the spleen *in vivo*. The plates were incubated for two hours, covered with guinea pig serum as a source of hemolytic complement, and reincubated. At the end of the second incubation, we counted "hemolytic areas" of hemolysis; that is, a hemolytic area was a group of two or more adjacent spleen fragments with surrounding hemolysis. Each one of these active areas presumably reflected a unit number of antibody-forming precursors transferred from the donor which had matured into a clone of antibody forming cells. This experimental design is shown in Fig. 1.

THE INVESTIGATORS

I was a young assistant professor, busy doing research and seeing patients. Edward A. Chaperon was a postdoctoral fellow who had just received his Ph.D. from the University of Wisconsin. R. Faser Triplett was a clinical fellow in pediatric allergy. Each experiment had two days of hard work, the beginning and the end. Chaperon and I irradiated the mice on day 0 and infused spleen, thymus or marrow cells i.v. On day 1, we injected the antigen SRBC. At the end of the experiment on day 5, all three of us sacrificed the mice and plated out the spleen fragments on petri dishes. I coded the plates, put the code in my wallet and went to clinic or the library. After incubation with complement, Chaperon examined the plates, indicated the hemolytic areas per plate and counted them. Then I broke the code and Chaperon compiled the data for each group and did the statistics.

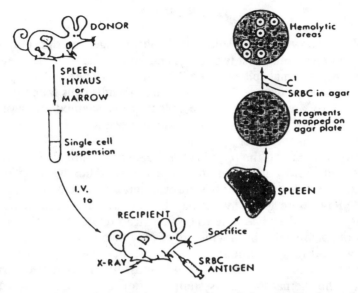

Fig. 1. The hemolytic assay for antibody production by cells from healthy donors injected into irradiated recipients which then receive sheep RBC antigen. A hemolytic area in the spleen fragments of the recipient represents a unit number of transferred immunocompetent cells [reproduced from ref.[8] with permission].

Table 1

Production of Active Areas of Hemolysis in Spleens of CBA Mice which were Irradiated and Injected with Spleen or Thymus Cells on Day 0, Given Sheep Erythrocytes on Day 1 and Sacrificed on Day 5

Cells injected	No. of cells ($\times 10^6$)	Active areas per spleen	Mean	
Normal spleen	2	00111112	.87	
Normal spleen	5	111122222222 334444		2.3
Immune spleen	.5	00113	.80	
Immune spleen	5	****	*	
Normal thymus	20	00000002	.25	
Normal thymus	50	0000	.0	
Normal thymus	90	00011	.40	
Immune thymus	100	000	.0	
Control	0	0000000000 0000001111	.2	

*Too many active areas to count accurately

THE RESULTS

As Table 1 shows, normal spleen cells plus antigen produced antibody in the irradiated recipients (first two rows), and immune spleen made even more (rows 3 and 4). Normal spleen made 2.3 active areas per 5×10^6 spleen cells transferred, while as many as 100×10^6 normal thymus cells failed to produce even one active area. Thus, while spleen cells seemed to have all the machinery for making antibody in an irradiated recipient, thymus cells did not. No progress had been made.

BUT...we wondered if the thymus cells, being immature, needed more time to mature and more antigen to stimulate them. Thus we lengthened the experiment to 8 days. Recipients were irradiated and cells were transferred on day 0, SRBC were given i.v. on day 1, a booster injection of SRBC was given on day 4 and the mice were to be sacrificed on day 8. This was fine for recipients of spleen cells, but recipients of only thymus cells died before day 8, and so we had no experiment. However, we persevered. If the irradiated recipients of only thymus cells died, it was most likely because of irradiation damage to the hematopoietic system. After all, the spleen contained hematopoietic cell precursors but the thymus did not. Therefore, to enable the "thymus only" group to get two injections of antigen and to reach day 8, we added some bone marrow cells to the thymus inoculum. This infusion of hematopoietic stem cells saved the lives of the mice. To our surprise, this group produced lots of antibody by day 8!

However, this experiment was difficult to interpret. In the thymus-marrow mixtures there might be antibody production by thymus cells, marrow cells or by both. We still needed "thymus only" and "marrow only" groups. By adjusting cell and irradiation doses and later changing mouse strains, we were able to show that antibody was produced by spleen cell populations and by thymus-plus-marrow populations but not by thymus or marrow populations alone. Fig. 2 shows the purpose of a key experiment, TT-15 (i.e., TT for "thymus transfer"). It was a check on a previous experiment which was suggestive that thymus and marrow cells act synergistically. Fig. 3 shows a "Playfair" plate with the spleen from a recipient who received thymus only cut in pieces and plated out in the hop half and another in the bottom half. Hemolysis around the pieces, indicating antibody production was scored 0-4. We also changed the data analysis method and counted hemolysis around each fragment. The percentage of all fragments with hemolysis ("specific activity") was 18.75% in the top thymus and 37.84% in the bottom (Fig. 4), shows a spleen from a mouse which received thymus plus marrow on the top (B) and a spleen from a mouse which received bone marrow only on the bottom (C). Fig. 5 shows the conclusion.

A more complete experiment is shown in Table 2. The specific activity (antibody production) of thymus and marrow (70.7%) is clearly greater than the sum of thymus alone (12.3% and and marrow alone (1.6%). Thymus marrow synergism was established and published ([8]).

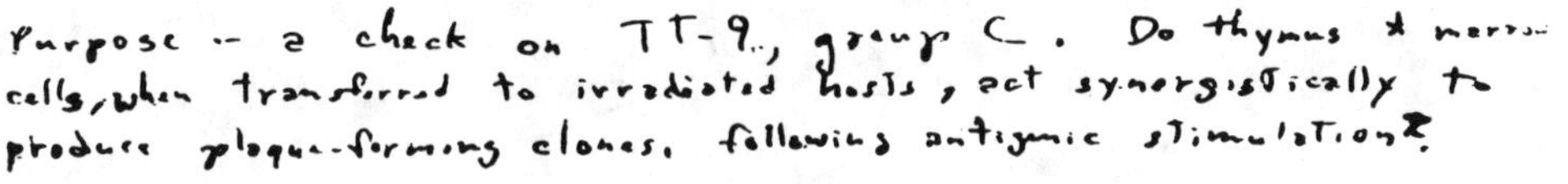

Purpose -- a check on TT-9, group C. Do thymus & marrow cells, when transferred to irradiated hosts, act synergistically to produce plaque-forming clones, following antigenic stimulation?

Fig. 2. The purpose of experiment TT-15.

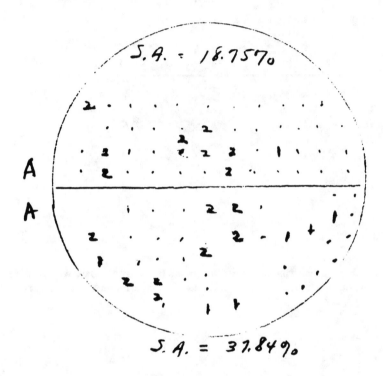

Fig. 3. A "Playfair plate" showing the spleen fragments from a mouse which had received only thymus cells and sheep RBC. S.A. = specific activity (i.e., percent of spleen fragments with hemolysis).

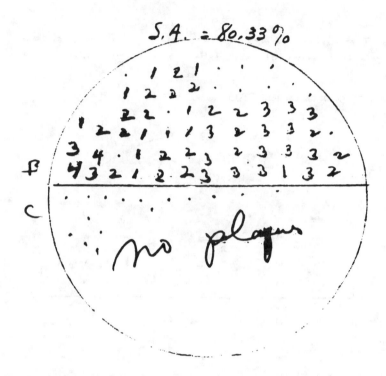

Fig. 4. A "Playfair plate" showing the spleen fragments from (B), a mouse which had received thymus plus bone marrow cells and sheep RBC, and (C) a mouse which had received only bone marrow cells and sheep RBC.

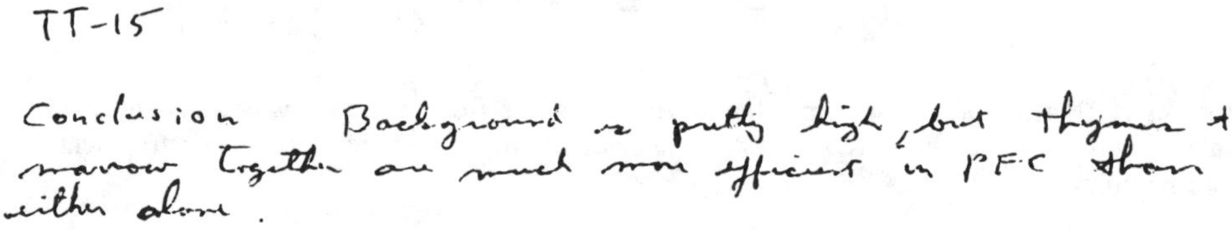

TT-15

Conclusion   Background is pretty high, but thymus + marrow together are much more efficient in PFC than either alone.

Fig. 5. The conclusion of experiment TT-15 in Ed Chaperon's hand. "Background is pretty high, but thymus and marrow together are much more efficient in PFC than either alone."

Table 2
Hemolytic Activity in Spleens of CBA Mice Which Were Irradiated and Injected with Spleen, Thymus, and/or Marrow Cells on Day 0, Given Sheep Erythrocytes (i.v. on Day 1 and i.p. on Day 4) and Sacrificed on Day 8

Cells injected	No. of cells (x 10^6)	Active areas per spleen	Mean active areas	Mean specific activity (% ± S.E.)
Thymus	35-50	{ 00011111 2333	1.3	12.3 ± 3.9
Marrow	10	{ 0000000000 01111122	.5	1.6 ± .5
Thymus + marrow	50 } 10 }	{ 1334** ******	>3.0	70.7 ± 3.3
Spleen	5	{ 12334* *****	>3.0	66.1 ± 9.0
None		{ 000000000 111112	.5	7.4 ± 2.9

*Too many active areas to count accurately

THE INTERPRETATION

Which cell, thymus or marrow, made the antibody (i.e., was the "effector cell") and which was the "auxiliary cell?" We had a 50-50 chance of being correct if we guessed. We leaned on some data from other investigators and said that the bone marrow cells made the antibody and the thymus cells were the auxiliaries.

We were correct (and lucky).

THE RECEPTION OF THIS WORK

To be quite honest, **nobody**, (not even us) realized the general importance of this experimental approach and these results. One colleague even suggested that this was an artifact! In short, it was not a bombshell.

Why did we publish a paper in *Proceedings of the Society for Experimental Biology and Medicine* (referred to as "Proc. Soc." or "blue bits")? At that time this was a very widely read journal. Furthermore, it had contained such immunological milestones as the first transfer of delayed hypersensitivity with cells (Landsteiner and Chase) and the induction of tolerance with oral DNCB (Chase). Finally, I had recently had a paper refused by *Science* and was angry at that journal.

AFTERMATH

The problem of which cell made the antibody was soon solved in elegant experiments by Miller and colleagues.[9] It was, as we had guessed, the bone marrow cell. As for my laboratory, we had become caught up in some parent-F_1 combinations which involved (unbeknownst to us) hybrid resistance[10] and we never made any headway. Soon after that, Mosier showed that a third cell, of macrophage phenotype, was needed in addition to T cells and B cells for optimal antibody production to SRBC.[11] Later, T cell subset immunology delineated cells with T helper function and work on the T cell receptor told us how T cells recognize antigen.

Not long after, I left this area to others and returned to questions of tolerance. The precise mechanism by which T cells "help" B cells make antibody has been investigated in many hundreds of papers involving *in vitro* and *in vivo* work. As our knowledge of lymphokines becomes sophisticated, it appears that these molecules are at the heart of the T-B cell collaboration.[12]

ACKNOWLEDGMENTS

Fig. 1 and Tables 1 and 2 are reprinted from Claman, Chaperon and Triplett, 1966.[8] I appreciate the help and collaboration of many people who helped in this early work--Drs. David Talmage, Edward A. Chaperon, R.F. Triplett III, Miss Jean Baughman and Mr. Terrill Smith. The National Institutes of Health supported this work from the beginning and the grant is now in its 24th year.

REFERENCES

1. **Miller, J.F.A.P.,** Immunological functions of the thymus, *Lancet,* 2, 748, 1961.
2. **Archer, O. and Pierce, J.C.,** Role of the thymus in development of the immune response, *Fed. Proc.,* 20, 26, 1961 (abstract).
3. **Good, R.A. and Gabrielsen, A.,** Eds, *The Thymus in Immunobiology,* Hoeber-Harper, New York, 1964.
4. **Claman, H.N. and Talmage, D.W.,** Thymectomy: Prolongation of immunological tolerance in the adult mouse, *Science,* 141, 1193, 1963.
5. **Clark, S.J., Jr.,** The penetration of proteins and colloidal materials into the thymus from the bloodstream, in The Thymus, D. Defendi and D. Metcalfe, Eds., Wistar Institute Press, Philadelphia, 1964.
6. **Jerne, N.K. and Nordin, A.A.,** Plaque formation in agar by single antibody-producing cells, *Science,* 140, 405, 1963.
7. **Playfair, J.H.L., Papermaster, B.W., and Cole, L.J.,** Focal antibody production by transferred spleen cells in irradiated mice, *Science,* 149, 998, 1965.
8. **Claman, H.N., Chaperon, E.A. and Triplett, R.F.,** Thymus-marrow cell combinations: synergism in antibody production, *Proc. Soc. Exptl. Biol. Med.,* 122, 1167, 1966.
9. **Mitchell, G.F. and Miller, J.F.A.P.,** Cell to cell interaction in the immune response. II. The source of hemolysin-forming cells in irradiated mice given bone marrow and thymus or thoracic duct lymphocytes, *J. Exp. Med.,* 128, 821, 1968.
10. **Cudkowicz, G.,** The immunogenetic basis of hybrid resistance to parental marrow grafts, *Wistar Inst. Symp. Monograph,* 3, 37, 1965.
11. **Mosier, D.E. and Coppleson, L.W.,** A three-cell interaction required for the induction of the primary immune response *in vitro, Proc. Natl. Acad. Sci. U.S.A.,* 61, 542, 1968.
12. **Singer, A. and Hodes, R.J.,** Mechanisms of T-cell, B-cell interaction, *Ann. Rev. Immunol.,* 1, 211, 1984.

Chapter 12

WILL THE REAL ANTIGEN-PRESENTING CELL PLEASE STAND UP?

Maxwell Richter

PROLOGUE

I was pleased when I received an invitation from Drs. Szentivanyi and Friedman to contribute an article to *The Immunological Revolution: Facts and Witnesses*. However, I must admit that it came as a shock to be informed that I qualified for this honor as I had carried out major research sufficiently long ago, the 1950s and the early 1960s, to ensure that today's young investigators would be totally unaware of it. Furthermore, if these investigators wish to read the published papers, they will not be able to find them in the bound journals on the "current" library shelves as they will have been put in storage "a long time ago" or "before I became a librarian here." Such a scenario is not very ego satisfying and encourages nostalgic reminiscence by those of us who labored in immunology research at a time when ideas shared with our colleagues and peers were paramount and the technology rather primitive by today's standards.

In the intervening years, the think tank has been transformed into the equipment room brimming with highly sophisticated apparatus. In the late 1970s, the technology to create hybridoma cells which can spew out specific monoclonal antibodies for individual investigators was introduced. Researchers can therefore carry out investigations without the possibility of verification by their peers since the immunological reagents used are the property of the investigators. This "personalization" of research had added a new troublesome variable to the research equation.

Another factor which, in my opinion, is hindering research today is the large number of papers published compared with the 1950s and the 1960s. So many papers are currently published in immunology yearly (the figure of 50,000 papers was brought up at the 6th International Congress held in Toronto, 1986) that it is not possible for investigators to assimilate more than a small fraction of the literature. Many young investigators are therefore "rediscovering the wheel" in many areas of research since they are ignorant of much of the research which predated their entry into the field.

A major goal of this book is to enlighten today's investigators about the not-so-recent contemporary investigations which laid the foundation for the current thinking in immunology. I have refrained from listing references since most authors list only those references which support their views. It is more instructive, and educational, for the serious reader to investigate the literature on his/her own. The results are often most satisfying and the individual feels that he/she has learned something in the process. On the other hand, my peers who have been in immunology since the 1950s are fully aware of the literature relevant to the topic of this paper and do not need direction from me in this regard. My objectives in this exercise are two-fold: 1) to present a unified picture of the mechanism of activation of the immune system by antigen to the young investigator in the hope that he/she will be sufficiently interested in this area of immunology to investigate the extensive literature

0-8493-4722-X/94/$0.00 + $.50

PREAMBLE

A major problem encountered in any attempt to understand the mechanism of activation of the immune system by antigen is the diversity of antigens used by different investigators. On the other hand, individual investigators tend to use a single "pet" antigen and a single inbred strain of mouse for an entire investigation. Their results cannot therefore be generalized to all antigens; they may, in fact, be valid only for the single antigen and the strain of mouse used by the investigator and may represent an attempt by the immune system to improvise a response rather than respond in the normal fashion. Furthermore, the results may be an artifact since they are frequently obtained under highly contrived conditions *in vitro* using suspensions of cells which are normally accustomed to a very precise functional relationship with each other within the tissues and organs.

The majority of researchers utilize soluble, simple, low molecular weight, non-toxic antigens which are frequently highly purified or synthetic. They blissfully forget that the immune system evolved to provide resistance to virulent pathogenic bacteria, as Friedman preached 30 years ago, and therefore to respond to complex high molecular weight, often toxic, antigens. Therefore, any mechanism proposed for the stimulation of the immune system by antigen must function for the induction of immunity to the most ubiquitous pathogens, the particulate bacteria. Ideally, the proposed mechanism should function in the identical manner for all randomly selected antigens which should include particulate antigens (microbial and non-microbial, i.e., erythrocytes) and soluble antigens (toxins and innocuous soluble proteins, i.e., serum proteins).

Antigens were classified into two broad categories in the late 1960s and early 1970s--the T-dependent antigens and the T-independent antigens. The term "T-dependent" was originally used to designate those antigens which must first react with the antigen-specific surface membrane receptors on a T cell as they cannot stimulate the antibody-forming cells in their native state. The T-independent antigens are those which do not require initial interaction with T cells to induce an immune response as they can stimulate the antibody-forming cells directly.

However, it was not appreciated at the time of the classification of antigens into T-dependent and T-independent that the cells which regulate the immune response are also T cells. The regulatory cells consist of the antigen-specific T helper cells and T suppressor cells which were discovered in the early 1970s. Since these T helper and T suppressor cells regulate the immune responses to both T-dependent and T-independent antigens, it is obvious that both of these classes of antigens are, in fact, T dependent. However, the terms T-dependent and T-independent antigens have been retained since antigens classified in these two categories differ in composition, structure and antigen-receptor specificity. The T-dependent antigens are characterized by flexible carriers to which are attached determinants with different specificities whereas the T-independent antigens are characterized by rigid carriers with numerous repeating identical antigenic determinants. The great majority of microbial-derived antigens are T dependent and only a small minority of the antigens normally encountered are T-independent.

BACKGROUND

Prior to 1965 it had been recognized that antibody formation takes place primarily in the spleen and that the antibody forming cell or AFC is a lymphocyte. The conventional wisdom of the day was that a single lymphoid cell could be "turned on" by the antigen to become an antibody synthesizing cell, a concept originated by Paul Ehrlich in 1894.

Investigations in the 1930s and 1940s strongly suggested a role for the macrophage since it was recognized that large particulate antigens, i.e. bacteria, require breakdown and degradation into small, soluble immunogenic constituents which react with and activate the precursors of the AFC resulting in antibody synthesis. Furthermore, blockade of the reticuloendothelial system, primarily the macrophages, by the injection of carbon particles (India ink) prevented an immune response to the injected antigen. The macrophage therefore appeared to be involved in the immune response and had to be incorporated into any proposed mechanism culminating in immune cell activation and antibody synthesis.

However, a question which was not posed at the time was what "informs" the macrophage that it may totally degrade one part of the antigen, the carrier, to its constituent amino acids and simple sugars, which at the same time ensure the preservation of the antigenic determinants (or epitopes) of the antigen. A system as essential as the immune system for the survival of the host and species cannot function on the basis of serendipity. Survival cannot depend upon random degradation of the antigen by the macrophage with the retention of the intact antigenic determinants left strictly to chance. There must be an infallible mechanism which ensures the integrity of the antigenic determinant(s) while permitting degradation of the carrier constituent of the antigen in a random, indiscriminate manner.

In 1965, a milestone discovery by Claman and his colleagues laid to rest the single lymphocyte model for antibody synthesis and provided an insight into how the macrophage could be programmed to degrade the carrier portion of the antigen while preserving the antigenic determinants. Claman et al. demonstrated that antibody synthesis in the rodent required interaction between a thymus-derived lymphocyte, the T cell, and a bone marrow-derived lymphocyte, the B cell. It was subsequently demonstrated and confirmed by Miller, Mitchell, Nossal and their colleagues that the T cell and B cell are separate lineages of cells and that one does not convert into the other. Furthermore, they demonstrated that the role of the T cell is to recognize (or cognize) the antigen, and that the role of the B cell is to synthesize antibodies. These T and B cells were therefore referred to on a functional basis as antigen-receptor bearing cells (or antigen-reactive cells) or ARC, and antibody-forming cells or AFC, respectively. It was established that the ARC cells are clonally preselected since they possess surface membrane receptors committed to interact with the antigenic determinants or epitopes upon initial exposure to them. Singhal and Richter demonstrated that the ARC obtained from the unimmunized rabbit respond with blastogenesis and mitosis following initial exposure to the unaltered native antigen *in vitro*. The pre-AFC B cells obtained from the unimmunized rabbit did not respond with blastogenesis and mitosis following culture with antigen. Richter also demonstrated by radioautography that radioactively labelled antigens adhered in high concentration to the ARC cells of an unimmunized rabbit following short-term incubation of the cells with the antigen. The pre-AFC B cells obtained from the unimmunized rabbit failed to interact with antigen following short-term incubation with the antigen. Abdou and Richter concluded that the ARC in the naive unimmunized rabbit are precommitted, clonally selected, unipotent or monogamous cells and not pluripotent polygamous cells; that is, the receptors on any one ARC are all directed toward the same antigenic determinant and not toward different determinants. The pre-AFC B cells, on the other hand, were considered to be uncommitted pluripotent cells which only become committed following their activation into antibody synthesis. Abdou and Richter also demonstrated that the ARC and AFC cells in the rabbit, as in the rodent, are separate lineages of cells which do not convert one into the other.

The pre-AFC B cell is activated by an antigenic signal resulting from the sequential interactions of the antigen with the ARC and the macrophage. These B cells transform first into medium, then large lymphocytes which dedifferentiate into undifferentiated blast cells. These latter cells proliferate into more blast cells which differentiate into antibody synthesizing and secreting lymphoblasts and plasmablasts. All of these steps are reversible. The plasmablast can now take two different directions--one is reversible transformation into the moribund plasma cell (life span 3-5 days) and the other is to back-track on all of the above transformation and proliferation stages and end up as a small mature memory lymphocyte. The memory lymphocytes cannot be distinguished morphologically from other mature lymphocytes. However, they possess complete or incomplete IgG antibodies on the surface membrane which can interact with the antigenic determinants of the specific antigen. If the antigen is an erythrocyte, then the memory cells form rosettes with the erythrocytes and can thereby be isolated from the other lymphocytes. If the memory cells are incubated in culture with the antigen, they undergo blastogenesis and mitosis, followed by their transformation into antibody synthesizing lymphoblasts and plasmablasts.

THE PROBLEM

Today we recognize that the induction of the antibody immune response is much more complex than was originally considered in the sense that there are more players than was previously envisioned. If we assume that all of the participants have *bona fide* roles, it is necessary to consider that antibody synthesis involves contributions from each of the following:

      1. The AFC B effector cell. This is the terminal cell in the activation of the immune system. It synthesizes and secretes the antibodies.

      2. The obligatory participating cells. These are the macrophage and the ARC cells.

      3. The regulatory cells. These are the antigen-specific T helper and T suppressor cells.

      4. The interleukins, primarily IL-1, IL-2, B cell growth factor (BCGF) and B cell differentiation factor (BCDF). The BCGF and BCDF may constitute what is also referred to as B cell stimulatory factors I and II (BSF-1 and BSF II).

      5. The HLA Class II antigens.

The transplantation or histocompatibility antigens, referred to today as the human leukocyte antigens or HLA antigens, were discovered and described in the late 1960s and early 1970s. It was demonstrated that immunization with leukocytes of the organ donor prior to implantation of the allograft resulted in rapid rejection of the allograft. It was then shown that the HLA antigens are highly heterogeneous, the products of a number of polymorphic genetic loci each of which is multiallelic. The HLA antigens were classified according to their position on the short arm of chromosome 6 - A, B, C and D(DR). HLA-A, B and C antigens are present on all nucleated cells whereas HLA-D(DR) antigen is present primarily on resting B cells, resting macrophages and activated T cells, not resting T cells. The HLA-A, B, C and DR antigens are serologically defined in the sense that individuals exposed to these antigens generate antibodies to them. In contradistinction, the HLA-D antigens are lymphocyte-defined since exposure to these antigens induces blastogenesis and mitosis of T cells, a reaction referred to as the mixed lymphocyte culture reaction or the MLR reaction. The HLA-A, B and C antigens differ from the HLA-D(DR) in their molecular configuration and composition. The HLA-A, B and C antigens are referred to collectively as Class I antigens and the HLA-D(DR) antigens are referred to as the Class II antigens.

The discovery of the HLA antigens was seized by immunologists as an opportunity to establish a role for these antigens in the normal immune response. After all, it was argued, the HLA antigens not have evolved for the sole purpose of sensitizing a host's immune system to antigens in an allograft resulting in the rejection of the allograft. The grafting of organs or tissues from one individual to another individual is not a physiological occurrence and the evolving immune system could not have ever anticipated it. Rosenthal and Shavach, in 1973, reported that immune guinea pig T cells could undergo blastogenesis to antigen stimulation only if "presented" with the antigen bound to autologous macrophages and not allogeneic macrophages. The investigators did not go beyond the blastogenic response of immune T cells of one animal species to antigen stimulation. The response is a secondary immune response. Nevertheless, this finding was immediately hailed as an example of an HLA restricted *primary* immune response in which an individual's naive immunocompetent cells can only respond to an antigen provided the antigen is complexed with autologous HLA antigens. However, the investigators who support the role of the HLA Class II antigens in antigen presentation and the induction of antibody synthesis have not taken into account the fact that T-independent antigens can activate the pre-AFC B cells without being linked to HLA antigens. Furthermore, they seem to have forgotten that Sell and Gell, in the mid-1960s, demonstrated that anti-Ig immunoglobulins can activate the B cells into blastogenesis and mitosis without the requirement of other cells and, by inference, without the requirement of HLA antigens to initiate this response. As was discussed above, Singhal and Richter demonstrated that rabbit ARC cells obtained from unimmunized rabbits responded with blastogenesis and mitosis upon exposure to the native antigen.

If we consider that antigen can only be recognized by the appropriate immunocompetent cell if it is complexed to autologous Class II HLA antigens, it follows that the immunocompetent cell has receptors for *both* autologous Class II HLA antigens(s) and the antigenic determinant on the exogenous antigen. It is behooven upon the investigator to ask him/herself "what could happen but must not happen if such a circumstance were to prevail?" The existence *in vivo* of immunocompetent cells capable of recognizing and reacting with autologous antigens constitutes a most hazardous situation for the host. What would prevent the immunocompetent cells from mounting an immune response against the autoantigen and thereby initiate an autoimmune disease? In order to obviate this possibility, it is essential that the immunocompetent cell which recognizes and is stimulated by the antigenic determinant complexed to the Class II HLA antigens not give rise to or transform into an effector cell, i.e., an antibody synthesizing cell, a cytotoxic cell or a lymphokine-secreting sensitized infiltrating delayed hypersensitivity cell. Such a situation dictates that two functionally distinct cells must participate in the immune response--the first an antigen-recognizing cell (ARC) which responds to antigenic stimulation and the second the precursor of the AFC effector cell which is activated by a product of the reaction between the antigen and the ARC cell. Thus, the finding initially made by Claman and his associates of the obligatory participation of ARC and AFC cells in the immune response to T dependent antigens finds a rational justification as a result of the incorporation of Class II HLA antigens into the mechanism of AFC activation.

THE RATIONALE

I would not like to turn to the main topic of this paper which is the delineation of the mechanism whereby the T dependent antigen is processed, transformed, degraded, and reduced to the entity which initiates the sequence of intercellular and intracellular reactions in the pre-AFC B cell which culminates in antibody synthesis and secretion. It has been postulated that this ultimate immunogenic entity is bound to a cell which "presents" it to the appropriate responding immunocompetent cell, presumably the pre-AFC cell. This cell is therefore referred to as the "antigen presenting cell" or APC. The process is euphemistically referred to as "antigen presentation."

"Antigen presentation" is, however, a very vague term since it does not indicate 1) the relationship of the antigen with the cell doing the presenting; 2) the cell the antigen is being presented to; and 3) the state of immune system activation. Macrophages, T lymphocytes and B lymphocytes have variously been described as antigen presenting cells. Nature is not so fickle or capricious as to "choose" three different cells to carry out a single function. It selects, through the process evolution, the single most direct, efficient and effective means to ensure that an immune response will occur. The term antigen presentation is an exercise in linguistic gymnastics to convince the reader that it represents progress in our understanding of the mechanism of antigen handling and processing by the appropriate cell(s) and the transmission of the antigenic message to the pre-AFC B cell.

Any serious proposal for the mechanism of activation of the immune system by antigen must take the following into account:

1. Class II HLA antigens are present primarily, if not only, on macrophages, B cells, and activated T cells.
2. The autologous MLR, or AMLR, is a reaction in which some T cells respond with blastogenesis and mitosis when confronted with *autologous* macrophages or B cells. This response suggests that these T cells possess receptors to *autologous* Class II HLA antigens.
3. The demonstration in the mid-1960s by Claman, Miller, Mitchell and Taylor that T ARC cells in the rodent react with the antigen before the AFC receive the "message" to enter the cycle of transformation-proliferation-differentiation into AFC. Richter and Singhal showed that the ARC cells in the rabbit respond with blastogene-

sis and mitosis when confronted with randomly selected undegraded antigens not complexed to any cell. These antigens included ovalbumin, human serum albumin, bovine gamma globulin, keyhole limpet hemocyanin and sheep and horse erythrocytes. There was no requirement for linkage between the antigen and HLA Class II antigen. Furthermore, the T-independent antigens can activate the pre-AFC B cells directly, and they certainly do not exhibit HLA antigens. Also, as will be discussed below, allogeneic anti-Ig immunoglobulins can also activate the B cells without the requirement of HLA Class II antigens.

4. Antigens are totally degraded following their phagocytosis by macrophages *in vitro*. Therefore, there must be an infallible mechanism to preserve the antigenic determinants following phagocytosis of the antigen *in vivo*. It simply cannot be left to chance to ensure that the antigenic determinants, required for the induction of an immune response, be preserved during the degradation of the antigen by the macrophage.

THE HYPOTHESIS

The three cells which participate directly in the induction of antibody synthesis to T-dependent antigens are the AFC, ARC and macrophage. We can hypothesize seven different sequences of reactions involving these three cells and the antigen (Fig. 1). The question is which of these sequences, if any, is the one which the immune system utilizes? Obviously any mechanism in which the AFC participates prior to the involvement of the other two cells can be dismissed since there would be no need for the ARC and the macrophage (sequences 3 and 5). Similarly, any reaction sequences in which the AFC is not the final cell can also be rejected (sequences 4 and 6). Sequence 2 can be seriously questioned since it involves the macrophage prior to the ARC in the processing of the antigen. As was discussed above, the macrophage cannot be left to its own devices to determine what part of the antigen will be degraded totally (the carrier) and what part of it will be retained intact [the antigenic determinant(s)]. It must receive specific instructions from another cell. Therefore, sequence 2 can also be discarded. That leaves sequences 1 and 7 to choose between as the one adopted by the immune system. In both of these reaction sequences, the antigenic determinant on the antigen reacts initially with the specific receptor on the precommitted ARC cell. If the receptor, still attached to the antigen, is then shed by the ARC cell, it will form an autologous protein coat (on the assumption that the receptor is a protein) on the antigenic determinant protecting it from degradation by the macrophage following phagocytosis of the antigen. The undegraded antigenic determinant can then be:

a) displayed on the surface of the macrophage adjacent or juxtaposed to HLA Class II antigen,

b) secreted into the circulation where it may attach to B cells and activate them, or

c) transferred from the macrophage back to the "denuded" ARC which will now display the antigenic determinants very prominently and in high density on its surface. This "reconstituted" ARC is the antigen presenting cell or APC (sequence 7 in Fig. 1).

It is proposed (Fig. 2) that the quiescent pre-AFC B cell exposed to the APC is activated by a "hot spot" on the APC composed of repeating sequences of the same antigenic determinant. The T-independent antigen with its linear arrangement of repeating units of the same antigenic determinant can activate the pre-AFC B cell in its native state, thereby bypassing the ARC and macrophage.

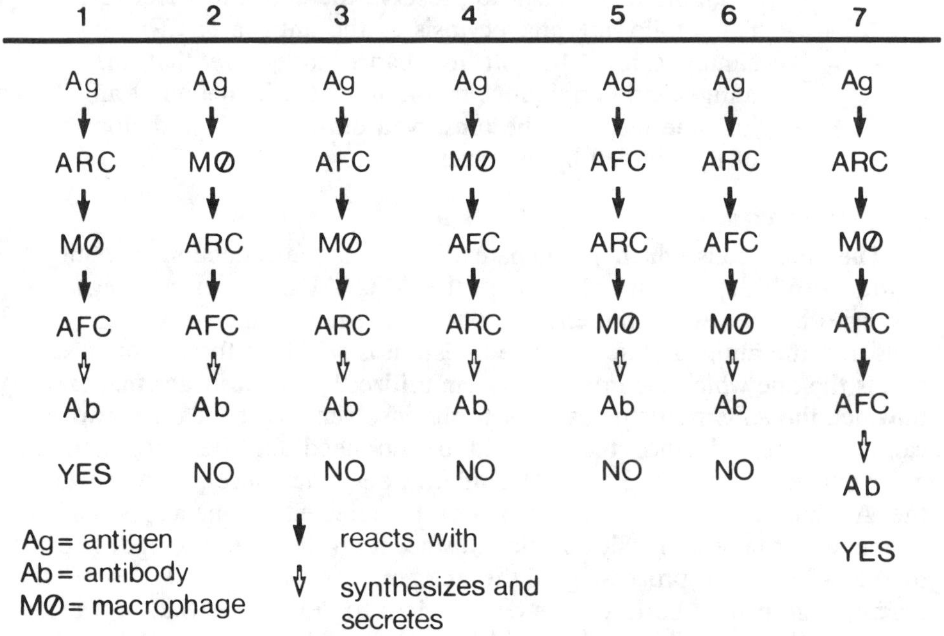

1	2	3	4	5	6	7
Ag	Ag	Ag	Ag	Ag	Ag	Ag
↓	↓	↓	↓	↓	↓	↓
ARC	MØ	AFC	MØ	AFC	ARC	ARC
↓	↓	↓	↓	↓	↓	↓
MØ	ARC	MØ	AFC	ARC	AFC	MØ
↓	↓	↓	↓	↓	↓	↓
AFC	AFC	ARC	ARC	MØ	MØ	ARC
⇓	⇓	⇓	⇓	⇓	⇓	↓
Ab	Ab	Ab	Ab	Ab	Ab	AFC
						⇓
YES	NO	NO	NO	NO	NO	Ab
						YES

Ag = antigen
Ab = antibody
MØ = macrophage

↓ reacts with
⇓ synthesizes and secretes

Fig. 1. The possible sequences of interactions between the antigen, the macrophage, the ARC and the AFC which lead to antibody synthesis.

However, this mechanism has a major shortcoming--it does not take into account the HLA Class II antigens. This author is not convinced, on the basis of the existing evidence, that the HLA antigens are involved in the activation of the antibody immune response. Nevertheless, the mechanism presented in Fig. 3 incorporates the HLA antigens in the induction of the antibody immune response. The antigenic determinants on the antigen react first with the specific receptors on the precommitted ARC. The receptors are shed from the ARC and protect the antigenic determinants from degradation following phagocytosis of the antigen by the macrophage. The positioning of the antigenic determinants adjacent to the HLA Class II antigens on the macrophage surface is, however, a random occurrence. Presumably, if sufficient antigen is processed by the macrophage, some antigen would, by chance, be deposited on the cell surface adjacent to the HLA antigens. A relatively large quantity of the antigen must therefore be injected to ensure the deposition of a sufficient number of antigen determinants adjacent to the

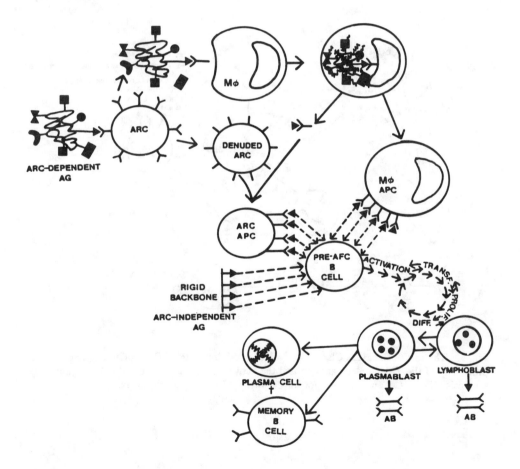

Fig. 2. The roles of the ARC and the macrophage in the processing of the T-dependent antigen and the presentation of the antigen to the pre-AFC B cell. The relationship of T-dependent and T-independent antigens.

HLA Class II antigens on the macrophage surface to activate the pre-AFC B cell. This may be the condition which determines the minimal amount of antigen that must be administered *in vivo* in order for antibody synthesis to take place.

A slightly different version of the mechanism presented in Figure 3 is presented diagrammatically in Figure 4. Here, the HLA antigen constitutes part of the antigen receptor. This ensures that the peripheralized antigenic determinant on the macrophage cell surface, following phagocytosis and degradation of the antigen-receptor complex and the preservation of the antigenic determinant, will always be adjacent to or contiguous with the HLA Class II antigen on the macrophage surface.

A number of investigators have proposed that the B cell itself is the antigen presenting cell. The majority of these investigators used a) cells of previously immunized animals and/or; b) allogeneic anti-immunoglobulin (anti-Ig) antibodies as the antigen; these antibodies can react with the surface membrane immunoglobulins (smIg) on the B cell and/or; c) selected antigens

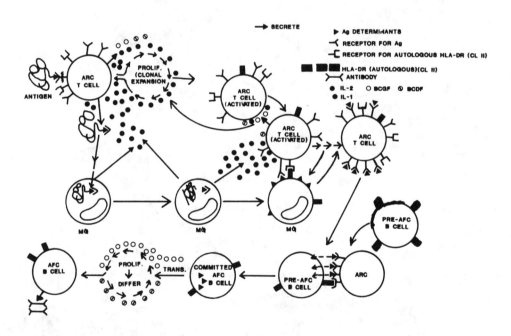

Fig. 3. The role of the HLA Class II antigens, in addition to the ARC and macrophage, in the processing of the T-dependent antigen and the activation of the pre-AFC B cell into antibody synthesis. The HLA antigens are not linked to the ARC antigen receptors.

which can inherently interact with certain unidentified constituents on the B cell surface. In the case of the previously immunized animal, it is universally accepted that the memory cells possess antibody molecules on their surface capable of interacting with the immunizing antigen and becoming activated by it. The memory B cell can also react with any antigens which cross-react with the immunizing antigen. However, it will not react with other randomly selected antigens.

Allogeneic (i.e., goat) anti-Ig antibodies used as the antigen bind to B cells which possess smIg. The allogeneic (goat) anti-Ig antibodies are all identical in structure and composition and they line up along the B cell surface membrane. The cross-linking of the smIg by the allogeneic (goat) anti-Ig antibodies may trigger the B cell to undergo blastogenesis and mitosis and/or to synthesize antibodies to goat Ig. Furthermore, the antigen (the allogeneic goat anti-Ig antibodies) bound in high density to the B cell may confer APC

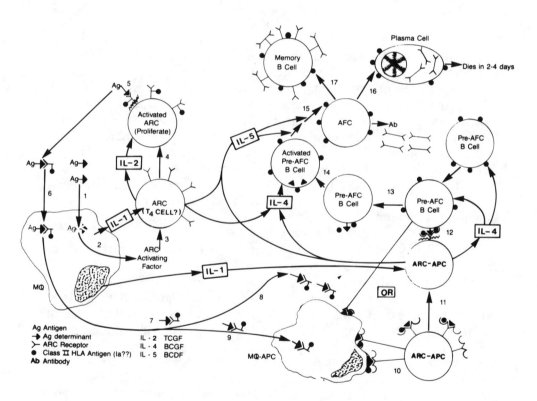

Fig. 4. The role of the HLA Class II antigens, in addition to the ARC and macrophage, in the processing of the T-dependent antigen and the activation of the pre-AFC B cell into antibody synthesis. The HLA antigens are linked to the ARC antigen receptors.

properties to it; the B cell may activate a second B cell into antibody synthesisin much the same way as T-independent antigens are able to activate B cells directly (Fig. 2). In both cases, the antigenic determinants are identical in composition and specificity. In both cases, the antigen activates the B cells without the intervention of other cells and without the need for HLA Class II antigens.

The mechanism of direct B cell activation functions only with respect to ligands which are capable of cross-linking specific cell-surface constituents on the B cell thereby inducing the necessary surface membrane changes which fool the B cell into becoming activated. It is instructive to note that allogeneic (goat) *non-antibody* Ig cannot trigger the B cells as it does not react with the B cells. Since the B cells neither react with nor are activated by randomly selected antigens, one should consider those instances of direct B cell interaction with specific antigens to be specific exceptions rather than the rule.

SUMMARY

I have presented a single, all-encompassing mechanism for the activation of the immune system and the induction of antibody synthesis by the antigen. I have proceeded on the assumption that the immune system has attained a high degree of evolution and that nature, in its wisdom, has selected only one mechanism to activate the immune system, a mechanism which is efficient, infallible, and sufficiently flexible to accommodate all of the different antigens in our environment. The approach which I rejected is that there exist different mechanisms for the activation of the immune system depending upon the antigen on the proposition that the immune system is still evolving. I cannot believe that a system as essential for the survival of the host as the immune system would not have reached a level of evolution today comparable to that of other systems in the body.

The difficulty in accepting a single mechanism emanates from the different results which investigators have obtained. This state of affairs may be attributed to investigators using different naturally-occurring and synthetic antigens in *in vitro* culture. It is essential to realize that the immune system evolved to process and react with antigens *in vivo*, under conditions quite different from those imposed on the immune cells dispersed in culture medium *in vitro*. *In vitro* investigations should be used primarily to confirm findings obtained *in vivo*, and not vice versa. Unquestionably, the plethora of investigations carried out *in vitro* are based on the mistaken belief that results are more dependable when they are obtained in a clean, well defined, isolated *in vitro* system than when they are obtained in uncontrolled experiments *in vivo*. Nevertheless, the results obtained *in vivo* must be considered to be the benchmark or standard with which results obtained *in vitro* should be compared. The mechanism of activation of the AFC by antigen which I have presented is based in large part on investigations in the immunized animal which may or may not have been irradiated or thymectomized prior to the administration of syngeneic or hemi-allogeneic cells in order to assess the contributions of the different cells in the induction of the antibody immune response. Although the animals have been manipulated, this approach is far more physiological than any *in vitro* system.

Any mechanism proposed for AFC activation must ensure the immune response to microbial antigens which is the reason for the evolution of the immune system in the first place. Particulate antigens must be at least partially degraded and must liberate their antigenic determinants intact. In order to ensure that the macrophage does not degrade the antigenic determinants while it is degrading everything else, the determinants must be protected from degradation. This protection is best provided by autologous receptors carried by the precommitted ARC cells.

The HLA Class II antigens have been incorporated into the general unified scheme since it is universally considered that they are essential in the stimulation of the antibody immune response. Arguments have been presented by many investigators in favor of an essential role for the HLA antigens; however, the evidence which they are based upon is neither impressive nor convincing. Numerous exceptions to the requirement for HLA antigens exist and have been referred to in the text. It is essential to show that HLA co-recognition by the immunocompetent cells is required for antibody synthesis to take place, not for blastogenesis or the secretion of interleukins, in order for the HLA antigens to be considered to have an obligatory role in antibody synthesis.

The arguments and mechanism which I have proposed for the activation of the immune system and the induction of antibody synthesis by the antigen are philosophically compatible with the considered requirements for the infallible activation of the immune system to the exclusion of randomness. Whether they will withstand the test of time is another matter. I am fully cognizant of the fact that progress in medical research dictates that a great deal of what is accepted to be true today is shown to be false tomorrow.

Chapter 13

IMMUNITY AND THE SISYPHUS EFFECT

Herman Friedman

HISTORICAL INTRODUCTION AND BACKGROUND

I was graduated from Temple University with an A.B. and decided to pursue my interests in the area of biomedical sciences, principally in the study of host immunity as the protector against bacterial infections. This interest was instilled by Dr. James Harrison, Professor of Bacteriology at Temple University in Philadelphia and a graduate of the University of Chicago.

After receiving my bachelor's degree I was honed by Dr. T. N. Harris at Children's Hospital at the University of Pennsylvania in Philadelphia. In my opinion, he is one of the most underrated immunologists in the modern era. Tzvi Harris, together with his wife, Shoshana, and a small group of investigators had been studying the role of lymphocytes in immunity. In the late 1940's he wrote that the riddle of immunity would not be readily solved because no one could separate antibody forming tissue from the whole individual and all experimental models being used at that time, such as x-radiation or drugs, not only wiped out the lymphoid system but also affected many other tissues. Nevertheless, in the early 1950's, Dr. Harris and his associates showed that cells obtained from the popliteal lymph nodes of rabbits could transfer the ability to produce antibody to Shigella in immuno-suppressed irradiated recipient rabbits.

Prior to my joining his laboratory, he had already shown that only organs rich in lymphocytes, e.g., cells from a draining lymph node, were capable of transferring such immunity. The thymus, however, was also rich in lympho-cytes but could not accomplish this feat. In experiments conducted in the 1950's he surgically removed the thymus, hypothesizing that this lymphoid organ may be important in immunity despite the conventional wisdom at the time. Although he thymectomized rabbits as young as 5 days of age, he failed to affect development of immunity to Shigella. We now know that similar experiments using neonatal rabbits could have shown an effect. Current immunobiologic studies now stress the importance of the thymus in developing immunity. Nevertheless, Harris showed 30 years ago that the transfer of lymph nodes rich in lymphocytes from immune donor rabbits could provide immunity in irradiated recipients. He also showed that antigen must be "processed" in the irradiated recipients and this might be due to radiation-resistant macrophages. He could immunize recipients to Shigella antigen even by giving cells from donors that had been immunized less than one day prior to the transfer. At the same time harris was also attempting to "immunize" normal lymphocytes *in vitro* using Shigella antigen, but was unable to do so, probably because he used a level of antigen that was too high and induced tolerance or the synthesis of antibody was masked.

During that period Harris published a paper with the whimsical title "Sisyphus effect" in which he reported that lymph node cells from donor rabbits given together with antigen would rapidly produce antibody to Shigella when transferred to animals, but when the same cells were not primed with antigen, but cultured first for a few days *in vitro* and then transferred to the irradiated rabbits, the cells, even though still viable, failed to produce

0-8493-4722-X/94/$0.00 + $.50

antibody immediately. There was a lag of several days before antibody was detected in the recipients. Control studies indicated irradiated rabbits receiving no cells or dead cells failed to produce antibody. Thus the transferred cells, when stimulated immediately with antigen, were activated to produce antibody, but if they were not treated with antigen for several days, they would lose their "activated state" and apparently had to begin again the process leading to activation and antibody production from the beginning, i.e., the sisyphus effect.

Modern immunology has made much of this sisyphus effect. As we learned in the 1950s, immunology has many peaks and valleys and while investigators are constantly in the process of filling in the valleys, the peaks have remained essentially unchanged from those first described 50-100 years ago. Thus, it seems valuable to review historical aspects of the development of the field of immunology from the perspectives of the 1950s and 1960s as a foundation of continuing excitement about advances being made in our understanding of antibody formation and immunity to microbes.

ANTIBACTERIAL IMMUNITY

Because of the AIDS epidemic, there is now a resurgence in interest concerning immune responses to infectious agents. However, it should be noted that from the 1950s to the 1970s and in the early 1980s, it was felt by many there was little need to delve into the nature and mechanisms governing resistance to infections "since all bacterial infections could be handled by antibiotics," an idea popularized in medical circles in the 1950s. However, it is blatantly apparent that defects in the immune response system or the development of an infection with an immunosuppressive agent, e.g., HIV infection, results in many common opportunistic infectious agents causing extensive morbidity and mortality. Investigators now acknowledge we need to know much more about immunity to all types of microbes to complement our understanding of the nature and mechanisms associated with immune responses to synthetic antigens, to tumor antigens or to antigens involved in autoimmunity.

Early studies on microbial immunity were a harbinger of much subsequent work in the 1950s and 1970s concerning the nature and mechanism of immune responses or the lack thereof. Nevertheless, many immunochemists and immunobiologists believed that work with "dirty," microbial agents, i.e., mixture of immunogens as they exist on a bacterium could not lead to an understanding of the immune response system. It seems important to note that among the first indications of immunological tolerance were studies dealing with LCM virus performed in the 1930s. Immune tolerance or paralysis to pneumococcal polysaccharides was first described in the 1940s and is still a major enigma. It was at this time that Dr. Merrill Chase in New York City initiated studies leading to important concepts of cellular immunity by showing that tuberculin skin reactivity in guinea pigs could be transferred only by lymphoid cells from TB-sensitized donor animals. Passive transfer of serum failed to transfer skin reactivity. It is now recognized that such transfer of TB "hypersensitivity" was really a manifestation of cellular immunity, dependent upon the transfer of T lymphocytes.

Dr. Tzvi Harris, in the early 1950s, was the first to show that the ability to produce antibody could be transferred by transferring lymphocytes, as described above. Dr. Gus Nossal, in Australia in the early 1960's, also found that lymphocytes were important in producing antibody to Salmonella and conclusively showed that a single lymphocyte was responsible for producing a single class of specific antibody, again using Salmonella as the model antigen. Dr. Nossal and his colleagues, including Gordon Ada, Chris Parrish, and others in Australia, focused attention on induction as well as mechanisms of immunological tolerance to a bacterial protein antigen derived from Salmonella, i.e., flagellin. Thus, by the 1950s and early 1960s studies employing bacteria and bacterial antigens were integrally associated with probing investigations of the nature and mechanism of immune responses to bacterial antigens.

Studies on RNA in Immunity

It is of interest to recall that Dr. Felix Horwitz and others in the United States as well as abroad strongly believed that subcellular factors could be involved in the development of or regulating immune responses. Prior to the theories and the work of Dr. Niels Jerne, Dr. David Talmage and Sir MacFarlane Burnett, a "lock and key" hypothesis was proposed to be responsible for the tremendous diversity in antibodies produced in response to the multitude of antigens known to exist. This was related to suggestions by Dr. Linus Pauling and his associates, including Dr. Dan Campbell, proposing that immunoglobulins could be "folded" around antigenic determinants and antibody would then be formed. Since it was recognized that lasting immunity continued long after antigen was undetectable, an indirect enzymatic mechanism for antibody production was proposed. This was followed by a modified template theory, whereby antigen combined with RNA served as an "immune stimulus" and such RNA-antigen complexes could be involved in antibody formation.

Although modern molecular biologic techniques and genetic analyses have shown it unlikely that RNA is responsible for antibody formation as per the indirect template hypothesis, studies in the 1960s and 1970s in a number of laboratories, including ours, were compatible with the notion that RNA-antigen complexes played a role, perhaps as a potent adjuvant whereby small amounts of antigens could persist and induce a secondary immune response. In early experiments in the 1950s and 1960s, Dr. Felix Horwitz showed that relatively small amounts of antigen injected into an animal would persist for long periods of time, essentially for years, and that the antigen was a conjugate of RNA-antigen. The later studies of Dr. Marvin Fishman and Dr. Frank Adler and associates in the 1960s indicated that RNA-antigen complex activity could be inhibited by a specific antibody.

Studies in this laboratory showed that the immune response to bacterial antigens could be transferred to virgin mice or could be initiated in spleen cell cultures by exposing the animal or cells to an RNA-rich extract obtained from donor mice immunized with Shigella. The spleen obtained from these animals was extracted with phenol water resulting in an RNA-rich protein extract. Relatively small amounts of this material, when injected into normal irradiated recipient mice, induced a specific antibody response to Shigella. Once the *in vitro* antibody plaque assay for sheep erythrocytes was popularized by Niels Jerne in the 1960s, similar studies were performed completely *in vitro*, since the plaque assay was a more sensitive system than serum antibody titrations. The sheep red blood cell (SRBC) antigens, when added to normal mouse spleen cells, produced an RNA-SRBC complex after several days which, when extracted with phenol water and added to normal mouse spleen cells *in vitro*, would induce specific antibody responses to the RBCs within a few days. The activity of the RNA-antigen complex could be inhibited by treatment with RNAse, but not DNAse or other enzymes. It was also blocked by anti-SRBC antibody, but not normal serum or antibody to other antigens. If recipients were already primed to SRBC antigens, the RNA-rich extract from SRBC immunized donors would induce a secondary antibody response. Unfortunately, reports from major laboratories that claimed that donor anti-sheep RBC immunoglobulin allotype appeared in genetically distinct recipients with a different immunoglobulin allotype, suggesting that the RNA not only was a carrier of the antigen, but also "converted" recipient cells to produce antibody of donor rather than recipient allotype, dampened investigations in this area. These reports remain unconfirmed.

Early studies examining the biological activity of what were eventually called cytokines, including the lymphokines, monokines, tumor necrosis factor, and the interleukins molecules involved in immunoregulation, were performed using similarly "dirty" or crude extracts of lymphoid cells or supernatants from cell cultures. In recent years, the advent of molecular biologic techniques has resulted in the availability of highly purified lymphokines for studies on immune regulation. In a similar sense, the advent of hybridoma technology in the 1970s, providing individual clones of antibody producing cell populations, resulted in the availability of model systems that relegated the proposed RNA-antigen complexes into obsoleteness. However, the early studies involving RNA-antigen complexes in immunity provided much intellectual excitement and many model systems that continue to be important for studying the nature and mechanisms of immunity.

Retroviruses and Immunosuppression

Development of the concept that viruses can be immunosuppressive agents is an interesting story that provides additional insights which advanced our knowledge about the immune mechanism. For over 60 years from the early 1900s to the 1960s there were many observations that virus infection could depress immune responses. Dr. Claude von Pirquet, at the beginning of the century, observed that children infected with measles, known to be a virus infection, could lose pre-existing skin reactivity to tuberculin antigen. This reaction was considered an indication of immunity to mycobacteria. Immunity to this and other bacterial agents also were found depressed as a consequence of many different viral infections, but the depression was usually finite in nature and short-lived. However, leukemia virus infection of experimental animals resulted in a prolonged and more pronounced immunodeficiency which progressed with the disease state.

The murine leukemia viruses were discovered during the 1950s and 1960s. There was intense interest in uncovering mechanisms whereby these viruses induced malignancy. A complication of these studies was death of experimental animals resulting often from a simple microbial infection, a problem of studying leukemia viruses *in vivo*. Shortly, however, it was recognized that leukemia virus infection of mice could serve as an important model to study virus-induced immunosuppression. The first publication regarding the effect of a murine leukemia virus on the immune response was a review in the *Annals of the New York Academy of Sciences*. This publication concerned itself only with the reticuloendothelial system, i.e., macrophages. The paper provided evidence of a depression of reticuloendothelial cell function in mice infected with the Friend virus, but failed to discuss this observation. Subsequent to this publication, several groups, including ours, almost simultaneously reported that mice infected with murine leukemogenic viruses evinced a marked immunosuppression long before development of overt leukemia.

The immunodepressive nature of these viruses did not appear due to the displacement of normal, functional lymphocytes with non-functional leukemic cells. Subsequent work in this and other laboratories showed that mice infected with these leukemogenic viruses develop a marked immune deficiency, including alteration in T cells, B cells and macrophage function, as well as lymphokine production. This completely deranged the immune response to test antigens and resistance to infectious agents such as other viruses, bacteria and fungi. These studies employing leukemogenic retroviruses preceded by several decades current passions involving the nature and mechanism whereby lentiretroviruses, principally HIV, induce immunodeficiency and affect an individual's ability to resist subsequent infections by opportunistic microbes which normally would not result in morbidity and/or mortality in non-immunocompromised hosts.

It is important to note that the experimental models discussed above employed erythroleukemia viruses which, although retroviruses, are not lentiviruses, the subgroup to which HIV belongs. There are genetic differences between these retroviral agents. Nevertheless, the murine leukemia virus studies permitted dissection of how an RNA retrovirus blocked the immune response system and was an important forerunner along with other retrovirus- animal model systems to yield technical approaches utilized presently to study HIV.

Because advances made concerning the mechanism whereby HIV suppresses immunity in man seem to be extensions of earlier investigations employing animal model systems, as discussed above, it seems appropriate to review briefly the historical aspects of how our group began the study of retrovirus-induced immunosuppression. In those early experiments we were preparing RNA-rich extracts from the spleens of mice previously immunized with sheep red cells and transferring this RNA preparation to irradiated recipient mice. At the same time and in the institution where our work was being conducted, Dr. Marvin Rich, head of the Tumor Virology Laboratory, was studying Friend virus leukemogenesis. This strain of virus, isolated by Dr. Charlotte Friend in New York City in the 1950s, was shown to induce leukemia in adult Swiss Webster mice. Dr. Ludwig Gross, also in New York City had earlier isolated a virus preparation called Gross passage A agent (at the time no one wished to go out on a limb stating that a virus was the cause of leukemia) which could induce leukemia in newborn mice. Dr. Friend subsequently did the same thing in adult mice. Marvin Rich, in cooperation with Dr. Friend, continued investigating the biochemical events associated with Friend virus-induced leukemia.

One day Dr. Rich showed me the spleen from a virus-infected mouse. It weighed over 2 g. A normal mouse, even after immunization with sheep red blood cells, had a spleen size in the range of 150-200 mg. Since mouse spleens from leukemic mice were approximately ten times larger than normal spleens, we reasoned that an RNA-antigen extract prepared from leukemic animals would yield greater quantities of RNA for studies on the adoptive transfer of "immune RNA." This made sense because Dr. Rich was sure that a leukemic mouse was immunologically "normal." In our first collaborative experiments with Dr. Rich, we found not only that the leukemic mice could not produce antibody, but that RNA extracts prepared from antigen-immunized leukemic mice failed to transfer antibody formation to that antigen. We tested and found that spleen cells from leukemic mice were markedly immunosuppressed and when normal, but infected animals received those cells, they failed to respond to an immunizing dose of a third party antigen. The immunosuppressive activity was found to be directly related to the virus itself. Thus, our discovery of the immunosuppression model using Friend virus was "accidental" and as serendipitous as many other discoveries in science.

Studies of the nature and mechanism whereby Friend virus affects the immune response showed that the virus infected both B and T cells, as well as macrophages, and depressed the ability of these cells to produce immuno-regulatory lymphokines. More recent studies showed that addition of these lymphokines to infected spleen cells *in vitro* or administration to infected animals restored some of the immune functions of the animals. Such studies restoring function to the immune system continues, especially in light of the new interest concerning retrovirus induced immunosuppression because of the AIDS epidemic.

SUBSTANCE ABUSE DRUGS, IMMUNODEFICIENCY AND PSYCHONEUROIMMUNOLOGY

A concept has emerged based upon work from a number of laboratories which indicates neurohumoral control of some immune functions and, furthermore, that immune factors and immunity itself may influence behavior. This concept is based upon a neuroimmune axis and its study has been termed "psychoneuroimmunology." We entered this area of immunology in the 1980s when we began to study the immunomodulatory effects of drugs of abuse, i.e., substances which have psychoactive effects and are used by individuals to alter "mood" and to produce a "high." In the 1970s reports appeared that peripheral blood lymphocytes from heavy marijuana smokers had markedly depressed blastogenic responses to mitogens. Furthermore, peripheral lymphocytes from marijuana smokers showed markedly depressed RNA, DNA and protein metabolism when stimulated *in vitro*. These reports were contested by other investigators who failed to observe consistent effects on lymphocyte function in marijuana smokers or users of other drugs such as heroin or cocaine. Thus, a controversy developed regarding whether drugs of abuse affected the immune response system.

With the advent of interest in psychoneuroimmunology, it was believed by some investigators that drugs of abuse such as marijuana and cocaine may affect the immune response indirectly by first interacting with the nervous system. This interaction would result in production of hormones, neurotrans-mitters, and other biologically active substances which could then affect immunity. Among these candidate substances were specific neurohormones, steroids, etc. However, immunologists soon discovered that drugs such as marijuana and cocaine as well as opiates could directly affect cells of the immune system such as B and T cells by interfering with their responsiveness to stimuli such as mitogens or antigens. Drug treatment could indirectly affect the immune system *in vivo* by exerting biological pressure on the neurological system which via immunoregulator substances resulted in altered immunity. Furthermore, laboratory animals treated with such drugs did not respond immunologically in a typical manner.

Over 200 years ago a prominent physician noted that alcoholics were more susceptible to consumption, i.e., tuberculosis, than "teetotalers." There have been many similar observations regarding altered resistance to a wide array of infectious agents in people who abuse drugs other than alcohol. Altered resistance to viral infections is even more noteworthy since i.v. drug abusers account for about one-third of AIDS patients in the United States. Drugs, such as heroin and other opiates, are now known to suppress the immune response and, in conjunction with exposure to an immunosuppressive virus, may promote the development of AIDS. This notion is fostered by the lifestyle activities of many AIDS victims, and it is apparent that many use drugs such as marijuana and cocaine.

In the early 1980s we were able to determine that the major psychogenic component of marijuana, i.e., tetrahydrocannabinol (THC), had a direct effect on the immune response system. In addition, mice injected with THC had a markedly depressed ability to respond when their lymphoid cells were stimulated *in vitro* with mitogens such as phytohemagglutinin and/or bacterial lipopolysaccharide. The ability of these lymphoid cells to produce interferon as well as other cytokines was also depressed as were the number and function of macrophages. To examine the mechanisms involved, studies were performed completely *in vitro*. We discovered that the toxic level of THC was at least 4-5 times higher than that which modulated lymphocyte function. Relatively low doses of THC, when added to human or mouse lymphoid cell cultures, markedly depressed a variety of functions including phagocytosis and cell spreading by macrophages, NK activity by peripheral blood or spleen cells, and CTL activity by T cells. Furthermore, IL-2 production, as well as synthesis of its cell surface receptor and the messenger RNA to synthesize the receptors, were also profoundly depressed in cells incubated with relatively low concentrations of THC. Thus, it was apparent that a drug such as marijuana and its components affected immune cell function *in vitro* at nontoxic doses.

Additional studies in our laboratory focused on susceptibility of mice to infectious agents including opportunistic fungi, viruses, and bacteria after treatment with THC. Our studies indicated that drug-treated animals have reduced functional activity of lymphocytes and macrophages to the bacterium Legionella, to herpes simplex virus, and to *Candida albicans*, all opportunistic pathogens. Injection of THC into mice made them more susceptible to lethal infection by these microbes as compared to control animals. In addition, recent studies demonstrated that mice injected with THC showed only a minimal alteration in susceptibility to Friend leukemia virus. However, these animals displayed a significantly pronounced susceptibility when infected with the Friend virus, given THC, and then exposed to an opportunistic virus, i.e., herpes simplex virus (type 2). It is possible that a drug of abuse such as marijuana may be a co-factor that alters the innate susceptibility in retrovirus-infected individuals to opportunistic microorganisms which normally would not be lethal. Studies encompassing drugs of abuse, psychoneuroimmunology and AIDS have a great deal of relevance to immunology and show once again that divergent fields of science may come together under the aegis of immunology when there is a convergence of interest and technology.

CONCLUSIONS

The Sisyphus effect implies there is no end, that the task cannot be accomplished. Along these lines, many investigators during the last few decades have found that much of the new immunology in essence is a revisitation of the old immunology. The mountain peaks or major questions remain despite lifetimes spent in developing answers. We always seem to be starting over again, using newer approaches and technical refinements to achieve the same goal, i.e., understanding the nature and mechanism of an extremely important biological system. Much of what we have accomplished this past decade, i.e., developing better cell culture procedures, further study of immunity to infectious agents, etc., started at the beginning of this century with what we consider crude methods and little or no understanding of the field. Now, following the development of more sophisticated technological approaches we find ourselves asking many of the same questions that were asked the beginning and middle of this century, only now we are faced with the urgency of an epidemic by an infectious agent which destroys our immunity and increases our susceptibility to opportunistic and environmental microorganisms. Yet we take solace in realizing that the cause of the AIDS epidemic brings with it the blessing of opportunity--in the form of a challenge- -to decipher and understand how the immune system is regulated and how we can regulate it, which will provide benefits to all those stricken with infectious diseases of all sorts throughout the world.

Chapter 14

ADVENTURES IN CELLULAR AND HUMORAL IMMUNOLOGY

Abram B. Stavitsky

INTRODUCTION

In retrospect, I began research at a particularly favorable time. For one thing as Nevill Mott, Nobel laureate in physics in 1977, has remarked of his career, "it was the most fortunate time to start research in theoretical physics because there were so many easy problems to solve.[1] There were not only many easy problems but many important ones which were susceptible to solution with the systems and techniques then available. Landsteiner's *The Specificity of Serological Reactions* (1954 edition) summarizes what was known of immunochemistry then and Topley and Wilson's *Principles of Bacteriology and Immunity* (1946 edition) reviews the immunobiology of that era. Students will be surprised to learn how much was known of the kinetics, memory, regulation, organ, and cellular sites of antibody production; about the heterogeneity, specificity, chemistry, and catabolism of antibodies; the chemistry and specificity of haptens; the chemistry and functions of the complement components; the effector functions of antibodies in host resistance. Much less was known about cellular immunity, but already there were some important insights into this subject as well.

Inasmuch as memory is naturally selective and imperfect and I have been charged with emphasizing my research, this account is biased toward my own contributions. However, with the help of textbooks and papers of those earlier times I have partially reconstructed the frame of knowledge within which my work was done. I have organized the discussion around some broad questions or recurring themes which were of interest to me and to other investigators and which still engage our attention. I hope the notion that science is largely a group rather than an individual effort comes through. I have had my share of good and bad fortune in my research and have benefited from serendipitous discoveries, felicitous and productive collaborations, and above all, from a very stimulating and free intellectual ambiance at this university for almost 50 years.

BACKGROUND

A productive career depends upon many elements including formal education, postdoctoral training, fellowships, graduate students, postdoctoral fellows, a stimulating intellectual environment, collaborators, service on active and productive committees, and a modicum of teaching. I have been fortunate to have had the advantages of all of these elements.

Education

Upon graduation from the University of Michigan in 1939, I began graduate work in bacteriology and immunology there. I investigated the role of mucins in enhancing the pathogenicity of *Klebsiella pneumoniae* with Dr. Walter Nungester. I was first exposed to the history of bacteriology and immunology in exciting courses in pathogenic bacteriology taught by Dr. Byron Soule. There was even a living link to the origins of bacteriology. Dr. Frederick Novy, then in his 80's, a student of Robert Koch, a pioneer

0-8493-4722-X/94/$0.00 + $.50
© 1994 by CRC Press, Inc.

virologist, bacteriologist and protozoologist, said to be the model for Sinclair Lewis' Arrowsmith in the novel of the same name, still roamed the halls. As a member of the BX (before xeroxing) generation, I did a lot of reading in the excellent university library, taking voluminous notes on index cards. I received the M.S. in 1940.

I decided to go farther west for the Ph.D., to the University of Minnesota, which had one of the outstanding departments of bacteriology in the country. I did my research with Dr. Robert Green on the pathogenesis and host resistance in leptospirosis. I learned a great deal of bacterial physiology, immunology, mycology, physiological chemistry, and pathology from an excellent faculty. As a sideline, I did some research on *Brucellosis* at the farm campus and thus became fascinated by comparative pathology and immunology. I became interested in the subject of antibody formation by preparing seminars on theories of antibody production. Thus, I first became acquainted with the side chain theory of Ehrlich;[2] the template theories of Alexander,[3] Mudd;[4] Breinl and Haurowitz;[5] and especially, the recent theory of Pauling.[6*] The theory proposed by Ehrlich was presented in a classical paper in the *Proceedings of the Royal Society* as his Croonian Lecture to the Royal Society.** This paper was and perhaps still is the most provocative one I have read as it was full of brilliant insights and ideas; e.g., the utilization of enzymes as antigens so that the persistence of antigen could be followed by monitoring enzyme activity. As a graduate student, I also became acquainted with the work of Heidelberger's group on immunochemistry, with the aforementioned book by Landsteiner, and a new book by Marrack on immunochemistry.

Because of my interest in comparative pathology and immunology, after receiving my Ph.D. degree in 1943, I embarked on the study of veterinary medicine at the University of Pennsylvania. This proved to be an excellent choice because not only was I educated in some areas of medical science for the first time, but I was exposed to a number of first-rate investigators and thinkers in bacteriology, immunology, and pathology. I was fortunate to have a part-time job at the Phipps Institute associated with the university where I spent a lot of time talking with Dr. Max B. Lurie who was then engaged in his classical genetic, immunological, and pathological studies of the role of mononuclear cells in the destruction of tubercle bacilli as part of the immune response in tuberculosis.[7] I also became acquainted with the important studies at the medical school by Ehrlich and Harris[8] on the role of lymph nodes and lymphocytes in the antibody response to particulate antigens. During my stay in Philadelphia, the seminal studies of Chase[9] on the passive

---

*Soon after going to the University of Pennsylvania, I met Dr. Stuart Mudd who was the Chairman of the Department of Bacteriology. While at Cal Tech one day a tall man showed up at my laboratory. It was Jerome Alexander. Of course, Pauling was there as well. Some years later I got to know Felix Haurowitz, MacFarlane Burnet, David Talmage, and Niels Jerne. Thus in my lifetime, I became acquainted with almost all of the people who contributed seminal theories of antibody formation. This just shows how new our field still is.

**Almost 60 years later, while on sabbatical leave in London, I was privileged to hear Sir MacFarlane Burnet, attired in black robes, present his theory of antibody formation at the 1959 Croonian Lecture to the Royal Society.

transfer of delayed hypersensitivity to tubercle bacilli drew my attention to the role of lymphocytes in cellular immunity and to the utility of the passive transfer technique for the study of immune phenomena *in vivo*.

Upon graduation from the University of Pennsylvania in 1946, I was fortunate to be accepted for postdoctoral training with Dr. Dan Campbell at Cal Tech. There I unsuccessfully attempted to repeat the experiments of Pauling and Campbell[10] on the production of specific antibodies *in vitro*—an experiment suggested by Pauling's theory of antibody formation.[6] I spent most of the year and a half there repeating the classical experiment of Landsteiner and Chase on the passive transfer of delayed hypersensitivity to tuberculin with lymph node and spleen cells of sensitized guinea pigs.[11] I also developed a technique for surgical removal of the popliteal lymph node in rabbits which I later utilized in numerous experiments.

In the fall of 1947, I began my academic career as an assistant professor of immunology in the Department of Pathology at Western Reserve University, a university which already had a thirty year old tradition of research in immunology under the direction of Dr. Enrique E. Ecker. With his students, most notably Louis Pillemer, Ecker had done and was doing outstanding research on complement activation. I did some research on *in vivo* complement fixation.[12] Although I did not work with Pillemer, I frequently talked to him and found him very stimulating.

In 1948 I joined the new Department of Microbiology there under the chairmanship of Lester O. Krampitz. Krampitz was one of the Iowa State College group which came to Western Reserve including Harland G. Wood, the first chairman of Biochemistry, and Merton Utter, who was to succeed him as chairman. This group was one of the pioneering groups in the world in the field of intermediary metabolism and quickly formed the nucleus of an exciting biochemistry department. The new microbiology department also featured intermediary metabolism but soon added an excellent microbial geneticist, Charles Yanofsky, who was very influential in my career. Resisting a number of offers to become a departmental chairman, I have remained at this university since saving a great deal of time that would have been consumed in moving and getting reestablished. In the meanwhile, the department has changed around me and has continued to be a very exciting place. In 1981, Dr. Fritz Rottman, a molecular biologist, became chairman and the name has been changed to the Department of Molecular Biology and Microbiology. The same year, Michael Lamm, an immunologist, became chairman of the Department of Pathology and has recruited a number of active and productive immunologists so that the environment for me is better than ever.

Fellowships

I spent the 1958-59 academic year at the National Institute for Medical Research with Drs. John Humphrey and Ita Askonas, two excellent immunologists. Although nothing publishable resulted from that year, I learned a great deal and met a number of stimulating people both in Britain and on the continent.

I spent the summer of 1965 in the laboratory of Olli Makela in Helsinki to learn single cell techniques. Our research resulted in a joint paper in 1967.[12]

Teaching-Research Interface

This university has always emphasized high quality teaching. I was deeply involved in the 1952 revision of the medical curriculum which resulted in an integrated curriculum taught by interdepartmental committees. Irwin Lepow and I completely overhauled the curriculum in pathology and immunology to emphasize the many common cellular and humoral elements and the many interfaces between these subjects.

I have found the teaching of medical, graduate, and postdoctoral students a helpful adjunct to research because it requires integration of large amounts of information, clarity of thinking, and the answering of many questions. I have taught an advanced course in immunology here since 1950. We have always had one or more outstanding visitors for a day or two in connection with this course, a feature which has provided me and my students with a great deal of up-to-date information as well as provocative discussions and a diversity of opinions.

A TEMPORARY FIXATION ON COMPLEMENT

I originally came to Western Reserve University in 1947 to work with Dr. E. E. Ecker on some aspect of complement. I decided to try to determine whether fixation of complement by an antigen-antibody reaction occurred *in vivo*.[11] It was known that there was a marked decrease in hemolytic complement activity during anaphylaxis, serum sickness and in the course of certain infectious diseases. It has been assumed that this loss of activity was due to fixation of complement *in vivo* similar to its fixation *in vitro*. M'Gowan[13] found that the intravenous injection of ox blood corpuscles into normal rabbits produced a diminution of complement activity; whereas, inoculation of ox erythrocytes into rabbit immunized to these cells produced a marked decrease in complement. Two other groups had observed a fall in complement following the injection of sensitized erythrocytes[14] and of tetanus toxin and antitoxin[15] into guinea pigs. We observed a marked diminution in complement as well as marked decrease in the number of granulocytes in the peripheral blood in rabbits after reinjection with the same antigen.[11] The reduction in granulocytes occurred almost immediately. The reduction in complement occurred 30 to 60 minutes following the injection of antigen and the level was restored in an hour or two.[11] The fixation of complement *in vivo* was a general phenomenon; it occurred following the reinjection of protein, carbohydrate, and bacterial antigens. Mainly the C'2 and C'4 components were implicated.

It then occurred to me that advantage could be taken of this method of reducing complement levels *in vivo* to determine whether complement was required for certain reactions *in vivo*. This possibility was tested by the study of clearance of bacteria from the blood of rabbits in which complement was reduced by the reinjection of bovine gamma globulin 15 minutes before the inoculation of the bacteria—at a time when the complement level in the blood was very low.[16] Compared to normal rabbits which rapidly cleared the blood of bacteria, the reimmunized animals accomplished this reduction much more slowly and only incompletely. However, it was not possible to link the inhibition of clearance directly with the drop in complement; alternative explanations were possible.

I then turned to the first of my collaborations with Walter Heymann, a nephrologist-pediatrician at this university who had produced kidney damage in rats by the administration of rabbit anti-kidney sera.[17] He was interested in this model disease because it resembled the nephrotic syndrome in infants and children. It was my aim to determine whether complement fixation occurred *in vivo* following the injection of these sera. In our first study we found a reduction in serum complement 30 minutes after the injection of this serum into rats.[18] However, complement was also decreased after the injection of this antiserum to bilaterally nephrectomized rats, indicating that antibodies to extra-renal tissues present in this antiserum could also fix complement. We found subsequently that complement fixation also took place when a duck anti-rat kidney serum was injected into rats, but there was no correlation between the time of complement fixation and the onset of renal disease.[19] Finally, no correlation was observed between the nephrotoxicity of rabbit anti-rat kidney sera and their hemagglutinating antibody titers against kidney antigens adsorbed to red cells.[20]

These experiments had not revealed whether or not complement was involved in the kidney damage caused by the injection of anti-kidney sera. I was not discouraged but felt we had not yet done the proper experiment. I wanted purposely to reduce complement levels before the administration of the anti-kidney sera to see whether this would prevent the kidney damage. Unfortunately, my collaborator did not want to do these experiments and, lacking both funds and personnel, I could not do these experiments unless I was to drop my studies of the antibody response which were already ongoing and yielding interesting results. This was a big disappointment as within a few years other investigators were able to show an important role of complement in the pathogenesis of kidney disease and in the pathogenesis of other types of lesions caused by immune complexes.[21]

HUMORAL IMMUNITY AS SEEN THROUGH THE KEYHOLE— LIMPET HEMOCYANIN

I began my studies on the antibody response in 1948 when I joined the Department of Microbiology at Western Reserve University. I was especially influenced by the doctoral thesis of Astrid Fagraeus[22] which appeared that year and presented evidence for the role of the spleen and plasma cells within that organ in the production of antibodies to *Salmonella*. However, my initial efforts were hampered by the lack of suitable systems and assays with which to approach a number of important basic questions. Fortunately a number of laboratories became interested in these questions about the same time and contributed greatly to their study.

Development of Systems and Assays for the Study of Antibody Production

We and others employed the transplantation of cells from antibody forming to normal animals to study a number of aspects of the antibody response until *in vitro* systems and sensitive antibody assays were developed. I became aware of the potent immunogenicity of key hole limpet hemocyanin as a postdoctoral fellow at Cal Tech through Dan Campbell's experience with this highly polymerized protein and was eventually to use it in many types of experiments.

In our initial *in vitro* studies, spleen, lymph nodes, lung, bone marrow and liver from immunized animals were cut into small fragments or slices with scissors or scalpel and incubated in suitable media. Provided the tissue was not badly macerated during preparation, antibody was synthesized.[23,24,25] Treatment or disruption of antibody-forming tissues by heating, freezing and thawing, autolysis, incubation in distilled water, or homogenization resulted in the loss of much if not all capacity to synthesize antibody *in vitro*.[22,23,26] Finally, cells were isolated from lymph nodes and shown to produce antibody in suitable media *in vitro*.[27,28] The most important factor affecting antibody synthesis *in vitro* was the presence of optimal concentrations of certain amino acids.[29,30,31] Tissue fragment cells from antibody-forming organs embedded in plasma clots or agar were shown to continue to produce antibodies for several weeks.[32,33,34,35] Various types of chambers for the maintenance of antibody-producing cells and tissues have been described.[36,37,38,39]

The passive hemagglutination procedure of Boyden[40] as modified in this[41] and other laboratories was useful, especially for the detection of 19S (IgM) antibodies to soluble proteins. The incorporation of radioactive amino acids into antibody[42] proved to be a very sensitive and useful assay for the study of methods including the development by a postdoctoral fellow, Colin Self, of an assay for radiolabeled antibody by antigen attached to a solid matrix.[43]

Further progress in the elucidation of the mechanisms of the antibody response required the development of suitable *in vitro* systems, purified antigens, purified cell populations, and additional assays for antibody. A postdoctoral fellow, Herbert Herscowitz, developed an *in vitro* anamnestic antibody response system to KLH.[44] A graduate student, George Manderino, developed methods for the preparation of KLH-primed T and B memory cells on anti-Fab' affinity columns.[45] He then prepared KLH-primed B memory cells by rosetting with complexes of erythrocyte-antibody to erythrocyte-complement complexes to remove complement-receptor bearing B cells and subsequent Ficoll-Hypaque centrifugation.[46] Another graduate student, Edward Arquilla, developed a hemolysis assay for the measurement of antibodies to insulin and other proteins.[47] Herscowitz purified KLH to a state of near homogeneity.[48]

Sites and Localization of Antibody Response

The seminal studies of McMaster and Hudack[49] suggested that lymph nodes were an important source of antibody to locally introduced antigen. Subsequently Fagraeus[50] pointed to the spleen as the organ which produced antibody following the subcutaneous introduction of antigen. Numerous studies in which different lymphoid organs were extirpated and the distribution of antibody in these organs was studied and pointed in the same direction. In one of our own early studies diphtheria toxoid was injected into the hind foot pad of rabbits and removal of the draining lymph node resulted in a much diminished antibody response to a second local injection of toxoid.[51]

In 1951 Chase[52] reported that the transfer of lymph node and spleen cells of guinea pigs highly sensitive to picryl chloride to normal guinea pigs led to the development of contact sensitivity and circulating antibody to this drug. At about the same time the Harrises[53] observed that the injection into normal rabbits of lymph node cells from rabbits injected with *Shigella* led to the appearance of agglutinins in the recipient. In both studies the transfer of antibody or antigen with the transferred cells was eliminated and *de novo* synthesis of antibody was strongly supported. In some of our experiments[51] rabbits were injected twice with diphtheria toxoid in the hind foot pads and 3 days later the cells were adoptively transferred into normal rabbits which developed a significant hemagglutination titer within the next week. In a similar experiment, we found that S_{35} L-methionine was incorporated into the antibody which appeared in the recipient, clearly showing *de novo* synthesis of antibody.[51] Taliaferro and Talmage also showed *de novo* synthesis of antibody by this criterion following the adoptive transfer of cells from immunized to non-immunized animals.[54]

Subsequently, it occurred to us that the role of antigen transferred with the cells in inducing antibody could be excluded by utilizing as recipients animals which were rendered incapable of responding to antigen by virtue of a profound nutritional deficiency. These experiments were done in collaboration with Abe Axelrod, a biochemist and nutritionist then on the faculty of this university. Rats were immunized with alum-diphtheria toxoid on days 1 and 21. On day 28, the spleen cells from 20 immunized donors were pooled and half of the pool injected into deficient recipients. The other half of the pool was injected into control rats. Hemagglutinating antibody was produced in the deficient as well as in the normal recipients.[55] At about the same time the Harrises did a similar experiment in which the capacity of the recipients to respond to carried over antigen was eliminated by x-irradiation.[56]

The criterion of incorporation of radioactive amino acids into newly synthesized antibody by different lymphoid cell preparations was then employed to study the organ sites of antibody production. Keston and Katchen[57] observed antibody production in spleen, popliteal lymph nodes, lung and liver of rabbits immunized with bovine gamma globulin. Following a single injection of ovalbumin into the foot pads of guinea pigs, Askonas and White[25] measured antibody production mainly in the draining lymph node but also in the spleen and bone marrow. In similar experiments in the rabbit, Askonas and Humphrey[26] observed antibody production in the local lymph node, and following intravenous injection of antigen in the spleen, lung, and bone marrow. Hyperimmunization of rabbits with Type 3 pneumococci by Humphrey and Sulitzeanu resulted in antibody synthesis in the lungs, bone marrow, spleen, lymph nodes and appendix, but not liver or kidneys.[58]

Over a period of years we and others have determined whether and, if so, how long the antibody response, including immunological memory, is confined to the lymphoid organ(s) draining the site(s) of introduction of antigen. These experiments tried to account for the observation that antibody synthesis continued for months or even years after the introduction of antigen. Several types of evidence suggested that continued antibody production depended upon the persistence of antigen in the tissues. Based on the assumption that the residual immunogen would function even *in vitro*, an *in vitro* system was developed by John Tew, a postdoctoral fellow in my laboratory.[59] He injected rabbits in the hind foot pads with glutaraldehydepolymerized human serum albumin (POL-HSA). Months later, the draining nodes were removed, cell suspensions were prepared and cultured in the absence of additional antigen but in the presence of ^{14}C-leucine. Appreciable incorporation of radiolabel into IgG antibody to HSA occurred after a lag of only several days, suggesting that—without further addition of antigen—an *in vitro* anamnestic antibody response had been induced. Dr. Tew and others have subsequently presented strong evidence that residual antigen associated with follicular dendritic cells is responsible for the maintenance of immunologic memory and for the induction of this spontaneous antibody response.[60]

Experiments were designed to determine if the spontaneous antibody response is greater in the antigen draining than in the more distal lymphoid organs. Rabbits were injected with POL-HSA into the left hind foot pad and months later cell cultures were prepared from the draining (DLN) and nondraining (NDLN) as well as from other lymphoid organs and the blood. In a typical experiment the spontaneous antibody response was strikingly localized in the DLN and did not occur in cultures from the NDLN, appendix, spleen, blood, thymus, and cervical or mesenteric lymph nodes.[59]

Another fellow in the laboratory, James Folds, investigated the degree and duration of localization of persistent antibody synthesis and immunologic memory as a function of the site of introduction of antigen. There was relatively little information about the comparative localization of the cells involved in the antibody synthesis and in immunologic memory. Vischer and Stastny[61] had injected keyhole limpet hemocyanin (KLH) into rabbits and employed the incorporation of ^{3}H-thymidine into DNA as a measure of immunologic memory. Upon addition of KLH to cells, by this criterion, memory was detected mainly in the cells of the popliteal lymph node which drained the site of injection or in the cells of the spleen after intravenous injection. Jacobsen and Thorbecke[62] injected diphtheria toxoid into one hind foot pad of rabbits and at various times removed the draining contralateral nodes for the preparation of fragments which were challenged with antigen *in vitro*. The draining nodes were much more active in the anamnestic synthesis of antibody than the contralateral nodes. This difference waned with time but was still evident 3 to 4 months after the initial injection of antigen.

We then examined the extent of the primary and anamnestic antibody responses in the draining and nondraining lymph nodes following local injection of KLH.[63] The primary response was restricted to the draining nodes as were the increases in DNA and RNA synthesis when the nodes were sampled 4, 8, 14, 30, and 43 days after immunization. The anamnestic response was also predominantly confined to the draining lymph nodes (Table 1). Cells of the right nodes were reinjected 8 or 14 days after priming of the left node (rabbits 118 and 123) incorporated about 2.5 times as much radioactivity into antibody (3,244 and 3,139 cpm, respectively) as the right node cells of control rabbit 65 (1,371 cpm) which was injected 4 days earlier for the first time with 1 mg alum-KLH. Cells of the right node reinjected 8 or 14 days after priming of the opposite node (rabbits 11 and 123) did not incorporate much radioactivity nor DNA or RNA (data not shown). However, cells of the contralateral nodes (rabbits 270, 380, and 506) synthesized much more antibody than control cells when antigen was reinjected 30 or more days after priming of the opposite node. Despite the gradual appearance in the non-draining node of immunologic memory, even 120 and 240 days after priming, a larger amount of antibody synthesis occurred in the draining nodes (rabbits 380 and 506). Over 85% of the antibody synthesized in these cultures was found to be IgG. This finding, together with the kinetics of the responses, clearly indicate that they were anamnestic in nature. Similar results were obtained with an *in vitro* model of the anamnestic antibody response to KLH in which cells from the draining and nondraining nodes were challenged *in vitro*.[44] In a subsequent study,[64] immunologic memory to sperm whale myoglobulin (Mb) peptides was demonstrated 175 days after the injection of this antigen by removal of the draining lymph node, preparation of cell suspensions, and induction of synthesis of antibody to Mb upon addition of small peptides to these cells. Still later, continued synthesis of antibody to soluble egg antigens was demonstrated in spleen cell and isolated hepatic granuloma preparations from mice infected for a number of months with *Schistosoma japonicum*.[65]

Table 1.
Antibody Synthesis During Secondary Responses by Cells of Lymph Nodes Draining and not Draining the Site of Primary Injection of KLH[***] [****]

Exp. No.	Day[c]	Lymph node	Cell no.[a]		CPM in Antibody[d]		
			$\times 10^8$	S.I.	/2 $\times 10^7$ cells	Total	S.I.
118	8	Left	11.7		144	8,410	
		Right	6.3	1.86	103	3,244	2.6
123	14	Left	13.5		180	12,150	
		Right	9.95	6.9	322	3,139	3.87
270	30	Left	9.0		1,892	85,000	
		Right	3.6	2.5	2,990	54,000	1.57
380	120	Left	14.0		1,198	83,860	
		Right	5.4	2.6	1,672	45,144	1.8
506	240	Left	5.4		7,000	189,000	
		Right	3.6	1.5	5,130	97,470	1.9

[a] From Stavitsky & Folds (1972) with permission of the Journal of Immunology.
[b] All of the rabbits were primed by the injection of 1.0 mg of alum-precipitated KLH into the left hind foot pad and reinjected on the designated days with 1.0 mg of the same antigen preparation. Popliteal lymph node cells were removed for culture 4 days later.
[c] Day after priming when reinjections of antigen were given.

Kinetics of the Antibody Response

Dixon et al.[66] determined the kinetics of the primary, secondary, and tertiary antibody responses of rabbits to bovine gamma globulin. They found similar rates of decline for all of the responses. The rates increased while antigen was circulating and began to decline rapidly after elimination of circulating antigen as though this antigen was required for persistence of antibody production. Askonas and Humphrey[26] found a delay of about 30 minutes in the labelling of extracellular antibody in perfused lungs of rabbits hyperimmunized with type 3 pneumococci. This delay was attributed to the time required for newly synthesized antibody to be released from the microsomes and for the process of secretion to occur. We studied the kinetics of the anamnestic production of antibody by lymph node cells of rabbits immunized with KLH.[67] Maximum intracellular immunofluorescence for antibody to KLH and the greatest incorporation of ^{14}C-labelled amino acids into antibody occurred between the third and fourth days after a second local injection of KLH. This was followed by an abrupt decline in the synthesis of antibody within the next day or two.

Evidence for the Immunogenicity of Peptides

As a consequence of the interest in the role of antigen envisioned by the various template theories, many studies were done in the 1950's to follow the localization and fate of antigen following introduction both *in vitro* and *in vivo*. Antigen was detected in a variety of subcellular sites in reticular cells,

***From Stavitsky and Folds (1972) with permission of the *Journal of Immunology*.

****All of the rabbits were primed by injection of 1.0 mg of alum-precipitated KLH into the left hind foot pad and reinjected on the designated days with 1.0 mg of the same antigen preparation. Popliteal lymph node cells were removed for culture 4 days later.

macrophages, lymphocytes, and plasma cells minutes or hours after the injection of viruses,[68] proteins,[69] labelled proteins,[70] and bacterial polysaccharides.[71] However, only occasionally was immunogenically-active[72] or serologically-active antigen[73] detected in the tissues.

Early experiments of Landsteiner[74] indicated that peptides could serve as immunogenic determinants when coupled to proteins. Our own interest in peptides was stimulated by the observations that enzymatic hydrolysis of several non-globular proteins such as silk fibroin,[75] lens crystallin,[76] oxidized ribonuclease[77] and tobacco mosaic virus[78] resulted in the appearance of small antigenically active peptides and antigenic fragments of serum albumin[79,80] and thyroglobulin[81] were prepared. A graduate student, David Bing, isolated and characterized antigenically active peptides from bovine ß-lacto globulin-A, a small globular protein found in cow's milk.[82] This protein was hydrolyzed with trypsin to yield a mixture of peptides which would not precipitate with rabbit antibody against the native protein, but would still inhibit the lactoglobulin-antibody reaction.[83] The hydrolysate was fractionated by ion exchange chromatography and found to contain seven antigenically active fractions. Two of these fractions were found to be homogeneous peptides. Each inhibited the reaction of antigen with antibody against the intact protein in hemagglutination, flocculation and passive cutaneous anaphylaxis reactions. One of the peptides had a molecular weight of 950 and the other had a molecular weight of 575. Both contained equal numbers of polar and apolar amino acids.

About ten years later we made another attempt to demonstrate the immunogenicity of peptides. We took advantage of our development of an *in vitro* anamnestic antibody response system and the demonstration by Atassi[84] that sperm whale myoglobin (Mb) contains five antigenic regions. In collaboration with Atassi in our initial study[64] rabbits were injected in the hind foot pads with Mb in complete Freund's adjuvant. At least 30 days later the draining popliteal lymph nodes were removed for the preparation of cell cultures which were challenged for 24 hrs with different concentrations of either Mb or synthetic Mb peptides. The medium collected after 24 hours of culture was assayed for macrophage inhibitory factor (MIF). ^{14}C-Leucine was added to the cells during 72-120 hrs of culture to radioactively label newly synthesized antibody to Mb. Synthetic Mb peptides representing sequences 1-6, 15-22, 15-23, 16-22, 54-62, 56-62, 6 = 57-63, 95-100, 113-119, and 146-151 induced the Mb-primed lymph node cell cultures to produce antibody to Mb. Peptides from all of these regions—except 1-6—induced these cultures to produce MIF. In a subsequent study,[85] IgG, protein, DNA and RNA syntheses were induced upon addition of each one of these peptides to Mb-primed lymph node cells. It was postulated that these univalent peptide determinants became immunogenic by becoming effectively multivalent through expression on lymphocytes, macrophages, and/or dendritic cells. However, for some reason(s)—perhaps because it was too early—"time was out of joint" for our work on the immunogenicity of peptides and it has received little attention in the literature. However, the field has come back strong in the 1980's, especially with respect to the subject of the processing of proteins by macrophages to yield peptides which bind to class II MHC molecules, a complex which is then recognized by T cells.

In the early 1960's our attention was diverted for a number of years in what turned out to be a fruitless endeavor to show that macrophages contributed to the antibody response by their processing of antigen to yield informational RNA-antigen complexes. This diversion was induced by a report by Fishman and Adler.[86] They incubated bacteriophage T2 and rat peritoneal exudate cells, then prepared an RNA fraction from these cells and added this fraction to rat lymph node cells in culture. Within a week specific neutralizing antibodies to the phage appeared in the medium. Since ribonuclease rendered this homogenate inactive it was assumed that RNA was the active factor in the homogenate. Doubt was cast on this interpretation by the finding in Askonas' laboratory[87] and in my laboratory by Friedman[88] that the RNA was contaminated with antigen, some of it clearly degraded. However, these studies renewed interest in the role of the macrophage in the immune response. Unanue et al.[89] found that some of the antigen taken up by the macrophages was more immunogenic than free antigen both *in vitro* and *in vivo*.[90] Moreover, clusters of macrophages and lymphocytes were observed. Therefore, it was soon postulated that the first phase of the immune response consisted of the uptake of antigen by macrophages, its processing and then display of processed antigen on the surface of this cell where it was available for interaction with and stimulation of lymphocytes—a prescient suggestion.

Antibody Synthesis from Free Amino Acids Rather Than From an Intracellular High Molecular Weight Precursor

As early as 1900, analogy was drawn between antibody formation and adaptive enzyme formation in microorganisms.[91] Fifty years later the question was raised whether the enzyme(s) induced in bacteria and the antibodies induced in mammalian hosts were produced from high molecular weight intracellular precursors or from free amino acids. Heidelberger et al.[92] in 1942 showed that actively synthesized antibody, but not passive antibody, was derived from free amino acids. However, the template theories postulated that antigen somehow converted a gamma globulin precursor to antibody. My initial study of this question was inspired by the report[93] that the antibody which appeared during the anamnestic antibody response was a secondary effect of the lysis of lymphocytes by adrenal cortical hormones with the release of preformed antibody. In our study, despite the production of a profound lymphocytopenia following the injection of adrenal cortical extracts into immunized rabbits, we failed to observe an increase in antibody.[94] Subsequently, the development of methods for studying the incorporation of radiolabelled amino acids into antibody permitted a more direct examination of this possibility. In a number of studies from this[30] and other laboratories[25,26,54,57,58] the incorporation of free amino acids into antibody was demonstrated and a great deal of evidence was presented to prove that there was no appreciable amount of intracellular precursor which was converted to antibody. Corresponding studies on enzymatic induction in bacteria reached similar conclusions.[95]

Biochemistry of the Antibody Response

Over the years we studied various other aspects of the biochemistry of the antibody response, including its induction as well as its regulation. In our first study,[96] different concentrations of actinomycin D were added to cultured lymph node or spleen cells or fragments which were prepared at the height of the anamnestic antibody response to proteins. Some concentrations of this antibiotic completely inhibited the synthesis of RNA, DNA, antibody, and nonantibody proteins. At lower concentrations DNA and RNA synthesis were inhibited completely, but considerable antibody synthesis continued for a day. Still lower concentrations inhibited DNA and RNA synthesis partially and occasionally stimulated or inhibited antibody synthesis partially. It was postulated that stable mRNA mediated the synthesis of antibody in the absence of DNA and RNA synthesis. Short-lived mRNA was implicated in the antibody synthesis which was inhibited by actinomycin. We then observed that the *in vitro* antibody response to KLH was inhibited by mitomycin C added at the same time as antigen, but this synthesis was inhibited only 40% if it was added 24 hr after antigen.[97] 5-Bromodeoxyuridine inhibited antibody production 50%, the incorporation of ^{14}C-thymidine into DNA 90% and RNA synthesis not at all. Interpretation of these results was difficult because of the heterogeneity of the cell populations, including lymphocytes, macrophages, blast cells and plasma cells, but they indicated an early phase dependent upon both DNA and RNA synthesis.

The abundant evidence that cyclic AMP was involved in immune phenomena as a possible second messenger or regulation of diverse events prompted a series of studies of regulation of the *in vitro* anamnestic antibody response by cyclic AMP. In the first study, by a graduate student, Richard Cook,[98] the additions of cholera toxin (CT) or dibutyryl cyclic AMP (DbcAMP) to KLH-primed rabbit lymph node cells for the first 24 hrs with KLH consistently enhanced the ensuing antibody synthesis 2 to 5 fold. (Addition of CT or DbcAMP to the medium during the productive phase (72-120 hrs) consistently inhibited this response). Both the IgM and IgG antibody responses were potentiated. CT and DbcAMP modulated only antibody synthesis—not protein synthesis in general. In the next study,[99] a dichotomy between the induction by KLH and regulation by CT or DbcAMP of antibody production was suggested. This dichotomy was studied further by omitting Ca^{2+} from the medium for the first 24 hrs of the culture. The absence of this cation during induction did not alter the KLH-induced response, but did abolish its enhancement by CT and DbcAMP. Alternative to the dichotomy between induction and regulation is the possibility that CT or DbcAMP enhance antibody production through the inactivation of suppressor cells. Inasmuch as these studies indicated that agents such as CT and DbcAMP which modulate cAMP levels enhance the antibody response, attention was then turned to the prostaglandins[100] because it had been shown that PGE's activate adenylate cyclase and thereby elevate intracellular cAMP in lymphocytes.[101] Moreover, *in vitro* addition of PGE1 prevented tolerization of mouse splenocytes when these cells were transferred to a host and then challenged with (T,G)-Pro-L.[102] Optimal concentrations of PGE1 or PGE2, but not PGEα, enhanced the KLH-stimulated *in vitro* anamnestic antibody synthesis two- to six-fold[100] In a subsequent study,[103] inhibitors of PG synthesis such as indomethacin inhibited the KLH-induced antibody response. Finally, it was found that the modulation of antibody synthesis by CT is mediated by CT-induced soluble factors.[104] Taken together, these findings strongly implicated the cyclic AMP pathway in the regulation of the antibody response. More recent studies with a graduate student, James Dasch, and a colleague, Lazarus Astrachan, have also implicated calmodulin[105] and the phosphorylation of cytoplasmic proteins, including at least one associated with the cytoskeleton, in the early steps of activation of both T and B lymphocytes by mitogens and B cell activation by antibody to immunoglobulin.[106]

19S and 7S Antibodies to Proteins, Bacterial and Phage Antigens, and Haptens—Serendipity Rewarded

In the fall of 1959 I had just returned from a year of sabbatical leave at the National Institute of Medical Research with Drs. Askonas and Humphrey. A new postdoctoral fellow, Dietrich Bauer from Michigan State University, joined the laboratory. I was altogether refreshed and ready for a new approach to research. We decided to try to enhance the primary antibody response to facilitate its study.[107] We used diphtheria toxoid, a poor immunogen, which induced a rather minimal antibody response and *Salmonella typhosa* as a source of endotoxin which was already known to promote antibody production. The hemagglutination method was employed to titrate the sera. In the initial experiment, as shown in Fig. 1, the sera from the *Salmonella*-primed rabbits showed a biphasic response with peak titers at about 9 and 15 days after the injection of toxoid. Moreover, the antibody which appeared first consistently lost most of its activity upon storage at +50°C or even -20°C, but the antibody which appeared later did not lose activity in the cold. The observation of two types of antibody by the criterion of cold-sensitivity led ut to postulate that two different populations of antibody molecules were represented in the two curves. The early response sera were fractionated by zone electrophoresis which revealed that the initial antibody had the mobility of a gamma-1 globulin, whereas the antibody which appeared later had the mobility of a gamma-2 golublin. The findings of gamma-1 and gamma-2 antibodies to diphtheria toxoid recalled the observation by Stelos and Talmage[108] first of gamma-1 and then gamma-2 globulin antibodies in rabbits injected repeatedly with sheep red cell antigens. The observation of two forms of antibody globulin in response to a single inoculation of diphtheria toxoid prompted us to examine the possibility that these two species of antibody were formed consistently in response to a single injection of a variety of antigens in the rabbit. Eventually it was found that the injection of proteins other than diphtheria toxoid into normal rabbits also resulted first in the production of antibodies with the mobility of gamma-1 globulins. Figure 2 shows the results of an electrophoretic separation of a 5-day antiserum to KLH in which hemagglutinating antibody to KLH is present in the faster migrating gamma-1 globulin fraction. Three days later some gamma-2 globulin antibody was demonstrable. By ultracentrifugation in a sucrose gradient it was shown that the antibody which appeared first was a macroglobulin. In subsequent studies it was shown that the antibody response to T2 bacteriophage and *Salmonella typhosa* H antigen was initially macroglobulin[109] and that both high and low molecular weight antibodies were produced to the DNP and NIP determinants.[12] However, upon a second injection of antigen the response was shown to be predominantly low molecular weight and gamma-2 (Fig. 3).[109]

Benedict[110] confirmed these findings with respect to antibody production to human serum albumin. Svehag subsequently found the antibody

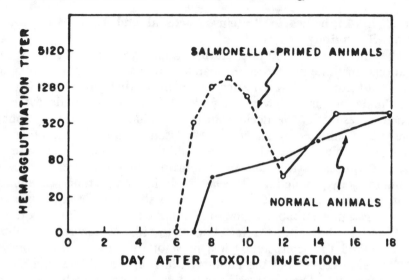

Fig. 1. The effect of prior injection of *Salmonella* vaccine of the primary antibody response to diphtheria toxoid. The data represent the average response of 12 rabbits treated with Salmonella vaccine and 6 rabbits which received only the toxoid. The dashed line represents the antibody formed which lost its hemagglutinating activity during *in vitro* storage in the cold and the solid line that antibody which did not lose this activity under these circumstances. (Reproduced with permission from D.C. Bauer and A. B. Stavitsky. *Proc. Natl. Acad. Sci.* (USA) 47: 1667, 1961)

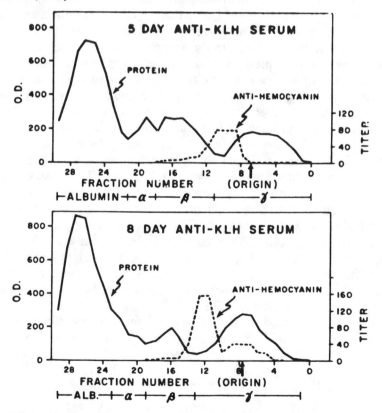

Fig. 2. Zone electrophoresis of primary response antisera to hemocyanin five and eight days after a single injection of antigen. Five ml serum electrophoresced for 21 hr at 400 voluts. One cpm strips eluted with 5 ml 0.15 M phosphate buffered saline, pH 7.2. (Reproduced with permission from D. C. Bauer and A. B. Stavitsky. *Proc. Natl. Acad. Sci* (USA) 47: 1667, 1961).

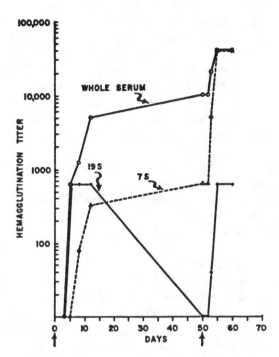

Fig. 3. Distribution of hemagglutinating activity for hemocyanin-conjugated erythrocytes among fractions prepared by sucrose density ultracentrifugation of rabbit sera obtained at various times after a primary and secondary injection of 4 mg of alum-precipitated hemocyanin into hind foot pads. Only peak hemagglutinating titer of bottom (19S) or upper (7S) fractions are shown so that 19S and 7S titers for a particular day need not add up to the serum titer on that day. The actual titer is plotted on a logarithmic scale so as to accomodate the wide spread in titers. (Reproduced with permission from Bauer, D.C., M. J. Mathies and A. B. Stavitsky, *J. Exp. Med.* 117, 889, 1963).

response to polio virus also consisted of these two molecular species and also found differences in antigen dose requirements for their sustained synthesis, anamnesis, and sensitivity to x-irradiation; the secondary response reflecting memory was predominantly of S and x-irradiation sensitive.[111] Uhr made similar observations with respect to the antibody response of the guinea pig to the phage ØX 174.[112] When he found that the goldfish showed similar heterogeneity he made the prescient suggestion that the 19S antibody response preceded the 7S response phylogenetically.

Our finding of the 19S and 7S antibodies to a variety of antigens was clearly serendipitous. However, we were also very fortunate in a number of respects. First, we employed hemagglutination and it was later shown that this assay is very sensitive for the detection of the 19S antibody which is present in lower concentration than the 7S antibody. Second, the cold-sensitivity of the first antibody and the cold-insensitivity of the second antibody suggested the production of two distinct species of antibodies, whereas subsequent immunization of non-*Salmonella*-primed rabbits did not result in the synthesis of cold-sensitive antibodies. Third, the antibody response to diphtheria toxoid was enhanced by priming with *Salmonella*, but attempts to promote the antibody production to other proteins by this type of priming did not yield consistent results. Fourth, we employed the rabbit rather than the mouse which makes much less 19S antibody than the rabbit. Fifth, our work was preceded by the demonstration of high molecular weight antibodies to non-protein antigens.

We suggested that different cells might be involved in the synthesis of 19S and 7S antibodies, but also considered the possibility that a single cell might embark on the synthesis of 19S and then switch to the production of 7S antibody[107]—the first suggestion of an "isotype shift." The latter possibility was shown to be correct by the studies of Nossal on antibody production in microdroplets by single cells from the popliteal lymph nodes of rats immunized with flagella from *Salmonella*.[113] Double producers of 19S and 7S antibodies were frequent when the switchover from 19S to 7S antibody was occurring.

During the early 1960's, as a member of the Microbiology Fellowship Review Committee at NIH, I saw a large number of applications which proposed to examine the 19S and 7S antibody responses to a variety of antigens in a variety of species! 19S and 7S antibodies were certainly in fashion. Scientists are not so different after all!

THE IMMUNOLOGY OF INFECTIOUS DISEASES REVISITED

In my first published paper in 1943, I described a method for producing skin infections in guinea pigs with *Staphylococcus aureus*.[114] My doctoral research dealt with the mechanisms of immune pathogenesis and host resistance to *Leptospira icterohemorrhagica*.[115] During this research and research in my "spare time" on Brucellosis, I became interested in comparative pathology and immunology and, therefore, undertook the study of veterinary medicine at the University of Pennsylvania. As I have already indicated, my sojourn at the university was productive and stimulating in that I became acquainted with the research of Drs. Lurie, Ehrich, and Harris. I also did some research on chick embryo infection with *Mycobacterium johnei*, the causative agent of Johne's disease.[116]

Upon graduation from veterinary school in 1946, I returned to the study of immunology as a postdoctoral fellow at Cal Tech. From 1946 until 1978, I largely worked on some of the model systems I have described. However, beginning in 1954, I gradually became interested in schistosomiasis. My initial research was on the production of antibodies to a lactic dehydrogenase of *Schistosoma mansoni*.[117] Another hiatus followed until the late 1960's when I began to play squash with Kenneth Warren of this medical school who was doing some interesting and important research on schistosomiasis both in man and in animal models. Over a period of years I learned a great deal about this fascinating disease from him, from one of my Ph.D. students, Ronald Pelley, who went to work with Warren, and from Dov Boros, a postdoctoral fellow with Warren, now professor of microbiology and immunology at Wayne State University School of Medicine. Warren left here in 1977 to become director of health sciences for The Rockefeller Foundation and was succeeded as head of the Division of Geographic Medicine in the Department of Medicine by Adel Mahmoud. Finally, in the late 1970's I decided to embark with Mahmoud on a study of immune pathogenesis and immune regulation of the disease caused in mice by *Schistosoma japonicum*. I was attracted to this disease because it had not been studied as extensively and intensively as the disease caused by *Schistosoma mansoni* and it seemed ideal because it consists of essentially one lesion, the hepatic granuloma, and of sequelae of granulomatous inflammation, including the rise in portal pressure and esophageal varices, all of which are spontaneously down-regulated. During the past decade we have enjoyed working with this disease and have made some interesting observations about the role of cellular immunity in the pathogenesis of the disease and about both cellular and humoral regulation of the granulomatous inflammation.[118,119,120,121] These experiments involved not only Mahmoud and myself but also the collaboration of Keith Garb, an M.D./Ph.D. student, and an immunoparasitologist/physician; and G.R. Olds, who recently became head of the Division of Geographic Medicine at Brown University. After 40 years I finally returned to the study of the immunology of infectious diseases. After years of working with artificial systems and non-replicating antigens, it feels good to be examining a dynamic, real infection again.

EPILOGUE

Present Status of Our Knowledge

Enormous progress has been made in the study of many of the classical questions in immunology. There has been an especially large gain in knowledge of the molecular biology, molecular genetics, and cell biology of immune and non-immune systems. I am delighted that there is a return to the study of *in vivo* models of immunologic disease and of their immune pathogenetic and immune regulatory mechanisms; in the past there has been disproportionate emphasis on *in vitro* models which are sometimes of dubious relevance to the *in vivo* situation. The numerous and sharp tools of molecular biology—such as *in situ* hybridization—can now be applied to intact cells and intact organs to provide useful information about the cellular architecture and functions of these cells in these organs *in vivo*.

Numerous studies of the immune response have revealed its beautiful symmetry, e.g., the similarities between cellular and humoral immunity, including the structural and functional analogies between T and B cell receptors. Another interesting and exciting analogy which has been revealed and is now undergoing extensive investigation is between the immune and nervous systems. Indeed the many interfaces and similarities which have been revealed among the various elements of the immune system and between the immune and non-immune systems such as the nervous system indicate that "The web of our life is of a mingled yarn."

Outlook for the Future

Despite the impressive progress, many important immunological questions are only partially answered or not answered at all. A partial list which occurs to me is as follows:

> 1. How does the immune system function in health and disease in the intact host? The system has been dissected in great deal on the basis of *in vitro* responses, but there is little appreciation of whether and, if so, how these cellular, genetic, and humoral elements interact *in vivo*.
>
> 2. How are the various cellular participants in the immune system activated? This includes the cells, whose variety is continually increasing, which can function to process and/or present antigen to T lymphocytes as well as cells such as dendritic cells which do not seem to be able to process antigen; knowledge of the possible role of oncogenes; the role of cell proliferation as there often seems to be a dichotomy between activation as expressed in cellular proliferation and in lymphokine production; finally, the mechanisms of signal transduction.

3. How are the various cellular participants in the immune system regulated? This includes a number of possibilities such as actual absence of certain populations; defects in the functions of populations; active regulation (suppression) of the functions of these populations by nonspecific cells (macrophages) or specific suppressor cells; regulation by specific antibodies or anti-idiotypic antibodies. Regulation may be positive or negative.

4. How do the various organ microenvironments contribute to the overall immune responses? For instance, what accounts for the differences in the types of immune responses supported upon introduction of antigen into different organs: differences in isotypes; cellular vs. humoral immunity; the persistence and localization of these responses; the magnitude of the responses. On the basis of recent studies, these differences may depend to some extent on the efficiency of antigen-presentation in these environments as well as the capacity of the cells in these microenvironments to produce chemotactic factors for cells for which they can then mount local cellular and/or humoral immune responses.

5. What is the role of persistent antigen, e.g., on follicular dendritic cells, in the maintenance of cellular and humoral immunity through complexing to I-A-like determinants and induction of continued cell proliferation and differentiation and the maintenance of immunologic memory?

6. How is immune deviation, that is the reduced cellular immunity and enhanced humoral immunity seen in many infections, explained? Recent studies suggest a division of labor among T cells subsets, some of them producing lymphokines and others providing help for B cells and antibody production. If the former subset is absent or defective, it is conceivable that cellular immunity will be reduced or absent and the antibody response still active. However, to return to the first question, this mechanism or other mechanisms to account for immune deviation *in vivo* must be studied and validated.

7. What is the nature of immunologic memory and how is it regulated? Immunologic memory is a well-authenticated phenomenon, but its mechanisms are not understood. This question is related to all of the previous ones.

8. How is the isotype shift regulated? For instance, how do antigen concentration, the chemical nature of the antigen, and the microenvironment into which the antigen is introduced determine which isotype(s) of antibody are synthesized and for how long do these syntheses persist.

9. How do the cellular and humoral immune responses to genetically engineered or synthetic peptide vaccines compare to these immune responses to live vaccines or following recovery from infections? Live vaccines or recovery from infection often induces a high level of long-lasting cellular and/or humoral immunity, presumably owing to the persistence of relevant immunogenic fragments of virus or other microorganisms. The answer to this question presumably encompasses the answers to

most of the previous questions, especially with respect to the efficiency with which these antigens are processed, presented and the extent and duration of their persistence in immunogenic form.

10. How does nutrition affect the immune response? There is a great deal of evidence that proper nutrition, including amino acids, vitamins and other factors, is required for the proper functioning of the immune response. However, much of this evidence is derived either from *in vitro* experiments or from poorly designed *in vivo* experiments. A fresh start on this important question is urgently needed as the answers impinge on other problems such as the role of nutrition in the development of immunity to tumors.

Most of these questions are under intensive study. With the continuous development of more sophisticated tools for their analysis, undoubtedly progress in their solution will accelerate.

ACKNOWLEDGMENTS

I am grateful to the late Dr. Lester O. Krampitz, Chairman of the Department of Microbiology, Case Western Reserve University, for providing me with a stimulating intellectual environment, unlimited freedom, and financial and psychological support for 30 yrs. I also want to express my gratitude for the devoted and intelligent support I have received from Mr. Weldon W. Harold, my research assistant for almost 30 yrs. I greatly appreciate the support I have received from the National Institutes of Health for over 30 yrs.

REFERENCES

1. Mott, N., *A Life in Science*, Taylor and Francis, Philadelphia, 1986.
2. Ehrlich, P., *Proc. Roy. Soc. (London)*, B66, 424, 1900.
3. Alexander, J., *Protoplasma*, 14, 302, 1932.
4. Mudd, S.J., *Immunol.*, 23, 423, 1932.
5. Breinl, F. and Haurowitz, F. *Zeit.*, *Physiol. Chem.*, 192, 45, 1930.
6. Pauling, L., *J. Amer. Chem. Soc.*, 62, 2643, 1940.
7. Lurie, M.B., *J. Exp. Med.*, 75, 247, 1942.
8. Ehrich, W.E. and Harris, T.N., *J. Exp. Med.*, 76, 335, 1942.
9. Chase, M.W., *Proc. Soc. Exp. Biol. Med.*, 59, 134, 1945.
10. Pauling, L. and Campbell, D.H., *J. Exp. Med.*, 76, 211, 1942.
11. Stavitsky, A.B., Stavitsky, R., and Ecker, E.E., *J. Immunol.*, 63, 389, 1949.
12. Plotkin, D.H., Kontiainen, S., Stavitsky, A.B., and Makela, O., *Immunology*, 15, 799, 1968.
13. M'Gowan, J.P., *J. Path. Bact.*, 12, 519 (1908).
14. Loeffler, F. C., *Ztschr. F. Immunitatsforsch. u. Exper. Therap.*, 8, 129, 1910.
15. Magher, G. and Maghers, A., *Compt. rend. Soc. de Biol.*, 101, 206, 1929.
16. Stavitsky, A.B., *Science*, 113, 520, 1951.
17. Heymann, W. and Lund, H.Z., *Pediatrics*, 7, 691, 1951.
18. Stavitsky, A.B., Hackel, D.B., and Heymann, W., *Proc. Soc. Exp. Bio. Med.*, 85, 593, 1954.
19. Stavitsky, A.B., Heymann, W., and Hackel, D.B., *J. Lab. Clin. Med.*, 47, 349, 1956.
20. Rothenberg, M.B., Stavitsky, A.B., and Heymann, W., *Pediatrics*, 18, 455, 1956.
21. Unanue, E.R. and Dixon, F.J., *Adv. Immunol.*, 6, 1, 1967.

22. Fagraeus, A., Antibody production in relation to the development of plasma cells, Stockholm, 1948.
23. Thorbecke, G.J. and Keuning, F.J., *J. Immunol.*, 70, 129, 1953.
24. Stavitsky, A.B., *J. Immunol.*, 75, 234, 1955.
25. Askonas, B.A.and White, R.G., *Brit. J. Exp. Path.*, 37, 61, 1956.
26. Askonas, B.A. and Humphrey, J.H., *Biochem. J.*, 68, 252, 1956.
27. Stavitsky, A.B., *Brit. J. Exp. Path.*, 39, 46, 1958.
28. Stavitsky, A.B., *Brit. J. Exp. Path.*, 39, 661, 1958.
29. Mountain, I.M., *J. Immunol.*, 74, 270, 1955.
30. Wolf, B. and Stavitsky, A.B., *J. Immunol.*, 81, 404, 1958.
31. Vaugh, J.H., Dutton, A.H., Dutton, R.W., George, M., and Marston, R.Q., *J. Immunol.*, 84, 258, 1960.
32. Michaelides, M.C., *Fed. Proc.*, 16, 416, 1957.
33. Askonas, B.A. and Stavitsky, A.B., Unpublished data.
34. Grabar, P. and Corvazier, A., in Ciba Foundation, Symposium on Cellular Aspects of Immunity, pp. 198-206, 1960.
35. Bauer, D.C. and Stavitsky, A.B., Unpublished data.
36. Steiner, D.F. and Anker, H.S., *Proc. Natl. Acad. Sci. USA*, 42, 580, 1956.
37. Ainis, H., Personal communication.
38. Trowell, O.A., *Expt. Cell Res.*, 16, 118, 1959.
39. LeVia, M.F., Uriu, S.A. and Ferguson, L.A. , *J. Immunol.*, 84, 48, 1960.
40. Boyden, S.V., *J. Exp. Med.*, 93, 107, 1951.
41. Stavitsky, A. B., *J. Immunol.*, 72, 360, 1954.
42. Ranney, H.M. and London, I.M., *Fed. Proc.*, 10, 562, 1951.
43. Self, G.H., Tew, J.G., Cook, R.G. and Stavitsky, A.B., *Immunochem.*, 11, 227, 1974.
44. Herscowitz, H.B. and Stavitsky, A.B., *J. Immunol.*, 105, 1389, 1970.
45. Manderino, G.L., Gooch, G.T., and Stavitsky, A.B., *Cell. Immunol.*, 41, 265, 1978.
46. Manderino, G.L. and Stavitsky, A.B., *Cell. Immunol.*, 41, 276, 1978.
47. Stavitsky, A.B. and Arquilla, E.R., *Int. Arch. Allergy Applied Immunol.*, 13, 1, 1958.
48. Herscowitz, H.B., Harold, W.W., and Stavitsky, A.B., *Immunology*, 22, 51, 1972.
49. McMaster, P.D. and Hudack, S., *J. Exp. Med.*, 61, 783, 1935.
50. Fagraeus, A., *J. Immunol.*, 67, 281, 1948.
51. Stavitsky, A.B., *Fed. Proc.*, 16, 652, 1957.
52. Chase, M.W., *Fed. Prod.*, 10, 404, 1951.
53. Harris, S., Harris, T.N., Ogburn, C.A. and Farber, N.B., *J. Exp. Med.*, 10, 409, 1951.
54. Taliaferro, W.J. and Talmage, D.W., *J. Infect. Dis.*, 97, 88, 1955.
55. Stavitsky, A.B., Axelrod, A.E. and Pruzansky, J., *J. Immunol.* 79, 200, 1957.
56. Harris, S., Harris, T.N., Ogburn, C.A. and Farber, N.B., *J. Exp. Med.*, 104, 645, 1956.
57. Keston, A.S. and Katchen, B., *J. Immunol.* 76, 253, 1956.
58. Humphrey, J.H. and Sulitzeanu, B.D., *Biochem. J.*, 68, 145, 1958.
59. Tew, J.G., Self, C.H., Harold, W.W., and Stavitsky, A.B., *J. Immunol.*, 111, 416, 1973.
60. Tew, J.G., Phipps, R.P., and Mandel, T.E., *Immunol. Rev.*, 53, 175, 1980.
61. Vischer, t.L. and Stastny, P., *Immunology*, 12, 675, 1966.
62. Jacobson, E.B. and Thorbecke, G.J., *J. Exp. Med.*, 130, 387, 1969.
63. Stavitsky, A.B. and Folde, J.D., *J. Immunol.*, 108, 152, 1972.
64. Stavitsky, A.B., Stassi, M.Z., Gooch, G.T., Pelley, H.P., and Harold, W.W., *Immunochemistry*, 12, 959, 1975.
65. Stavitsky, A.B. and Garb, K.S., *Infect. Immun.*, 46, 276, 1985.
66. Dixon, F.J., Maurer, P.H., Weigle, W.O., and Deichmiller, M.P., *J. Exp. Med.*, 103, 425, 1956.
67. Schoenberg, M.D., Moore, R.D., Stavitsky, A.B. and Gusdon, J.P., *J. Cell. Physiol.*, 71, 133, 1968.
68. Cavosto, F. and Ficq, A., *Nature*, 172, 406, 1953.
69. Coons, A.H., Leduc, E.H. and Kaplan, M.H., *J. Exp. Med.*, 93, 173, 1951.
70. Sabin, F.R., *J. Exp. Med.*, 70, 67, 1939.
71. Hill, a.G.S., Deane, H.W. and Coons, A.H., *J. Exp. Med.*, 92, 35, 1950.
72. Stavitsky, A.B., Unpublished data.
73. Garvey, J.S. and Campbell, D.H., *J. Immunol.*, 72, 131, 1954.
74. Landsteiner, K., *The Specificity of Serological Reactions*, Harvard University, Cambridge, Massachusetts, p. 178, 1947.

75. Cebra, J., *J. Immunol.*, 86, 205, 1960.
76. Hara, T., *Jap. J. Biochem.*, 43, 263, 1956.
77. Brown, R., *J. Biol. Chem.*, 237, 1162, 1962.
78. Young, J.D., Benjamini, E., Shimizu, M. and Leung, C.Y., *Biochemistry*, 5, 1481, 1966.
79. Press, E.M. and Porter, R.R., *Biochem. J.*, 83, 172, 1960.
80. Richard, A.J., Beck, S. and Hock, H., *Arch. Biochem. Biophys.*, 90, 309, 1960.
81. Metzger, H., Sharp, G.C., and Edelhoch, H., *Biochemistry*, 1, 205, 1962.
82. Bell, K. and McKenzie, H.A., *Nature*, 207, 1275, 1964.
83. Bing, D.H. and Stavitsky, A.B., *Immunology*, 15, 305, 1968.
84. Atassi, M.Z., *Immunochemistry*, 12, 423, 1975.
85. Stavitsky, A.B., Atassi, M.Z., Gooch, G.T., Manderino, G.L., Harold, W.W., and Pelley, R.P., in *Immunobiology of Proteins and Peptides*, M.Z. Atassi, and A.B. Stavitsky, eds., Plenum Press, New York, 1978.
86. Fishman, M. and Adler, F.L., *J. Exp. Med.*, 117, 595, 1963.
87. Askonas, B.A. and Rhodes, J.M., *Nature*, 205, 470, 1965.
88. Friedman, H.P., Stavitsky, A.B. and Solomon, J.M., *Science*, 149, 1106, 1965.
89. Unanue, E.R., Gerottini, J.-C. and Bedford, M., *Nature*, 222, 1193, 1969.
90. Unanue, E.R., *Adv. Immunol.*, 15, 95, 1972.
91. Dienert, F., *J. Microbiol.*, 40, 140, 1900.
92. Heidelberger, M, Treffers, H.P., Schoenheimer, R., Ratner, S. and Rittenberg, D. *J., Biol. Chem.*, 144, 555, 1942.
93. Chase, J.H., White, A., and Dougherty, T.F., *J. Immunol.*, 52, 101, 1946.
94. Stavitsky, A.B., *J. Inf. Dis.*, 93, 130, 1953.
95. Hogness, D.S., Cohn, M. and Monod, J., *Biochem. Biophys. Acta.*, 16, 99, 1955.
96. Stavitsky, A.B. and Gusdon, J.P., *Bact. Rev.*, 30, 418, 1966.
97. Herscowtiz, H.B., Stavitsky, A.B., and Tew. J.G., *Cell. Immunol.*, 2, 259, 1971.
98. Cook, R.G., Stavitsky, A.B., and Schoenber, M.D., *J. Immunol.*, 114, 426, 1975.
99. Cook, R.G. and Stavitsky, A.B., *Cell. Immunol.*, 24, 336, 1976.
100. Cook, R.G. and Stavitsky,
101. Bach, M.D., *J. Clin. Invest.*, 55, 1074, 1975.
102. Mozes, E., Shearer, G.M., Melmon, K.L. and Bourne, H.R., *Cell. Immunol.*, 9, 226, 1973.
103. Gerblich, A.A. and Stavitsky, A.B., *Cell. Immunol.*, 48, P 318, 1979.
104. Sanford, L.P., Stavitsky, A.B. and Cook, R.G., *Cell. Immunol.*, 48, 182, 1979.
105. Stavitsky, A.B., Dasch, J.R. and Astrachan, L., *Cell. Immunol.*, 87, 411, 1984.
106. Dasch, J.R. and Stavitsky, A.B., *Molec. Immunol.*, 22, 379, 1985.
107. Bauer, D.C. and Stavitsky, A.B., *Proc. Natl. Acad. Sci. USA*, 47, 1667, 1961.
108. Stelos, P. and Talmage, D.W., *J. Inf. Dis.*, 100, 126, 1957.
109. Bauer, D.C., Mathies, M.J. and Stavitsky, A.B., *J. Exp. Med.*, 117, 889, 1963.
110. Benedict, A.A., Brown, R.J. and Ayengar, R.J., *J. Exp. Med.*, 115, 195, 1962.
111. Svehag, S.-E. and Mandel, B., *J. Exp. Med.*, 119, 21, 1964.
112. Uhr, J.W. and Finkelstein, M.S., *J. Exp. Med.*, 117, 457, 1963.
113. Nossal, G.J.V., Szenberg, A., Ada, G.L., and Austin, C.M., *J. Exp. Med.*, 119, 485, 1964.
114. Clark, W.G. and Stavitsky, A.B., *Proc. Soc. Exptl. Biol. Med.*, 52, 168, 1943.
115. Stavitsky, A.B., *Bact. Rev.*, 12, 203, 1948.
116. Lee, H.F. and Stavitsky, A.B., *Amer. Rev. Tuberculosis*, 55, 262, 1947.
117. Mansour, T.E, Bueding, E. and Stavitsky, A.B., *Brit. J. Pharmacol. Chemotherap.*, 9, 182, 1954.
118. Garb, K.S., Stavitsky, A.B. and Mahmoud, A.A.F., *J. Immunol.*, 127, 115, 1981.
119. Garb,K.S., Stavitsky, A.B., Olds, G.R., Tracy, J.W. and Mahmoud, A.A.F., *J. Immunol.*, 129, 2752, 1982.
120. Stavitsky, A.B., Olds, G.R. and Peterson, L.B., *Infect. Immun.*, 49, 635, 1985.
121. Olds, G.R. and Stavitsky, A.B., *Infect. Immun.*, 52, 513, 1986.

Chapter 15

ANTIGENICITY OF ANTIBODIES

Felix Milgrom

In this chapter, I will use the term anti-antibody (A-A) in a broad sense, referring to all possible antibodies combining with other antibodies, the latter acting as antigens. This also will include antibodies against immunoglobulins of unknown antibody specificity. The very first attempts at A-A production stemmed from the statement of Ehrlich and Morgenroth[1] that formation of anti-autohemolysins may be a homeostatic mechanisms preventing the formation of autohemolysins that would destroy the individual's own erythrocytes. In a rather unambiguous way, Ehrlich and Morgenroth theorized about the formation of A-A directed against the antibody combining site that Ehrlich called cytophilic site, referring to hemolysins.

Studies conducted by Ehrlich and Morgenroth,[2] by Bordet,[3] and by Ehrlich and Sachs[4] dealt with immunization of animals of a foreign species with antibody-containing sera. It was soon realized that A-A resulting from such immunization did not react with the antibody combining site, but with another part of the antibody molecule. Furthermore, similar antibodies could be elicited by immunization with normal sera. Since interaction with such A-A prevented binding of complement, Ehrlich presented an extensive dissertation about their reaction with the complementophilic group of antibody, which we would call today Fc fragment. This notion was essentially correct.

ANTI-ANTIBODIES TO NATIVE ANTIBODY MOLECULE BUT NOT TO ITS COMBINING SITE

The above quoted studies of Ehrlich and his associates[2,4] and of Bordet[3] were the very first experiments on what we call today antibodies to immuno-globulins. As mentioned, in these studies the reaction of A-A could be detected by means of inhibition of the complement binding by the antibody acting as an antigen. A few years later (1908), Moreschi[5] used non-agglutinating, incomplete antibodies for studies on A-A. He showed that rabbit erythrocytes sensitized by incomplete antibodies of goat origin would undergo agglutination when exposed to a rabbit antiserum against goat serum proteins. This was the first description of what we call today anti-globulin tests which were introduced into laboratory practice by Coombs and his associates[6,7,8] which found most important applications in routine laboratory practice (see review by Dunsford.[9] A-A active in these reactions are primarily directed against the Fc fragment of the IgG antibody molecule, but also A-A to F(ab')$_2$ fragment are active and occasionally employed. Various methods have been used for the preparation of anti-globulin sera; most of them involve isolation of immunoglobulins by physicochemical procedures and immunization of an animal of a foreign species with such isolated proteins. In our first study on the antigenicity of antibodies published in 1956,[10] a procedure was described in which rabbit erythrocytes were agglutinated by natural antibodies of a pooled normal human serum and the washed agglutinates were injected back into a rabbit. A-A obtained in this way did not have any affinity for the antibody combining site, but the anti-globulin reagents obtained by this procedure proved very good and are still used by several laboratories.

0-8493-4722-X/94/$0.00 + $.50

Immunoglobulins carry inherited alloantigens, referred to as allotypes. These structures can seldom be recognized by an animal of a foreign species and are usually studied by means of A-A from the same species. In human, A-A with allotypic specificities were first described by Grubb and Laurell.[11] They are formed under natural and pathological conditions and the stimulus responsible for their formation is usually only poorly recognized. In rabbits, antibodies to allotypes may be produced by intentional immunization, as shown in 1957 by Oudin at the Pasteur Institute in Paris[12] and by Dubiski in my Polish laboratory.[13,14]

Allotypes serve as important markers for various studies. This may be exemplified by research conducted very recently in our laboratory.[15] Rabbits injected with cationized IgG of rabbit origin produced granular immune deposits in glomeruli. It was interesting to learn whether the cationized IgG may be demonstrated in the deposits. To this end, rabbits of b4 allotype were injected with cationized IgG or b4 or b9 allotype. Both groups of animals showed granular deposits of IgG along the glomerular basement membrane. In both groups, immunofluorescence staining for b4, but not for b9, allotype could be demonstrated. This suggested strongly that the injected cationized IgG set in motion an immunological process to formation of autologous immune deposits, however, the cationized IgG played an insignificant, if any, role in the formation of deposits.

ANTI-ANTIBODIES TO ALTERED ANTIBODY MOLECULES

The thesis that antibody molecule undergoes molecular transformation in the course of its reaction with the antigen was advocated by Bordet at the turn of the century.[16,17] Up to the mid-1950s, however, this was a controversial issue, not substantiated experimentally. In 1956, we[18,19] advanced a thesis that antibody undergoes molecular transformation in the serological reaction and that such transformation may expose or create new antigenic sites which are not present on the unaltered antibody molecule. Still, as mentioned before, our study on immunization of rabbits with human antibodies attached to rabbit erythrocytes led to formation of A-A that showed just properties of antiglobulin antibodies. We reasoned that in this experiment, the rabbit was "overwhelmed" by strongly immunogenic sites on antibody molecules of a foreign species and did not "notice" the subtle antigenic difference resulting from the alteration of the antibody in the serological reaction. We suggested that such differences would be noticeable by an animal challenged with antigens complexed with the antibody of the animal's own species and, still more so, by an animal challenged by antigen-antibody complexes which had been formed in its own body and contained autologous antibodies. In following this reasoning, we screened many human sera by means of human Rh+ erythrocytes sensitized by incomplete Rh antibodies. We anticipated that as a result of chronic exposure to antigen-antibody complexes, some individuals would have antibodies combining specifically with the antigenic sites which were exposed or created on Rh antibodies in the course of their reaction with Rh+ erythrocytes. Indeed, we found that a small proportion of human sera tested, considerably less than 1%, had such antibodies. These were IgM antibodies which combined with IgG antibodies complexed with their antigen but not with such antibodies in solution. Kunkel and Tan[20] named this A-A the Milgrom factor. Since this factor clearly distinguished the IgG antibody bound to the antigen from the free antibody in the solution, it provided evidence for the molecular transformation of antibody by the impact of serological reaction. A study by Ishizaka and Campbell[21] further supported this thesis by demonstration of changes in the optical rotation of antibodies after the reaction with their antigens.

The advent of serology of rheumatoid arthritis had a great impact on the discussed topic. Rheumatoid factor (for references see[22,23] is an antibody with broader specificity than the above discussed factor. Rheumatoid factor reacts with IgG not only of human but also of animal origin. By the generally accepted definition, rheumatoid factor combines with the Fc fragment of IgG, C_H2 and C_H3 domains.

In studying rheumatoid sera reacting with human and rabbit IgG, we[24] demonstrated the existence of three separate factors: 1) factor reacting with human IgG; 2) factor reacting with both human and rabbit IgG; and 3) factor reacting with rabbit IgG. At that time, we theorized that the factor 2 may be a multispecific antibody as defined by us[25,26] in the 1950s, i.e., have separate combining sites for human and rabbit IgG. Recent studies along these lines were conducted by me in collaboration with Dr. Z. Swierczynska of Warsaw, Poland. Using monoclonal human rheumatoid factor[27] obtained from Dr. M. Steinitz of Jerusalem, we presented evidence for the multispecific nature of the rheumatoid factor. These findings have interesting implications in relation to rheumatoid factors which, in addition to IgG, combine with such unrelated antigens such as DNA or cardiolipin.

Many investigators called rheumatoid factors autoantibodies. This obviously is an incorrect term to denote a factor that reacts with IgG of animal origin. On the other hand, the factor combining with human IgG can be called autoantibody only if it reacts with the patient's own native IgG. In my opinion, most of the presently available evidence indicates that rheumatoid factors react predominantly, if not exclusively, with allogeneic or otherwise with altered autologous IgG and accordingly are not autoantibodies.

The mode of formation of rheumatoid factors is still a matter of controversy. Some investigators consider that non-specific stimulation of B cells with mitogens may play a major role in the formation of this factor. Other investigators present valid arguments that in human diseases, rheumatoid factor is formed due to antigen-driven stimulation. Our experiments supported this latter contention. Rabbits exposed to immunization with each animal's own IgG, denatured by isolation and preservation procedures formed antiglobulin antibodies resembling the rheumatoid factor.[28] Furthermore, we and other investigators demonstrated that animals exposed for several months to immunization with any strong antigen would form antibodies which resembled the rheumatoid factor and which were apparently formed in response to a stimulus exerted by IgG antibodies altered during *in vivo* reaction with their antigens (for references, see Ref. [23]. In other words, the rheumatoid factor represents a stereotype of immune response of man or animals exposed to prolonged contact with an antigen and the resulting immune complexes.

Most of our early studies dealt with IgM rheumatoid factor and only in the last years, the IgG factors elicited attention. Pope[29] has shown that self-polymerization of IgG rheumatoid factors occurs in such a way that each molecule of the factor acts as a bivalent antigen, through its Fc fragment, and as a bivalent antibody through its $F(ab')_2$ fragment.

In a rather unexpected way, the pathogenic role of rheumatoid factors became more obvious in various human glomerulonephritides than in rheumatoid arthritis.   We[30] studied dissociation of immune deposits in human kidneys by exposing kidney sections to aggregated human IgG which was expected to exert dissociating effect of antigen excess.   Dissociation of immune deposits was recognized by the disappearance of immunofluorescent staining of section for IgG and C3.   By means of this procedure we dissolved immune deposits in glomerulonephritides associated with SLE, idiopathic membranous nephropathy and streptococcal infections.   Subsequently, studies of Sugisaki in our laboratory brought similar results on dispersion of immune deposits accumulated in human renal allografts.[31]   We concluded that IgG rheumatoid factor is an integral and frequently the most important component of nephritogenic immune complexes deposited in kidneys.

ANTI-ANTIBODIES TO THE ANTIBODY COMBINING SITES

As stated before, Ehrlich and Morgenroth[1] were the first to propose that A-A directed against what we call today antibody combining site may be formed and that such antibodies may exert a regulatory role.   Numerous experiments were undertaken to produce such "true anti-antibodies."   These studies dealt mostly with immunization of an animal of a foreign species with crude or purified preparations of antibodies.   In all these experiments, including our own studies,[10] the resulting A-A did not recognize the antibody combining site but they had properties of anti-immunoglobulins. Landsteiner[32] summarized some of these studies by concluding that "there is no evidence for the existence of true anti-antibodies which would bear a relation to the specific antibody function."   In spite of these discouraging data, we continued our studies on "true anti-antibodies."   In contrast to previous investigations, we conducted immunization within the species; in 1957, we[33] immunized rabbits with rabbit antibodies against Proteus and against Escherichia bacilli.   The rabbits formed antibodies of the type of "true anti-antibodies" in that they clearly distinguished Proteus antibodies from Escherichia antibodies.   Subsequent studies conducted in the 1960s by Oudin and Michel[34] and by Kunkel et al.[35] were very much consistent with this observation.   To denote the antigenic specificity detected by such "true anti-antibodies," the term idiotypic specificity was used.

However, idiotypic specificity is not completely identical with the specificity of the combining site.   It is well known that immunization with even a simple hapten gives an immune response with heterogenicity of antibodies. Therefore, even antibodies directed against a very simple epitope may differ in their idiotypic specificity.   Furthermore, idiotypic specificity is always situated in the proximity of the antibody combining site, but is not necessarily within this site and this may again account for variable idiotypic specificity of antibodies combining with the same antigen.   Conversely, very similar amino acid sequences may be used for the assembly of two or more different antibody combining sites.   This would account for idiotypic identity or similarity of antibodies with different serological specificities.

The hypothesis of Jerne[36] about the existence of idiotype networks and their regulatory mechanisms need not be reiterated here.   The fascinating consequence of this theory is the concept of "internal images."   There is evidence indicating that idiotypic A-A resemble the structure of the original antigen and accordingly be used in its stead to induced protective immunity whenever the original antigen is a noxious agent.   A great deal of experimentation along these lines is conducted at present.   Definite results of these studies are eagerly awaited.

REFERENCES

1. Ehrlich, P. und Morgenroth, J., *Übrt Hämolysine. Dritte Mittheilung. Berl. klin. Wschr.*, 37, 453, 1900.
2. Ehrlich, P. und Morgenroth, J., *Über Haemolysine. Sechste Mitteilung. Berl. klin. Wschr.*, 1901.
3. Bordet, J., Les proprietés des antisensibilisatrices et les théories chimiques de l'imunité, *Ann. Inst. Pasteur*, 18, 1904.
4. Ehrlich, P. und Sachs, H., *Über den Mechanismus der Antiamboceptorwirkung, Ber. klin. Wschr.*, 1905.
5. Moreschi, C., Neue Tatschen über die Blutkörperchenagglutination, *Centralbl. Bakt. I. Orig.*, 46, 49, 1908.
6. Coombs, R.R.A., Mourant, A.E., and Race, R.R., A new test for the detection of weak and "incomplete" Rh agglutinins, *Brit. J. Exp. Path.*, 26, 255, 1945.
7. Coombs, R.R.A., Mourant, A.E., and Race, R.R., Detection of weak and "incomplete" Rh agglutinations: a new test, *Lancet II*, 15, 1945.
8. Coombs, R.R.A., Mourant, A.E., and Race, R.R., In vivo isosensitization of red cells in babies with haemolytic disease, *Lancet I*, 264, 1946.
9. Dunsford, I. and Grant, J., The Anti-Globulin (Coombs) Test in Laboratory Practice, Oliver and Boyd, London, 1959.
10. Milgrom, F., Luszczynski, T., and Dubiski, S., Preparation of antiglobulin sera, *Nature*, 177, 329, 1956.
11. Grubb, R. and Laurell, A.B., Hereditary serological human serum groups, *Acta. Path. Microbiol. Scand.*, 39, 390, 1956.
12. Oudin, J., *C.R. Acad. Sci.*, 242, 2606, 1956.
13. Dubiski, S., Badania nad Aglutynacja Lancuchowa, Ph.D. Dissertation, *Silessian School of Medicine, Zabrze-Rokitnica:Poland*, 1957.
14. Dubiski, S., Dudziak, Z., Skalba, D., and Dubiska, A., *Immunology*, 2, 84, 1959.
15. Cavalot, F., Miyata, M., Dubiski, S., Terranova, V.P., Vladutiu, A., Brentjens, J., Andres, G., and Milgrom, F., Nephropathy in the rabbit induced by injection of homologous cationized IgG (cIgG), *FASEB J.*, 3(4), A1121, Abst. No. 5198.
16. Bordet, J., Le Mécanisme de l'agglutination, *Ann. Inst. Pasteur*, 13, 225, 1899.
17. Bordet, J., Traite de l'immunite dans les maladies infectieuses, 2nd ed., Masson, Paris, 1939.
18. Milgrom, F., Dubiski, S., and Wozniczko, G., Human sera with "anti-antibody," *Vox Sand*, 1, 172, 1956.
19. Milgrom, F., Dubiski, S., and Wozniczko, G., A simple method of Rh determination, *Nature*, 178, 539, 1956.
20. Kunkel, H.G. and Tan, E.M., Autoantibodies and disease, *Adv. Immunol.*, 4, 351, 1964.
21. Ishizaka, K. and Campbell, D.H., Biological activity of soluble antigen-antibody complexes, V. Changes of optical rotation by the formation of skin reactive complexes, *J. Immunol.*, 83, 318, 1959.
22. Mannik, M., Rheumatoid factors, in *Arthritis and Allied Conditions. A Textbook of Rheumatology*, D.J. McCarty, Ed., Lea and Febiger, Philadelphia, 1985, p. 660.
23. Milgrom, F., Development of rheumatoid factor research through 50 years, Scand. *J. Rheumatol.*, 17(Suppl. 75), 1988.
24. Milgrom, F., Witebsky, E., Goldstein, R., and Loza, U., Studies on the rheumatoid and related serum factors, II. Relation of anti-human and anti-rabbit gamma globulin factors in rheumatoid arthritis serums, *JAMA*, 181, 476, 1962.
25. Milgrom, F., Studies on structure of antibodies (Polish), *Panstwowy Zaklad Wydawnictw Lekarskich:Warszawa*, 1950.
26. Milgrom, F., Recherches sur la structure des isoanticorps groupaus, *Reveu Immunol.*, 16, 86, 1952.
27. Steinitz, M., Klein, G., Koskimies, S., and Makel, O., EB virus-induced B lymphocyte cell lines producing specific antibody, *Nature*, 269, 420, 1977.
28. Milgrom, F. and Witebsky, E., Studies on the rheumatoid and related serum factors. I. Autoimmunization of rabbits with gamma globulin, *JAMA*, 174, 56, 1960.
29. Pope, R.M., Teller, D.C., and Mannik, M., The molecular basis of self-association of IgG rheumatoid factors, *J. Immunol.*, 115, 365, 1975.

30. **Penner, E., Albini, B., Glurich, I., Andres, G.A., and Milgrom, F.,** Dissociation of immune complexes in tissue sections by excess of antigen, *Int. Arch. Allergy Appl. Immunol.*, 67, 245, 1982.

31. **Sugisaki, T., Kano, K., Brentjens, J.R., Anthone, S., Anthone, R., Andres, G.A., and Milgrom, F.,** Immune complexes in renal allograft with *de novo* membranous nephropathy, *Transplantation*, 34, 90, 1982.

32. **Landsteiner, K.,** *The Specificity of Serological Reactions,* Harvard University Press, Cambridge, Mass., 1946.

33. **Milgrom, F. and Dubiski, S.,** Antigenicity of antibodies of the same species, *Nature*, 179, 1351, 1957.

34. **Oudin, J., and Michel, M.,** Une nouvelle forme d'allotypie des globulines gamma du sérum de Lapin apparemment liée à la fonction et à la spécificité anticorps, *Compt. Rend.*, 267: 805, 1963.

35. **Kunkel, H.G., Mannik, M., and Williams, R.C.,** Individual antigenic specificity of isolated antibodies, *Science*, 140, 1218, 1963.

36. **Jerne, N.K.,** Idiotypic networks and other preconceived ideas, *Immunol. Reviews,* No. 79, Munksgaard, Copenhagen, 1984, p. 5.

Chapter 16

ON THE THRESHOLD OF THE DOOR OF "NO ADMITTANCE"

Joseph G. Sinkovics

I. QUESTIONS WITHOUT ANSWERS

A. Idealism and Romanticism

In 1946-50, my main motive for the study of microbiology, especially virology, was to understand how primitive life originated on Earth in ancient times. In 1946, the committee that investigated all university students individually, established that I did not collaborate with the German occupational forces and their extreme rightist Hungarian puppets; and, that I extended help to those whose lives were threatened. Therefore, I received the stamp "Igazolt" ("investigated and found clean") in my student book and was back to classes of my medical school where I first enrolled in 1942. During my last years as a medical student at the renowned Péter Pázmány University in Budapest, I had gained permission from Professor Sándor Belák (who envisioned a connection between the nervous system and immune functions) to work without stipend at the Institute of Microbiology and Pathophysiology in a marvelous old building under Hőgyes Endre Street 9. Decades earlier those laboratories housed Professor Hugó Preisz and his cultures referred to as "Pettenkoferia" which were really the first protoplasts and L-forms of bacteria as I will have had come to recognize this relationship many years later. In a city devastated by war and at an impoverished university of magnificent past, we were bursting with ideas and energy and were hoping for a good relationship with the western world and its scientific leadership that we admired.

Adjunct professor Dr. László Berta took over my education in research. He failed to obtain a fellowship to the west but instead received and completed one in the Soviet Union where he learned the basics of contemporary virology. Laci Berta was a wonderful man, teacher and investigator; he died young but he made an indelible impression of the best kind on those who worked with him. Imagination was encouraged, day-dreaming was forbidden. Basic virologic techniques (autopsies of inoculated mice, preparation of tissue extracts, titrations, and calculations) had to be done precisely, accurately and repeatedly. I was impatient and in a hurry. He was circumspect, meticulous and deliberate. I dreamed about photosynthesis as the clue to the origin of life on Earth and wrote my first (unpublished) manuscript on the subject, not knowing then of the magnificent advances that occurred much later. These new developments such as the biochemistry of *Rhodopseudomonas* utilizing chlorophyll but not releasing O_2 thus utilizing photons from the sun as the most primitive "bacteria" must have done three billion years ago living in the anaerobic environment of the archaic Earth, I still read with great interest. Higher plants created our atmosphere and vascular plants — angiogenesis is so primitive that it occurs in plants — acquisitioned two photosynthetic cell types.

Then I splenectomized rats to induce bartonellosis, dreaming that I would induce vascular tumors (on the analogy of *verruga peruana*) like Kaposi's sarcoma but induced only hemolytic anemia. This was my second unpublished

0-8493-4722-X/94/$0.00 + $.50
© 1994 by CRC Press, Inc.

manuscript; these manuscripts were not rejected by some journals, they were never submitted for publication. In 1948, Laci made me work on a project of antiviral immunity. This work was readily and immediately published. We "blockaded the reticuloendothelial system" of mice with intravenous colloid copper and found that small doses of intranasally instilled influenza A viruses (strains received from Dr. Smorodincev from Moscow and Dr. Andrewes from London) caused large and rapidly fatal hemorrhagic pneumonias, concluding that immunosuppression increased susceptibility to viral infections. The work was done precisely and it was readily reproducible. Yet, it was a primitive work by today's standards: we knew nothing about interferons; did not know that NK cells without MHC-restriction and immune T lymphocytes with MHC-restriction kill virus-carrier host cells; had no idea that in some virus-host systems (lymphocytic choriomeningitis) tolerance meant disease-free state despite replicating virus, whereas immunity to virus and to virus-carrier cells meant fatal illness. The wealth of information concerning separate antibody- and cell-mediated immune reactions to subviral components (neuraminidase; hemagglutinin, etc.) was entirely unknown to us. Perhaps we blocked a very early step in immune reactivity, i.e., viral antigen presentation by dendritic macrophages to lymphocytes, and thus abrogated antiviral immunity, allowing for unopposed viral replication and direct cytotoxicity to alveolar cells of the lung. I wish Laci had lived to see how far the science of immunology developed. Had he been able to survive a devastating illness, he certainly would have mightily contributed to the knowledge of antiviral immunity.

After Professor Belák's death, his institute was divided into Medical Microbiology and Pathophysiology and Professor Ferenc Faragó became chairman of the Medical Microbiology Department. Laci Berta, in the last year of his life, and I joined Professor Faragó. Professor Faragó was a former Rockefeller fellow, maintained extensive correspondence with English and U.S. professors and remained strongly pro-western during the communist takeover of Hungary. He assembled a very fine group of young investigators working remarkably well together despite wide political discrepancies: we openly opposed to communism; others opposed to communism but playacting out of fear or opportunism as if they were willing to go along with it; and those actually representing the communist party within our ranks. We feared this latter group but there is no evidence that they went as far as to report on us; as a matter of fact today I somehow believe that none of them was a true communist and that they secretly envied us who dared to express opposition and probably even covered up for us. Observing our polarization, Professor Faragó engaged an English (briefly) and a Russian (more persistently) language teacher for us.

There was no work on tumor virology in post-war Hungary where Marek left his blazing trail by describing decades earlier the chicken leukosis now known to be caused by a unique herpes virus. Professor József Baló resumed quite erratically some evening classes of virology, including the chicken leukemias and Rous sarcoma. He was a famous pathologist whom I once inadvertently angered beyond measure when for my own studies I sliced up a pair of lungs filled with abscesses that he wanted to photograph but I thought the organ was set aside for disposal. On one of these evenings, I first met György Klein who served as instructor of pathological anatomy at Professor Baló's institution. Soon Gyuri confided to me that he obtained exit permit and visa to Sweden on a fellowship and that he will not return. I wished him well and in a kind way envied his intelligence and skill. When I saw him next in the 1960s in Stockholm, he was Professor George Klein, Director of the Institute of Tumor Biology at Karolinska that he and his wife, Eva, made world famous.[*]

In those years, lymphocyte function was also uncharted territory and Fagraeus in Sweden was yet to report high immune globulin content in plasmacyte-rich nasal polyps. Professor Faragó was fascinated and frequently urged me: "Joe, work with lymphocytes!" "Joe, study the lymphocytes!" I wish he had survived to hear that a decade or so later in a splendid American laboratory Joe was setting lymphocytes after cancer cells, observing with great amazement how the patient's own lymphocytes could kill autologous cancer (chondrosarcoma) cells (*Cancer* 27:782-93, 1971).

In 1948, I became doctor of medicine *summa cum laude*. Professor of neurology and psychiatry, Béla Horányi, whom we admired for his intelligence, factual knowledge and whose lectures we never missed, offered me a position at his clinics. He explained to me ideas that had not been conceived anywhere else in those days and were named later as "neurooncology, neurovirology, neuroimmunology." He indicated to me that in his judgment I would be good at working on those ideas. At the same time, I had another idol, professor of internal medicine, Imre Haynal, who took interest in me during some colloquia concerning a patient with "Drüsenfieber" (infectious mononucleosis). This was a great opportunity for me to elaborate on viruses (the viral etiology for infectious mononucleosis was discovered decades later by Drs. Gertrude and Werner Henle). I especially admired Professor Haynal for his firm and courageous stand against "cult of personality." One particular communist leader of an especially vicious and vindictive disposition ("the great Stalin's best Hungarian pupil" he wanted himself to be referred to) liked his photographs posted everywhere, including classrooms. Some communist medical students decorated Professor Haynal's classroom provocatively with Party insignia, among them large posters showing this evil man in glorious postures. The professor, without displaying any emotion, removed these posters one by one and started putting up his own illustrations of high level cardiology. He received an applause and foot-stomping that would not stop for a long time. This was in 1947. In the 1950s, the evil man became the Communist dictator of Hungary, relying on a police force so brutal that such a free display of feelings would have resulted in a blood bath.

After the communist takeover of Hungary, some publications were found containing Professor Huzella's early recognition what monsters of history Hitler and Stalin together really were. This view was first presented in confidence to a few of us young medical students in the early 1940s by Dr. Tivadar Huzella, professor of histology and ontology (embryology). Professor Huzella was a master of tissue culture work in an era when no antibiotics existed and quick, precise and sterile work and meticulous attention was essential. I read and re-read his book, *The Organization of the Cell Community* (Budapest, 1942), several times. My copy of his book signed by him perished during the war, but recently I succeeded in obtaining another copy. In re-reading the book now, with amazement and fascination I see how his observations on his live cultures pre-dated the discovery of the cell skeleton

---

[*]After completing this chapter, excerpts of the autobiography of the Drs. Klein appeared (*Ann. Rev. Immunol.* 7, 1-33, 1989). The Kleins shine with unparalleled brilliance. I am happy that I knew Gyuri as a young man seeking his way in the "vast oceans of science over which the sun never sets."

and its dynamic interaction with the extracellular stroma or matrix. No one before Professor Huzella emphasized the profound influence the extracellular matrix exerts on the shape, locomotion and function of the cells overriding it. Now we know that integrins function as cell receptors for fibronectin, thus connecting the cytoskeleton's actin, talin and vinculin with the extracellular matrix. Similar relationship exists between another major matrix protein laminin and its receptor and between the cell adhesion proteins (uvomorulins, cadherins, cognins) and their cell receptors. These interactions guide the locomotion of cells during embryogenesis, histogenesis, regeneration, wound healing and cancer invasion or metastasis. The sequence L-arg-glyc-L-asp in the cell binding domain of fibronectin is specifically recognized by cell receptors. Reading Professor Huzella's "cytostromal unity" and "elasto-motor" mechanism of cell activity, I wish that his texts were written in English. He published in German in Virchow's Archivs für Pathologie und Physiolgie in 1932; in Archivs für experimentelle Zellforschung and in the Wiener klinische Wochenschrift in 1937 describing his "Zellenlehre und Zwischenzellenstruktur" well but not as eloquently as in his Hungarian monograph.

In 1946, Professor Huzella was ordered by Communist functionaries to withdraw his statements on Stalin, "repent" (exercise strong "self-criticism") and write some sort of high praise on Stalin and submit it for publication. Courageously, Professor Huzella refused. Promptly, he was dismissed as professor and chairman, threatened and harassed, but to my knowledge escaped arrest. He died soon thereafter. In 1986, during the International Cancer Congress held in Budapest, Hungary, Professor Huzella was rehabilitated. On this occasion, Dr. George Klein of the Karolinska Institute remembered Professor Huzella. We must remember that György Klein, medical student in post-war Hungary, received his fellowship enabling him to begin his work in Stockholm in 1947-48 because of what he learned from Professor Huzella in 1946 about the techniques of tissue cultures.

At the Institute of Microbiology under Hőgyes Endre Street 9 we found refuge from political turmoil of the outside world. Professor Faragó invited me to be his adjunct professor to develop a section of virology, and this position I gladly accepted. I was allowed a brief visit with Professor Dionyz Blaskovics in Bratislava (formerly Pozsony, where Hungarian kings used to be crowned hundreds of years earlier). Professor Blaskovics received me very kindly. He learned virology under Drs. Gertrude and Werner Henle in Philadelphia. He now serves as director of Czechoslovakian Institute of Virology. Comparing his education to that of Laci Berta, I clearly recognized what I really wanted: a fellowship in virology, immunology and infectious diseases in the United States, but by then there was no way for a noncommunist to get a passport out of the country: the iron curtain was slowly and heavily descending. Back at our Institute of Microbiology, we were successful in isolating Newcastle disease (ND), influenza, mumps and lymphocytic choriomeningitis viruses from patients. The mumps virus I isolated from saliva in the amnion cavity of embryonated chicken eggs after I learned the technique from Beveridge's and Burnet's book without anybody actually showing me the tricks of this procedure.

From Denmark we obtained poliomyelitis virus strains (the Brunhilde and Lansing viruses) to practice their passage and observe their pathogenicity. We observed viral interference between NDV and influenza viruses (both A and B, the PR8 and Lee strains) in the mouse lung. During our debates concerning the mechanism of viral interference, we concluded that the first virus destroyed cell receptors for the second virus and thus entirely missed the concept of interferon production (to be discovered by Isaacs and Lindenmann in England some six years later).

I clearly recall how we debated if antibodies were antigenic and what would happen if we produced antibodies against antibodies. Young Drs. István Vass and Szilárd Bognár argued a great deal about this. Later, Vass became professor and chairman of McGill's microbiology department of Montreal, Canada. Again, in the late 1940s, the crucial experiment in which the second antibody (antibody against an antiviral antibody) could pose as an antigen for the production of a third antibody that would not only react with the second antibody but also with the virus that induced the production of the first antibody, eluded us. What a consolation it was for me when I observed with amazement and fascination more than 20 years later in works of Drs. Gordon Dreesman and Joseph Melnick of the Department of Virology and Epidemiology of Baylor College of Medicine, documentation for these series of events in the case of hepatitis B virus. In 1948-50, we had a section of virology at the Institute of Microbiology in Budapest that was active, fully operational and productive, arising on the ruins of the war and blossoming in a most repressive and frightening political atmosphere. Our young inquisitive group tackled some of the most fundamental questions of modern immunology (lymphokines; idiotypic immunization) but without being able to carry out the crucial experiments. In 1950-1, under immense political pressure, the membership of this institute was dispersed. Dr. Ilona Szeri (whom I introduced into the art and science of virology) and Dr. István Nász (who now is the director) remained.

B. Harsh Lessons in Realism

In the summer of 1950 my work and life suffered a major break. Professor Faragó, a healthy man in his late 40s was arrested by the political police and died in prison within weeks. He was accused of producing a hyperimmune antipertussis serum tainted with tetanus toxin due to negligence or deliberate act of sabotage (!?). Infants receiving the serum died. This was horrible news to me. Being isolated in my virology section at one geographic end of the department, I was not involved at all with the other end, where bacteriology, vaccine development and passive immunization were major topics under study with the personal guidance and supervision of Dr. Faragó. Nevertheless, a few days later, plainclothesmen and uniformed men of the secret police (AVH = Police of State Security) arrested me at 2 A.M. In no time I was declared "enemy of the people" and "lackey of the imperialists." I spent some time in the wet, cold, blood- and excrement-stained cellars of Secret Police Headquarters at Andrássy Boulevard 60, deep underground. There I saw Professor Faragó's swollen and bruised face once more for the last time. Thereafter, I was taken to the prison of Markó Street, the place where I believe Professor Faragó must have died (his body was never given out to his family). Alapi, the murderous chief prosecutor for State Security pressed for a "confession" that we were spreading bacteria in Hungary in order to undermine the achievements of communism and that Professor Faragó received his orders from the capitalists. After Professor Faragó's death, Alapi never interrogated me again, thus my denials remained unbroken.** My nightmare is that I knew that with more time and intensification of their interrogative technology, Alapi's mentally deranged team could have obtained this "confession"! I was then kept (always in solitary confinement) in the notorious "Small Prison" of the huge Collecting Prison at the outskirts of Budapest in a bedbug-infested cell. Death row was on the first floor. I was on the second floor and overheard and witnessed brutal beatings and executions by hanging. The Korean War was on and the communist regime was determined to liquidate all its internal opponents. Without Professor Faragó, the State had no case against us. They could have possibly accused him of being a western spy and saboteur but we, his young associates, simply did not have credible connections to the west. Soon I was transferred to the worst political prison of the country at the township of Vác on the mighty river Danube where I was contemplating a jump into the icy waters, a long underwater swim and a long float toward the south to Yugoslavia and on foot to Italy (Laci Berta failed to discipline all dreaming out of me). This prison was called "Punitive Institution of State Security." Here I survived massive, repeated exposures to tuberculosis from fellow prisoners without falling ill, as I was assigned physician to the prison hospital. There I received extra food, could frequently shower (sometimes my face was splattered with cough and blood droplets from the dying I attended) and change into clean garments. I could walk and exercise in a small courtyard surrounded by high walls covered by electrified barbed wires.

A most paradoxical situation developed between the chief prison physician and me. This man was the major of the secret police and came in two to three times a week. He declared that I committed no crime and that he will set up a virus laboratory in the prison hospital (with the consent of his superiors) for me to continue my work. He started bringing in English, French, German and Russian articles from the Medical School's library for one-week time loan, all checked out for his own use under his name.

Last year medical student György Markos, instructor at the Faragó Institute, was also arrested. He was brought to the hospital to assist me and work with me. We discussed the physician-in-chief's possible motivations. We thought I might eventually be taken to a secret lab somewhere and be forced to work on biological warfare; I had nightmares about that, too (fortunately it did not happen). Incredibly, Gyuri Markos (now a vascular surgeon in Aachen, Germany) and I worked in the prison lab on photodynamic inactivation of influenza viruses and on their immunogenic potency as vaccines. Much later, in the USA, I used the same techniques to prepare a mouse leukemia virus vaccine (*Cancer Research* 25:624-7, 1965). Drs. Wallis and Melnick of Baylor, in their work written on photodynamically inactivated virus vaccines, gave us credit for our early work carried out in the laboratories of a prison hospital.

It was in 1953, after the death of Stalin, that the situation temporarily improved in Hungary. We in the prison celebrated his death. Rákosi, the communist dictator, who liked to execute his fellow-communist rivals, was temporarily demoted and replaced by Imre Nagy, a "communist with a human

---

**Long after the completion of this manuscript, I read with great amazement the book of Professor Yakov Rapoport on "The Doctors' Plot" (Harvard University Press, 1991). In the Soviet Union in the early 1950s, outstanding and innocent physicians were arrested and executed as saboteurs and murderers (and rehabilitated decades later often posthumously).

face." On the eve of December 27, 1953, I was suddenly released in my mold-smelling thin summer suit in which I was arrested in the summer of 1950. Minister of Health Zsoldos and Minister of Justice Erdei requested my release for open trial. A few friends of mine (Dr. László Erdős rendering expert testimony; Dr. Laci Csatáry and many others) found a way to reopen the case.

In a sack I had my manuscript of a virology textbook that was published later in 1955 in Hungarian and in 1956 in German and a little dog called Bundzsi, slightly drugged to keep her quiet. I acquired her as a puppy and hid her for a year or so in my cell and in the courtyard, sharing my food and my bed with her. This little white and black dog of mixed breed displayed the most profound understanding of life: she greeted and delighted all fellow prisoners exultantly dancing and jumping around them but growled at guards without fail displaying her sharp, white teeth. The guards periodically hunted down all dogs that took up temporary shelter somewhere in the prison, chased them in playing a wild game, laughing and yelling and in the end clubbed the frightened animals to death. Maybe this was part of the prison guards' curriculum to make them good guards for the system they guarded. It was a matter of life or death for the little dog that I hid her; and I did get her out of there, too! Of course, some of the guards knew that I had a dog. However, this subhuman species of prison guards relied on me for their concealed treatment of gonorrhea, soft chancres and the like which they feared to disclose to their superiors.

I climbed on an ice cold freight train to Budapest and just after midnight I was back in my mother's apartment eating a good home-cooked meal that she could put together as quickly and as well as the circumstances permitted. In a few days I married Dr. Erzsébet Molnár, a former member of the Faragó Institute (who escaped arrest), now a virologist at the State Institute of Hygiene (Public Health). A year later she gave birth to the twins, Géza, a son, and Eszter, a daughter.

Within a few months I stood trial and had the luxury of a fine defense attorney. However, the new State prosecutor dropped all accusations. I was acquitted. Until this day I possess documents typed on poor quality paper which state "acquitted because he committed no crime." Within a few days I also became a virologist at the Department of Virology of the State Institute of Public Health.

A few weeks later I was summoned to the Parliament building. There in the basement sat a corpulent man in shirt sleeves, his voluminous trousers held up by suspenders. He tossed a bundle of cash on the table. "Sign," he said. I signed a paper under the statement, "I accept this compensation from the People's Democracy and have no further claims." It was almost 10,000 forints—worth three to four months' earnings in Hungary; worthless, anywhere else.

The editors who did not dare, or were forbidden to, publish three of my manuscripts in 1950 while I was a "nonperson" (see Orwell: "1984"), now published them in 1954. With amazement I observed that they remained up-to-date.

My work continued along theoretical and practical lines. I was attracted by the idea that some viruses evolved from bacteria through retrograde evolution and sensed some analogy between filterable L forms and large "viruses" (psittacosis and trachoma agents; vaccinia; and down on the scale through herpesviruses to myxoviruses). Most of my evidence was morphological and not biochemical. Professor Miklós Melczer knew how to grow *Streptobacillus moniliformis* and pleuropneumonia microorganisms. At his department in the city of Pécs he taught me this art quickly and generously. I maintained and observed these fascinating microorganisms for the years to come and enjoyed this work immensely. I observed the fusion and regeneration of filterable spheroplasts into vegetative bacteria (*Nature* 181:566-7, 1958). A.J. Salle's textbook *Fundamentals of Bacteriology* (McGraw Hill, N.Y., 1961, p. 77) quotes these observations in good details. When Burnet recombined influenza viruses, it had come so quickly to me to envision genetic recombinations between unrelated viruses and between viruses and host cell genes. Laci Berta's advice to me was self-restraint and caution; I obeyed (and I am sorry that I did).

In my book, *Die Grundlagen der Virusforschung* (1956), I had forcefully restrained my imagination in my discussions (pp. 122-124; 141-147; 156-200) how host cells and viruses or bacteria and viruses may exchange genetic materials. I spoke of "Kernsubstanzaustausch," the exchange of genetic material and was quite liberal about it. The "Möglichkeit" (possibility) was there and if it happened, the genetic consequences were enormous. Now (in the 1980s) we know of pseudovirions incorporating host cell genome fragments and/or gene products, *v*-oncogenes that were transduced from host cells by retroviruses; and of plasmid constructs (of retroviruses) for the transfer of genetic material from cell to cell. I conclude that I had a vivid imagination as a young man but was not courageous enough to expound my ideas fully in public.

From early 1954 to late 1956, I worked on the eclipse phenomenon of influenza virus replication (discovered by the Henles) and on the phenotypic recombination of influenza and other viruses (as practiced by Sir MacFarlane Burnet). From Stockholm, Dr. George Klein sent us the Ehrlich ascites tumor line. I inoculated mice intraperitoneally with NDV and stopped the growth of these cancer cells. NDV strains adapted to the brain of newborn mice were the most effective "carcinostatic" agents.[1,2] Levaditi and Nicolau in France, Lindenmann in Switzerland, and Ackermann and Kurtz and Cassell in the United States performed similar experiments, but I did not have ready access to the U.S. literature in those years.

We lived in great excitement in those days. Dr. André Lwoff, at the Institut Pasteur in Paris succeeded in activating phage nucleic acids to encode the synthesis of lysogenic phages and in this we saw analogy with viral carcinogenesis. Dr. Ludwik Gross in New York claimed first the isolation of a mouse leukemia virus. At about this time a young oncologist (while the clinical science "oncology" did not exist as yet), Dr. Sándor Eckhardt came to me to propose cooperation in research. He is now the renowned director of the Hungarian National Institute of Oncology. He provided me with chemicals (alkylating agents) and I tested them against tumors in laboratory mice. In order to make the project more acceptable for a virologist working with state funds, I included a study on "activation of latent oncogenic viruses after exposure of Ehrlich ascites carcinoma cells to chemicals." We simply tried to induce tumors in mice with cell-free filtrates of the ascites. In our primitive way of thinking we expected the growth of solid tumors (not unlike what Rous sarcoma virus would induce in the wing web of chickens) but this never happened. I overlooked and left without proper investigation a few mice with large spleens. These large spleens remained photographed in my mind and tormented me for years to come. By then I was at Rutgers in New

Brunswick, New Jersey, and became acquainted with the legendary work of Dr. Charlotte Friend of the Sloan-Kettering Institute. She isolated a unique mouse leukemia virus (different from the Gross virus) from such large spleens. The bitter fact remains: I did not pursue the lead of the large spleens in 1955.

In 1954, I passed subspecialty examinations in clinical pathology (laboratory medicine). In 1956, my book appeared in German. I requested an English publication but I was overruled. The book was published under the title *Die Grundlagen der Virusforschung* in 420 pages, and it contained 150 figures and tables and 1488 worldwide references. Akadémia Kiadó (Budapest), the publisher, marketed it in Europe. It received the finest recensions in the European journals, from Professor Zhdanov (whom I met later in Chicago in a Soviet Science exhibit in 1960 where he expressed to me his regrets for the invasion of Hungary in 1956 by the Soviet Union) in Voprosi Virusologiya, to the Italian and German book reviews. French, British and American virologists replied individually. Letters came from Drs. C. Andrewes, Buddingh, Melnick, Sabin, Shope, Theiler and arrived to my address at the State Institute in Budapest (a dangerous sign of being "pro-western" in those days). The most extensive quotations I received in *Die Viruskrankheiten der Haut* by A. Marchionini and Th. Nasemann, Springer Verlag, Berlin, 1961. These nice people had, of course, no idea that the first manuscript of this exemplary virus book was written in prison.

On October 23, 1956, the Hungarian nation fearlessly rose in unison against the terror and tyranny imposed on it by puppets of an immense foreign power. By November 5, after a glorious week resembling "freedom," this nation that had served as a bastion and bled for the freedom of its western neighbors many times during its 1,100 year history, was brutally crushed again and it received no help whatsoever from the west. I did not bear arms during the Hungarian uprising, but I expressed elation and happiness over the utter disintegration of a rotten and criminal regime. To avoid another imprisonment, as this regime quickly re-established itself in full power, late in November, through dangerous and guarded passages, I escaped to Austria.

C. Solitary Confinement in a Prison Cell May not Form Man Out of a Boy: Internship at Cook County Hospital Does

In cold Vienna, now illuminated and ready for the Christmas of 1956, I had a thin overcoat and no money (Hungarian forints were worthless in the west). Herr Votruba, the great sculptor, let me sleep on a cot in his studio; he and his beautiful wife had me for a sumptuous dinner in their elegant home. I sat there in my clothes, badly needing repair and showing all the signs of escape through rough terrain a few days earlier. The Austrian Medical Association gave all Hungarian doctors $25. I used the small change to buy oranges from a Street vendor. Oranges I had not seen, smelled or tasted since my childhood; I ate them on the Street, peels and everything. Then I sent a telegram to Dr. Albert Sabin in Cincinnati, U.S.A., asking for his help to get a U.S. fellowship in virology. Months earlier, while still in Budapest, I received a letter from Dr. Sabin who received a complimentary copy of my virus book; he replied in the nicest of terms (later I learned how difficult it was to extract praise from Dr. Sabin). While waiting for something to happen, I visited Dr. Moritsch, adjunct professor of virology at Professor Bieling's institute. He worked with herpes viruses and was friendly toward me (he later died of herpes virus encephalitis probably acquired in the lab) but Professor Bieling felt that I should have cited his works in my book and resented the omission. I humbly apologized.

Tens of thousands of Hungarian refugees surrounded the U.S. Embassy in Vienna from daybreak to evening every day and there was no way to even get close to it as it was guarded by marines. At the street corners we got a cup of hot soup, crackers and cubes of cheese from friendly volunteer ladies and there we milled and waited. When the Mariahilferstrasse and the shopping centers lit up in the afternoon, we dispersed to reassemble there again in the darkness and cold of the next morning. One morning the loud speakers blared: "Doktor Sinkoviks! Doktor Sinkoviks!" "Here, here," I replied in Hungarian and German. "Let me get through, open up, they are calling me, let me pass," I said as I pushed forward. Inside the embassy, Ambassador Llewelyn Thompson held a telegram he received that morning. It read "Request special visa for outstanding young Hungarian virologist Joseph Sinkovics, M.D. Stipend guaranteed. Sabin." I was processed on the spot: interview, physical exam, chest X-ray, etc. A distinguished gentleman gave me his card: "Meyer, Rockefeller Foundation, New York" and invited me for an interview in the lobby of the Grand Hotel that evening.

On that evening I passed through the lines of crisp and immaculate porters, bellhops and londiners in my outfit clearly showing that I was not a paying guest of their suites. Mr. Meyer, representing the Rockefeller Foundation and offering fellowships to selected Hungarian scientists, was to interview me in English. I was confident and elated. In my teens I learned Latin, some ancient Greek, Italian and German; later French and Russian (enough to translate from medical books like the Prakticheskaya Virusologiya). English? I kept an English-Hungarian dictionary hidden in the prison and memorized its entire vocabulary from aardvark to zyzzle. However, I never learned grammar and pronunciation (except for a few hours at the Faragó Institute) and was deprived of English broadcasts and movies for a decade or so. I trusted, as I shook hands with Mr. Meyer, that my formidable vocabulary which enabled me to read and understand English publications of virology and medicine would not fail me now. Mr. Meyer spoke and slowly repeated his sentences: he spoke in a language I could not understand. Then I formulated my prepared introductory statements. Mr. Meyer's eyes popped out: he understood not one word. I stood there annihilated. Suddenly an idea lit up in my head. On a piece of paper with perfect English spelling I composed a few sentences (maybe not in perfect grammatical order). Mr. Meyer grinned broadly. He replied in writing: "I understand perfectly." In a rapid pace we exchanged written notes, first mutely, later him reading out loud what he wrote. I was sorry to follow suit: my pronunciation was atrocious. We had a fine interview to the great amazement of people passing by us. Right there, I received my Rockefeller fellowship. In a few days I was driven by bus to Munich and from there flown through stops in Ireland and Newfoundland to Camp Kilmer, New Jersey.***
A couple of days later I sat across the desk of Mr. Dean Rusk and Dr. G. Pomerat in the New York skyscraper of the Rockefeller Foundation where I

***Now I know a fine retired gentleman here in Florida. His wife is my patient. He was the captain of pilots who flew the aircrafts filled with Hungarian refugees from Munich to New Jersey in 1956.

received an "advance stipend," was checked into Hotel Abbey, purchased some new garments and was set free to roam the streets of Manhattan. There I had a most memorable evening when I met in person my scientific heroes, whose publications I used to practically memorize (but not pronounce): Drs. Werner Henle, Hilary Koprowski and Vincent Groupé. I was given a dry martini by Vince; I did not exactly know what it was and drank it up. The effects were devastating on me but exhilarating to my new friends who helped me home to my hotel.

The year 1957 I spent at Vince's department at Rutgers' Waksman Institute. Dr. S. Waksman was the director and the antibiotic brewery was in full operation. It was a very good year. My stipend was $100 per month. I rode the bus or the Pientas gave me a ride. I lived in a rented room in New Brunswick. My suits came from the Salvation Army; they were of the finest material and cost a few dollars only (I only had to conceal or cover up a small cigar burn here and there). Outstanding young men and women were studying under Vince for Ph.D. in virology: we became life-long friends. Bob Dougherty, Virginia Dunkel, Bob Manaker, Roman Pienta, Dick Rauscher, Robert Simpson and Bert Spencer were among them.

Rockefeller's travel allowance was most generous. I visited with Drs. John Buddingh (New Orleans), Leon Dmochowski (Houston), Charles Evans (Seattle), Albert Sabin (Cincinnati), Jerome Syverton (Minneapolis), Lawrence Kilham (Bethesda), Richard Shope and Max Theiler (New York), and Paul Szanto (Chicago). Fine positions of associate and adjunct professorships were offered to me: all research and teaching. Quickly I learned that a foreign-trained medical doctor could not attend patients in the U.S. unless he served at least one year internship and passed state board examinations in medicine, from basic science on to all clinical disciplines. Suddenly I found myself at the most important dividing line of my new life: staying in pure medical research and giving up the practice of medicine but retaining a decoratory M.D. title by accepting a university position, or serving a year of approved internship and then passing the board examinations.

Thinking back about why I elected to take the second choice, I can list the following main reasons: 1. I idealized, loved and knew quite well clinical medicine, especially as it pertained to infectious and tropical diseases; 2. I believed that after securing my M.D. degree in the U.S., I could go back to research and/or I could ideally combine medical research with the practice of clinical medicine, especially in the university environment; and 3. the project I was working on at Rutgers was not with tumor viruses after all. I hoped for a project with chicken or mouse leukemia-sarcoma viruses but instead Vince wanted me to continue to work with NDV, especially its incomplete replication in the mouse brain. This project was just not attractive enough to hold me in the lab when recertification of my M.D. degree was at stake.

On the eve of December 31, 1957, I was admitting new patients straight from the emergency room to the medical wards of the immense Cook County Hospital in Chicago. Dr. Blaha assigned me to the job. The next morning one of my attending physicians made rounds listening to my report. During the night I had to work-up, at least tentatively diagnose, and start treatment of eight new patients while I inherited eight additional former patients already admitted by the intern on call the previous days who rotated to another service on January 1. What patients these people were! These were men and women of the skid row, deathly ill and ravaged with alcoholism, congestive heart failure, pneumonias, hypertensive crises, diabetic coma, myocardial infarcts, strokes, emboli and assorted bizarre infections. We interns collected the blood samples, inoculated the media, pushed the stretchers to diagnostic X-ray and back, set the IVs (preparing cut-downs), placed catheters, performed thora- and paracenteses and spinal taps and did minor biopsies. Drs. William Hardy and E. Krasnow were the chief resident physicians to whom I reported; above them were the attending physicians. An intern was easily responsible for 16 to 18 very ill patients with complex problems. The morale of my fellow interns was incredibly high: we helped each other, worked easily 16 hours or more per day and it never occurred to us to strike and demand better hours, longer vacations and higher pay. Teaching was outstanding; the experience and knowledge of my resident and attending physicians were far above anything that I ever was exposed to. My Hungarian medical school training was good but highly theoretical: it appeared now as child's play to a front-line soldier. I utterly lacked the practical knowledge that was essential for my job. I constantly looked up solutions to problems in textbooks that I carried with me in a satchel on the job; I learned the techniques from my fellow interns who were ahead of me four months (starting their service on September 1). I had to steal hours from my well-deserved sleeping time for more studies. We were housed and fed very well. There were separate bedrooms for each of us, sharing a bathroom in between; the Chicago winter howled outside my sixth floor window. Food was good, plentiful and cold cuts were served for a midnight snack. It was an unforgettable year: before that year I believed I was a grown up man, seasoned, though, and capable of original ideas. At Cook County Hospital I learned first how it is to be at the mercy of the elements for the seriously ill, what a life-saving value it is to have a devoted physician standing by and what an overwhelming, triumphant emotion for the doctor it is to sort out the correct diagnosis from a most complex presentation, promptly institute treatment, reverse the relentless course of a process overnight and have an afebrile and compensated patient 24-48 hrs later. Clinical medicine emerged to give me this triumphant new emotion equal or superior (?) to a scientific discovery in the lab. This new emotion was among the greatest we human beings may experience that makes our lives worth living on this cruel Earth. Research appeared now as a plaything; the challenge was to conquer an illness that was presented to me in its complexity daily. Failures and defeats were unbearable and served as most powerful motivations for more studies, tireless efforts, cutting hours from time assigned for rest or recreation: work replaced recreation.

D. Research in Cancer Virology and Immunology in its Infancy

When I first visited the University of Texas M.D. Anderson Hospital in 1957, Dr. Leon Dmochowski was section chief of virology. He was jovial, anecdotal and friendly. Dr. Clifton Dexter Howe was head of the Department of Medicine; he had served in Africa as liaison officer with the British during the war and knew a great deal of tropical diseases (later on we diagnosed leprosy cases at M.D. Anderson). He and Dr. Ed White, head of the Surgical Department, took me for lunch to the Doctors' Club. We were served by black waiters wearing white gloves. After New York and Chicago, Houston was still deep South. On that occasion both men were more interested in politics than in medicine. Both served in World War II and wanted to know how the U.S. could lose World War II to its "ally," the Soviet Union. Dr.

Howe for many years to come referred to my comments, declaring them most eye-opening to him; it was I who first explained to him the enormous rift that existed between the Soviet Union and China. We took great mutual liking in each other. When I outlined my desires to do clinical medicine and research under the same roof, Dr. Howe described M.D. Anderson as the ideal place for such a combination. There was no problem with research: I could immediately take a position with Dr. Dmochowski. However, without internship and license, I could not do any clinical work. This conversation contributed to my leaving Rutgers at the end of the year and serving one year rotating internship at Cook County Hospital in 1958. As my year at Cook County was coming to its end, I wrote Dr. Howe. By return mail I received an appointment starting January 1, 1959, for one year research fellowship in virology and residency in medicine at M.D. Anderson Hospital.

The third year in the U.S.A. was another very good year. I had a decent furnished apartment and purchased my first car, a second-hand big Packard with a swan on the top of the hood. In buying this car I was influenced by the description of a scene in World War II, Moscow, when Commissar of Foreign Affairs Molotov was driven to diplomatic meetings in a big Packard; now I owned one and Molotov was deposed.

Half day I worked with Dr. Howe at outpatient clinics and with hospitalized patients. The afternoons and evenings I spent in the lab where I quickly learned that it was Dr. John Sykes who was master of all technology. John and his wonderful wife, Mary, accepted me in a peculiar way; they had three small sons and treated me as son number four (even though John was only 12 years older than I). My projects were 1. to grow human leukemia and lymphoma cells in tissue culture; the original tissues and the cultured cells were compared by Dr. Dmochowski's technicians in electron microscopy for the number of type C virus particles; and 2. to inoculate thousands of suckling mice with supernatant fluids of these cultures for observation of leukemia, lymphoma or solid tumor induction. I dissected all sick or dead mice and observed the healthy-appearing animals until the end of the year.

By the end of 1959, I wanted to take the specialty board examination in internal medicine. To my consternation, I learned that I had to serve three years in an approved residency program and M.D. Anderson was entitled to give me only one year. January 1, 1960 found me again in Chicago at Cook County Hospital as a second-year resident physician in medicine receiving room and board and a stipend of $100/month. There I served two full years, completing my three-year residency training by December 31, 1961.

At the Hektoen Institute of Medical Research affiliated with Cook County Hospital, unprecedented discoveries were claimed in 1960 by the chief of hematology service (a most reputable clinician) and his technologist: they repeatedly reported the isolation of mouse and human leukemia viruses from the brain but not from the leukemic tissues of mice and men! Dr. Bill Maduros, chief resident in hematology, and I received permission to work on this project. The Rockefeller Foundation supported my work on the project. I started out with faith, great elation and deep gratitude to the chief that I might become part of an epoch making discovery. Bill and I worked "double-blind": brain extracts prepared by me were inoculated by Bill and vice versa. He did not know the origin of the extracts (leukemic or control) and I did not know which groups of animals were inoculated with leukemic or control brain extracts, and vice versa. We repeatedly and utterly failed to isolate leukemia viruses from the brains of leukemic human beings. The chief angrily demanded that we uncode the experiments. We refused. Bill and I were fired on the spot and threatened with severe repercussions for undermining the discovery. Then the chief hired two PhD virologists-immunologists (Drs. Lea Sekely and Eric Brown) who also failed to isolate leukemia viruses from the brains of leukemic patients. Then, the technologist was fired. To my best knowledge, the publications describing the original "discovery" were never retracted. Hospital medical directors (Drs. Kushner, Hoffman and Szanto) fully supported Bill and me. I completed my residency training with the best of credentials. To this day the memories of this experience fill me with disbelief (that it could have happened) and sorrow. After reading the book *Betrayers of Truth* (Wm. Broad & N. Wade. Simon & Schuster, N.Y. 1982) some 20 years later, I realize that laboratory work may be subject to accidental or deliberate distortions.

During this time (and later) I passed examinations for licensure in the U.S. starting with the exam given by the Education Council for Foreign-Trained Physicians. In all I scored high (98%), especially in the basic sciences in Seattle. In Indiana, I scored the highest in my group: 98.8% and was put on the "honor roll." Later I repeated this feat in Florida (where I made a 98.6% in medicine) and received a complimentary letter from the director of the board. (I was tempted to reply that I did not make 100% because some of the questions were faulty, but I restrained myself.)

On January 1, 1962, I was back at M.D. Anderson and started on the staff as assistant professor of medicine. This is the year I became a naturalized citizen.

In the 12 years that followed I worked very hard, achieving a great deal. In this decade I proved that it was possible to practice high level clinical medicine and conduct productive laboratory research at the same time. My clinical work was at the "solid tumor clinics" where most sarcoma and melanoma patients were referred; I founded this service at M.D. Anderson. Fellows in training rotated through this service and many of them now fill distinguished positions at M.D. Anderson and at other institutions in the U.S. or abroad. Many publications and chapters reflect the work of this clinical service. I was an invited lecturer at M.D. Anderson Hospital Symposia, the Chicago Tumor Conferences and at international cancer conferences in Africa, Canada, Europe, Japan, Mexico, South America and in the U.S.A. The trip to Africa in January 1966 was most remarkable; so much so that I was again tempted to join the East African Virus Research Institute in Entebbe, Uganda. My curriculum vitae rapidly grew to a thick volume due to all presentations (abstracts), papers and chapters listed in it.

In 1964, I passed the oral specialty board exam in internal medicine at New Orleans' Charity Hospital where I felt at home: it looked like Cook County Hospital. Passing this exam at Charity Hospital in 1964 was of great satisfaction to me. In 1957, I had applied for internship at Charity Hospital (while visiting with virologist Dr. Buddingh). Hospital administrator Flores addressed me pointedly as "mister," declared that my medical education, as far as he was concerned, came from a second rate medical school and advised me to go elsewhere. I also became diplomat of the American Academy of Microbiology in laboratory virology and public health. In the 1970s, I passed subspecialty exams in infectious diseases and in medical oncology-hematology, thus raising my specialty board examinations, fitting to a true academician, to 5!

Back to research. Immediately in 1962 I obtained National Cancer Institute research grants and furbished my own small laboratory which later developed into a complex of several very well-equipped laboratories called Section of Clinical Tumor Virology and Immunology, Department of Medicine. It housed three M.D. investigators and myself, one PhD immunologist and eight technicians and aides, all paid from funds I raised mainly as NCI research grants and contracts. Project site visitor Dr. Ray Bryan of the old NCI staff supported me and helped me to gain independence from Dr. Dmochowski's morphology-oriented department; I am grateful to him.

In the mid-1960s we worked with mouse leukemia viruses. From the late 1960s on we worked with human lymphocytes and tissue cultures of tumors, actually establishing a human tumor cell bank. The mouse leukemia work was most interesting and rewarding but not in terms of recognition or monetary gains: I just immensely enjoyed making indentations by biological interventions on the relentless course of leukemia, such as slowing its course, preventing it by immunization and actually curing it by radiotherapy and adoptive immunization. First (1964-5) we showed that "chimeric" mice with graft-versus-host disease were less susceptible to viral leukemia.[3-5] Even though our papers were the first to show the "graft-vs-leukemia" reaction in mice, when this phenomenon was rediscovered in patients showing reduced relapse rates of leukemia after allogeneic bone marrow transplantation, if they also withstood a low degree of graft-versus-host disease, our early papers somehow were not remembered.

We then actively immunized mice against viral mouse leukemia with an attenuated mouse leukemia virus or with photodynamically inactivated mouse leukemia virus.[6] Spleen and lymph node cells of immune mice protected recipient mice against leukemia transferred either by virus or leukemic cells. Immune mice possessed mouse leukemia virus-neutralizing antibodies, complement-fixing antibodies lytic to leukemia cells and lymphocytes cytotoxic to mesenchymal tumor (sarcoma) cells induced in mice with a mouse leukemia virus.[7,8] We also showed that adoptive immunization against virally induced leukemia was most effective when leukemia-immune donor cells were inoculated into recipients rendered tolerant to the donor cells, but it was irrelevant whether or not the donor cells were tolerant to the recipient; thus, allogeneic disease was not essential for the antileukemia effect.[9,10] We recorded 8 to 25% leukemia-free survival when we treated leukemic mice with lethal radiotherapy and rescued them with spleen, lymph node and bone marrow cells of mice immune to mouse leukemia virus and/or cells.[11]

We speculated a great deal (1966-67) that the attenuated but immunizing mouse leukemia virus lost a gene on which leukemogenesis depended and showed that the attenuated virus could re-acquisition this gene from highly diluted preparations of virulent virus through "multiplicity reactivation".[12] These speculations however did not carry us far enough; we fell short of referring to these genes as "oncogenes" and did not have the knowledge to clone them and compare their base sequence with that of genes taken from mammalian cells. The epoch-making suggestion of Drs. Bishop and Varmus that oncogenes of retroviruses derived from protooncogenes of mammalian cells did not answer the question we were interested in: where did the genuine viral genes env, pol, and gag derive from? Were these also escaped cellular genes? All viruses derived from cellular genes (the "endogenous" derivation theory) or could self-replicating viruses have existed before cells on Earth (similar to the "large viruses" or psittacosis agents)? Have intracellular parasitism reduced them to what they are today through "retrograde evolution" (the "exogenous" derivation theory)? If I re-wrote those chapters dealing with these problems in my *Die Grundlagen der Virusforschung* of 1956 today, I still could not answer these basic questions. If I started again anew, I would search for archaic retroviral genes in Drosophila. There the copia-sequences behave like transposable elements ready to break loose transcribed into polyadenylated RNA strands equipped with coding sequences for reverse transcriptase: a good case for endogenous origin of a retrovirus (as DJ Finnegan proposed it in 1983). The incomplete intracisternal type A retroviruses of mammals are also candidates for endogenous origin. Still someone may immediately argue that the copia-sequences had derived from ancient exogenous retroviruses incorporated by the insect cells eons earlier.

The mouse leukemia work culminated in an observation without precedent that we repeatedly reported in the late 1960s. This unprecedented phenomenon consisted of the fusion of a mouse leukemia virus-producer and thus immortalized diploid lymphoma cell with a plasma cell making mouse leukemia virus-neutralizing antibodies.[13-20] We maintained the tetraploid fusion products in suspension cultures or as tetraploid ascitic leukemia cells for a decade. During this time it continued the production of specific mouse leukemia virus-neutralizing antibodies. We missed the opportunity to call these cells "hybridomas" and the immune globulins "monoclonal antibodies."

Dr. Jerome Vaeth of San Francisco gave me the opportunity to present and overview once more our 20-year-old mouse leukemia virus work for the audience of the 24th San Francisco Cancer Symposium.[21]

II. ANSWERS ARE COMING IN
E. Discovery of the "Hybridoma Principle" in 1968-69

It was in 1967-68 when we recognized that fusion must have occurred between diploid murine lymphoma cells and splenic plasma cells. The lymphoma cells replicated budding mouse leukemia virus particles. The spleen cells produced specific neutralizing antibodies to the mouse leukemia virus. In 1968 we envisioned the fusion as consequential to a specific immune reaction between the budding virus still embedded in the cell membrane and the antibodies retained before their release on the surface of the immune spleen cells (Fig. 1).

We considered the phenomenon an exceptional one occurring under special conditions only. We theorized that it occurs in nature during the course of lymphoreticular malignancies and it serves the neoplastic cell to escape further immune recognition as self-immunoglobulins now cover alien (the viral) antigens. We named Burkitt's lymphoma cells, Hodgkin's Reed-Sternberg cells and the large Sezary cells as possible examples. The fused tetraploid cells were certainly more pathogenic than the original diploid cells.

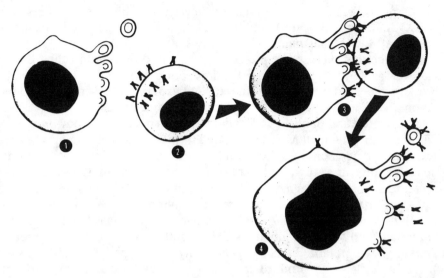

Fig. 1. The hybridoma principle as envisioned in 1968: 1) diploid, leukemia virus-producer lymphoma cell; 2) leukemia virus-neutralizing antibody-producer plasma cell; 3) juxtaposition of 1 and 2 due to antigen-antibody reaction; 4) fusion of 1 and 2 resulting in tetraploid cell retaining malignancy (immortality) and specific antibody production. This slide was shown and explained as above at five international conferences in 1968-70. No questions or comments were made by large audiences. The publisher of *Leukemia-Lymphoma* (1970), Year Book Medical Publishers, reprinted it on the outside front cover of the book; it also appeared in our text on page 60.[16]

The diploid cells grew as solid tumors; the fused tetraploid cells grew as ascites tumors. Large cell numbers of the antigenic diploid cells were needed for inocula to take, whereas the fused tetraploid cells grew out from a few inoculated cells and were rapidly fatal. The fused tetraploid cells grew in suspension cultures for years and continued producing specific mouse leukemia virus-neutralizing antibodies. In one single experiment these antibodies did not inhibit (rather slightly enhanced) the growth of both the diploid and tetraploid lymphoma cells. We could not clearly see practical (therapeutic) use for the phenomenon: the fused cells were producers of leukemia virus (deformed particles coated by antibodies) and the antibodies did not inhibit the growth of these cells.[13-21]

In the late 1960s, Dr. Eiichi Shirato (now in Japan) produced rabbit antibodies against these cells. Dr. Jose Trujillo (currently head of the Department of Laboratory Medicine at M.D. Anderson) maintained these cells in culture for years and showed that the same cell produced both virus and antibody, and that the original lymphoma cells were of diploid, and the fused cells were of tetraploid chromosomal mode. Dr. Roman Pienta (now at the Dynamac Corporation in Rockville, Maryland) purified the antibody produced by the fused cells and participated in our virus-neutralizing experiments. Dr. Benjamin Drewinko (deceased) showed that when we co-cultivated antibody-producer plasma cells and diploid lymphoma cells, a race of new cells emerged with diameters and volumes at least twice of either one of the parent cells. Dr. Michael Ahearn (now at the office of Vice President of M.D. Anderson Hospital) and Dr. Donald Pinkel (now Distinguished Professor at the Department of Pediatrics at M.D. Anderson Hospital) produced electron microscopic pictures of the fused tetraploid cells. Dr. H. David Kay (now at the Veterans Administration Medical Center, Omaha, Nebraska) repeated successfully the fusion experiments with the diploid lymphoma cells and specific antibody-producing spleen cells.[19]

We presented and published[15,19,20] data on our specific antibody-producing fused cells in the biannual M.D. Anderson Hospital Research Reports 1970-4; at two M.D. Anderson Hospital symposia in 1969; at three international conferences, one in Perugia and one in Ciudad Mexico in 1969 and at the International Cancer Congress in Houston. In the *Lancet* in 1969 we wrote "we propose that tetraploid immunoresistant lymphoma cells in the mouse emerge by fusion of the diploid, virus-producing lymphoma cell with a plasma cell producing virus-specific globulins. The resulting tetraploid cell will retain malignant growth potential and the genetically determined committedness of both parent cells — to produce leukemia virus as coded for by the viral genome within the neoplastic cell and to synthesize virus-specific globulins, as coded for by the genome of the plasma cell".[17] Our presentation in 1969 at the 2nd M.D. Anderson Hospital Symposium appeared in the volume, *Leukemia-Lymphoma* by the Year Book Medical Publishers of Chicago in 1970.[16] The publisher chose our figure for the outside cover of the volume.

Deep silence characterized the response from the scientific community. In the *Lancet* no correspondence followed. At the international meetings nobody rose to say, "This phenomenon will revolutionize immunity: clone your fused cells and you can now make monoclonal antibodies." Dr. Trujillo and I appreciated that within the fused cells "immortalized" antibody production became operational. We were first amazed, then devastated by the indifference with which this discovery was received and by the fact that our grants were not funded by the new NCI after the enactment of the "Conquest of Cancer" National Cancer Act. When the first conference was assembled on lymphocyte hybridomas in 1979, we were not invited to present our material and have it criticized or accepted, and our work was not even mentioned in the volume of that conference (*Lymphocyte Hybridomas*, F. Melchers, M. Potter and N. Warner, eds., Springer-Verlag, 1979).

When I presented this material in 1969 in Perugia[15] no questions concerning this material were addressed to me. A bus took us back to the hotel. I sat in the first row next to the window behind the driver. Sir Macfarlane Burnet climbed in the bus and took the seat next to me. He recalled that in 1956 or 1957 he received a copy of my virus book. He then clearly showed that he fully grasped the meaning of my presentation and said, "In those fusion experiments, if accurate cloning is performed, the clonal selection theory could receive most powerful support." I was very pleased because from the 1950s on, Dr. Burnet was my greatest hero in virology and immunology.

It took no time for us to recognize the importance of fused cells formed naturally during the course of neoplastic cell proliferations. Dr. Peter Clifford (whom I had the good fortune to personally visit in 1966 in Africa and who visited me later in Houston) published together with the Kleins (in the *Lancet* in 1968) that primary Burkitt lymphomas consisted of diploid neoplastic cells; when after remission the disease relapsed in immunoreactive patients, the neoplastic cell proliferation consisted of tetraploid cells. What if the diploid BL cell fused with a reactive B cell making antibody against EBV structural proteins expressed in the BL cell? — I speculated. Thereafter the large fused cell would conceal its neoantigens by a self-antibody coat, thus escaping immune rejection (except for macrophages which recognize antigen-antibody complexes and phagocytize these cells: hence, the "starry sky" histologic pattern of this lymphoma). In our paper[17] we drew an analogy between our #620 and #818 murine lymphoma and African BL based on these considerations. In the early 1970s, Reed-Sternberg (RS) cells of Hodgkin's disease (HD) emerged as an even more attractive subject matter for these speculations. Hematology fellow in training, Dr. Francisco Gonzalez (now professor of medicine and hematology at the University of South Carolina, Columbia, South Carolina) asked me for a research project. Promptly I designed some experiments that he diligently carried out with research technicians Keith Mollohan and Sandra Tzobari-Schneider. In these experiments, an envelope-gene defective spleen focus-forming murine leukemia virus appeared to accept a helper virus from HD tissue extracts and cells that were not pathogenic by themselves in mice but were able to significantly alter (frequently increase; rarely decrease) the focus-forming activity of the murine virus. On top of it, some sera of patients with HD neutralized this effect while these sera never could neutralize focus formation by the murine viruses injected alone. This was good indirect evidence for the existence of a retrovirus in HD tissues. I hand-carried mouse spleens and patients' sera to Dr. Ferenc Györkey at the Veterans Medical Center for immune electron microscopy studies aimed to show attachment of human antibodies to virions budding in the spleen cells of mice coinoculated with the spleen focus-forming murine virus and HD cells, but no attachment of these antibodies to virions budding in spleen cells of mice inoculated with the spleen focus-forming murine virus alone. On one occasion our vision appears to have been confirmed by Ferenc but the work was not continued thereafter. We then obtained a most precious gift from Mr. Leo Lippman in memory of Mrs. Bertha Lippman in the form of an electron microscope. Just as we were to set up our immune electron microscopy studies (we were not trained in this technology but were determined to learn it), the vice president of our institution declared that, in his opinion, we did not need an electron microscope and ordered me to dismount this magnificent equipment that was already installed for our use, and to transfer it to the Department of Anatomical Pathology, now being reorganized under its new chairman who later rose to be the director of research for the entire institution. It was consolation to me that an expert electron microscopist, Dr. Bruce Mackay, was put in charge of "our" electron microscope thereafter. We never completed the immune electron microscopy studies. After presenting two abstracts of his work,[23,24] Dr. Gonzalez completed his training and left the institute.

Thereafter Dr. H. Thota and I reproduced some of the neutralization studies and observed soluble substances in HD tissue extracts interfering with lymphocyte blastogenesis.[25]   Lack of funds for salary and supplies at our research section forced Dr. Thota to switch to Dr. B. Drewinko's section at the Department of Laboratory Medicine and Clinical Pathology where he worked until his death on projects unrelated to our studies on RS cells as natural hybridomas, but managed to "sneak" back to our lab now and then for an extra hour or two of work on his favored projects.

Not in the laboratory but in my mind, this project remains active up to this day.   Repeatedly, I proposed that RS cells are natural hybridomas of the mononuclear HD cells fusing with B and/or T cells reactive to retroviral antigens the HD cell expresses.   Most recently I was invited to give grand rounds on this subject at M.D. Anderson Hospital.   In addition, I plan to review our early work on the notion that natural hybridomas are formed in the course of neoplastic cell proliferations.   My conclusions will be that the neoplastic cell can subvert the defensive cell by fusing with it and thus gaining a degree of immunoresistance.[****]

In 1980, I attended the 18th annual meeting of the Infectious Diseases Society of America in New Orleans.   I felt utterly abandoned as my research career ended; I was unrecognized and lonely in a large crowd.   In the huge and packed conference room Dr. Scharff reviewed monoclonal antibodies. Somewhere at the end of his lecture I suddenly heard him mention my name. He said something like this, "But really this hybridoma phenomenon was discovered and described first by a man, Sinkovics, some six years before Kohler and Milstein.   Sinkovics showed that..."   And he went ahead to describe our work in a few sentences.   I had not received much credit for my work before and hardly could believe my ears.   Thereafter there were questions and answers.   I was sitting in one of the last rows.   I raised my hand but the chairman overlooked me and did not call on me.   Finally, he said, "One more, the last question, way back there."   I rose and said, "I am that man Sinkovics."   I walked to the next microphone, said a few sentences about our obscure work quite unknown to this audience.   I drew a lengthy applause, the meeting adjourned and people came to me from all directions for a hand shake and tap on my back: old friends whom I had not seen for years (Dr. Joseph Ury, Dr. Stuart Levin and many others) were there to say hello. When Dr. Scharff's presentation appeared in print in 1981, the anecdote about our work was left out.   But in another previous publication written for biochemists in 1981, Drs. Yelton and Scharff did list our data as the first example of hybridoma work.   In a hybridoma conference (National Symposium on Hybridomas and Cellular Immortality) in Houston in 1981, Dr. Baldwin Tom gave us credit "as a footnote" for observing and working with fused cells that were clearly hybridomas by modern terminology.

In 1980, I asked the editors of *Cancer Research* to publish a brief account of our work with the fused cells producing specific antibodies for so many years when grown as ascites tumors or in suspension cultures.   For their perusal I submitted material: contemporary laboratory documents and annual

---

[****]Long after the completion of this manuscript, this work appeared in print (*Critical Reviews Immunology* 11:33-63, 1991).

research reports, abstracts, manuscripts, photographs from the 1960s and actual publications. *Cancer Research* sent me copies of the reviewers' comments according to which I presented convincing evidence that I produced and worked with the first "hybridoma" in the late 1960s. Our report was published.[22] Dr. Cesar Milstein wrote me politely that he was unaware of our work when he and Dr. Georg Kohler reported their hybridoma work in 1975. A few years later the front page of *Cancer Research* celebrated Kohler and Milstein for the 1975 discovery of hybridomas and monoclonal antibodies and the awarding of the Nobel Prize. Our simple work was not mentioned, not even in a footnote.

By the late 1970s, my idealism and faith in the fairness of the great grant-providing institutions and the scientific establishment, in general, was somewhat shaken. I put the antibody-producer fused tetraploid cells in 10% glycerol and tissue culture medium and froze them in liquid nitrogen for storage forever at a temperature of the outer space. These momentous events took place in laboratories 347-8.

F. Adolescence of Cancer Research (in Basic and Applied Immunology): In the Front Lines Without Even Knowing It

By the early 1970s my motivations to translate research results from mouse to man had become quite strong. We started out with tissue cultures of human bone marrow, lymph nodes and solid tumors (mainly sarcoma and melanoma) in the late 1960s. Now we had accelerated the pace of this simple work.[26-30] Immediately, we were captivated by the interrelationship of lymphocytes and malignant cells. We observed how lymphocytes explored the surface membrane of other cells, even appeared to pass through them without harming them. Some lymphocytes existed and multiplied within fibroblast-like cells and received cytoplasmic granules from them. Other lymphocytes killed their target cells. Many ways of killing a target cell were observed and photographed in my lab in the early 1970s. Most lymphocytes killed by lysing the cytoplasm of the target cell. Smaller lymphocytes with dark nuclei killed autologous tumor cells; larger lymphocytes with pale nuclei and granular cytoplasm killed allogeneic tumor cells. Small lymphocytes killed target cells without lysing the cytoplasm: the nuclear chromatin of target cells broke down very rapidly. The ficoll-hypaque technique existed for lymphocyte purification but no monoclonal antibodies for lymphocyte typing were available. We were working with overlapping and not yet discovered and defined subclasses of lymphocytes producing results difficult to reproduce even in our own laboratory. Nevertheless, in our hands, two major findings emerged: 1) patients with tumors possessed lymphocytes cytotoxic to tumor

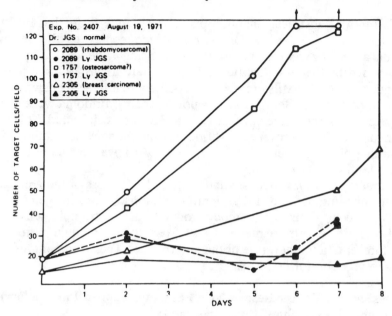

Fig. 2. My buffy coat lymphocytes as tested on August 19, 1971, strongly inhibit the growth of allogeneic sarcoma and breast carcinoma cell lines. When observed in 1971, we referred to the phenomenon as "immune surveillance at work"[38] and wondered if a medical oncologist could develop "immunity" to some cancers to which he is repeatedly exposed in his professional life. This observation sharply contradicted the doctrine emanating from Seattle according to which patients with cancer circulated lymphocytes cytotoxic only to their tumor cells and healthy donors served as their negative controls. It was at the NCI where the lymphocyte population responsible for this type of cytotoxicity was later called that of "natural killer cells" (Herberman, R.B., Djeu, J. Y., Kay, H. D., et al., *Immunol. Rev.* 44:43, 1979).

cells identical with and entirely different from the patient's histologic tumor type; and 2) healthy donors (among them myself in 1971) circulated lymphocytes readily cytotoxic to a battery of tumor cells.[28-35] (Fig. 2). Both findings contradicted the ruling tenet of times, what we had been referring to as the "Hellström doctrine." According to this doctrine, patients circulated lymphocytes cytotoxic to their histologic type of tumor and not to other histologic types of tumors and healthy donors could be used as "negative controls" for not possessing such cytotoxic lymphocytes.

These findings turned out to be quite disastrous to our welfare. We were working on one of the best NCI contracts I have ever received: some $225,000 per annum. Prior to the National Cancer Act, an investigator named his/her topic, outlined the research plan, was checked out by project site visitors and support was forthcoming without delay as grant funds (however seldom exceeding $75,000 per year). After passage of the National Cancer Act, the NCI in its immense wisdom determined research priorities ("targeted research"), hired intra- and extramural principal investigators and instead of grants, gave out large contracts to these principal investigators who then hired the best personnel (PhDs, technicians, etc.) to carry out the work. Fabulous "overhead expense accounts" made these contracts very attractive to university-affiliated hospitals and research institutions which immediately started hiring principal investigators able to attract NCI contracts. New wings were built in rapid succession to house these projects and an unprecedented rapid development of cancer research became clearly visible. Failure of the new system could have meant discontinuation or reduction of cancer research funds that were to be re-approved annually by Congress. Successes and "breakthroughs" (cure of acute leukemia; isolation of human leukemia virus ESP-1 for vaccine production, etc.) were reported daily in the media; publicity-seeking and self-praise replaced modesty and caution. Those investigators, who previously were recipients of small individual grant funds, were suddenly left out of the new arrangement. They either surrendered to a new and more influential principal investigator (often abandoning their own projects) or perished from the field. Many of the new principal investigators also served as project site visitors; it appeared as if they project site-visited and supported each other. It also appeared (at least from my angle) that one had to be part of this insider network playing the game of publicity-seeking and promising results before the actual work was done in order to secure continuous high level support. Apparently the Congress went along with the new line of doing research because NCI funds soon doubled to exceed one billion dollars per year.

In this atmosphere I certainly was not ready to perish but I did not want to pay the price of giving up my principles of scientific conduct. I could not promise results in advance and shied away from press conferences announcing what we planned to discover. As my mouse leukemia grant applications in this new era were considered to be of "low priority" and thus received no support ("approved without funding": the profoundly despised terminology of the new NCI that I was to hear more and more often), I submitted to the NCI in "a letter of intention" the description of a technique by which autologous and allogeneic lymphocytes cytotoxic to tumor cells could be quantitatively measured (our Lab-Tek chamber-slide assay).[33,35] In no time I received forms for the submission of a contract application. Drs. Paul Levine and Gary Pearson specified that the target of the contract is a lymphocyte-mediated, tumor-specific cytotoxicity assay. Quickly we received funds. I thought I received a very generous contract, but soon I learned from my administrative superiors that in comparison to other NCI contracts (those received by the new Department of Virology for the ESP-1 virus which soon turned out to be not the "first human leukemia-lymphoma virus" as it was claimed but the result of sloppy work: a contaminant mouse leukemia virus; or the new Department of Developmental Therapeutics) my contract still was rather limited.

I had reasons to believe that my relationship with my administrative superiors was not good. I was given an NCI research career award with a very modest salary. Embarrassed, Dr. Howe explained that the hospital needed outside funds for salaries and I readily qualified for a research career award while other members did not: would I please accept just for a few years? I accepted.

I made some other mistakes in institutional politics. For example, once soon after establishment of the National Cancer Act, I was summoned to the director's office. He requested that I immediately apply for a large NCI contract for research on mycoplasma as an etiologic agent in leukemia. He received confidential information that the NCI (again in its immense wisdom) had put a huge sum of money aside for the project after a Dr. Negroni in England isolated mycoplasma from the bone marrow of leukemic patients. I was astonished: "Why me?" He replied that the bibliography of the staff was searched and I was the only one who had worked with mycoplasmas and pleuropneumonia-like organisms (PPLO). It was true. In the 1950s, I worked with and published in German on these delightfully capricious micro-organisms.[36] One of my papers appeared in *Nature.*[37] Most unfortunately for my future career, the offer elicited the wrong reaction in me. I pleaded to be released of this task and requested his support for my own ideas (among them a grant application in which I would isolate common viruses such as influenza, adeno-, herpes- and others from naturally infected cancer patients to see if these viruses picked up and propagated a "cancer gene." I still have a copy of this grant application which later was "approved without funding"). The director insisted on the mycoplasmas. After three days of thinking time (he frowned when I requested this) during which time I expressed my opposition to the mycoplasma project to my friends, among them Drs. Howe, Fletcher, Shullenberger and Tessmer, who however unanimously advised me not to resist but accept, I accepted, submitted the application and promptly received a contract for $195,000 per year. Dr. Fletcher started to call me (and still does) "PPLO Joe."

Together with a very able technologist, recruited from New Orleans, we quickly equipped a new laboratory with brand new equipment and I provided her daily with fresh specimens of coded bone marrow aspirates that were meticulously and expertly set into cultures. By the year's end, I concluded in my report that the mycoplasma isolates from human malignancies did not fulfill Koch's postulates to be regarded as of any etiologic significance in leukemia: 8-12% of all people with malignancies and fevers (sometimes without fevers) yielded them and their isolation was not limited to leukemics. The mistake was that I proposed discontinuation of the project. What I did not realize was that as yet unspent millions were earmarked up there somewhere at the new NCI for the mycoplasma project. Under the electron microscope some mycoplasmas or PPLO contained phage-like particles; now this was new and interesting and this I would have spent some money on (how these phages get in there without cell membranes and receptors?), but to continue on the false route in search of a leukemogenic mycoplasma or PPLO, I considered futile. After omitting in my report that "further studies were needed," the project was taken from me. It was transferred to the Department of Virology (unfortunately, as the technologist had to go with the project), where it was pursued for some three more years, reaching the same conclusion that I had presented after the first year, but after its substantial budget was used up in its entirety.

Now my "grantsmanship" was restored to some extent as I was again principal investigator of another contract on cytotoxic lymphocytes. The trouble was that the lymphocytes did not obey the contracting agency. They expressed cytotoxicity towards targets they were not supposed to affect and I faithfully (and fatefully) reported this to the contracting agency. If tumor-specific reactions emerged[27] they were rare and difficult to document repeatedly at will. Some target tumor cells susceptible to lymphocyte-mediated cytotoxicity could gain resistance (Figure 3). No amount of discussions on the merits of an altered "target," i.e., change from tumor-specific to nonspecific lymphocytes, worked. The contract was "phased out." As gently as he could, Paul Levine broke the news to me over a drink we had at the Shamrock Hotel (by now demolished); the glass fell from my hand and its contents spilled over us.

The momentum carried us in the lab for another few years. We tried to correlate lymphocyte-mediated cytotoxicity with clinical course of our patients with sarcomas yielding the lymphocytes and concluded that most (but not all) patients possessing lymphocytes strongly cytotoxic to sarcoma cells lived longer tumor-free, especially if they also circulated serum factors (antibodies) potentiating this effect. Admittedly, our technology appears now primitive after precise lymphocyte subtyping technology developed. Yet it hurt me deeply that our work received no citation at all when many years later with more advanced techniques and sophistication Drs. F. Vanky and Eva Klein at the Karolinska Institute in Stockholm reached practically the same conclusion (they used immune T lymphocytes against autologous sarcomas) (Tables 1 and 2).

I lost two of my finest research associates: Dr. H. David Kay[38-41] went to work on "natural killer cells" with Dr. R. Herberman when we lost funding for his salary. It was a great pleasure for me to see David's name among the co-authors of Hilary Koprowski in a recent paper in PNAS describing the idiotypic cascade in a patient with colon cancer. The patient was treated with Wistar Institute's monoclonal antibody Co-17-1A (Ab1) and developed anti-idiotype antibodies against these antibodies (Ab2). Ab2 imitated the tumor antigen and induced the production of further antibodies (Ab3). Ab3 exerted antitumor cytotoxicity reactions similar to Ab1. One now wonders about antitumor antibodies produced by B lymphocytes-plasma cells in the regional lymph nodes of tumors or in patients receiving active tumor-specific immunization with viral oncolysates. These antibody-producing B lymphocytes-plasma cells can be rescued by fusion with a human lymphoma-myeloma cell and thus immortalized. Their antibody (Ab1) can be used for passive antitumor immunotherapy. The variable regions of these immunoglobulins induce the production of antibodies (Ab2) that imitate tumor antigens that originally induced Ab1. Ab2 further immunizes the host as if it were a tumor antigen leading to the production of antibodies (Ab3). Ab3 act as Ab1 and react with the original genuine tumor antigens.

Table 1.
Clinical Correlations with Cytotoxic Lymphocytes

Subjects Tested		Average % Reduction of Growth of Allogeneic	
		Sarcoma Cells	Carcinoma Cells
Long NED	Ly	44-52	24-29
Sarcoma Survivors	SeLy	80-82	37-45
Pts with Metastatic Sarcomas	Ly	27-35	18-20
	SeLy	20-40	15-29
Healthy Donors	Ly	32-37	28-33
	SeLy	44-48	27-32

NED = no evidence of disease
Ly = lymphocytes
Se = serum (heat inactivated)

References: *Sinkovics et al*. Front Rad Ther Oncol 7:141-154, 1972; in *Immunological Aspects of Neoplasia*, 1973, Williams & Wilkins, Baltimore, pp. 367-401, 1965; Bibl Haematol 43:281-284, 1976; in *Tumor Progression*, Elsevier N Holland, pp. 316-318, 1980.

Table 2
Clinical Correlations with Cytotoxic Lymphocytes

Autologous Sarcoma Cells Blastogenesis to		(%)	Lysis of	(%)	NED Survival/Death (mean, mo) Blastogenesis		Lysis	
Osteo	13 r	(65)	8 r	(44)	6 s	(71)	3 s	(>36)
	7 nr/20	(35)	10 nr/18	(56)	6 d	(<18)	9 d	(<30)
Soft Tissue	6 r	(46)	7 r	(37)	6 s	(48)	7 s	(40)
	7 nr/13	(54)	12 nr/13	(63)	7 d	(<30)	12 d	(<24)

r = reactive; nr = nonreactive; s = survivor; d= dead
Vánky et al.; *Cancer Immunol. Immun. Ther.* 16:11-16, 1983; 21:69-76, 1986

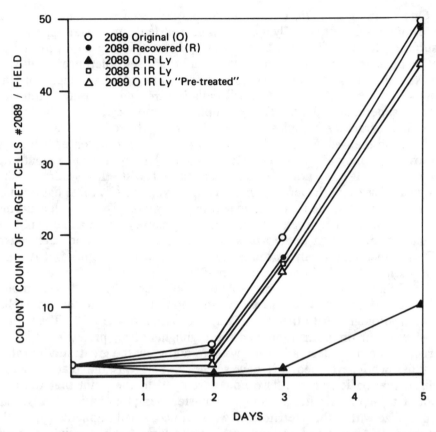

Fig. 3. Graph first presented in 1970 in San Francisco showing that a rhabdomyosarcoma cell line resistant to cytotoxic lymphocytes releases soluble substances that render cytotoxicity-susceptible rhabdomyosarcoma cells cytotoxicity-resistant ("pretreated"). Lymphocyte donor patient IR came to me in 1968 with rhabdomyosarcoma stage IV (with bone marrow involvement). He entered complete remission on chemotherapy and possessed lymphocytes strongly cytotoxic to sarcoma cells and serum factors (antibodies) potentiating this effect. He is alive, free of disease over 20 years in Abbeville, Louisiana.[50,52,77]

Going back to my associates, Dr. Harikishan Thota,[42,43] a genius in sorting out comparable subgroups from a large conglomerate of data and applying statistics to compare these subgroups, also lost his funding and soon committed suicide. Clinical fellows assigned to my service also had to leave the lab (due to lack of research funds) but they at least could complete their training in clinical oncology; one of them became a most prominent practitioner of oncology in Houston, Texas.

From laboratory research I had to return to speculations. In the *Lancet* and in the *British Journal of Medicine* I proposed that suppressor cells and blocking-enhancing antibodies evolved with placentation to accommodate the allograft fetus (expressing paternal antigens but escaping rejection).[44,45] When science writer Patrick McGrady asked me how I arrived at this thought, I explained that I was restricted to thinking because I had no research grants to work on. "I would periodically keep all scientists on water and bread," he replied. He once also said, "If you must have cancer, have it *in vitro*." Unfortunately he died of cancer later.

One morning in 1970, Dr. C. Shullenberger and I were making rounds. We examined a man with "lymphosarcoma cell leukemia" who appeared as if suffering from graft-versus host disease. I was thinking aloud presuming that neoplastic lymphocytes lost the faculty of "self-tolerance" and were attacking their host. Within days we found that the patient's "lymphosarcoma cells" killed a battery of tumor target cells *in vitro* and released "cytotoxins" in their supernatant fluid. Those neoplastic lymphocytes were large with azurophilic granular cytoplasm. Our letter to the editor was promptly published in the *New England Journal of Medicine* and I presented a "case of cytotoxic lymphoma" in Milan, Italy at an international hematology congress.[46,47] I have not seen another patient with this syndrome, but malignant disease of the large granular lymphocytes (or NK cells) has become well documented in the literature in subsequent years. The idea that normal molecular mediators are released in excess and cause disease appears not too far fetched now, when endotoxin shock, cerebral malaria and cachexia of AIDS are mediated partly by tumor necrosis factor (cachectin); but it was a good original thought from our part in 1970.

Dr. John B. Moloney (who isolated and characterized a new mouse leukemia and sarcoma virus at NCI) continued to invite me to the assemblies of tumor virologists with the Virus Cancer Program of the NCI. These once or twice a year programs remained the highlights of my professional life: I learned modern (molecular) virology there and grew the greatest admiration for those who developed this new science. This was the place where I realized that basic sciences have now developed to the point that full-time devotion to them was still not enough to master them; that basic scientists had to specialize within their territory to well-defined, small segments (the DNA virus and RNA virus people; and within these large fields, specialists in just one or two viruses emerged). Very likely the oncogene work of the 1980s developed as a spin-off from the Virus Cancer Program of the NCI (but I have not heard the promoters of the oncogene work speak at meetings of the Virus Cancer Program). I am grateful to John Moloney for having allowed me to be there and observe even after I lost my NCI research support.

By now I was full professor and extricated myself from the need for a research career award as a source of income. However, it was not really my own doing that my cancer research career award was not renewed after some five years. Hungarian-born Dr. Jacob Furth came for a project site visit. We had a great day together. My admiration for him was very well founded. He worked with malignant tumors that remained under the hormonal influence of their host until they succeeded through sequential steps in gaining complete autonomy and full growth potential independent from hormonal influences of the host. Late afternoon I drove Dr. Furth to the airport. He appeared elderly and frail but very pleased and animated. I felt certain that my lab and clinics, operating side-by-side and supplementing each other in a most ideal fashion for clinically oriented research, impressed him quite favorably. In my mind I was looking forward to the renewal of my award with mixed feelings: increasing scientific reputation to me, great satisfaction to my administrative superiors that a staff salary once again has been secured from outside funds, versus continuation of my low salaried status in comparison with my peers. Again, in my mind, I accepted. Close to the airport at a red light stop Dr. Furth suddenly turned toward me, looked into my eye and said, "I shall not support the continuation of your award." He then in friendly and somewhat paternal terms (adding a Hungarian word to it here and there) explained that this was in my best interest. My work has now become so demanding, so complex and so sophisticated both at the bedside and in the lab that I shall not be able to pay meticulous attention to details and practice the highest clinical and laboratory skills at the same time. He advised me to choose between either one of the two (leaning toward research) but not try to pursue both. Taken by surprise I stuttered a few misconstructed sentences about my work habits, that I can go on 16-hour days for weeks or months without a break, that I can read a complex article once and recite it, methodology included, that I have unquenchable drive to find out new things about cancer, that the two fields interdigitate and are really one and indivisible, that I can give new ideas to work on to ten people in the lab, and that all I need are some grant funds to hire assistance and so on. He gave me a handshake and repeated his advice: seek the highest possible knowledge in just one field, and departed. I did not write him. Early in the day I was already entertaining the thought of correspondence with him and returning his visit: what a most precious acquaintance and friendship will develop, I mused. I never saw him again. My career award was not renewed. I continued to pursue both clinical medicine and research as long as I could and my salary now came from my state hospital. Today I feel Dr. Furth's advice was motivated by goodwill. Recently, George and Eva Klein reviewed Furth's work in *Cancer Research* giving him full credit for the fundamental concepts in the evolution of tumor autonomy that he (and Dr. L. Foulds) developed in 1950s.

In the meantime my clinical service referred to as "Solid Tumor Clinics and Service" continued to enlarge. Most of our patients had sarcomas or melanomas. Fellows and residents in training passed through this service for six to 12 months: many fine oncologists whom I had the privilege to assist and educate and learn from are now in practice or are working in academic medicine. I also served as consultant for infectious diseases for the departments of gynecologic oncology, medicine and surgery. In this area endotoxin shock was my main challenge and remains that up to this date.[48]

Our Department of Medicine was undergoing some unfair downgrading in comparison to the lavish funding and support a newly established Department for Development Therapeutics enjoyed. I was privileged to make friends with two members of that new department: Dr. Jules E. Harris would visit with me in my lab just for "discussions." One day he invited me to co-author the book he planned to write, *The Immunology of Malignant Disease* (first and second editions, 1972 and 1976). I know we will remain friends as long as I live. Dr. Jeffrey Gottlieb sought cooperation with me for clinical trials of adriamycin-based chemotherapy regimens on patients we attended at our service. He invited me to present some of our cases at their departmental meeting, where I expected some condescending remarks. Instead, he introduced me by saying, "I invited Joe because his patient care is the best and we can learn exemplary patient care from him." We worked together until his death.[49] I shall always remember him with gratitude for those remarks made in an unfriendly atmosphere that prevailed between our departments.

My relationship to chemotherapy did not develop easily. While I knew that chemotherapy was the only means to induce a remission, I was hesitant to expose my patients to its toxicity. Many years earlier I saw the World War II English movie, *The Cruel Sea*. One of the two warships was torpedoed, and as it was sinking the sailors abandoned ship and were vigorously paddling in floats toward the other ship to be rescued. Suddenly, Sam Hawkins, captain of the other ship, found the German submarine hiding under his ship. He was to throw deep charges as his fellow sailors were approaching, begging for rescue. He threw the deep charges. His fellow sailors perished with the submarine. What would I have done? Probably I would have rescued the sailors while the submarine maneuvered itself into a position to torpedo me also. For years I thought of this movie (its story might have been somewhat altered in my memory). Our patients were randomized into treatment groups; while one group perished (due to their malignancy), the other group did better. However, in those early protocols no switch from the doomed treatment arm to the effective treatment could be done: that was violation of the protocol, contrary to statistical requirement for proper evaluation. To gain a little in one group, those pioneer oncologists sacrificed the other group. Whenever I see the famous graph depicting clearly that continuous intravenous cytosine arabinoside is much more effective in inducing remissions in acute leukemia than bolus conventional dose cytosine arabinoside, I consider the utter abandonment of those patients who were randomized into the bolus group where they rapidly perished (due to their disease but nevertheless practically left untreated). Again, I probably would have violated the protocol and have transferred all patients into the group receiving continuous administration after the first hint that it was working better. It was not easy for me to reconcile my feelings with clinical research on randomized patients.

With this attitude, how could I have made any discoveries of significance in the chemotherapy of cancer in clinical oncology? Well, I did not. But my patients demanded treatment and I delivered, without randomization, the best individualized treatment that I could marshal, including chemotherapy in full dose. I was not cut out to experiment on randomized groups of patients. My Department of Medicine not only tolerated but appreciated this philosophy. Another department that was designed to develop newer and newer protocols and whose financial support in contract funds depended on this type of clinical research could not have accepted this attitude. As highly effective antibiotics and supportive care (blood products, anti-nausea medications, leucovorin, mannitol and other protective agents) became available, I have become very aggressive with chemotherapy and scored many fine durable complete remissions and some cures even in metastatic disease.[50]

Up to this date I have not settled in my mind where to place those physicians who became famous through designing combination chemotherapy protocols in an era when no blood products (platelets, granulocytes) and no truly broad spectrum bactericidal antibiotics were available. They must have experienced the triumph of inducing complete remission in acute childhood leukemia followed by the devastation in observing deaths due to myelosuppression, infections and hemorrhage. However, frequently those who designed the protocol did not actually work at clinics (fellows in training did); so they probably did not actually see patients with devastating toxicity. The medical profession honors them highly together with those who described new pathological entities caused by the treatment they designed (example: candidiasis of the endocardium in myelosuppressed patients and the like). I certainly give them credit for not retreating at that point and tenaciously remaining on the job as they feverishly developed the supportive measures that should have been available from the beginning.

Back to the early 1970s. Adriamycin appeared on the scene and it was effective for sarcomas but not for melanomas. Using Dr. Gottlieb's CYVADIC protocol, we induced durable remissions in our patients with sarcomas but the relapse rate was still unacceptably high. Influenced by some earlier mouse work of spectacular success (oncolytic viruses eradicating ascites tumors in mice), I envisioned and designed a chemoimmunotherapy protocol utilizing viral oncolysates for active tumor-specific immunotherapy. We had all the ingredients needed for a most accurate clinical trial: large numbers of patients with excellent supportive services (diagnostics, pathology, blood banking, etc.); an excellent laboratory fully equipped for tissue culture work, my experience, enthusiasm, and endurance to hard labor. I put this into a contract application addressed to Dr. William Terry of the NCI. The application was rejected without a project site visit (Figure 4). I was shaken and discouraged but did not lose faith in reason. I knew we had proposed a superb, original project reinforced with laboratory measurements of tumor specific and other immune responses before, during and after immunotherapy. We reapplied within a year. No project site visitors came but a letter came from Dr. Terry. Our application now was "approved without funding" due to low priority assigned to it by the NCI. To our amazement and consternation we found that NCI had spent a few million dollars on scarifying BCG into patients during those years. This "breakthrough" received publicity in the daily press. We had initiated then some frantic efforts to raise a "shoestring" budget for the work outside the aegis of the NCI. The Kelsey-Leary Fund, Dr. C.D. Howe Fund, the Lippman Fund and above all the Don and Sybill Harrington Fund and the Baker and Taylor Drilling Company Fund of Amarillo, Texas helped. I wish these donors could truly sense my deep gratitude. Dr. William Cassel visited from Atlanta. He had similar ideas. He later used viral oncolysates made from autologous melanoma cells with NDV and reduced postoperative relapse rate from untreated 67% to 17% in treated patients. He observed our techniques in growing established sarcoma, melanoma, kidney carcinoma cell lines, their infection with influenza A PR8 virus (grown in the allantoic cavity of leukosis virus-free embryonated eggs), lysing of the cells and separation of cell membranes with budding virus, inactivation of virus by UV-light and storage of the preparation in small aliquots deep frozen. Dr. Cassel could not raise NCI support either and did his work in Atlanta supported by small private donations. It never occurred to me that we competed for priority or fame: we continued to exchange ideas and remain friends up to this date. As reported in abstracts of lectures, chapters and papers, we succeeded in stabilizing metastatic disease, induced higher remission rates and documented *in vitro* some very favorable immunological changes (developing cytotoxic lymphocytes and serum factors intensifying this effect) in the immunized patient.[51-63]

CHEMOIMMUNOTHERAPY FOR SARCOMAS

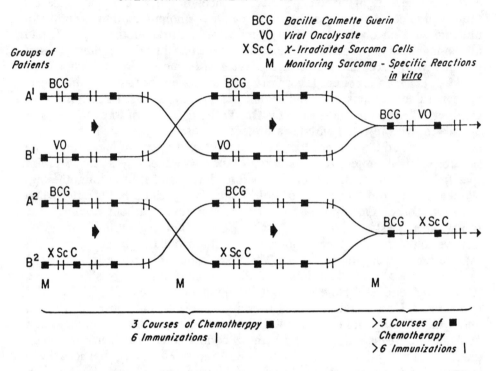

Fig. 4. The design of our chemoimmunotherapy protocol in the early 1970s (that was not funded by NCI) utilizing the CYVADIC regimen plus BCG scarifications and x-ray irradiated allogeneic sarcoma cells (produced from established cell lines) and *in vitro* monitoring for immune responses (cytotoxic lymphocytes and serum factors blocking or intensifying lymphocyte-mediated cytotoxicity). In a later (1973) modification of the protocol, instead of x-ray irradiated sarcoma cells, viral oncolysates were used (not funded by NCI).[52-64]

When the Wistar Institute produced viral oncolysates with vaccinia virus for the treatment of melanoma and colon carcinoma (and patented the procedure which did not occur to either Dr. Cassel or us), in their first report in *Cancer* in 1977, they referred to a "novel approach" and made no reference to our prior pioneering work. However, Dr. William Cassel and Dr. Ralph Freedman in the U.S. and Dr. Peter Hersey in Australia gave us credit for something original and worthy. Our work at M.D. Anderson under much improved conditions is being pursued further in the 1980s for the immunotherapy of gynecologic tumors by Drs. James Bowen, R. Freedman, C. Ioannides and Eva Lotzová. They use our basic techniques and monitor immunized patients for clinical response, skin test reactivity and *in vitro* detectable changes of their antitumor reactivity. They certainly added sophistication to the project.

In 1978, at the International Cancer Congress in Buenos Aires, I proposed a new protocol that has not as yet been implemented. The rationale was again based on some earlier mouse experiments. Viable embryonal cells were injected first, presuming that one of the physiologic functions of carcinoembryonic antigens is the activation of tumor-protective suppressor cells. Then cyclophosphamide (or methotrexate) was given to eradicate expanding (replicating) clones of these suppressor cells; then the tumor-bearing host, deprived of these suppressor cells, was either observed for unopposed antitumor immune response of its own or was to be actively immunized with viral oncolysates to induce unopposed antitumor immunity. Just now, in 1988, I read about clinical trials of active tumor-specific immunization against melanoma conducted in Philadelphia and in Los Angeles with potentiating effect added by the coadministration of cyclophosphamide aimed at the elimination of suppressor cells. I wonder if the efficacy of this intervention could be further intensified by applying also our first step (the stimulation of suppressor cells by fetal antigens to replicate and expand, thus increasing their vulnerability to alkylating agents or folic acid antagonists).[64]

In the second half of the 1970s, our large and well-equipped laboratory space was not well utilized anymore. The medical fellows, PhDs and most of the technicians left due to lack of support and funding. We launched extraordinary efforts to still raise ACS and NCI grant funds for the continuous growth and study of human normal and neoplastic lymphocytes and for the study of the resistance human tumor cells acquire against cytotoxic lymphocytes. Included in both projects were the study of cell-free supernatants for molecular mediators; study of a chondrosarcoma cell line undergoing differentiations toward fibroblast-like cells under the effect of a normal lymphocyte population; "immunovirological" characterization of 48 established human tumor cell lines as accounted for in *Methods of Cancer Research*;[65] and effects of human interferon on the growth curves of these cell lines *in vitro*. All efforts failed as our applications were again "approved without funding." Rereading these old grant applications today, they still appear quite viable. What a gold mine those cell lines would be today for the study of oncogenes and growth factors! I am at a loss to explain how the wealthy NCI could allow to drop us from its work force. Could two unusually malicious project site visitors have had such a powerful influence on the once noble institution?

Some nice speaking engagements in the late 1970s, on special invitation (at McGill in Montreal for a series of three lectures; by the College of Royal Surgeons to osteosarcoma conference in Ottawa, Canada for two lectures; at the University of Wisconsin in Milwaukee for a series of three lectures; at Rush-Presbyterian in Chicago where I received the Wadsworth Award; at the new Medical College of the Mexican Military Academy as inaugural speaker in Mexico City; at the University of Chicago for a dinner lecture on "immunoresistant tumors"); and an invitation from Dean Blunt to develop a comprehensive cancer center for the state of Mississippi in Jackson, were of little consolation since without funds I could not generate new data in the laboratory to present to these audiences. Fortunately, our material remained up-to-date until the early 1980s but I could not add anything new (except for some original thinking and interpretations).

In 1978, Dr. Joseph Bellanti, director of the International Center for Interdisciplinary Studies of Immunology at Georgetown University Medical School in Washington, D.C. gave me the Ignaz Philipp Semmelweis Award for advancing the knowledge of tumor immunology and immunotherapy. Hungarian born Dr. László Tauber who co-signed the certificate offered to equip research laboratories at his private hospital, Jefferson Memorial Hospital, if I worked there full-time. He would not hear of supporting my work at M.D. Anderson in Houston. Not being able to receive a written contract outlining my authority over the laboratory, I turned down this very fine but verbal offer.

In the late 1970s, Dr. Dmochowski suffered a near fatal coronary occlusion and retired soon thereafter. Dr. Howe developed squamous cell carcinoma of the lung and Dr. Shullenberger, not far from his retirement, became acting head of our department. While I have not fostered plans for high positions and feared the administrative duties of these big jobs, now suddenly I realized that if either one of the two positions, thus vacated, were offered to me, I would gratefully accept either one. First, I could have stayed in academic medicine. Second, fate would have decided for me. If I fill the virology position, I can pursue all those projects that I conceived, started but never could complete because of clinical duties and demands and lack of funds for assistance. I could convert the virology department from an old-fashioned morphology-oriented establishment into a biologically oriented multidisciplinary research faculty, I fantasized. Third, if I am to serve as head of the medical department, I shall prove that research and clinical medicine are not in an irreconcilable schism (not as Dr. Furth had suggested to me just a few years earlier) but can be well integrated: I shall see to it that each subspecialty service within the department will have its research laboratories serving immediate (and not so immediate) clinical needs, thus building a good infrastructure for clinical developments.

Soon the highest leadership had made its decision known. The department of virology was dismounted, its sections were absorbed up by other research departments, and several of its members were summarily dismissed. The chief of the nuclear medicine section was nominated head of the department of medicine with instructions from the executive vice president to have our department be absorbed up into the then most powerful department of developmental therapeutics. Shaken by disbelief, I asked vice presidential candidate, Dr. Fred Conrad, for his interpretation. Confidentially and in the friendliest of terms, this outstanding ex-military physician explained to me that without million dollar NCI contracts and grants, I never will have a chance for a promotion and that he would have supported the department of medicine at the expense of the department of developmental therapeutics if he had the power to act. He was killed in his office a few years later.

The department of medicine, however, was saved by the new president of the institution who in 1980 nominated Dr. Irv Krakoff to head the division of medicine. From them I receive an annually renewed nomination for consultant professorship at M.D. Anderson for which I am most grateful: I can go "home" for frequent visits to the hospital where I served so devotedly and idealistically in my best younger years. There I now see a powerful Division of Medicine; fast moving clinics; individualized care; flexible protocols allowing for escalation and de-escalation of drug dosages; innovative combinations of chemotherapeuticals with biologicals; may attend the finest conferences in basic sciences and clinical oncology; and I receive friendly greetings from the staff, my old and new friends.

III. EPILOGUE
G. Physically I am in Private Practice but my Mind is Still in Academic Medicine

To train myself for private practice, I summarized medical oncology-hematology for my own use. It happened so that Marcel Dekker Publishers approached me to write a volume of my choice. I gave them the manuscript under the title, *Medical Oncology, An Advanced Course*. It appeared in print in 1979 and quickly became quite popular among the younger generations of oncologists-hematologists.

In 1979 I went to Fort Lauderdale to work in private practice at the best clinics of that city as a *locum tenens* for Dr. R. Ferrayorni. He was a gentle physician of great practical knowledge and possessed the highest human values. He was ill with cancer. I resigned my position at M.D. Anderson but returned to Houston in 1980 for the private practice of oncology at the greatest private hospitals of that city in association with Drs. L.T. Campos and V. Collins. I enjoyed the hard work very much; it fully restored my self-esteem.

As I resigned from M.D. Anderson after some two decades of devoted and meritorious work there, I felt the great void of no more medical research but not too long. A helpful arm reached out to me right away: it was Dr. Joseph Melnick's arm. Dr. Melnick with a warm smile and with the finest compliments invited me to serve as visiting professor of virology at his Department of Virology and Epidemiology at Baylor University. Dr. Ferenc Györkey worked with Dr. Melnick for some time now and I knew Ferenc well from previous cooperation with him in the co-discovery of lupus erythematosus' tubuloreticular structures.[66-72] What a very nice editorial Dr. Dorothea Zucker-Franklin wrote in 1983 in the *New England Journal of Medicine* about our discovery of these structures!

A strange new disease was appearing in a few middle-aged veterans at Houston's VA Hospital and Dr. Györkey found cytomegalovirus (CMV), herpesvirus, papovavirus and retrovirus particles in the electron microscope (EM) in their tissue sections and tubuloreticular structures in their lesions that resembled Kaposi's sarcoma. An enormous challenge was rising. After rounds (sometimes in six Houston hospitals and clinics), I was back in the lab returning evening pagings from nurses from there, while I was poring over EM sections and tissue cultures. I told Ferenc (whose main interest lay in CMV), "forget about the other viruses and concentrate on the retrovirus-like particles."

Not unexpectedly, another friend emerged. As Dr. R. Lee Clark, M.D. Anderson's president, was preparing to retire, Dr. Fred Conrad was recruited for a high position. Fred called me into his office many times. He was appalled by the injustice and predicament befalling me and promised to "restore me in glory" as he strengthened his position in about two years' time. In less than two years thereafter, a hired (?) assassin killed him from behind, in his office, with several pistol shots.

At about the same time when I left Houston for Tampa, at the 1983 Los Angeles meeting of the American Association for Cancer Research (which I did not attend that year), my death was announced to some 3,500 members who then stood silently for a minute (except for Charlotte Friend who cried). It felt unusually good to be alive, when I heard the news of my premature death.

In 1983, I moved to Tampa to become medical director at St. Joseph's Hospital's Community Cancer Center (CCC). In 1983-84 my clinical service was small. Quickly I revised *Medical Oncology, An Advanced Course*. It appeared again by Marcel Dekker in 1986, spanning now 2,200 pages and incorporating 25,000 references. I have them stockpiled in large boxes; point out in the text which one you want, I will pull it for you!

My goals here are to render the highest quality of clinical service beyond the call of duty to those in need. Cooperation with the University of South Florida (USF) College of Medicine is my privilege: I have professorial appointments in the Departments of Medicine and Medical Microbiology, serve as a consultant at teaching hospital Bay Pines VA Medical Center and contribute to symposia and conferences organized by the USF faculty. Here I learn from and exchange ideas with scholars of the highest order (Drs. H. Azar, R. Good, H. Friedman, J. Szakacs, A. Szentivanyi and many others).

At the CCC we are developing laboratories for patient-oriented clinical services beyond standard care: 1. high dose chemotherapy with autologous stem cell reinfusion; 2. expansion of tumor infiltrating lymphocytes with interleukin-2 for reinfusion into patients with melanoma and kidney carcinoma; 3. probably development of monoclonal antibodies; and 4. active tumor specific immunotherapy (for melanoma first). I hope that work here will develop into another story to be presented ten years from now.

My old friends remember me and invite me. I was presenting my ideas on the combination of interferon and chemotherapy for the treatment of melanomas and sarcomas in Fort Lauderdale in 1980 on the occasion of receiving the Faillace Award from the L. Goodwin Cancer Institute, presented by director of the institute, Dr. Joel Warren; our pioneering viral oncolysate work in Los Angeles, 1982; and in Vienna, 1983; our retrovirus work including a review of oncogenes in Buenos Aires, 1984; our Kaposi sarcoma experience in Cairo, 1985; in Quebec, 1986; in Budapest, 1986; our early work on AIDS in Vienna, 1983; and Belem, 1986.

Dr. Robert Gallo, sitting in the front row, attentively listened to my lecture given in Vienna in 1983, where I showed EM pictures of "retroviruses" in lymphocytes and macrophages, vascular endothelial cells, platelets and brain cells of AIDS patients from the material of Houston's VA Hospital and Baylor's Department of Virology. After some delay, Dr. Györkey permitted me to publish one of these pictures.[73] As I returned to Tampa, an invitation from Bob Gallo was waiting for me to go to Bethesda and deliver the same lecture to members of his large and multinational department. His was the most advanced and most crowded virology department I have ever seen and Bob Gallo liked the looks of the retrovirus particles I showed.

Recently, I presented a paper on oncogenes, antioncogenes and virus therapy of cancer at the European Association of Cancer Research.[74] I am a founding member of the Inter-American Society for Chemotherapy. My first lecture at their charter conference in 1984 was entitled: "Patients Cured of Metastatic and/or Locally Advanced (Inoperable) Sarcomas." Our CCC at St. Joseph's Hospital organized two fine cancer conferences here for our third and fifth anniversaries.

From 1984 to 1988 on assignment by Secretary of Health, Margaret M. Heckler, I served four years on the Advisory Council to NIH's National Institute of Allergy and Infectious Diseases under Dr. Anthony Fauci (who attends patients and does high level clinical research in immunology of AIDS). Here I met outstanding Council members and observed and practiced the distribution of funds for research. This Council labored to be fair and treat the applicant investigators respectfully. It was a breath of fresh air after what I experienced down under at the receiving end from another NIH agency in the mid-1970s.

Now I know both worlds: academic medicine in all of its shades (splendor in the high ranks — a little bit; and the subdued existence down under — a great deal) and the practice of medicine: I am now a "health care provider" in clinical oncology. Very few among us spanned these distant points being actually involved in full in all states as I have been. The most outstanding investigators do superb work in the laboratory but they never experience the demand, tension and satisfaction of bedside practice of medicine. I am pleased that I did.

Among many similar items I am looking at now is one randomly chosen: "Chemotherapy, Tumor Immunology and Virology Seminar," sponsored by the American Cancer Society in Lafayette, Louisiana, on September 6 and 7, 1974. Of the five speakers, one advanced to exceptional altitudes, received high national and international awards, directed the national cancer program in the U.S. and now serves as physician-in-chief at the Sloan-Kettering Memorial Hospital, but never worked in laboratory research. Another one became a highly respected director of two comprehensive cancer centers (and once considered me to be his deputy); he also worked only in clinical medicine. One abandoned oncology altogether and sails around the world. Two left academic medicine and practice medical oncology (one in New Orleans, one in Tampa). The practicing oncologist in Tampa (myself) is the only one who did extensive work in basic laboratory research. The door to the highest and sustained academic recognition opened up for only two of the five selected speakers of year 1974.

In comparing myself to others, I am not really sorry that both major sustained academic recognition and substantial wealth bypassed me. What I really and deeply regret is that I could not remain on board to be part of, and contribute to, the great developments that have taken place from the early 1980s on. We are now deciphering the language of the cell and have already been communicating with our own cells in monosyllables. The time will come when we shall construct full sentences by administering biological response modifiers in the proper dosage and sequence. Even immortalized cells are expected to respond and return to the normal pathway of differentiation.

H. Cytocidal and Biological Therapy: the Winning Combination

Neither chemotherapy, nor biological therapy alone score high in remission induction in patients with metastatic tumors. There are most remarkable early reports suggesting a potentiation effect when these two modalities of treatment are combined. One can envision a scenario in which biologicals induce differentiation and a resting stage of formerly malignant cells which now escape cycle-specific cytocidal chemotherapy, whereas malignant cells that continue to remain undifferentiated and replicating succumb to cytocidal chemotherapy. Thus, removal of neoplastic cells from the tumor cell population proceeds along two different pathways. A good example is the combination of chemotherapy and interferon (Hu-rIFN-α2a) for the treatment of multiple myeloma as given by Oken and associates at the 1988 ASCO meeting: the VBMCP chemotherapy regimen induces 19%, the MP chemotherapy regimen, 11% CR rate; however, when Hu-rIFN-α2a was used in combination with VBMCP, the rate of sustained CR reached 41%.

Over ten years ago at the Solid Tumor (now Melanoma-Sarcoma) Service of M.D. Anderson Hospital we struggled desperately to improve remission induction in metastatic melanomas by adding active tumor-specific immunization with melanoma viral oncolysates and nonspecific immunization with BCG to dacarbazine-based chemotherapy.[62]

In 1978-9, we were first to propose a combined natural interferon-ß and hydroxyurea regimen for melanomas resistant to standard chemotherapy. Our protocol was approved at M.D. Anderson Hospital but was considered much too premature at the NCI and was not implemented. I received the Faillace Award from the Goodwin Cancer Institute in 1980 in Fort Lauderdale just for the thought and rationale of it. With this award I am in the very best company: Drs. Koprowski and Sabin are also recipients of this award!

While the newer chemotherapeutic agents tested against melanoma continue to score low (detrorubicin, dibromodulcitol, taxol, vindesine, etc.), a phenomenal body of new knowledge is emerging in relation to the biology of melanoma cells incorporating hormones and their receptors, growth factors and their receptors interacting and regulating mitosis and differentiation of these cells (Table 3). These cells also express new or amplified normal antigens (products of activated protooncogenes-oncogenes) against which monoclonal antibodies (and immunotoxins) can be produced with profound effect on the life and demise of these cells. Melanomas produce growth factors affecting unrelated benign skin tumors (acrochordons, acanthomas, seborrheic proliferations of Leser-Trelat, etc.).

This particular tumor (that I was set against as a much younger man to overcome) continues to remain quite unmanageable. At the same time, this tumor displays biological features that render it most susceptible to differentiation induction and/or to immune attack by its host. Interleukin-2 (IL-2) and LAK (lymphokine-activated killer) cells, cyclophosphamide, and TIL (tumor-infiltrating lymphocytes) suppress its growth or are cytocidal to it (Table 3) even though the induction of durable complete remission remains most elusive even by these means.

Table 3
Biology and Biotherapy of Human Melanoma

Molecular Mediators	Biological Effects/Therapeutic Results
Estrogens (E) and antiestrogens	Growth stimulation and inhibition independent from ER expression. E induced EGF and TGF-α.
Androgens and antiandrogens	Prognosis worse in men than in women. Testosterone and cyproterone have no *in vitro* effects.
Corticosteroids (CS)	Receptor (R) expression up to 86% of melanomas. Act through progesterone receptors. Gluco-CS-R homologous to v-erbA oncogene product. Antagonize proliferative effect of insulin and transferrin.
Insulin (I) and I-like GF	Mitogenic to melanoma cells.
Prostaglandins	Growth inhibitory. Synergistic with CS.

Table 3 continued

Melanocyte stimulating hormone (MSH)	Dopa isomers increase MSH-R expression. Induces melanin formation (differentiation).
Melatonin and pineal extracts (Bartsch)	Growth inhibitory to melanocytes and melanoma cells.
Melanoma growth stimulatory activity (MGSA) (Richmond)	Product of melanocytes/melanoma cells. Homologous to platelet-derived thromboglobulin B.
Transforming GF-α	Uses EGF-R. Melanoma-derived TGF-α induced growth of benign tumors (acrochordons, acanthosis nigricans, seborrheic keratosis L-T) (Ellis)
Transforming GF-ß	Growth (colony) inhibitor.
Epidermal GF	EGF-R expression amplified when extra copies of chromosome 7 are present (Koprowski). Expression correlates with amelanotic, epithelioid phenotype (pigmented, spindle-shaped melanoma cells are EGF-R⁻) (Real). EGF-R is homologous to v-erbB oncogene product.
Platelet-derived GF (Westermark) and thrombospondin (Roberts)	Produced by melanoma cells, not by melanocytes. Promoter of attachment and spreading of melanoma cells.
Nerve GF (Fabricant, DeLarco, Todaro)	NGF-R receptor expressed by melanoma cells as detected by anti-R monoclonal antibody (Koprowski).
Basic fibroblast GF (Richmond)	Mitogenic to both melanocytes and melanoma cells. Produced by melanoma cells (not melanocytes). Natural mitogen for melanocytes (Halaban).
Transferrin (Tf)	Mitogenic. Melanoma cell surface glycoprotein p97 is homologous to Tf.
Products of oncogenes H-ras, N-ras, c-mel	Oncogenes extracted for transfection studies: transforming
c-myc	Downregulates class I HLA expression: dedifferentiation.

Table 3 continued

e-<u>erb</u>B	EGF-R amplified with aneuploidy of chromosome 7(locus 7p11-13) (Koprowski).
<u>hst</u>/<u>int</u> 2 (Adelaide)	Locus 11q13. Co-amplified in melanoma. Gene product: bFGF family.
Hu-rIFN-α2a DTIC (Thomson)	7 CR 9 PR/ 51 pts
Hu-rIL-2, TIL CTX (Rosenberg)	1 CR 10 PR/ 20 pts
Allogeneic melanoma cells, Detox, CTX (Mitchell)	2 CR 3 PR/ 17 pts
Autologous melanoma cells, CTX (Berd & Mastrangelo)	3 CR 2 PR/ 35 pts
Viral oncolysates (Cassel, Hersey, Sinkovics, Wallack)	Prevention of relapse after resection (Cassel & Murray: 67% → 15%)
Monoclonal antibodies & immunotoxins (Goodman, Houghton, Lichtin, Oldham, Spitler)	8 responses/ 103 pts
EBV-transformed lymphocyte-derived Hu-n IL-1 (Bertoglio)	Direct cytotoxicity to melanoma cells (promoted growth of astrocytoma cells)

bFGF	=	basic fibroblast growth factor
CR	=	complete remission
CTX	=	cyclophosphamide (Cytoxan)
DTIC	=	dimethyl triazeno imidazole carboxamide
EBV	=	Epstein Barr virus
EGF	=	epidermal growth factor
ER	=	estrogen receptor
IL-1,2	=	interleukin
L-T	=	Leser-Trelat
PR	=	partial remission
TGF	=	transforming growth factor
TIL	=	tumor infiltrating lymphocytes

Active tumor-specific immunization (with nonspecific immunostimulants of bacterial origin: detoxified endotoxin; with cyclophosphamide to eliminate suppressor cells) induces substantial remission rate. Even today (1989), x-ray irradiated tumor cells and BCG are used together. These preparations cause granulomatous inflammation at the site of inoculation. Our viral oncolysates were injected intra- or subcutaneously in the mid-1970s and the sites were scarified over with BCG: no long-term oozing granulomas were formed by this technique. Interferon (Hu-rIFN-α2a) and dacarbazine induce more remissions than either one of these two agents alone. With these brilliant leads, realistic opportunities emerge for us who work now in the front lines of oncology practice to induce truly meaningful remissions both in high rate, duration and quality.

This vicious and unpredictable tumor teaches us many useful lessons as it gradually gives away several of its secrets. Lessons one and two are in prevention (sun screens and avoidance of sun exposure) and early diagnosis (shallow lesions are close to 100% curable, deep lesions close to 100% fatal). Lesson three entails the unusual susceptibility of this chemo- and radiotherapy-resistant tumor to biologicals: nonspecific immunostimulation, interferons and interleukin-2, LAK and TIL cells expanded by IL-2, monoclonal antibodies and immunotoxins. Even patients with metastatic tumors may respond to active tumor-specific immunization with melanoma cell (autologous or allogeneic) or melanoma cell membrane (lysate) vaccines if host suppressor cells counteracting tumor-specific immune T cells are killed by the co-administration of cyclophosphamide. In a previous era, less sophisticated attempts at active tumor-specific immunization resulted in tumor enhancement due to the production of antibodies blocking cytotoxic lymphocytes. While cyclophosphamide helps by eliminating suppressor cells of tumor-specific T lymphocytes, low dose cytosine arabinoside appears to have eliminated blocking antibodies (our own observation).[75] Lesson four: chemotherapy and biologicals are rather additive and synergistic than antagonistic. Examples are the above-mentioned cyclophosphamide or cytosine arabinoside with active tumor-specific immunization or interferon and dacarbazine. Lesson five is the applicability of various means of immunization with or without chemotherapy for the prevention of relapse, i.e., immunobiological elimination of micrometastases that exist in an undetectable form at the time of diagnosis or after excision of primary tumor and/or its regional lymph node metastases.

The other tumors I spent considerable time studying, both in tissue cultures and in patients, were sarcomas. We established cell lines and produced virus-modified sarcoma cell membrane preparations ("viral oncolysates"). We immunized patients with these preparations and scarified BCG over the immunization site (while patients with metastatic disease also received chemotherapy).[58,59] Durable remissions were induced and progression of disease was halted in more patients than in the control group receiving standard chemotherapy only. Now we hear that in Boston the combination of MAID chemotherapy (mesna, adriamycin, ifosfamide, dacarbazine) and GM-CSF induced less myelosuppression and higher response rate than chemotherapy alone. Sarcoma cells express receptors for GM-CSF which might stimulate their growth by recruiting resting tumor cells in the cell cycle and rendering them more vulnerable to cytotoxic chemotherapy. In addition, GM-CSF stimulates granulocytopoiesis, thus reducing the myelosuppressive effect of chemotherapy, perhaps allowing for higher doses of chemotherapy to be given.

On invitation by the Royal College of Surgeons in Ottawa, Canada in 1976, I reported that our lymphocyte- and antibody-mediated cytotoxicity assay picked up cross-reactions between osteo- and chondrosarcomas but not between these tumors and Ewing's sarcoma.[60] Now very recently we learn that Ewing's sarcoma is in the class of primitive neuroectodermal tumors! Thus, our conjecture that we dealt with tumors of different histogenesis and antigenicity proves to be correct, giving additional credibility to other results that we obtained with our assay. I wish NCI supported our work with this assay!

As to oncolytic viruses and viral oncolysates, the simplistic practice to inject (instill, inhale or give for ingestion) viruses into tumor-bearing patients will probably be abandoned as primitive and outdated. The first administration may induce occasionally partial tumor regressions but repeated administrations are expected to meet strong antibody response resulting in viral antigen-antibody complexes of no benefit (but perhaps causing glomerulonephritis, synovitis and other consequences of immune complex deposits). The emergence of some quite bizarre recombinant viruses is also remotely possible when live attenuated veterinary virus vaccines are inoculated into human beings harboring latent viruses of their own. Still attractive viral agents for this practice are parvoviruses (not those strains that cause crises of aplastic anemia), because these viruses replicate only in dividing cells and spare resting cells. Viral oncolysates remain promising for active tumor-specific immunization. They induce tumor-specific cell- and anti-body-mediated immune reactions and the release of host interferon, tumor necrosis factor and interleukin-2. However, the new developments of great potential therapeutic value are the gene transfer experiments. Retroviral plasmid vectors not only could return the retinoblastoma gene into retinoblastoma (and osteosarcoma) cells, thus rendering these cells non-oncogenic; plasmid vectors can deposit functional viral genes in cells and endow the cell with highly immunogenic new surface antigens. Viral envelope antigens or influenza virus' nucleoprotein or hemagglutinin antigens can thus be expressed by tumor cells. These "xenogenized" tumor cells elicit tumor-specific, histocompatibility antigen-restricted cytotoxic T lymphocyte responses so powerful that tumor rejection results. The host remains immune thereafter to challenge with tumor cells. This approach was not yet tested *in vivo*; that is, a growing tumor *in vivo* was not yet shown to take up new genes transfected by viral plasmid vectors and thus induce in the tumor-bearing host an immune reaction that would result in the rejection of a growing neoplasm. No technical or theoretical reasons are evident that would speak against this possibility. I expect that Dr. Townsend in Oxford, England, Dr. Itoyo in Sapporo, Japan (or at M.D. Anderson Cancer Center in Houston, Texas) or Dr. Huang in San Diego, California are in the process of conceiving and designing such clinically applicable experiments at this time.

More lessons are to be learned as the status of protooncogenes-oncogenes and their growth factors becomes known in the process of tumor growth, differentiation and dedifferentiation.[76]   Oncosuppressor genes may be introduced by harmless retroviral vectors. Oncogene product polypeptides may be neutralized by monoclonal antibodies which abrogate their action. Using one example, malignant melanoma, there is no doubt that a new era is dawning in human tumor biology and biological therapy. The lessons learned by deciphering the secrets of melanoma will be useful to use in the design of treatment protocols for many other major tumors. And beyond that, we shall learn how organized cell growth is regulated. The rules and regulations of embryogenesis can teach us about cancer more than the study of any individual cancer in itself. When insects resolved the problem of metamorphosis (envision for a moment the precise clockwork of molecular mediators switched on and off in the right dose at the right time and in the right combinations), the road was open for the accomplishment of practically any task by the living matter.

REFERENCES

1. **Sinkovics, J.,** Studies on the biological characteristics of the Newcastle disease virus adapted to the brain of newborn mice, *Arch. ges. Virusforschung* 7, 403, 1957.

2. **Sinkovics, J.,** The human pathogenicity and biological characteristics of Newcastle disease virus, *Arch. ges. Virusforschung,* 7, 242, 403, 1957.

3. **Sinkovics, J.G., Shullenberger, C.C. and Howe, C.D.,** Prolongation and prevention of Rauscher virus mouse leukemia by spleen cells of naturally resistant or actively immunized mice, *Clin. Res.* 13(1), 36, 1965.

4. **Sinkovics, J.G., Shullenberger, C.C. and Howe, C.D.,** Immunological functions of homologous spleen cells in viral mouse leukemia, *Texas Reports Biol. Med.,* 23, 94, 1965.

5. **Sinkovics, J.G. and Shullenberger, C.C.,** Effect of hematopoietic chimerism on the course of Rauscher's viral mouse leukemia, *Proc. Am. Assoc. Cancer Res.,* 4(1), 62, 1963.

6. **Sinkovics, J.G., Bertin, B.A. and Howe, C.D.,** Some properties of the photodynamically inactivated Rauscher mouse leukemia virus, *Cancer Res.,* 25, 624, 1965.

7. **Sinkovics, J.G., Pienta, R.J. Fiorentino, M. and Bertin, B.A.,** Neutralization of sublines of a mouse leukemia virus with murine antibody as measured by the spleen focus assay, *Cancer Res.,* 27, 88, 1967.

8. **Sinkovics, J.G.,** Modalities of immunotherapy for virally induced murine neoplasms, *Ann. N.Y. Acad. Sci.,* 276, 557, 1976.

9. **Sinkovics, J.G., Shullenberger, C.C., Howe, C.D. and Bertin, B.A.,** Treatment of leukemic mice with irradiation and adoptive immunization, *Proc. Am. Assoc. Cancer Res.,* 7, 65, 1966.

10. **Sinkovics, J.G., Ahearn, M.J., Shirato, E. and Shullenberger, C.C.,** Viral leukemogenesis in immunologically and hematologically altered mice, *RES, Journal of the Reticuloendothelial Society,* 8, 474, 1970.

11. **Sinkovics, J.G.,** The causative viruses of murine leukemia and their identification through immune responses of the host, in *Carcinogenesis: A Broad Critique,* Williams and Wilkins, Baltimore, MD, 1967, pp. 157-175.

12. **Sinkovics, J.G., Bertin, B.A. and Howe, C.D.,** Occurrence of low leukemogenic but immunizing mouse leukemia virus in tissue culture, *Natl. Cancer Inst. Monograph,* 22, 349, 1966.

13. **Sinkovics, J.G., Groves, F.B., Bertin, B.A. and Shullenberger, C.C.,** A system of tissue cultures for the study of mouse leukemia virus, *J. Infect. Dis.,* 119, 19, 1969.

14. **Sinkovics, J.G., Pienta, J.R., Trujillo, J.M. and Ahearn, M.J.,** An immunological explanation for the starry sky histological pattern of a lymphoma, *J. Infect. Dis.,* 120, 250, 1969.

15. **Sinkovics, J.G., Pienta, R. J., Trujillo, J.M. and Ahearn, M.J.,** Leukemogenesis in mice immunologically altered at birth and immunocompetence of leukemic lymphoblasts, in *Immunity and Tolerance in Oncogenesis,* L. Severi, ed., Division of Cancer Research, Perugia, Italy, 1970, pp. 975-987.

16. **Sinkovics, J.G., Shirato, E., Györkey, F., Cabiness, J.R. and Howe, C.D.,** Relationship between lymphoid neoplasms and immunologic functions, in *Leukemia-Lymphoma,* Year Book Medical Publishers, Chicago, 1970, pp 53-92.

17. **Sinkovics, J.G., Drewinko, B. and Thornell, E.W.,** Immunoresistant tetraploid lymphoma cells, *Lancet i,* 139, 1970.

18. **Trujillo, J.M., Ahearn, M.J., Pienta, R.J., Gott, C. and Sinkovics, J.G.,** Immunocompetence of leukemic murine lymphoblasts: ultrastructure, virus and globulin production, *Cancer Res.,* 30, 540, 1970.

19. **Sinkovics, J.G.,** in *Research Report: M.D. Anderson Hospital,* The University of Texas Press, Austin, TX, 1970, pp 331-336; 1972, pp. 476-479; 1974, pp. 454-455.

20. **Sinkovics, J.G., Trujillo, J.M., Pienta, R.J. and Ahearn, M.J.,** Leukemogenesis stemming from autoimmune disease, in *Genetic Concepts and Neoplasia*, Williams and Wilkins, Baltimore, MD, 1970, pp, 138-190.

21. **Sinkovics, J.G.,** The earliest concept of the "hybridoma principle", in *Frontiers of Radiation Biology and Oncology: Monoclonal Antibodies*, J. Vaeth, ed., Vol. 24, 1990, pp. 18-31.

22. **Sinkovics, J.G.,** Early history of specific antibody-producing lymphocyte hybridomas, *Cancer Res.*, 41, 1246, 1981.

23. **Gonzalez, F., Mollohan, K.R., Györkey, F. and Sinkovics, J.G.,** Augmentation of, or interference with spleen foci of Rauscher virus in mice inoculated with cultured human neoplastic cells, *Proc. Am. Assoc. Cancer Res.*, 14, 118, 1973 (Abstract #472).

24. **Gonzalez, F., Tzobari, S., Sinkovics, J.G., Campos, L.T. and Howe, C.D.,** Immunological evidences for the viral etiology of human mesenchymal neoplasms, *Proc. Am. Assoc. Cancer Res.*, 15, 62, 1974 (Abstract 247).

25. **Sinkovics, J.G.,** in *Research Report: M.D. Anderson Hospital*, University of Texas Press, Houston, TX, 1974, pp. 447-454; 1976, pp 578-585; 1978, pp. 337-339.

26. **Sinkovics, J.G.,** Lymphoid cells in long-term cultures, *Med. Record Annals (Houston, TX)* 61, 50, 1968.

27. **Sinkovics, J.G., Tebbi, K. and Cabiness, J.R.,** Cytotoxicity of lymphocytes to established cultures of human tumors: evidences for specificity, *Nat. Cancer Inst. Monograph*, 37, 9, 1973.

28. **Sinkovics, J.G.,** Intracellular lymphocytes in leukemia, *Nature*, 196, 80, 1962.

29. **Sinkovics, J.G., Howe, C.D. and Shullenberger, C.C.,** Cellular activities in tissue cultures of leukemic human bone marrow, *Blood*, 24, 389, 1964.

30. **Sinkovics, J.G., Shullenberger, C.C. and Howe, C.D.,** Cell destruction by lymphocytes, *Lancet* i, 1215, 1966.

31. **Sinkovics, J.G., Reeves, W.J. and Cabiness, J.R.,** Cell- and antibody-mediated immune reactions of patients to cultured cells of breast carcinoma, *J. Nat. Cancer Inst.*, 48, 1145, 1972.

32. **Sinkovics, J.G., Shirato, E. Martin, R.G., Cabiness, J.R. and White, R.G.,** Chondrosarcoma. II. Immune reactions of a patient to autologous tumor, *Cancer*, 27, 782, 1971.

33. **Sinkovics, J.G., Campos, L.T., Kay, H.D., Cabiness, J.R., Gonzalez, F., Loh, K.K., Ervin, F. and Györkey, F.,** Immunological studies with human sarcomas: effects of immunization and chemotherapy on cell- and antibody-mediated immune reactions, in *Immunological Aspects of Neoplasia*, 26th Annual Symposium, M.D. Anderson Hospital. Williams & Wilkins, Baltimore, pp. 367-401, 1975.

34. **Sinkovics, J.G.,** A reappraisal of cytotoxic lymphocytes in human tumor immunology, in *Cancer Biology and Therapeutics*, J.G. Cory and A. Szentivanyi, eds., Plenum Press, New York, 1987, pp 225-253.

35. **Sinkovics, J.G.,** Cytotoxic lymphocytes, *Ann. Clin. Lab. Sci.*, 16, 488, 1986.

36. **Sinkovics, J.G.,** Pleuropneumonia-ähnliche Eigenheiten in alten *E. coli* Kulturen, *Acta Microbiol. Hungarica*, 4, 59, 1957.

37. **Sinkovics, J.G.,** Occurrence and filterability of protoplast-like elements in aged bacterial cultures, *Nature*, 181, 566, 1958.

38. **Kay, H.D., Sinkovics, J.G., Cabiness, J.R. and Carrier, S.K.,** The concept of immune surveillance and its experimental testing, *Clin. Res.*, 44A, 1974.

39. **Kay, H.D., Cabiness, J.R., Kitowski, T. and Sinkovics, J.G.,** Cytotoxicity to and immune stimulation of cultured tumor cells by normal human lymphocytes and serum factors, *Proc. Am. Assoc. Cancer Res.*, 15, 64, Abstract 254, 1974.

40. **Kay, H.D. and Sinkovics, J.G.,** Cytotoxic lymphocytes from normal donors, *Lancet*, ii, 296, 1974.

41. **Kay, H.D., Thota, H. and Sinkovics, J.G.,** A comparative study on *in vitro* cytotoxic reactions of lymphocytes from normal donors and patients with sarcomas to cultured tumor cells, *Clin. Immun. Immunopathol.*, 5, 218, 1976.

42. **Thota, H., Romero, J.J., Sinkovics, J.G., Carrier, S.K., Crawford, J. and Kay, H.D.,** Leukocytes of patients with sarcomas express significantly more cytotoxicity to cultured sarcoma cells than to carcinoma cells, *Ann. Meet. Am. Soc. Microbiol.*, 75, 69, Abstract E49, 1975.

43. **Thota, H., Sinkovics, J.G., Carrier, S.K., Romero, J.J., Kay, H.D.,** Cytotoxic lymphocytes. III. Cross-reactions between melanoma and sarcoma cells as expressed by lymphocytes and serum factors of patients with melanoma and sarcoma and of normal donors, in *Proceedings of the 9th International Pigment Cell Conference*, Karger, Basel, 1976, pp. 124-133.

44. **Sinkovics, J.G., DiSaia, P.J. and Rutledge, F.N.,** Tumor immunology and evolution of the placenta, *Lancet*, ii, 1190, 1970.

45. **Sinkovics, J.G.,** Suppressor cells in human malignant disease, *Brit. J. Med.*, 1, 1072, 1976.

46. **Shullenberger, C.C. and Sinkovics, J.G.,** Lymphocytic cytotoxins in wasting syndrome, *New Engl. J. Med.*, 283, 1348, 1970.

47. **Sinkovics, J.G. and Shullenberger, C.C.,** Cytotoxic lymphoma: do neoplastic lymphoid cells produce cytotoxins *in vivo*? in *Proceedings of the 1st Meeting of the European Division of the International Society of Hematology*, Milan, Italy, 1971, p. 273.

48. **Sinkovics, J.G.,** Clinical recognition and treatment of endotoxinemia. In: *Immunobiology and Immunopharmacology of Endotoxins*, H. Friedman and A. Szentivanyi, Eds., Plenum Presss, New York, 1986, pp. 269-279.

49. **Gottlieb, J.A., Bodey, G.P., Sinkovics, J.G., Rodriguez, V. and Burgess, M.A.,** An effective four-drug combination regimen (Cy-VA-DIC) for metastatic sarcomas, *Proc. Am. Soc. Clin. Oncol.*, 10, 162, 1974.

50. **Sinkovics, J.G.,** Complete remissions lasting over three years in adult patients treated for metastatic sarcoma, in *Tumor Progression*, R. Crispen, Ed., Developments in Cancer Research 2, Elsevier North Holland, 1980, pp. 315-331.

51. **Sinkovics, J.G., Williams, D.E., Kay, H.D., Campos, L.T. and Howe, C.D.,** Clinical settings favorable for immunotherapy of sarcomas, in *Interaction of Radiation and Host Immune Defense Mechanisms in Malignancy*, Brookhaven National Laboratory Report, BNL 50418, 1974, pp. 331-339.

52. **Sinkovics, J.G., Williams, D.E., Campos, L.T., Kay, H.D. and Romero, J.J.,** Intensification of immune reactions of patients to cultured sarcoma cells: attempts at monitored immunotherapy, *Seminars in Oncology*, 1, 351, 1974.

53. **Sinkovics, J.G., Thota, H., Kay, H.D., Loh, K.K., Williams, D.E., Howe, C.D. and Shullenberger, C.C.,** Intensification of immune reactions by immunotherapy: attempts at measuring sarcoma-specific reactions *in vitro*, in *Neoplasm Immunity: Theory and Application*, R. G. Crispen, ed., University of Illinois Chicago, pp. 137-152, 1974.

54. **Sinkovics, J.G., Thota, H., Loh, K.K., Gonzalez, F., Campos, L.T., Romero, J.J., Kay,, H.D. and King, D.,** Prospectives for immunotherapy of human sarcomas, in *Cancer Chemotherapy -- Fundamental Concepts and Recent Advances*, M.D. Anderson Hospital and Tumor Institute, Year Book Medical Publishers, Chicago, pp. 417-443, 1975.

55. **Sinkovics, J.G., Loh, K.K. and Shullenberger, C.C.,** Use of viral oncolysates for tumor-specific immunotherapy in man, in *Modulation of Host Immune Resistance in the Prevention or Treatment of Induced Neoplasias*, Fogarty International Center Proceedings, No. 28, 1974, 235-236.

56. **Sinkovics, J.G., Campos, L.T., Loh, K.K., Cormia, F., Velasquez, W. and Shullenberger, C.C.,** Chemoimmunotherapy for three categories of solid tumors (sarcoma, melanoma, lymphoma): the problem of immunoresistant tumors. In: *Neoplasm Immunity: Mechanisms*, R.G. Crispen, Ed., Institution for Tuberculosis Research. The University of Illinois at the Medical Center, Chicago, 1976, pp. 193-212.

57. **McMurtrey, M.J., Campos, L.T., Sinkovics, J.G., Romero, J.J., Loh, K.K. and Romsdahl, M.M.,** Chemoimmunotherapy for melanoma: preliminary clinical data and difficulties with *in vitro* monitoring of tumor-specific immune reactions, in *Neoplasms of the Skin and Malignant Melanoma*, The University of Texas System Cancer Center, M.D. Anderson Hospital and Tumor Institute, Year Book Medical Publishers, Inc., Chicago, 1976, pp. 471-484.

58. **Sinkovics, J.G.,** Immunotherapy of sarcomas with viral oncolysates, *J. Am. Med. Assoc.*, 237, 869, 1977.

59. **Sinkovics, J.G., Plager, C. and Romero, J.J.,** Immunology and immunotherapy of patients with sarcomas, in *Immunotherapy of Solid Tumors*, R. Crispen, ed., Franklin Institute Press, Philadelphia, PA., 1977, pp. 211-219.

60.   Sinkovics, J.G., Thota, H., Romero, J.J. and Waldinger, R., Bone sarcomas: etiology and immunology, *Canad. J. Surg.*, 20, 494, 1977.

61.   Sinkovics, J.G., Plager, C., McMurtrey, M.J., Romero, J.J. and Waldinger, R., Active immunization with viral oncolysates integrated in the chemoimmunotherapy of human tumors, in *Abstracts of Interscience Conference on Antimicrobial Agents and Chemotherapy*, New York, 1977, Abstract #460.

62.   Sinkovics, J.G., Plager, C., McMurtrey, M.J., Papadopoulos, N.E., Waldinger, R., Combs, S., Romero, J.J. and Romsdahl, M.M., Adjuvant chemoimmunotherapy for malignant melanoma, in *Neoplasm Immunity: Experimental and Clinical*, R.G. Crispen, ed., Elsevier N. Holland, 1980, pp 481-519.

63.   Sinkovics, J.G., Plager, C., Papadopoulos, N., McMurtrey, M.J., Romero, J.J., Waldinger, R.R. and Romsdahl, M.M., Immunology and immunotherapy of human sarcoma, in *Immunotherapy of Human Cancer*. The University of Texas M.D. Anderson Hospital and Tumor Institute, Raven Press, New York, 1978, pp. 267-288.

64.   Sinkovics, J.G., Plager, C. and McMurtrey, M.J., Chemoimmunotherapy: basic principles and clinical examples, in *Advances in Medical Oncology, Research and Education*, M. Moore, ed., Vol 6, Permagon Press, Oxford, England, 1979, pp. 121-129.

65.   Sinkovics, J.G., Györkey, F., Kusyk, C. and Siciliano, M.J., Growth of human tumor cells in established cultures, in *Methods Cancer Research* 14:243, 1978.

66.   Sinkovics, J.G., Györkey, F. and Thoma, G., A rapidly fatal case of systemic lupus erythematosus: structures resembling viral nucleoprotein strands in the kidney and activities of lymphocytes in culture, *Texas Reports on Biology and Medicine*, 27, 887, 1969.

67.   Sinkovics, J.G., Working hypothesis: viral etiology of autoimmune diseases (letter to editor), *New Engl. J. Med.*, 208, 903, 1969.

68.   Sinkovics, J.G., Virus-like particles in systemic lupus erythematosus (letter to editor), *New Engl. J. Med.*, 284, 107, 1971.

69.   Györkey, F., Sinkovics J. and Györkey, P., Electron microscopic observations on structures resembling myxovirus in human sarcomas, *Cancer*, 27, 1449, 1971.

70.   Györkey, F. and Sinkovics, J.G., Microtubules of systemic lupus erythematosus, *Lancet*, i, 131, 1971.

71.   Györkey, F., Sinkovics, J.G., Min, K.W. and Györkey, P., A morphological study on the occurrence and distribution of structures resembling viral nucleocapsids in collagen diseases, *Am. J. Med.*, 53, 148, 1972.

72.   Sinkovics, J.G., Tubuloreticular structures in hairy cell leukemia, *J. Biol. Resp. Modif.*, 6, 573, 1987.

73.   Sinkovics, J.G., Györkey, F., Melnick, J.L. and Györkey, P., Acquired immune deficiency syndrome (AIDS): speculations about its etiology and comparative immunology, *Rev. Inf. Dis.*, 6, 745, 1984.

74.   Sinkovics, J.G., Oncogenes, antioncogenes and virus therapy of cancer, *Anticancer Res.*, 9, 1281, 1989.

75.   Sinkovics, J.G., Cabiness, J.R. and Shullenberger, C.C., Disappearance after chemotherapy of blocking serum factors as measured *in vitro* with lymphocytes cytotoxic to tumor cells, *Cancer*, 30, 1428, 1972.

76.   Sinkovics, J.G., Oncogenes and growth factors, *CRC Critical Rev. Immunol.*, 8, 217, 1988.

77.   Sinkovics, J.G., Cabiness, J.R. and Shullenberger, C.C., Monitoring *in vitro* of immune reactions to solid tumors, *Frontiers Radiation Therapy & Oncology*, 7, 141, 1972.

Chapter 17

CONCEPTS OF DELAYED TYPE HYPERSENSITIVITY - HISTORICAL ASPECTS WITH SPECIAL REGARD TO THE '60's

Günther Gillissen

The discovery of bacterial cells by Louis Pasteur and Robert Koch in the last decades of the 19th century, satisfying the definition of a specific pathogen, i.e., isolation of identical form by growth on artificial media and experimental induction of characteristic infections, has been, together with the possibility of prophylactic immunization shown to be applicable in a number of infectious diseases, the landmark of the nascent immunological sciences [for reviews see Foster[1] and Silverstein].[2] Within the same period of time, a further remarkable advance was achieved by the findings of Emile Roux and Alexandre Yersin that typical diphtheria could be induced in animals not only by bacteria but also by a metabolic bacterial product, an exotoxin. It did not take long for von Behring and Kitasato (1890) to show that immunizing with diphtheria or tetanus toxoids resulted in the production of antitoxic entities, then called antibodies, which can be used effectively for antitoxic serotherapy. This was confirmed when Ehrlich demonstrated the formation of neutralizing antitoxins by immunization with plant toxins.

The discovery of specific bacterial agglutination by Gruber and Durham (1896) applied to erythrocytes by Bordet and that of precipitin reactions by Kraus (1897) opened the way to study the antigen-antibody reactions *in vitro*. It was Paul Ehrlich (1897) who quantitatively measured diphtheria antisera by their reaction with toxin and defined specificity by chemical composition and molecular orientation. He recognized different functional domains on the toxin (as the haptophore and the toxophore groupings) and on the antibody (as for antigen binding and for other biological effects such as complement fixation). Only in the 1920's and '30's it was shown by Marrack and Heidelberger that antigen and antibody might combine in varying proportions.

Bordet claimed that the binding of antigen and antibody results in a change of configuration of the latter permitting a non-specific binding or activation of complement, a concept which was later confirmed. In the case of erythrocytes as antigen carriers, the antibody- and complement-mediated immune hemolysis was first introduced for diagnostic purposes in syphilis by August von Wassermann. The observation of erythrocyte agglutination or hemolysis by antibody and complement focused attention on red blood cells as antigens and it was Karl Landsteiner to whom we owe the discovery of human blood grouping system which he began to study in 1901.

Approximately within the same period, i.e., at the end of the last century, there was the beginning of the long-lasting controversies between humoral and cellular theories of immunity. The pivotal point was the discovery of the phagocytosis phenomenon by Metchnikoff in 1884. From there on it took a very long time to understand immunity as a network of cellular activities both for antibody and mediator production.

Based on early observation of Charles Richet and Paul Portier on systemic anaphylactic shock using primarily toxic substances, soon it was shown that this phenomenon could be induced by challenging appropriately sensitized organisms with corresponding nontoxic antigens. In contrast to this systemic reaction, a kind of local anaphylaxis was represented by the so-called Arthus

0-8493-4722-X/94/$0.00 + $.50

reaction (1903). It was induced by repeated intracutaneous injections of antigen. The local response increased with the number of applications and were characterized by polymorphonuclear leukocyte (PMN) infiltration and vasculonecrotic reactions. Later it was shown that immunocomplexes are involved in this anaphylactic reaction.

Another type of antibody-dependent reaction is the phenomenon of serum sickness discovered by Clemens von Pirquet and Bela Schick. It was observed after the injection of large quantities of foreign serum. Here again, antibodies specific for the injected proteins were shown to be the responsible agents.

The predominant role of antibodies for allergic sensitivity was demonstrated by passive transfer of antibody as in the reverse passive anaphylaxis discovered by Karl Prausnitz and Heinz Küstner (1921) or in the PCA-reaction in guinea pigs found by Ovary (1951). These observations were explained by the binding of a special class of antibodies, called cytophilic antibodies, on tissue or cell surfaces providing a local reactivity with the specific antigen on challenge. All typical anaphylactic reactions have in common their specificity, their passive transfer by serum, and in general, their quick appearance after challenge, called for this reason, immediate type reactions.

It is understandable that Robert Koch envisioned using tuberculin, the supernatant of boiled cultures of tubercle bacilli, for the cure or prevention of tuberculosis similarly as the specific protection against diphtheria by toxoid application or treatment by corresponding antibodies. However, tuberculin was not only ineffective prophylactically, but in patients with tuberculosis often led to severe systemic shock and even to an activation of otherwise quiescent foci. Locally, the ineffectiveness of the intradermal injection of tuberculin in naive organisms was followed by a marked local inflammatory reaction in tuberculous recipients with a delayed onset and a peak 24 to 48 hours later.

Subsequently, it could be shown in the 1920's by Dienes and colleagues that this type of reaction was also achieved in simple protein antigens if injected into tubercles. This was comparable to the assays of Ramon[3] who injected antigens into an area of local inflammation, and later used antigens together with adjuvant material;[4] in this way he was the forerunner of the use of Freund's adjuvant.[5]

Because of these and other experiments, two major points have to be remembered: the specificity of the reaction and the delayed onset of the reaction, which was for this reason called "delayed type hypersensitivity," included in the superior term of "cellular immunity."

Whereas the anaphylactic type of hypersensitivity could easily be transferred by serum this was not possible in the case of the delayed type.[6,7,8] In contrast, a passive transfer of tuberculin reactivity was shown to be possible by cells or tissues of sensitized donors. The first observation can be traced back to 1883[9] followed by comparable results obtained by Maksutow[10] and Bail (1910-1912)[11,12] which confirmed by many others.[13,14,15] Karl Landsteiner and Merrill Chase[16] showed in 1942 that the delayed type of specific hypersensitivity induced by simple chemicals could be transferred by white cells. This was demonstrated to apply for tuberculin sensitivity by Chase in 1945.[17] The extent of the passive sensitization by cells was dependent on the number of cells transferred, the degree of sensitization of the cell donors, and the viability of cells because dead cells were less effective. These results were largely confirmed.[18,19,20,21,22,23]   Even under clinical conditions, the possibility of a passive transfer of tuberculin sensitivity has to be considered as has been seen after blood transfusion or blood exchange transfusion[24,25,26] which could be explained by the transfer of white blood cells.

These results demonstrate clearly the cellular dependency of delayed type allergic reactions and their fundamental difference from anaphylaxis. Because both types of allergic reactions exhibit specificity to certain antigenic determinants, it was thought that antigen-binding structures on white cells were capable of transferring passively delayed type hypersensitivity (DTH). Therefore the antigen-binding property of DTH active cells was first one of the major problems and, in this context, the mechanism of the delayed onset of local allergic reactions.

The development of conclusive concepts were however, handicapped at that time by a lack of tools for differentiating lymphocyte classes and subpopulations. This meant that for examining lymphoid cells with respect to anaphylactic and particularly to DTH reactions, one had to use unseparated lymphocytes taken from organisms sensitized to exhibit the first or the latter kind of allergic reaction.

The first candidates for the study of antigen-binding capacity were plasma cells which secrete antibody as shown in 1954[27] and 1955.[28] On the other hand, humoral antibodies are apparently not responsible for the delayed type allergic reactivity. The derivation of plasma cells from lymphocytes was then discovered in 1962 by Gowans.[29] It was some years later that the two major differentiation pathways of lymphocytes were recognized. The one lineage of cells had its origin in the bursa Fabricii in chicken or in the bone marrow of mature mice and in the liver during embryonic life, respectively.[30,31,32,33,34,35,36] The other lineage derived from the thymus. For bursa-equivalent cells, the progenitors of antibody-secreting plasma cells, the term B-cells was coined; for the thymus-derived lineage, later shown to be responsible for specific DTH, the term T-cells was coined. It was first discovered that, early in their life history, B-cells produce membrane-bound antibodies with a hydrophobic transmembrane tail and antigen-binding sites facing outward from the cell membrane. These sIg+ B-cells[31] produce when newly formed both μ heavy and light chains.[37] It was, however, only in the 1980's that the problems of how T-cells recognize antigen and how the mechanism of the DTH-reaction works was elucidated (see Reference).[38] Most T-cells can recognize antigen only in combination with MHC-molecules, i.e., in the case of helper T-cells with MHC-class II and in that of cytotoxic T-cells with MHC-class I molecules (for review see Reference).[39]

Up to this time, at least up to the end of the 1960's, much work was done to elucidate the problem of DTH and it is tempting to review these experimental findings in comparison with our actual knowledge. The synopsis of data might, perhaps, even lead to an additional understanding of the *in vivo* phenomenon of DTH, if not only to further questions. Describing these assays, two major points have to be considered, i.e., the specificity of DTH-reactions and their delayed onset after challenge, both in connection with lymphocytes.

After the first experiments concerning a passive transfer of tuberculin allergy (see above), definite proof of a specific passive sensitization by cells was given by Landsteiner and Chase[16] and Chase[40] in 1942 and 1945, respectively. The efficacy seemed to depend on the number of cells transferred and the degree of sensitivity of the donors; heating of cells at

48°C for 30 min reduced the effect.[19,21,22] In contrast, the passive transfer of tuberculin hypersensitivity by cellular extracts (with one exception, see Reference)[41] could not—or at least not in a conclusive way—be achieved in animals.[17,40]   Lawrence[42,43,44] however, described in man a passive transfer with dead leukocytes, or cell extracts of tuberculin-sensitive donors treated by freezing and thawing or by distilled water.[42,45]   The responsible factor has been called "transfer factor" (TF) because most recipients become sensitized as early as 18 hrs later and remained reactive months or even up to 2 years later,[46,47,48] as if active and passive sensitization had been accomplished by the same extract.

The TF is dialysable (MW < 10,000), resistant to over 6 hrs of heating at 37°C and to treatment with DNAse, RNAse, or trypsin.[44,46,47] Lawrence[43] suggested that the TF had an affinity for cell surfaces as well as for the antigen or hapten which reminds some of the reaction between T-cells with their MHC restricted capacity for antigen-binding on the one hand, and with antigen bound to sIG^+ on B-cells on the other.[39,49,50,51] Although there were some reasons for postulating antigen-binding structures in/on leukocytes or TF positive extracts of cells from DTH positive donors, the assays to demonstrate these structures serologically failed.[44]

In 1927-1928, Rich and Lewis[52,53] observed a migration inhibition by tuberculin of leukocytes in tissue cultures and of spleen cells if tissues or cells were taken from tuberculous-infected animals, but inhibition did not occur in the case of normal ones. In this phenomenon, the interaction of humoral antibodies could be excluded.[22,54,55] The reaction (also demonstrable with tubercle bacilli) was apparently antigen specific. Here again it was suggested that the reaction was due to the binding of tuberculin on antigen-binding structures of leukocytes, some kind of sessile antibodies.[56]

Waksman[55,57] suggested that the specific induction of migration inhibition was followed by the release of immunologically nonspecific cellular factors directly responsible for this reaction, which was later defined as the lymphokine "migration inhibiting factor" (MIF). This migration inhibiting reaction is only demonstrable in DTH and is, therefore, a characteristic *in vitro* model for this kind of allergic reactivity.[57] In spite of its specificity, the compelling postulation of antigen-binding structures on leukocytes could not be serologically confirmed. Furthermore, the detection of the DTH characteristic MIF did not explain the delayed onset of the reaction either.

Another attempt to elucidate the problem of specificity of DTH-reactions was the idea that white blood cells might be sensitized for antigen by a special kind of antibody, called cytophilic antibody by Sorkin and Boyden.[58] It is present in serum of sensitized animals for some days after a booster injection of antigen,[59,60] differing from precipitating antibodies by its capacity to bind onto white cells mediated by thermolabile cell receptors.[60,61,62] These experiments were mainly done with serum proteins as antigens but assays with cells of tuberculin reactive animals failed to demonstrate antigen-binding. It is interesting to see that Boyden an Sorkin, as well as Lawrence and, already a decade earlier, Burnet and Fenner[63] postulated that for DTH reactions particular antibodies are involved with a special affinity for white cells. Therefore, attempts to demonstrate antigen binding structures on white cells of tuberculin reactive animals with different methods were resumed.

First, extracts from peritoneal exudate cells of highly tuberculin positive g.p (PEC) and cells of normal animals (control) were reacted with old tuberculin (OT)-sensitized sheep red blood cells ($SRBC_{OT}$). The PEC were composed of approximately 70% lymphocytes and 12% PMN cells. The extracts consisted of supernatants of PEC obtained after freezing and thawing or after treatment with histamine because it was shown[64] that certain concentrations of histamine may lead to the liberation of cell products.

In these direct assays, neither an agglutination nor an hemolysis could be seen.[65] On the other hand, using the Coombs technique, a rabbit-anti-g.p. serum globulin (inactivated and absorbed with dead H37Rv-tubercle bacilli) reacted with $SRBC_{OT}$ which pretreated with an extract of PEC from sensitized g.p., exposing a higher agglutination titer than the controls with an extract of PEC from normal animals. There was only a small difference in titers, but easily reproducible under identical conditions. The same results were obtained if $SRBC_{OT}$ were sequentially treated with an extract of PEC from sensitized g.p., with human complement (absorbed with SRBC) and afterwards with absorbed and inactivated rabbit-anti-human serum-globulin.[65]

By reason of the small differences in titers between assays and controls, the results had to be verified by other methods. Therefore, an attempt was made to demonstrate antigen binding on lymphocytes of PEC of sensitized g.p. with immunofluorescent techniques. For this purpose PEC fixed on slides were treated sequentially with OT, then with rabbit-anti-tuberculin antibodies, and finally with fluorescein-isothiocyanate (FIT) labeled gout-anti-rabbit serum antibody. The result was a bright fluorescence. In contrast, all controls were negative, whether OT was omitted in this system or the rabbit-anti-tuberculin antibodies were replaced by normal rabbit serum. With the same principle, complement binding could also be shown. Fixed PEC of sensitized g.p. were sequentially treated with OT, rabbit-anti-tuberculin antibodies, human complement, and FIT labeled rabbit-anti-human serum antibodies. Whereas this assay was positive, all the controls, i.e., PEC from normal animals, replacing active complement by an inactivated (30 min, 56°C) one or by the addition of EDTA to active complement[65] were again negative. Similar results were obtained by Freedman et al.,[66] in man with peripheral white blood cells or with transfer active cells of tuberculin positive rabbits.[67,68]

Up to that time, all assays to transfer systemic DTH to tuberculin with cell extracts of sensitized animals failed. Our own experiments in this sensitization using g.p. were also unsuccessful, but the possibility of a local sensitization was suggested.[69] PECs were, therefore, taken from g.p sensitized 12 to 14 days prior with 20 mg/wet weight of autoclaved tubercle bacilli H37Rv incubated with histamine (see below), and a supernatant (the cellular sediment for comparison) injected intracutaneously into the back of g.p. Two days later, animals were challenged with OT injected next to the extract application site. The area of local reaction was evaluated after 6 hrs, 1 day and 2 days. These experiments[69] showed a clear-cut positive reaction on day 1 with diameters between 10 and 12 mm, no effect at all after 6 hrs, and a reduced reactivity on the second day. Injection of the cellular sediment instead of the supernatant resulted in only a slight reactivity but it was not negative either. All controls with PEC of normal g.p. were completely negative. It was important to use a sufficiently high number of PEC, a high sensitivity to tuberculin of PEC donors, and a fairly short interval between extract injection and challenge. These results supported the idea of antigen-binding structures on white cells. The observation of the late local reaction (24 hrs) let us suppose that these structures are either not comparable with normal precipitating antibodies or that additional factors are released which are responsible for the delayed onset.

Proof of the presence of tuberculin-binding structures in PEC extracts (freezing and thawing) of tuberculin positive g.p. was furthermore sought using an extremely sensitive method known in virology.[70] The principle is the abolishment of the spontaneous aggregation of erythrocytes (in buffered glucose containing medium with low ionic strength) by tuberculin which can be reversed by antibodies.[71,72,73,74] By this method in PEC extracts of tuberculin positive g.p., antigen-binding activities directed against OT and PPD could be found.[74]

Already in the 1930's the tuberculin sensitivity of white cells from tuberculin-positive donors was observed.[53,54] Alteration of cells followed by cytolysis was then described in detail by Favour[75] which was confirmed by many other authors[64,76,77,78,79,80,81,82,83] but there were also contradictory results and interpretations.[47,84,85] Fremont-Smith and Favour[86] had the impression that the cytolytic effect of tuberculin would be C-dependent. Others observed such a cytolytic tuberculin effect on white cells of tuberculin negative patients sensitized by serum of tuberculin positive patients and explained it by an equally C-dependent plasma factor.[87] For this reason, Waksman suggested in 1953[55] that cytolysis might be compared with a Middlebrook-Dubos reaction. The tuberculin induced cytolysis has been demonstrated by changes in morphology[78,88,89] by the liberation of cell proteins[90] or by reduction in cell density.[89]

In spite of many comparable observations, not all of the results were unequivocal which might have been due to differences in methodology. Thus, Lawrence[43] did not see any cytolytic effect of tuberculin on the white cells of tuberculin-positive humans. In order to reproduce the tuberculin-induced cytolysis and for a better understanding of the phenomenon our experiments were extended. The results may be summarized as follows: Washed PEC or white blood cells taken from g.p. sensitized with autoclaved tubercle bacilli showed morphological alterations and subsequent lysis up to 25-32% after induction with OT in the absence of serum.[64,89,91] OT treated fixed cells of sensitized rabbits were capable of binding C as could be shown using g.p. complement and FIT labelled rabbit-anti-g.p. C.[68,92,93] All controls, i.e., assays with heat-inactivated C from g.p., with C in the presence of EDTA or with the addition of a non-labelled anti-C before the labelled preparation, were negative. White cells of non-sensitized normal g.p. showed neither OT nor C binding. This means that lymphocytes of tuberculin-positive g.p. are capable of binding OT, subsequently C and undergoing lysis but the lytic effect is not C dependent. In contrast, the effect of PPD on cytolysis is quite different.

PEC of BCG-sensitized g.p., but not those of normal animals–reacted with cytolysis after contact with PPD only in the presence of g.p. complement.[89] Decomplemented g.p. serum had no effect.[89] Cytolysis by PPD could be observed as early as 5 days after sensitization when the tuberculin skin reaction was still negative. The PPD induced cytolysis is therefore C-dependent whereas the OT dependent one is not.

In this context it seems of importance that the C-independent OT-cytolysis as well as the C-dependent PPD-cytolysis of lymphoid cells from specifically sensitized g.p. can be transferred passively into normal cells by cell extracts obtained by freezing/thawing.[94] There is apparently a tuberculin binding material on lymphoid cells which will be liberated by cell lysis into the extract.

This suggestion was confirmed by absorption assays. The material responsible for the C-independent OT-induced cytolysis could be absorbed by OT sensitized SRBC letting the transfer capacity of the extract for the C-dependent PPD induced cytolysis onto normal cells unchanged. An inverse effect was observed using for absorption PPD bound to tanned SRBC. Absorption with tubercle bacilli eliminated both kinds of cytolysis.[94]

An antigen-antibody reaction producing an anaphylactic type hypersensitivity is followed by liberation of histamine. Histamine is, therefore, one of the components for this type of allergic reactions. Conversely, it is generally admitted that in cellular immunity as in tuberculin skin reactions histamine does not play a role since antihistaminic treatment does not reduce the extent of a tuberculin reaction.[20,84] On the other hand, Inderbitzin[95] described the appearance or liberation of histamine at the site of tuberculin skin reactions.

Attempts were, therefore, made to elucidate the possible role of histamine in tuberculin cytolysis. It could be shown that the incubation of PEC from g.p. sensitized with tubercle bacilli (consisting of approximately 70% lymphoid cells, 13% PMN cells, 10% plasma cells and 2% monocytes) with OT but not those of normal animals resulted in a cytolysis of approximately 30%.[64,89] This effect could be abolished by a histamine inactivating preparation (toranti!, Hoechst Inc., F.R.G.).[96] From that observation it was concluded that the OT-induced cytolysis of sensitized cells is initiated by histamine. In the affirmative case the latter should also be able to induce lysis of normal cells which was indeed the case.[64]

Histamine release is regarded as the concomitant phenomenon of cell membrance alteration[97,98,99] as a consequence of an antigen-antibody reaction. Therefore, it is of interest that a histaminase preparation abolished the OT-cytolysis. It looks as if in the case of OT-cytolysis histamine liberation has no symptomatic effect but some pathogenic role of unclear significance. The histaminase effect is specific because the original OT-induced cytolysis could again be reconstituted by aminoguanidinosulfate a histaminase-blocking agent.[96]

The aim of these experiments was finally to get a better understanding of the mechanism of DTH-reactions. Convincingly and reproducibly it was shown that these reactions are immunologically specific and lymphocyte dependent: they are dependent on an antigen for induction and challenge, a passive transfer is only possible by lymphocytes of DTH-positive donors but not by humoral antibodies, and a tuberculin hypersensitivity could also be induced in congenitally agammaglobulinemic individuals.[100] For all these reasons, it is understandable that antigen binding sites on lymphocytes of DTH-positive donors were suggested. This idea was supported by several observations. One example is the specific migration inhibition of macrophages (MO) of tuberculous g.p. in tissue cultures after the addition of tuberculin which was first shown in 1932 by Rich and Lewis and confirmed very often with the same or modified methods (for overview see Reference.[101]

This phenomenon is characteristic for DTH[102,103] i.e., it cannot be shown with cells of anaphylactic donors and specific antigen. The responsible factor is produced by lymphocytes inhibiting the migration of macrophages. It is transferable onto normal cells. It is liberated by incubation of cells with antigen.[104,105,106,107,108] According to these observations the suggestion seemed to be justified that lymphoid cells of tuberculin-positive donors express antigen binding structures and produce, moreover, one or perhaps more, substances as the MIF characteristic for the DTH-phenomenon. Tuberculin-induced lymphocytolysis might similarly be related to DTH-reactions because cells, also taken from tuberculin-positive donors, reacted specifically with OT or PPD shown by microscopic evaluation, by liberation of cell protein and of LDH activity.[109]   This suggests that two antigen binding specificities are involved because the quantitative composition of OT and PPD is different.   Whereas OT contains predominantly tuberculo-polysaccharides, the main components of PPD are tuberculoproteins or protein derivatives, respectively.   Tuberculopolysaccharides are very easily bound to native SRBC by simple incubation[110,111] and PPD material to tanned erythrocytes.[112]

Different mechanisms of OT and PPD-induced cytolysis of lymphoid cells from tuberculin positive g.p. can be suggested by the fact that OT-cytolysis is independent of C-fixation, and may be abolished by histaminase, whereas PPD cytolysis is C-dependent.   The former effect may be due to antigen binding structures specific for polysaccharides and the latter to protein derivatives because the one or the other can be absorbed out of cell extracts specifically.

There are several reasons indicating that the OT-induced cytolysis is not directly related to the DTH-reactions: 1) for a given organism there is no correlation between the extent of OT-cytolysis and that of tuberculin skin reactions;[113,114] 2) histamine has been described to have no significance in DTH reactions[84,115] whereas OT-cytolysis is apparently histamine dependent;[64,96] 3) true DTH reactions to polysaccharide are not known; 4) immunization of g.p. with OT results in antibody production but not in DTH, and in a positive OT-cytolysis of lymphoid cells.[89,94] PPD-induced cytolysis appeared as early as a few days after sensitization with BCG and one week before the tuberculin skin test became positive.[89,92,110] In respect to the specificity of tuberculin skin reaction, PPD is superior to OT. For these reasons, and in the context of the observation of Rother[116] that genetically C3-deficient rabbits may produce humoral antibodies but are not qualified for eliciting DTH-skin reactions, a possible correlation of PPD cytolysis in DTH was hypothesized, but could not be confirmed. As to the immunological specificity of DTH reactions, specific antigen binding structures like antibodies on transfer active lymphoid cells were suggested. In this context two different terms for such structures were discussed, namely the cytophilic and sessile antibodies. The former was defined as antigen-binding structures with a considerable affinity (more than precipitating antibodies) for spleen, liver and kidney cells as well as for PMNs but not for erythrocytes.[59,60,117,118,119] The cell-fixed cytophilic antibodies are then capable of binding antigen. It is to be mentioned, however, that cytophilic antibodies are not found in g.p. or rabbits after sensitization with BCG or tuberculoprotein, whereas this kind of antibody could be demonstrated in DTH induced to other antigens.[61,62]

In tuberculin-positive animals, the so-called sessile antibodies are found on lymphoid cells demonstrable by different methods (see above). They were shown to be transferable by cell extracts to lymphoid cells of unsensitized animals[101] but they were also present on/in lymphoid cells of animals unsensitized in the sense of DTH.[89] That comparison may indicate that at least in the case of tuberculin, DTH cytophilic and sessile antibodies are not identical.[110]

In any case, antigen binding structures were demonstrated on/in lymphoid cells and their corresponding extracts. It is, however, difficult to understand why these structures alone should have a direct pathogenetic significance in contrast to serum antibodies because assays to transfer typical tuberculin hypersensitivity in animal models by lymphocytes or their extracts of tuberculin-positive donors in general failed.[17,40]

There were only a few experiments showing a local tuberculin reactivity of lymphoid cell extracts of g.p. sensitized with tubercle bacilli and challenged shortly thereafter by tuberculin.[69] A passive transfer of tuberculin sensitivity was also described in inbred g.p. by the application of cells from sensitized animals together with tuberculin,[120] so that a reaction similar to a booster effect was assumed.[121] Nevertheless, these assays did not give a sufficient and conclusive explanation for the typical delayed onset of tuberculin reaction as a special phenomenon of cellular immunity since not only locally but also systemically a certain delay can be observed relative to the anaphylactic type of hypersensitivity.

The delayed development of local tuberculin reactions was, at that time, attempted to be explained by the liberation of pharmacological mediators[113] whereby the immunological, i.e., specific, reactions would only serve as a trigger factor. This idea was quite understandable and led to the discovery of many immunological and pharmacological mediators produced as a consequence of antigen recognition by transfer active lymphoid cells, i.e., T-cells. But even now, when the mechanism of MHC-restricted binding of antigen on T-cell receptors has been elucidated by ingenious experimental designs (for review see Reference,[38] the explanation of the phenomenon of the delayed onset of DTH skin reactions is only based on the assumption that the slowly proliferating lymphocytes and macrophages had to be recruited by antigen. It might, however, be that this delay is due to cellular products or cell contents involved early after antigen application and capable to inhibit or to delay the development of allergic reactions of the anaphylactic type.

During the 60's, little was known about the identification of lymphocyte subpopulations by characteristic markers and, therefore, about their interactions either. For that reason, the problem of the mechanism of the delayed onset of local hypersensitivity was first tried to be elucidated by assays on anaphylactic reactions under the conditions of heterospecific DTH, by comparing the effect of cell extracts (PEC) from BCG-sensitized and normal g.p. on immune reactions *in vitro* and *in vivo* PCA reactions as well as by comparing the corresponding effects of isolated basic nucleoprotein fractions (histones) with cell factors described by others as the lymph node permeability factor (LNPF).

It could be shown in g.p. that the extent of PCA reaction (BSA-anti-BSA) is reduced in BCG or DNCB-sensitized animals relative to normal ones, but not in anaphylactic g.p. (HSA).[122] The same inhibition of PCA reactions (BSA-anti-BSA) was demonstrable if the anti-BSA was injected intra-cutaneously together with a cell extract of BCG-sensitized animals which did not occur using normal cell extracts or cell extracts of anaphylactic animals.[121] In the latter two cases there was rather an enhancement.

The inhibitory entity in cell extracts is sensitive to KJO_4 and cannot be dialysed.[121] If PCA reactions were performed with graduated doses of antibody injected intracutaneously with either cell extracts of non-sensitized or of tuberculin-positive g.p. and compared with reactions normally obtained without extracts, then, the cell extracts of non-sensitized animals were enhancing and that of BCG-sensitized ones were inhibiting.[123] These assays show a clear-cut difference between cell extracts of BCG-sensitized and normal animals. If the experimental design was changed so that the extract material was injected intravenously, i.e., by the same way as the antigen in the

PCA system, these differences between the two kinds of cell extracts could also be observed.[123]

Because of these results the possibility was tempting that by varying the intervals between extract application and challenge, the inhibition at the beginning could be reversed to an enhancement imitating by this way a delayed onset of local hypersensitivity. This was apparently the case: if challenge of PCA-reaction by antigen injection was done between 0 and 24 hours after intravenous application of extracts, the effect of the extracts from BCG-sensitized g.p. relative to those of normal animals showed an inhibition at 2 hrs followed by increasing values up to a maximum at 24 hrs.[123] This resembles the kinetics of a local DTH-reaction. In the case of an inverse PCA as experimental model both extracts had, however, similar effects.

In these experiments, cell extracts were prepared by PEC composed predominantly of PMN's. If PEC's consisting of mostly mononuclear cells were used for extract preparation, cell extracts of BCG-sensitized as well as of those of normal animals showed similar effects. Both were inhibitory up to an interval of 5 hrs between extract injection and challenge followed by an increase with a maximum at 24 hrs.[123] According to these experiments it seemed reasonable to conclude that the responsible factor is particularly present in lymphoid cells where it might be liberated from, e.g., by cytolysis. The mechanism of such an inhibitory factor in cell extracts could not be attributed to Ig's of the PCA system.[124] It should, therefore, act independently of the immune system used and should be demonstrable *in vitro*.

Assays in this respect showed that all results were in line with this suggestion: cell extracts inhibited agglutination of SRBC by rabbit-anti-Forssman-antibodies (A); the responsible factor was found predominantly in mononuclear cells and in cells of BCG-sensitized animals more than in that of normal ones; it was sensitive to KJO_4 and could not be dialyzed; it was not impaired by EDTA treatment; reacted only with fixed proteins and was not neutralized by soluble proteins; binding on SRBC-A-complexes was demonstrable by Coombs serum; thus the factor did not impair sensitization of SRBC but prevented agglutination.[124]

It was suggested as early as in 1962[125] that in the development of DTH specific cellular factor(s) might be involved. Subsequently much experience was gained by performing studies with this focus: a so-called lymph node permeability factor (LNPF) demonstrated biologically was described as a possible mediator of DTH reactions.[117,126,127,128,129,130] It was found in lymph node cells but also in spleen and liver cells of different species[125,126,131] were enriched in mononuclear cells of tuberculin-positive animals, or in skin sites of tuberculin or DNCB reactions,[132] but also to a lower degree in normal cells. LNPF increased vascular permeability for proteins, facilitated the emigration of PMN and mononuclear cells up to 45 min and 24 hrs after intracutaneous injection, respectively,[133] and induced locally the deposition of an eosinophilic, fibrinoid resembling material[134] imitating a DTH reaction without a particular immune system. The increase of permeability is abolished by local application of sodium salicylate or systemically by indomethacin.[126,135] LNPF was shown not be identical with known vascular permeability factors as histamine, substance P, globulin permeability factor and others.[135] The chemical nature of LNPF was not known, but in cell extracts it was apparently associated with macromolecular material, particularly complexed with albumin, less with gamma-globulin.[136]

LNPF activity was not only found in cell extracts of DTH-positive animals but, to a certain extent, also in that of normal animals of different species. For this reason, it was suggested that the LNPF might be attributed to the function of histones as regular components of cell nuclei. Histones apparently stabilize DNA structure[137,138] and regulate biosynthetic cell activities.[137,139,140,141,142,143,144] In cell-free systems, histone inhibits DNA-dependent RNA-synthesis[139,145,146,147] which was also shown when histone was added to cell cultures[148,149] for histones are able to penetrate cell membranes.[148]

If histones are identical or correlate with LNPF, it should be possible to demonstrate corresponding biological functions and particularly inhibition or delayed development of immune reaction. In this context, it was first shown in 1968 that histone application in mice resulted in a delay of homograft skin rejection.[150,151] Histones of calf thymus nuclei prepared as histone sulfate, preparation A, according to Murray[152] were somewhat less active than histones from mouse liver and spleen. The F3 fraction of calf thymus histone was generally more active than the F1 fraction or histone B.[153] It was also shown in mice that histones were able to depress antibody production to SRBC[154,155] as well as to viruses,22[156] and can easily be fixed on cell surfaces.[157] In further experiments it could be shown that histone B and the arginine rich F3 fraction of calf thymus histone adjusted to an equal nitrogen content inhibited the antibody-mediated agglutination of SRBC as well as the immune hemolysis.[158] Agglutination inhibition was due to a prevention of antibody binding (amboceptor A) by histone and inhibition of hemolysis by a reduced C1 fixation.[158] These observations suggested that the so-called mimicry effect of histone in the skin transplantation model, i.e., the increased survival time of skin homografts by histone treatment of graft donors[159,160] or the prevention of a second set reaction[161,162] might be explained by a reduced immunogenicity of histone-treated tissues. The possibility, therefore, may be considered that histones induce an early inhibitory effect on immune response either by immune suppression or by prevention of antigenicity.[160]

In contrast to the F3 fraction (see above) the F1 fraction rich in lysine abolished particularly the effect of F3 on agglutination but not that on hemolysis.[158] This result might explain the difference between extracts of native, unseparated LNPF active cell and histone in connection with hemagglutination.[124]

The inhibitory effect of histones on homograft rejection was to some degree comparable to that of cyclophosphamide. Histones however, did not cause leukocytopenia, and the "mimicry" effect (see above) induced by histone was not achievable by cyclophosphamide.[163]

Using tumor transplantation as an experimental model it could be shown that tumor growth was inhibited when tumor cells were exposed *in vitro* to histones prior to transplantation[144,145,164,165] but also by treating the tumor-bearing animals.[163,164] In contrast, a considerably enhanced tumor growth was seen when the prospective tumor recipients were pretreated with histone about two weeks before transplantation,[164] reminiscent of an immune suppression. According to these results, histone may act directly on tumor cells as well as on immune defense.

In the PCA model (BSA-anti-BSA rabbit serum) histones (F1, F3 histones of calf thymus nuclei, commercial histone sulfate of thymus, histone "B" of g.p. PEC) had also characteristic effects. An inhibition was observed if histones were injected locally together with the immune serum or systemically shortly preceding antigen injection.[166]   Increasing the interval between histone application and challenge, the reaction was inverse, i.e., the PCA-reaction was considerably more pronounced in the histone-treated animals than in the control group.[166] This result is comparable to that obtained by cell extracts of DTH-positive animals (see above).   In both cases an early inhibition was followed by a later or delayed maximum which might be correlated with the phenomenon of local DTH reactions.

One of the known phenomena of DTH is the disappearance of free macrophages (MDR) from glycogen-induced peritoneal exudate of DTH-positive animals after application of specific antigen.[167,168] It was possible to imitate this phenomenon in normal animals by intraperitoneal injection of total histone extracted from calf thymus nuclei. Comparable results were obtained by subcutaneous application.[169,170]

This means that also in this respect histones might be considered to function as mediators of the DTH phenomenon. In this context it was of interest whether histones correlate with LNPF also with respect to other biological functions of this factor. It could be shown that histones (F1 and F3 fractions and "histone B" from calf thymus nuclei) and LNPF containing cell extracts both increase vascular permeability for plasma proteins at 45 min but not at 24 hrs after intradermal injection. This is inhibited again in both cases by sodium salicylate.[171,172]

Leukocyte emigration is also enhanced after the intracutaneous injection of histones[133] or of LNPF[171] with predominantly PMN at 45 min and mononuclear cells at 24 hrs. Local formation and deposition of an eosinophil-ic, fibrinoid resembling material is in the case of histone less regular than after injection of LNPF containing extracts.[134,171] The regulation of gene functions by histones necessarily implicate reversible changes in histone composition. First it was supposed that this mechanism would be based on acetylation[173] because acetylated histones were not very effective as inhibi-tors and acetylation precedes RNA synthesis.[174,175] This concept, however, was not unequivocally held,[176] because in association with RNA synthesis a decreased rather than an increased histone acetylation was found.[177] Acetylated histone was, therefore, assayed in the homotransplantation model [total histone extracted from calf thymus nuclei, acetylated and dialysed against distilled water and freeze-dried].[178]   At equivalent amounts of histone nitrogen, it inhibited graft rejection similarly as the unacetylated one but to a smaller degree.[178] Sodium salicylate abolished this effect as it did with unacetylated histone or LNPF.[178] Taking these results together, it could be stated that essentially all biological effects of LNPF can be elicited equally with histones.

SUMMARY

The aim of this overview was to describe conceptual and experimental efforts made during the '60's for a better understanding of DTH reactions. This was all the more tempting because it was a relatively long period between the establishment and development of immunological sciences with major fundamental discoveries in the broad field of recognition of specific pathogens, of humoral and cellular defense mechanisms, of allergology and of immunochemistry on the one hand—and considerably later—the differentia-tion of lymphocyte classes and subpopulations by characteristic cell markers, the development of monoclonal antibodies, the discovery of pharmacological and immunological cellular mediators and particularly the revealing of MHC-restricted antigen recognition by lymphoid cells of animals with DTH (see Ref.[38] for review). It was the latter discovery providing the key to unlock the enigma of DTH-phenomena.

On the whole, during the '60's, it was well known that local DTH reactions, as the tuberculin reaction, are immunologically specific and can passively be transferred only by lymphocytes of sensitized donors.[16,23,40,179] This phenomenon, however, was poorly understood although it was recognized that specific antigen binding structures on lymphocytes are likely to be present which could indeed be demonstrated with a variety of methods.[65,67,68,69,74,180,181] For all these studies lymphocytes of DTH-positive animals were used. Soon it was, therefore, suggested that cells representing the active part of cellular immunity exhibit structures for binding native antigen. The antigen binding structures called "sessile antibodies" could equally be demonstrated by antigen-induced leukocytosis, a phenomenon which also could be transferred to normal cells by cell extracts.[94] Further experiments showed that leukocytosis can also be elicited with lymphoid cells of g.p. sensitized only with tuberculin instead of BCG.[89] For this reason, it seemed that these "sessile antibodies" are not typical for DTH. It cannot be excluded, and it is rather likely, that the native antigen binding cells are B-cells, because unseparated total lymphoid cells were used and defined as transfer active cells for DTH only by sensitization of cell donors with BCG. At that time a detailed differentiation of lymphoid populations by their markers were not yet available. This is in line with our modern knowledge of MHC-restricted antigen recognition according to which native antigen can only be bound to B-cells and in T-cells at most to Ts-cells.[182,183]

Also in the '60's the suggestion was raised that antigen-specific cell reaction might only be a trigger function for the development of DTH reaction. Besides the specific induction of DTH reaction the other characteristic phenomenon is the delayed onset and late maximum of this allergic reaction. In this sense, a mediator or mediators were postulated to be liberated by cells after cytolysis. In the affirmative case, such mediators should be expected to be found more or less in most cells or to be produced after cell contact with antigen and to produce phenomena similar to DTH reactions independent of specific sensitization.

Such a factor or mediator was described functionally as LNPF. It was particularly found in extracts of lymphoid cells or tissues of DTH-positive animals but also, though to a lesser extent, in cells of unsensitized animals (for review see Ref.)[131] This factor was able to produce intracutaneously the histological signs of a DTH reaction in the absence of a specific immunological system.[134] Comparing cell extracts of lymphoid cells from BCG-sensitized animals with that from unsensitized ones or from those immunized in the sense of an anaphylactic hypersensitivity, the following could be stated: Only the extract of BCG-sensitized g.p. was able to inhibit PCA reactions.[123] In contrast, an enhancement was seen when animals were challenged at a later time after extract application.[123] This looks like an imitation of a DTH reaction with anaphylactic antibodies, i.e., a delayed onset and a later maximum.

Histones as regular components of cell nuclei were thought to be responsible for these effects. The experiments performed in this respect with histone prepared from calf thymus nuclei or from lymphoid cells showed, indeed, that their biological effect is comparable with that of LNPF and/or extracts of lymphoid cells of DTH-positive animals. The F3 fraction seemed to be more active in this respect than the F1 fraction or histone "B".[153,171,184]   Histones delayed skin homograft rejection[151] and also PCA reactions,[123,166] they imitated a MDR, a characteristic phenomenon of DTH, in the absence of specific sensitization[169,170] and induced intracutaneously the typical histological signs of a local DTH reaction after 45 min and 24 hrs, respectively.[171] These observations might justify the idea that local DTH reactions are triggered by immunospecific phenomena but are actuated by cell contents such as histones. The delayed onset of the reaction was hitherto not regarded to be due to a particular mediating cell product. Even in the light of the actual knowledge of the mechanism of MHC-restricted antigen recognition by T-cells in DTH, the delayed onset of the local reaction is only explained by the time necessary to recruit slowly proliferating lymphocytes and macrophages.

The experiments described above suggest that intradermal antigen injection is followed by histone liberation as a consequence of cytolytic effects in which sIg exhibiting B-cells might be implicated as antigen-binding cells. The conception of histones as responsible mediators for DTH reactions seems to be all the more interesting as it allows also an explanation of systemic DTH-reactions whereby after antigen application no time is necessary for accumulating lymphocytes.

REFERENCES

1. Foster, W.D., *A History of Medical Bacteriology and Immunology*, Heinemann, London, 1970.
2. Silverstein, A.M., The history of immunology, in *Fundamental Immunology*, W.E. Paul, Ed., Raven Press, New York, 1984, pp. 23-40.
3. Ramon, G., Sur la production des antitoxines, *C.R. Acad. Sci. (Paris)*, 181, 157, 1925.
4. Ramon, G. and Lemétayer, E., Sur une méthode de production rapide et intensive de l'immunité et de l'antitoxine tétanique chez des animaux; son intéret pratique et théoretique, *C.R. Soc. Biol.*, 119, 248, 1935.
5. Freund, J. and McDermott, K., Sensitization to horse serum by means of adjuvants, *Proc. Soc. Exp. Biol.*, 49, 548, 1942.
6. Angevine, D.M., Comparison of cutaneous sensitization and antibody formation in rabbits immunized by intravenous or intradermal injections of indifferent or hemolytic streptococci and pneumococci, *J. Exp. Med.*, 73, 57, 1941.
7. Follis, Jr., R.H., Effect of preventing development of hypersensitivity in experimental tuberculosis, *Bull. Johns Hopkins Hosp.*, 63, 283, 1938.
8. Freund, J. and Opie, E.L., Experimental study of protective inoculation with heat-killed tubercle bacilli, *J. Exp. Med.*, 66, 761, 1937.
9. Falk, F., Beitrag zur Impf-Tuberkulose, *Berlin. Klin. Wochenschr.*, 772, 1883.
10. *Matsutow, Zbl. Bakter.*, 1897 as cited by F. Schmid, in, Handbuch der Tuberkulose, G. Thieme, Stuttgart, 1958.
11. Bail, O., Übertragung der Tuberkulinempfindlichkeit, *Z. Immunitätsforsch.*, I. Orig. 4, 470, 1910.
12. Bail, O., Weitere Versuche, betreffend die Übertragung der Tuberkulinempfindlichkeit, *Z. Immunitätsforsch.*, 12, 451, 1911-1912.
13. Onaka, M., Weitere Studien über die Übertragbarkeit der Tuberkulinempfindlichkeit, *Z. Immunit. Forsch.*, 7, 507, 1910.
14. McJunkin, F., Tuberculin hypersensitiveness in non-tuberculous guinea pigs enhanced by injections of bacillus-free filtrates, *J. Exp. Med.*, 33, 751, 1921.
15. Caspari, J., Zur Frage der Sensibilisierung gegen Tuberkulin, *Z. Tbk.*, 44, 447, 1926.

16. **Landsteiner, K. and Chase, M.W.,** Experiments on transfer of cutaneous sensitivity to simple compounds, *Proc. Soc. Exp. Biol.*, 49, 688, 1942.

17. **Chase, M.W.,** in *The Nature and Significance of Antibody Response*, A.M. Pappenheimer, Jr., Ed., Columbia University Press, New York, 1953.

18. **Censi, G.P. and Mangione, A.,** Aspetti des transporti passivo della allergia tubercolinica con essudate e poltiglie d'organo. Comportamento della leucolisi, della fenomeno di Koch, della reazione die Middlebrook-Dubos, *Riv. Inst. Sieroter. Ital.* 27, 134, 1952.

19. **Cummings, M.M., Petnode, R.A., and Hudgins, P.C.,** Passive transfer of tuberculin sensitivity in the guinea pig, *Pub. Health Rep.*, 62, 994, 1947.

20. **Kirchheimer, W.F. and Weiser, R.S.,** The tuberculin reaction. I. Passive transfer of tuberculin sensitivity with cells of tuberculous guinea pigs, *Proc. Soc. Exp. Biol. Med.*, 66, 166, 1947.

21. **Lawrence, H.S.,** The cellular transfer of cutaneous hypersensitivity to tuberculin in man, *Proc. Soc. Exp. Biol. Med.*, 71, 516, 1949.

22. **Schmid, F., Essler, H., and Hagge, W.,** Die Zellgebundenheit der Tuberkulinallergie, *Beitr. Klin. Tuberk.*, 108, 237, 1953.

23. **Wesslén, T.,** Passive transfer of tuberculin hypersensitivity by viable lymphocytes from the thoracic duct, *Acta. Tuberc. Scand.*, 26, 38, 1952.

24. **Schlange, H.,** Die passive Übertragung der Tuberkulinhautempfindlichkeit durch Blutaustauschtransfusionen und die Übertragbarkeit erworbener Tuberkulinnnegativität, *Arch. Kinderhk.*, 148, 12, 1954.

25. **Schlange, H.,** Die Übertragbarkeit der Tuberkulinhautempfindlichkeit von Kindern auf Meerschweinchen durch Cantharidenblasensedimente, *Z. Kinderhk.*, 76, 39, 1955.

26. **Stavitsky, A.B.,** Passive cellular transfer of tuberculin type of hypersensitivity, *Proc. Soc. Exp. Biol. Med.*, 67, 225, 1948.

27. **Good, R.A.,** Agammaglobulinemia, An experimental study, *Amer. J. Dis. Child.*, 88, 625, 1954.

28. **Coons, A.H., Leduc, E.H. and Connolly, J.M.,** Study on antibody production. I. A method for the histological demonstration of specific antibody and its application to a study of the hyperimmune rabbit, *J. Exp. Med.*, 102, 49, 1955.

29. **Gowans, J.L.,** The fate of parental strain small lymphocytes in F1 hybrid rats, *Ann. N.Y. Acad. Sci.*, 99, 432, 1962.

30. **Cooper, M.D., Cain, W.A., Van Alten, P.J. and Good, R.A.,** Development and function of the immunoglobulin-producing system, I. Effect of bursectomy at different stages of development on germinal centers, plasma cells, immunoglobulins and antibody production, *Inst. Arch. Allergy Appl. Immunol.*, 35, 242, 1969.

31. **Cooper, M.D., Kearney, J. and Scher, I.,** B Lymphocytes, in *Fundamental Immunology*, W.E. Paul, Ed., Raven Press, New York, 1984, pp. 43-55.

32. **Melchers, F., von Boehmer, H., and Phillips, R.A.,** B Lymphocyte subpopulations in the mouse. Organ distribution and ontogeny of immunoglobulin synthesizing and mitogen sensitive cells, *Transplant. Rev.*, 25, 26, 1975.

33. **Osmond, D.G. and Nossal, G.J.V.,** Differentiation of lymphocytes in mouse bone marrow. II. Kinetics of maturation and renewal of anti-globulin binding cells studied by double labeling, *Cell. Immunol.*, 13, 132, 1974.

34. **Owen, J.J.T., Cooper, M.D. and Raff, M.C.,** *In vitro* generation of B lymphocytes in mouse fetal liver: A mammalian "bursa equivalent," *Nature*, 249, 301, 1974.

35. **Warner, N.L.,** The immunological role of different lymphoid organs in the chicken, IV. Functional differences between thymic and bursal cells, *Aust. J. Exp. Biol. Med. Sci.*, 43, 439, 1965.

36. **Cooper, M.D., Peterson, R.D.A., South, M.A. and Good, R.A.,** The functions of the thymus system and the bursa system in the chicken, *J. Exp. Med.*, 123, 75, 1966.

37. **Lydyard, P.M., Grasi, C.E. and Cooper, M.D.,** Ontogeny of B cells in the chicken. I. Sequential development of clonal diversity in the bursa, *J. Exp. Med.*, 144, 79, 1976.

38. **Nossal, G.J.V.,** Triumphs and trials of immunology in the 1980's, *Immunology Today*, 9(10), 286, 1988.

39. **Male, D., Champion, B. and Cooke, A.,** *Advanced Immunology*, J.B. Lippincott Company, Philadelphia, 1987.

40. **Chase, M.W.,** The cellular transfer of cutaneous hypersensitivity to tuberculin, *Proc. Soc. Exp. Biol.*, 59, 134, 1945.

41.   **Jeter, W.S., Tremain, M. and Seebohm, P.M.,** Passive transfer of delayed hypersensitivity to 2,4-dinitrochlorobenzene in guinea pigs with leukocyte extracts, *Proc. Soc. Exp. Biol. Med.*, 86, 251, 1954.

42.   **Lawrence H.S.,** The transfer of generalized cutaneous hypersensitivity of the delayed tuberculin type in man by means of the constituents of disrupted leukocytes, *J. Clin. Invest,* 33, 951, 1954.

43.   **Lawrence H.S.,** The delayed type of allergic inflammatory response, *Amer. J. Med.,* 20, 428, 1956.

44.   **Lawrence, H.S.,** Some biological and immunological properties of transfer factor, in *Cellular Aspects of Immunity,* G.E. Wolstenholme and M. O'Connor, Eds., Ciba Foundation Symposium, J. and A. Churchill, Ltd., London, 1060.

45.   **Lawrence, H.S.,** The transfer in humans of delayed skin sensitivity to streptococcal M substance and to tuberculin with disrupted leukocytes, *J. Clin. Invest.,* 34, 219, 1955.

46.   **Lawrence, H.S.,** The transfer of hypersensitivity of the delayed type in man. , in *Cellular and Humoral Aspects of the Hypersensitive States,* H.P. Lawrence, Ed., Hoeber-Harper, New York, 1959, pp. 279-318.

47.   **Lawrence, H.S.,** in *Mechanisms of Hypersensitivity,* J.H. Shaffer, G.A. LoGrippo, and H.W. Chase, Eds., Little, Brown and Company, Boston, 1959.

48.   **Rapaport, F.T., Lawrence, H.S., Miller, J.W., Pappagianis, D., and Smith, C.F.,** Transfer of delayed coccidioidia hypersensitivity with leukocyte extracts in man, *Fed. Proc.,* 18, 593, 1959.

49.   **Chestnut, R.W., Colon, S.M. and Grey, H.M.,** Requirements for the processing of antigens by antigen-presenting B cells, Functional comparison of B cell tumors and macrophages, *J. Immunol.,* 129, 2382, 1982.

50.   **Lanzavecchia, A.,** Antigen specific interaction between T and B cells, *Nature,* 314, 537, 1985.

51.   **Manca, F., Fenoglio, D., Kunkl, A., Cambiaggi, C., LiPira, G., and Celada, F.,** Regulatory roles of surface and secreted immunoglobulins, *Immunology Today,* 9/10, 300, 1988.

52.   **Rich, A.R. and Lewis, M.R.,** Mechanism of allergy in tuberculosis, *Proc. Soc. Exp. Biol. Med.,* 25, 596, 1927.

53.   **Rich, A.R. and Lewis, M.R.,** The nature of allergy in tuberculosis by tissue culture studies, *Bull Johns Hopkins Hosp.,* 50, 115, 1932.

54.   **Moen, J.K. and Swift, H.K.,** Tissue culture studies on bacterial hypersensitivity. I. Tuberculin-sensitive tissues, *J. Exp. Med.* 64, 339, 1936.

55.   **Waksman, B.H.,** Studies of cellular lysis in tuberculin sensitivity, *Amer. Rev. Tbc.,* 68, 1002, 1954.

56.   **Aronson, J.D.,** Specific cytotoxic action of tuberculin in tissue culture, *J. Exp. Med.,* 54, 387, 1931.

57.   **Waksman, B.H.,** in *Cellular and Humoral Aspects of the Hypersensitivity States,* H.S. Lawrence, Ed., Hoeber, New York, 1959.

58.   **Sorkin, E.,** Zellfixierte Antikörper bei der Tuberkulose, *Allergie und Asthma,* 7, 79, 1961.

59.   **Boyden, St. V. and Sorkin, E.,** The adsorption of antigen by spleen cells previously treated with antiserum *in vitro, Immunology,* 3/3, 273, 1960.

60.   **Boyden, St. V. and Sorkin, E.,** The adsorption of antibody and antigen by spleen cells *in vitro,* Some further experiments, *Immunology,* 4/3, 244, 1961.

61.   **Boyden, St.V.,** Cytolytic antibody, in *Cell Bound Antibodies,* B. Amors and H. Koprowski, Eds., Wistar Institute Press, Philadelphia, 1963, pp. 7-14.

62.   **Boyden, St. V.,** Cytophilic antibody in guinea pigs with delayed hypersensitivity, *Immunology,* 7, 474, 1964.

63.   **Burnet, F.M. and Fenner, F.,** The production of antibodies, Mac Millan and Co., Lts., Melbourne, 1949.

64.   **Gillissen, G.,** Histamine and its possible role in cytolysis of white blood cells in guinea pigs sensitized with tubercle bacilli, *Nature* (London), 196, 590, 1962.

65.   **Gillissen, G.,** La définition sérologique des anticorps sessiles par rapport á la réaction tuberculinique, *Rev. Immunol.,* (Paris), 27, 43, 1963

66.   **Freedman, S.O., Turcotte, R., Fish, A. J., and Schon, A.H.,** The *in vitro* detection of "cell-fixed" hemagglutinating antibodies to tuberculin purified protein derivative (PPD) in humans, *J. Immunol.,* 90, 52, 1963.

67. Gillissen, G., Fluoreszenzserologische Darstellung der C'-Bindung durch sessile Antikörper, in *Second International Congress of Histo- and Cytochemistry,* Frankfurt/Main, Springer-Verlag, August 1964, Abstract p. 213.

68. Gillissen, G., Die fluoreszenzserologische Darstellung einer Komplementbindung durch zellständige Antikörper bei der Tuberkulose, *Z. Hyg.,* 150, 194, 1964.

69. Gillissen, G., Zellfrei Präparate des sog. Transfer-Faktors bei der Tuberkulinallergie beim Tier, *Zbl. Bakter.* I. Origin 191, 260, 1963.

70. Drescher, J. and Schrader, K., Titration of poliovirus and influenza virus by means of the hemaggregation test, *Amer. J. Hyg.,* 79, 218, 1964.

71. Drescher, J. and Gillissen, G., Die Titration von Tuberkulin u. Tuberkulinantikörpern mittels des photometrischen Haemaggregationstestes, I. Methodik der Tuberkul-intititration, *Zbl. Bakt.* I. Origin., 200, 480, 1966.

72. Drescher, J. and Gillissen, G., Essay of tuberculin antibody by means of the photometric hemaggregation test, I. Description of the method, *Amer. J. Epidemiol.,* 87(2), 329, 1968.

73. Gillissen, G. and Drescher, J., Die Titration von Tuberkulin und Tuberkulin-antiköpern mittels des photometrischen Haemaggregationstestes, II. Die Beziehung zwischen hemaggregationshemmender Aktivität (HIV) und Tuberkulin-Hauteinheiten (TE), *Zbl. Bakter.,* I. Orig., 201, 65, 1966.

74. Gillissen, G. and Drescher, J., Assay of tuberculin antibody by means of the photometric hemaggregation test, II. Comparative titration of antibody by hemaggre-gation test and by conventional techniques, *Amer. J. Epidemiol.,* 87, 339, 1968.

75. Favour, C.B., Lytic effect of bacterial products on lymphocytes of tuberculous animals, *Proc. Soc. Exp. Biol. Med.,* 65, 269, 1947.

76. Böke, W. and Diekhues, B., Experimentelle Tuberkulin Cytolyse isolierter Entzüunungszellen aus der Vorderkammer, *v. Graefe's Arch. f. Ophthalmologie,* 166, 28, 1963.

77. Fabrizio, A.M., Effect of purified fractions of tuberculin on leukocytes from normal and tuberculous animals in tissue cultures, *Amer. Rev. Tbc.,* 65, 250, 1952.

78. Gillissen, G., Der Ablauf der Leukocytolysreaktion im Verhältnis zur Zellart, *Z. Hyg.,* 149, 210, 1963.

79. Janicki, B.W. and Patnode, R.A., Enzymatic determination of *in vitro* lysis of leukocytes by tuberculin, *Proc. Soc. Exp. Biol. Med.,* 102, 311, 1959.

80. Raffel, S., Delayed hypersensitivities, *Prog. Allergy,* 4, 173, 1954.

81. Schmid, F., Die Tuberkulincytolyse, *Beitr. Klin. Tuberk.,* 109, 151, 1953.

82. Waksman, B.H. and Bocking, D., A comparison of leukocyte lysis with certain other immunologic phenomena demonstrable in sera of tuberculous rabbits, *Amer. Rev. Tbc.,* 69, 1002, 1954.

83. Witte, S., Morphologische und serologische Studien über Tuberkulinwirkungen an Leukocyten *in vitro, Beitr. Klin. Tbk.,* 104, 252, 1950.

84. Friedman, E and Silverman, I., The effect of antihistamine medication on the tuberculin reaction in children, *Amer. Rev. Tbc.,* 60, 354, 1949.

85. Kerby, G.P., Chaudhuri, S.N., and Durham, N.C., Plasma levels and the release of a lysozyme-like enzyme from tuberculin-exposed leukocytes of tuberculous and non-tuberculous human beings, *J. Lab. Clin. Med.,* 41, 632, 1953.

86. Fremont-Smith, P. and Favour, C.B., *In vitro* lysis of leukocytes from tuberculous humans by tuberculoprotein, *Proc. Soc. Exp. Biol. Med.,* 67, 502, 1948.

87. Miller, J.M., Vaughan, J.H., and Favour, C.B., The role of complement in the lysis of leukocytes by tuberculoprotein, *Proc. Soc. Exp. Biol. Med.,* 71, 287, 1949.

88. Bassermann, in Kolloquium über "Die Allergie bei der Tuberkulose," *Allergie und Asthma,* 7(1/2), 98, 1961.

89. Gillissen, G., Der Mechanismus der Tuberkulincytolyse, *Z. Hyg.,* 150, 239, 1964.

90. Gillissen, G., Der Nachweis freigesetzter Zellinhaltstoffe als Kriterium einer Cytolyse, *Z. Hyg.,* 149, 473, 1964.

91. Gillissen, G., Experimental studies concerning the mechanism of the tuberculin reaction, in, "Symposium d. Schweiz. Allergie-Gesellschaft über 'Delayed Type Hypersensitivity,'" Davos, 1964.

92. Gillissen, G., Immunologische Grundlagen der allergischen Spätreaktion, *Klin. Wschr.,* 43(11), 590, 1965.

93. **Gillissen, G.,** Immunohistological evaluation of sessile antibodies and the complement fixation on cellular immune complexes, *Path. Europ.*, I(3), 217, 1966.

94. **Gillissen, G.,** Die passive Sensibilisierung weisser Blutzellen mit zellulären Tuberkulinantikörpern, *Z. Hyg.*, 150, 251, 1964.

95. **Inderbitzin, Th.,** The effect of acute and delayed cutaneous allergic reactions on the amount of histamine in the skin, *Int. Arch. Allergy*, 7, 140, 1955.

96. **Gillissen, G.,** Die spezifitat einer Hemmung der Tuberkulincytolyse, *Naturwiss*, 50(11), 405, 1963.

97. **Katz, G.,** Histamine release from blood cells in anaphylaxis *in vitro*, *Science*, 91, 221, 1940.

98. **Kinsell, L.W., Kopeloff, L.M., Zwermer, R.L., and Kopeloff, N.,** Blood constituents during anaphylactic shock in the monkey, *J. Immunol.*, 42, 35, 1941.

99. **Rocha e Silva, M.,** Antihistamine agents in allergy. Role played by leukocytes and platelets in anaphylactic and peptone shock, *Ann. N.Y. Acad. Sci.*, 50, 1045, 1950.

100. **Porter, H.,** Congenital agammaglobulinemia: A sex-linked genetic trait and demonstration of delayed skin sensitivity, *Am. J. Dis. Child.*, 90, 617, 1955.

101. **Heilmann, D.H.,** Tissue culture methods for studying delayed allergy, A review, *Tex. Rep. Biol. Med.*, 21, 136, 1963.

102. **Carpenter, K.K.,** *In vitro* studies on cellular hypersensitivity, *J. Immunology*, 91, 803, 1963.

103. **Stinebring, W.R., Axelrod, A.E., and Trakatellis, A.C.,** *In vitro* testing for delayed hypersensitivity to proteins, protein derivatives, and peptides, *Fed. Proc.*, 22, 617, 1963.

104. **Bloom, B.R., and Bennett, B.,** Mechanism of a reaction *in vitro* associated with delayed type hypersensitivity, *Science*, 153, 80, 1966.

105. **David, J.R.,** Delayed hypersensitivity *in vitro*: its mediation by cell-free substance formed by lymphoid cell-antigen interaction, *Proc. Natl. Acad. Sci. USA*, 56, 72, 1966.

106. **David, J.R., Lawrence, H.S., and Thomas, L.,** Delayed hypersensitivity *in vitro*. II. Effect of sensitive cells on normal cells in the presence of antigen, *J. Immunol.*, 93, 274, 1964.

107. **David, J.R. and Peterson, Ph.Y.,** *In vitro* demonstration of cellular sensitivity in allergic encephalomyelitis, *J. Exp. Med.*, 122, 1161, 1965.

108. **Svejcar, J. and Jahanovsky, J.,** Demonstration of delayed (tuberculin) type hypersensitivity *in vitro*, I. Selection of methods, *A. Immunitätsforschg.*, 122, 398, 1961.

109. **Gillissen, G.,** Der Nachweis einer LDH-Aktivität als Ausdruck einer Schädigung weisser Blutzellen, *Z. Med. Mikrobiol. u. Immunol.*, 152, 134, 1966.

110. **Gillissen, G.,** Sessile Antikörper bei der tuberkulinallergie, *Current Topics Microbiol. Immunol.*, 45, 70, 1968.

111. **Takahashi, Y., Fujita, S., and Sasaki, A.,** The specificity of the passive hemagglutination methods used in serology of tuberculosis, *J. Exp. Med.*, 113, 1141, 1961.

112. **Boyden, St. V. and Sorkin, E.,** The adsorption of proteins on erythrocytes treated with tannic acid and subsequent hemagglutination by antiprotein sera, *J. Exp. Med.*, 93, 107, 1951.

113. **Schild, H.O.,** Pharmacologically active mediators in delayed hypersensitivity, in "Symposium der Schweiz. Allergie-Gesellschaft über 'Delayed Type Hypersensitivity,'", Davos, 1964.

114. **Waksman, B.H., Carrol, M.P., and Gaulitz, D.** Studies of cellular lysis in tuberculin sensitivity. *Amer. Rev. Tbc.* 68:746-759, 1953.

115. **Woodruff, C.E.,** Antihistaminics and the tuberculin reaction, *Amer. Rev. Tbc.*, 62, 555, 1950.

116. **Rother, K.,** The significance of the complement system for allergic reactions *in vivo*, *Int. Arch. Allergy*, 22, 322, 1963.

117. **Sorkin, E.,** Cytophilic antibody, in *The Nature and Origin of the Immunologically Competent Cell*, Ciba Foundation Study Group, J. and A. Churchill Ltd., London, 1963.

118. **Sorkin, E.,** On the cellular fixation of cytophilic antibody, *Int. Arch. Allergy*, 25, 129, 1964.

119. **Sorkin, E., Rhodes, J.M., and Boyden, St. V.,** Antibody synthesis in relation to levels of humoral and cell-fixed antibodies in rabbits, *J. Immunol.*, 80(1), 101, 1961.

120. **Blazkovec, A.A., Sorkin, E. and Türk, J.L.,** A study of the passive cellular transfer of local cutaneous hypersensitivity, *Int. Arch. Allergy*, 27, 289, 1965.

121. **Leskowitz, S.,** Mechanism of delayed reactions, *Science*, 155, 350, 1967.

122. Gillissen, G., Untersuchungen über den Mechanismus der allergischen Spätreaktion, I. Die Bedeutung der Reaktionsbereitschaft vom Spättyp für eine PCA-Reaktion, *Z. Med. Mikrobiol. u. Immunol.*, 152, 148, 1966.

123. Gillissen, G., Untersuchungen über den Mechanismus der allergischen Spätreaktion, III. Der Einfluß von Zellinhaltstoffen auf die PCA-REaktion, *Z. Med. Mikrobiol. u. Immunol.*, 154, 221, 1968.

124. Gillissen, G., Untersuchungen über den Mechanismus der allergischen Spätreaktion, II. Der Nachweis einer Agglutinationshemmung durch Zellfaktoren spätallergischer Tiere, *Z. Med. Mikrobiol. u. Immunol.*, 152, 216, 1966.

125. Willoughby, D.A., Spector, W.G., Schild, H.O., and Boughton, B., A vascular permeability factor extracted from normal and sensitized guinea pig cells, *Life Sci.*, 7, 347, 1962.

126. Walters, M.N.J. and Willoughby, D.A., The effect of tissue extracts on vascular permeability and leukocyte emigration, *J. Path. Bact.*, 89, 255, 1965.

127. Willoughby, D.A., The lymph node permeability factor: a possible mediator of delayed hypersensitivity reactions, *Bibl. Haemat.*, 29, 634, 1968.

128. Willoughby, D.A., Mediators of delayed hypersensitivity reactions, *Int. Arch. Allergy*, 36, 22, 1969.

129. Willoughby, D.A. and Spector, W.G., The lymph node permeability factor: a possible mediator of the delayed hypersensitivity reaction, *Ann. N.Y. Acad. Sci.*, 116, 874, 1964.

130. Willoughby, D.A., Spector, W.G., and Boughton, B., A lymph node permeability factor in the tuberculin reaction, *J. Path. Bact.*, 87, 353, 1964.

131. Schild, H.O. and Willoughby, D.A., Possible pharmacological mediators of delayed type hypersensitivity, *Brit. Med. Bull.*, 23(1), 46, 1967.

132. Willoughby, D.A., Waltes, M.N.I., and Spector, W.G., Lymph node permeability factor in the dinitrochlorobenzene skin hypersensitivity reaction in guinea pigs, *Immunology*, 8, 578, 1965.

133. Spector, W.G. and Willoughby, D.A., The effect of vascular permeability factors on the emigration of leukocytes, *J. Path. Bact.*, 87, 341, 1964.

134. Willoughby, D.A. and Spector, W.G., The production of eosinophilic deposits resembling fibrinoid by injections of lymph node extracts, *J. Path. Bact.*, 88, 557, 1964.

135. Willoughby, D.A., Boughton, B. and Schild, H.O., A factor capable of increasing vascular permeability present in lymph node cells, *Immunology*, 6, 484, 1963.

136. Meacock, S.C.R. and Willoughby, D.A., Purification of serum proteins from lymph node cell extracts with permeability activity characteristic of the lymph node permeability factor, *Immunology*, 15, 101, 1968.

137. Huang, R.C., Bonner, I., and Murray, K., Physical and biological properties of soluble nucleohistones, *J. Molec. Biol.*, 8, 54, 1964.

138. Littau, V.C., Burdick, C.J., Allfrey, V.G., and Mirsky, A.F., The role of histones in the maintenance of chromatin structure, *Proc. Natl. Acad. Sci.*, 54, 1204, 1965.

139. Allfrey, V.G., Observations on the mechanism and control of protein synthesis in the cell nucleus, in *Functional Biochemistry of Cell Structures*, O. Lindberg, ed., Pergamon Press, Oxford, 2, 127, 1961.

140. Bonner, J. and Ts's, P., *The Nucleohistones*, Holden-Day, Inc., San Francisco, 1964.

141. Busch, H., *Histones and Other Nuclear Proteins*, Academic Press, New York, 1965.

142. Huang, R.C. and Bonner, I., Histone, a suppressor of chromosomal RNA synthesis, *Proc. Natl. Acad. Sci.*, 48, 1216, 1962.

143. Vorobyev, V.I., The effect of histones on RNA and protein synthesis in sea urchin embryos at early stages of development, *Exp. Cell. Res.*, 55, 168, 1969.

144. Vorobyev, V.E. and Bresler, V.M., Unfractionated preparations of histones from normal mammalian tissues as agents inhibiting growth of transplanting tumors, *Nature*, 198, 545, 1963.

145. Johns, E.W. and Connors, T.A., Specific toxicity of histone fraction F2C against TLx5 lymphoma ascites cell *in vitro*, *Nature*, 228, 1201, 1970.

146. Król, B., Grabowska, M. and Chorazy, M., Effect of histones, poly-L-lysine and DNA on the mitotic activity of Chinese hamster fibroblasts, *Neoplasma*, 16(3), 265, 1969.

147. Yoshida, M. and Shimura, K., Specific repression of chromatin-dependent RNA-synthesis by silk gland histones, *J. Biochem.*, 67, 507, 1970.

148. Fischer, H. and Wagner, L., Die Wirkung niedermolekularer (basischer) Proteine auf Zellen und Organismen, *Naturwiss.*, 41, 532, 1954.

149.   **Pohjanpelto, P.,** Inhibition of growth of subtilis phage SP-50 by histones, *Nature*, 215, 439, 1967.

150.   **Gillissen, G.,** Die Hemmung einer Abstossung von Organtransplantaten. Neue Gesichtspunkte, in *Hochschulmitteilungen der Technischen Hochschule Aachen*, Bericht PM, 1968.

151.   **Gillissen, G. and Seifert, H.,** Verlängerte Haltbarkeit von Homotransplanttaten nach Histongaben, *Naturwiss*, 55(3), 137, 1968.

152.   **Murray, K.,** The heterogenicity of histone, in *The Nucleohistones*, J. Bonner and P. Ts'o, Eds., Holden-Day, San Francisco, 1964.

153.   **Gillissen, G.,** Untersuchungen über den Mechanismus der allergischen Spätreaktion. VI. Der Immunosuppressive Effekt von Histonen am Modell der Homo-Transplatations-Reaktion, *Zbl. Bakt. I.*, 212, 146, 1969.

154.   **Pelletier, M., Baxin, S. and Delaunay, A.,** Effet immunodépresseur exercé chez la souris par des histones totales et la fraction F1 de Johns, *Rev. Franc. Etud. Clin. Biol.*, 14, 663, 1969.

155.   **Pelletier, M. and Delaunay, A.,** Effet exercé par une fraction d'histone (PII) sur la formation des anticorps, *C.R. Acad. Sci.*, 266, 1540, 1968.

156.   **Drescher, J. and Gillissen, G.,** Influence of histones on the antibody response in guinea pigs to vaccination with A/Aichi/2/68 (H3 N2) influenza virus, *Infect. Immunity*, 8(4), 573, 1973.

157.   **Pelletier, M., Delaunay, A., and Bazin, S.,** Sur l'agglutination bactérienne produite par un complex polypeptidique extrait du thymus de veau avec ou sans traitement préalable par le lysozyme, la trypsine, le chlorure de calcium ou le polypeptide PII, *Path. er Biol.*, 13, 46, 1965.

158.   **Gillissen, G.,** Untersuchungen über den Mechanismus der allergischen Spätreaktion. IV. Der Einfluß von Histon-Präparationen aud die Haemagglutination und die Immunhaemolyse, *Z. Med. Mikrobiol. u. Immunol.*, 154, 349, 1969.

159.   **Gillissen, G. and Nehring, G.,** Beeinflussung der Homo-Transplantations-Reaktion durch Vorbehandlung der Transplantat-Spender, *Naturwiss.*, 8, 418, 1969.

160.   **Gillissen, G. and Nehring, G.,** Mimicry effect of histones in homograft tissue, *J. Reticuloentothel. Soc.*, 7(6), 700, 1970.

161.   **Gillissen, G.,** Die Haftung von Homotransplantaten unter Behandlung mit Histon, *Langenbecks Arch. Chirurgie*, 327, 278, 1970.

162.   **Gillissen, G.,** Der Effekt von Histon auf Immunreaktionen *in vivo*, in *Allergie und Immunitätsforschung*, Vol. III, F.K. Schattauer Verlag, Stuttgart, 1970, pp. 263-271.

163.   **Gillissen, G.,** Der immunosuppressive Effekt von Histon am Modell der Haut-Homotransplantation, Vergleichende Untersuchungen mit Cyclophosphamid, *Z. Ges. Exp. Med.*, 152, 335, 1970.

164.   **Gillissen, G. and Schweizer, K.,** Effect of histone on tumor growth and survival rate of tumor-bearing mice, in *Advances in Antimicrobial and Antineoplastic Chemotherapy. Proceedings of the VIIth International Congress of Chemotherapy*, Urban Schwarzenbeg, München, pp. 175-176, 1972.

165.   **Shah, V.C. and Reilly, P.,** Effects of histones, other basic proteins and some antibiotics on the transplantability of mouse mammary tumors, *Nature*, 213, 403, 1967.

166.   **Gillissen, G.,** Untersuchungnen über den Mechanismus der allergischen Spätreaktion, V. Die Beeinflussung allergischer Reaktionen durch Histone, *Zbl. Bakt. I.*, 212, 137, 1969.

167.   **Nelson, D.S. and Boyden, S.V.,** The loss of macrophages from peritoneal exudates following the injection of antigens into guinea pigs with delayed type hypersensitivity, *Immunology*, 6, 264, 1963.

168.   **Nelson, D.S. and North, R.J.,** The fate of peritoneal macrophages after the injection of antigen into guinea pigs with delayed type hypersensitivity, *Lab. Invest.*, 14, 89, 1965.

169.   **Bubenzer, B. and Gillissen, G.,** Die Dichte freier Makrophagen im Peritonealexsudat nichtimmunisierter und spätallergischer Tiere nach Histonbehandlung, *Zbl. Bakt. Abt. I.*, 214, 518, 1970.

170.   **Gillissen, G. and Bubenzer, B.,** Histone-induced macrophage disappearance reaction in normal guinea pigs, *Experientia*, 26, 781, 1970.

171.   **Gillissen, G. and Breining, H.,** Untrsuchungen über den Mechanismus der allergischen Spätreaktion, VII. Die funktionelle Beziehung zwischen LNPF (lymph node permeability factor) und Histonen, *Ärztl. Forschg.*, 23(8), 263, 1969.

172. Gillissen, G and Breining, H., Rapport fonctionnel entre le "LNPF" (facteur de perméabilité vasculaire des ganglions) et les histones, *C.R. Acad. Sci.*, 269, 281, 1969.
173. Phillips, D.M.P., The presence of acetyl groups in histones, *Biochem J.*, 87, 258, 1963.
174. Mukherjee, A.B. and Cohen, M.M., Histone acetylation: cytological evidence in human lymphocytes, *Exp. Cell Res.*, 54, 257, 1969.
175. Pogo, B.G.T., Allfrey, V.G., and Mirsky, A.E., RNA synthesis and histone acetylation during the course of gene activation in lymphocytes, *Proc. Natl. Acad. Sci. USA*, 55, 805, 1966.
176. Ellgaard, E.G., Gene activation without histone acetylation in *Drosophila melanogaster*, *Science*, 157, 1070, 1967.
177. Monjardino, J.P. and MacGillivray, A.J., RNA and histones metabolism in small lymphocytes stimulated by phytohemagglutinin, *Exp. Cell Res.*, 60, 1, 1970.
178. Gillissen, G., Influence of acetylation on biological effects of histones, *Z. Immun. Forsch.*, 141, 232, 1971.
179. Wesslén, T., A historical study of the tuberculin reaction in animals with passively transferred hypersensitivity, *Act. Tuberc. Scand.*, 26, 175, 1952.
180. Gillissen, G., Ist die Tuberkulinallergie Ausdruck einer Antigen-Antikörper-Reaktion? *Beitr. Klin. Tuberk.*, 127, 202 and 207, 1963.
181. Gillissen, G., Der zellständige Antikörper bei der Tuberkulose, in *5. Europ. Allergiekongr. Kongressbericht, Selbstverlag Schweiz. Allergieges*, Schwabe u. Co., Basel, 1963, pp. 276-277.
182. Cantor, H., T Lymphocytes, in *Fundamental Immunology*, W.E. Paul, Ed., Raven Press, New York, 1984, pp. 57-69.
183. Fresno, M., McVay, A., Bouderau, L. and Cantor, H., Antigen specific T lymphocyte clones, III. Papain splits purified T suppressor molecules into two functional domains, *J. Exp. Med.*, 155, 981, 1981.
184. Gillissen, G., Die Beeinflussung vom Immun-Reaktionen durch Histone unter besonderer Berücksichtigung der zellulären Immunität, *Eur. J. Immunol.*, 34, 1969.

Chapter 18

REMEMBRANCES OF THINGS PAST BY A PARTICIPATING WITNESS

Zoltan Ovary

My principal scientific interests have always been concerned with antibody production and regulation and *in vivo* antibody-antigen interactions leading to anaphylactic reactions. The reason for my interest was, that I became very allergic to cats and I wanted to find out more about allergic reactions. I started to do research after the Second World War at the Clinical Medica at the University of Roma, Italy. What was known about antibodies and allergic (anaphylactic) reactions in the late forties when I became actively involved in this field?

It was known that allergic reactions can be transmitted passively by serum (antibody) since in 1921 Prausnitz had shown passive sensitization in humans (the Prausnitz-Kustner reaction).[1] It was known that antibodies were not a "property" of the immune serum, but a substance, as Heidelberger had shown in 1935[2] that antibody can be specifically precipitated and weighed. It was known that antibodies are globulins as Tiselius and Kabat[3] had shown that they migrated with the globulins in electrophoresis. The sedimentation velocity was determined and from this, the molecular weight had been also calculated. Most of the antibodies had a MW of about 150,000 but some hemolysins in rabbit sera and some other antibodies in other species had a higher molecular weight (around 900,000).[4] Most antibodies had a valency of 2, i.e., one antibody molecule could combine with two molecules of the antigen (we would say now that one antibody molecule could combine with two epitopes of the same specificity). That was about all that was firmly established concerning antibodies. Not much, as we can see.

It was known that during anaphylactic reactions, smooth muscles contract. This had been shown by Sir Henry Dale (1936 Nobel Prize winner) using the Schultz-Dale test.[5,6] It was also known that this contractile action is due to the action of histamine, liberated during anaphylactic reactions. I wanted to investigate histamine liberation *in vivo* not *in vitro* like Dale, as I had learned a very sensitive new technique from the great Hungarian pharmacologist Jancso: the use of intravenous injection of India ink.[7] Jancso showed that if histamine is injected into the skin or liberated in the skin, then the intravenously injected India ink particles are phagocytosed by the endothelial cells of the small postcapillary venules. Although the action of histamine to increase the permeability of the small post-capillary venules was well known from the work of Lewis,[8] the accumulation of the India ink particles in the endothelial cells was a new phenomenon.

I wanted to learn more about anaphylactic reactions, as we did not know much about the fixation of antibody to the receptors in the tissues (i.e. on the cells). We did not known anything about the structure of antibody: what and where are the structures which react with the antigen and what and where were the structures which permit the fixation to the receptors. Last but not least, we did not know anything about the possible existence of different categories of antibodies (today we call them antibody classes or isotypes).

0-8493-4722-X/94/$0.00 + $.50

In my first experiments, I injected the antibody intradermally and challenged the animal intravenously with the mixture of antigen and India ink. The reasoning behind this idea was that if histamine is really liberated in these *in vivo* reactions, the fixation of India ink in the endothelial cells of the small venules would reveal the liberated histamine. I started to use the technique of Jancso (India ink) with Biozzi, who later, with Benacerraf used this technique for the study of the reticuloendothelial system.[9] Once I was certain that increased permeability of the venules was caused by histamine, I switched to the use of Evans blue as it was easier to manipulate.

In experimental animals (guinea pigs) Chase[10] had investigated anaphylactic reaction in the skin and got very interesting results showing a local inflammatory reaction. The novelty of the technique that I used was the use of the dye which permitted better visualization and especially an **easier quantitation** of the reaction.

Most experimentators used rabbit (sometimes horse) antibodies and the amount was usually determined by the Heidelberger-Kendall microprecipitin reaction.[2]

The emphasis in the late forties was on quantitation. Reactions obtained without the use of the dye were not easy to quantify as they were of short duration and slight redness was difficult to read with exactitude. I was therefore happy to be able to measure easily the precise amount of antibody necessary to provoke this *in vivo* reaction which I called passive cutaneous anaphylaxis (PCA).[11] PCA was first described in guinea pigs with rabbit antibodies. I was able to show that as little as 20 nanograms of antibody protein could be detected by PCA. With any other method in use at that time the minimal amount of detectable antibody was three orders higher.

We also showed that antibodies from some species (chicken, horse) were unable to sensitize the guinea pig, but when these antibodies were directed against rabbit IgG (as antigen) and the rabbit IgG was injected intradermally into guinea pigs these antibodies could give a reverse PCA reaction.

We established that a certain period was necessary after the intradermal injection of the antibody to sensitize for PCA reactions (sensitization period) and that an optimum period existed after which the reactions would be smaller and with limiting amounts of antibody, could not be obtained at all.[11]

Looking back after so many years on these early experiments, I am amazed by the serendipity and our luck and also by our great ignorance. Serendipity and luck: first, rabbit IgG (called then the 7S antibody) is not subdivided into subclasses (isotypes of IgG). Second, rabbit antibody can sensitize guinea pigs for anaphylactic reactions. Our ignorance: we did not know if the antibody from one species could sensitize the same species or also others. We knew nothing about the structure of antibodies and antibody isotypes and their biological activities. We were totally ignorant about the structures with permitted the antibody to get "fixed" and the "receptors" to which it got fixed. We could continue the list.

Using anti-lactoside antibodies, Fred Karush and I found[12] that a monovalent hapten (lactose in this case) would not elicit anaphylactic reactions. Using anti-dinitrophenyl (DNP) antibodies I could then show that the monovalent hapten εDNP-lysine was unable to provoke anaphylactic reactions. In fact it could even be used to prevent PCA by polyvalent DNP-proteins by competing with the polyvalent antigen. This was a logical and expected result from the experiments with the anti-lactoside antibodies. What was more interesting was the fact that the bivalent hapten α-ε-bis-DNP-Lysine was able to induce PCA reactions and liberate histamine in the skin of guinea pigs. This experiment with monovalent and bivalent haptens led me already in 1961 to propose the "bridging" or "crosslinking" hypothesis,[13] which I formulated later as follows: "A bridging of two combining sites of two different antibody molecules by two determinants on the same antigenic molecule is necessary and sufficient for obtention of PCA reactions".[14] The bridging or crosslinking hypothesis has been confirmed by many investigators. The most beautiful confirmation was by Teruko Ishizaka et al.,[15] who showed that antibodies against the receptors for IgE on mast cells can provoke mast cell degranulation and histamine release.

A great breakthrough came at this time (1959): Rodney Porter published his first results on papain digestion of rabbit gamma globulin.[16] He showed that two types of fragments can be obtained: the Fab fragment which could still combine with the antigen and another fragment which he called Fc as it was crystallizable. Nobody guessed then that this was because the Fc fragment was the same in all rabbit gamma globulin molecules but the Fab fragment varied from one molecule to the other. Yet, that a fragment was crystallizable already established that in all rabbit IgG molecules there is a portion which is constant.

With Fred Karush we showed that the Fab fragment cannot sensitize the guinea pig for PCA reactions, but using reverse PCA reactions we showed that the Fc fragment can "get fixed" to cellular receptors. When anti-rabbit gamma globulin was used for challenge, a reverse PCA reaction was obtained.[17] No complement fixation was obtained with the Fab fragments. Later Nisonoff digested the rabbit gamma globulin molecule with pepsin and obtained a bivalent fragment $F(ab')_2$ which could precipitate the polyvalent antigen.[18] We showed that this fragment, though it combines with the antigen, is still unable to sensitize the guinea pig for PCA reaction and cannot fix complement by the classical pathway. Our conclusion was that the Fc fragment carries the biological activities: i.e., the structures necessary for complement fixation by the classical pathway[19] and the structure for the fixation to cellular receptors on mast cells.

Porter continued his investigation of the rabbit IgG molecule and showed that each molecule is made up of two identical heavy (H) and two identical light (L) chains: the four chain model of Porter.[20] This work was rewarded with the Nobel prize. Shortly afterward, Hilschmann[21] showed that the L chain is divided in two portions of about the same size: the N terminal half is variable (V), but the C terminal half is constant (C) and identical from one myeloma protein to the other of the same type. It cannot be emphasized enough the tremendous impact that this discovery had on future investigations not only on immunoglobulins, but also on other molecules such as the Class I and Class II molecules coded for by the genes of the major histocompatibility complex and on the T cell receptors, to quote those which come immediately to mind. Shortly after this discovery it was shown that the H chain had also an N-terminal V and a C-terminal constant portion, but that the constant portion of the H chain is three times longer than the V portion. In retrospect the fact that the rabbit Fc fragment was crystallizable should have led us to an awareness of its constant structure.

Intrachain disulfide bonds delimit loops in each chain, called domains. It was then investigated if some functions could be assigned to separate domains. The site which reacts with the antigen is in the first domain made up by the two V portions of the H and L chains. I was concerned with the domains in the Fc fragment. We and others showed that the constant domain and specifically the first domain in the Fc fragment carries the structures reacting with the first component of complement (C1Q).[19] However, the domain concept does not hold for some of the other reactions. For example the fixation to macrophages necessitate the integrity of the Fc domain. We had shown with Lamm that when the last domain is separated neither the remainder of the IgG nor the separated last domain can fix to the macrophage receptor. Moreover the mixture of the two separated fragments is unable to inhibit the fixation of the intact molecule.[22] Quite recently in beautiful experiments Geha showed that the same is true for the IgE antibody fixation to the high affinity IgE mast cell receptor. Geha showed, that only those peptides in which the junction of the last two domains was present could inhibit the fixation of the intact IgE molecule.[23] Glowsky obtained the same results.[24]

From the studies of the immunoglobulin chains came a better knowledge concerning allotypes. From the study of the C portions of the H chains came the division of immunoglobulin molecules in classes and subclasses (isotypes).

In 1962 at NYU in collaboration with Benacerraf and Bloch we made an observation studying guinea pig antibodies: the guinea pig IgG can be subdivided into two classes: one, the electrophoretically faster moving IgG1 can sensitize the guinea pig for anaphylactic reactions, but does not fix complement by the classical pathway as it lacks structures to react with C1Q; the other, the electrophoretically slower moving IgG2 does not sensitize the guinea pig for PCA reaction but fixes complement by the classical pathway.[25,26,27,28]

These studies were confirmed by many investigators and were an impetus to study the heterogeneity of immunoglobulins in other species too. Different immunoglobulin isotypes were found in many species and it was confirmed, that different isotypes may carry different biological activities. We know now that the difference between the isotypes in a species is due to differences in amino acid sequences of the constant regions. As the Fc fragment is made up from the last domains of the two similar heavy chain constant regions, it is expected that different isotypes might carry different biological activities. These first observations made with the guinea pig IgG1 and IgG2 were thus important in view of the fact that the biological functions of antibodies could be better understood, and called attention to the importance of the different immunoglobulin isotypes.

I had shown that rabbit IgG can sensitize the guinea pig for PCA reactions, but not the rabbit for anaphylactic reactions and guinea pig IgG1 can sensitize the guinea pig, but not other species. At that time it was still not clear what is the isotype involved in human allergic reactions. First, it was thought, that it is the IgA isotype, but then Mary Loveless presented data on patients without IgA, who still had tremendous allergic reactions.[29] The Ishizakas with great effort and insight and marvelous work showed that the sensitizing antibody is not of the IgG isotype and called it IgE.[30,31]

Shortly afterward Johansson and Bennich in Sweden,[32] found an unusual human myeloma protein and it turned out that it was an IgE myeloma. The existence of a human IgE myeloma not only confirmed the existence of the IgE immunoglobulin class, but also made it possible to develop *in vitro* methods of human IgE determinations (such as the commercially available Pharmacia Phadebas Rast and Phadebas IgE tests). The importance of *in vitro* tests cannot be overestimated as today it would be impossible to use the Prausnitz-Kuestner test in view of the possibility of transmission of the hepatitis and AIDS viruses. IgE is present in very small amount in the serum (nanogram amounts); for this reason it was not discovered earlier. IgE is also present in experimental animals. Here too, it is present in nanogram amounts and here too, it sensitizes for anaphylactic reactions. However, in addition to IgE in experimental animals there is often a class (or subclass) of IgG (IgG1 in guinea pig) which is present in milligram amounts and can also sensitize for anaphylactic reactions.

IgE is heat labile in every species which permits its inactivation easily *in vitro* and for some time this inactivation was used to demonstrate its presence. IgE is heavier than IgG (MW about 180,000) as its heavy chain has four constant domains rather than three like IgG.

In mice where no IgE myeloma has been found, PCA reaction was for 20 years the only method by which IgE could be detected and quantitated. In 1975, Kohler and Milstein constructed the first monoclonal antibody producing hybridoma.[33] This work had a tremendous effect on the development of immunology as it was possible now to use this technique for precise analysis of many different immunological reactions and reactants. In 1980 we constructed the first hybridoma producing monoclonal anti-dinitrophenyl IgE antibody derived from cells of BALB/c mice.[34] Nearly at the same time, Z. Eshhar[35] and David Katz[36] also constructed anti-DNP IgE producing hybridomas from cells derived from different strains of mice. It was now possible to use radioimmune assays and ELISA[37] instead of PCA for many investigations. The construction of monoclonal anti-murine IgE antibodies[38,39] made ELISA a very sensitive, reliable method for IgE antibody determinations. It must be underlined, however, that tremendous progress was accomplished using the PCA reaction and, in fact, progress was made because of the use of PCA. For certain investigations even today PCA is very useful.

As mentioned above, the Fc fragment of IgE carries the structure which can bind to Fcε receptors (FcεR). The FcεR on mast cells are those which must be bridged[14] to initiate the cascade of reactions which culminates in mast cell degranulation and histamine release. This cascade is initiated by activation of a serine esterase followed by activation of adenylate cyclase, Ca^{++} influx, activation of methyltransferases and many other events, the last of which is histamine release (reviewed in Ref.)[40] The bridging hypothesis was not the only consequence of the work done using PCA. Another and very important problem was the anchorage of antibody molecules to cellular receptors. The receptors on cells which bind the Fc fragment have been studied by many investigators. Metzger and his collaborators showed that the mast cell IgE receptor is a multichain molecule[41] and is made up from one alpha, one beta and two gamma chains. It is the first domain of the alpha chain which reacts with the structure on the Fc fragment of IgE. The chains have been sequenced, but we don't know anything about the tertiary and quaternary structures of the molecule (Metzger, personal communication). It is called the high affinity Fcε receptor (affinity of 5×10^8 to $1 \times 10)^{10}$ and also FcεRI. A second type of receptor for the IgE molecule has also been described. This is the low affinity IgE FcR also called FcεRII. Its affinity is of several order lower than of the FcεRI. The gene for FcεRII was cloned simultaneously by Kishimoto[42] and by Yodoi.[43] It is composed of a single chain. It turned out that this molecule had already been identified on the surface of B cells and was called CD23. Interestingly, there are two different forms of human Fcε Receptor II, the C terminal extracellular portion is the same in both, but the N terminal intracellular portion is different. FcεR IIa is expressed constitutively only on B cell lines, whereas Fcε R IIb is detectable also on other cell types such as monocytes and eosinophils. Normally FcεRIIb is undetectable on B cells and monocytes, however, it can be induced in B cells and monocytes by interleukin-4.[44]

Finally, with Lynch and Mathur we described a third type of IgE binding receptor on Lyt-2[+] cells.[45] The phenotype of this T cell is that of the so-called cytotoxic/suppressor phenotype: Lyt-2[+]3[+] also called CD8 T cell. Mathur showed that these T cells suppress the synthesis of the messenger RNA for the ε chain, even in the IgE producing hybridoma cells.[46]

Receptors for IgE, excluding the high affinity receptor on mast cells (FcεRI) might have a regulatory role on IgE production. We have just seen that Lyt-2[+] T cells can inhibit the synthesis of the IgE molecule. The regulation of IgE production by IgE receptors and IgE binding factors was extensively studied in the laboratories of K. Ishizaka and David Katz (reviewed in References).[47,48] A review concerning the structure and function of Fc receptors for IgE on lymphocytes, monocytes, and macrophages was published by Spiegelberg in 1984.[49] We mentioned above that we had shown that the integrity of the Fc fragment is necessary for fixation to mast cells.[22] However, that antibodies might fix to cells was shown already earlier by Boyden and Sorkin.[50,51] These authors coined the term "cytophilic" for those antibodies which were capable to "passively sensitize" cells. Berken and Benacerraf showed that only guinea pig IgG2 and not IgG1 is cytophylic for guinea pig macrophages.[52] With Tigelaar and Vaz we showed that mouse mast cells possess receptors for IgG molecules.[53] Unkeles et al. wrote a chapter in *Annual Review of Immunology*[54] which reviews the Fcγ receptor.

In 1962 we observed that when haptenated proteins are used as antigens for secondary anti-hapten antibody production, it is necessary that the hapten be coupled to the same carrier that was used to induce the primary response; this was called the "carrier effect".[55] About seven years later, Claman,[56] Miller and Mitchell,[57] Szenberg and Warner[58] showed that the lymphocytes involved in antibody production are divided into two distinct families: the B cell which actually produces the antibody (in this case against the hapten as epitope) and the T cells which do not produce antibodies. Mitchison[59] and Rajewsky[60] then showed that a subpopulation of T cells (generally L3T4[+] in mouse and T4[+] in humans) later called T helper cells (Th) recognizes the carrier protein and then help the B cells to produce antibodies. The carrier effect is thus due to the recognition by Th cells of the carrier protein.

Many scientists worked then to discover how B and T cells recognize the epitope (hapten) and the carrier protein. It was readily understood that the immunoglobulin, anchored to the surface of the B cell, recognizes the antigen by its specific epitope (in this case the hapten). This involves the recognition of the surface configuration in natural proteins, therefore it can be a recognition of tertiary or quaternary structures which may not exist in the unfolded protein. However the recognition mechanism used by T cells was for a long time elusive. Finally Davis and Hedrick[61] were able to identify the genes encoding the T cell receptor by differential hybridization. It turned out that the T cell receptor for antigen is also a two chain molecule and has domains similar to the antibody molecule. The studies of Marrack et al.,[62] Rock and Benacerraf[63] and that of Lanzavecchia[64] have shown that T cell recognition is a complex phenomenon. For effective antibody production most of the time T cell help is needed. However, the Th cell does not recognize the antigen if it is not "processed" and presented in the context of a Class major histocompatibility molecule, the Ia molecule, on the surface of the antigen-presenting cell. The first step in this process is the internalization of the entire antigenic molecule, the second is the unfolding and partial breakdown of the polypeptide chain of the antigen, the third is the exposition of the processed molecule on the membrane of the antigen-presenting cell, in context of the Ia molecule.

The macrophage-type antigen presenting cell can internalize any antigenic molecule, the B cell internalizes only those molecules which have epitopes recognized by the surface-anchored antibody molecule of the B cell. Thus, the B cell has specificity in the recognition process, the macrophage-type antigen presenting cell has no specificity. The hapten fixed to the carrier molecule is the specific epitope which the B cell recognizes. In native proteins the epitope is a surface structure. As proteins are folded polypeptide chains, it is possible that the epitope is formed by juxtaposition of amino acids which are far away from each other in the polypeptide chain. The exact mechanism of the "antigen processing" is not yet known. It is thought that the processing is necessary because it unfolds the protein and T cells, unlike B cells, recognize sequential (contiguous) amino acid structures. The unfolding of protein (the carrier moiety of the antigen) exposes amino acids which are recognized by the T cell and also other amino acids which might interact with the Ia molecule.[65,66,67,68] -68). B cells might recognize tertiary or quaternary structures, T cells recognize portions of the unfolded polypeptide chain of the carrier protein.

When L3T4 (CD4) T cells recognize the processed antigen fragment + the MHC Class II molecule (Ia molecule) on the surface of the antigen presenting B cell, the T cell is activated and one of the important consequences of this activation is the production and secretion of interleukins. We still do not know how these processes come about.

These developments have, of course, been progressive, but have occurred in a relatively very short time. The enigma now is the processing and how the processed antigen is then placed so that the T cell receptor can recognize it together with the Class II (or Class I) MHC molecules. The antigen processing is such an important phenomenon* that in 1988 an entire issue of *Immunological Review* was dedicated to "antigen processing".[69] This example shows how we progressed from the simple observation of the carrier effect to a much better understanding of antibody production.

We mentioned above the domains of immunoglobulins and that some of the different biological functions might be localized to different domains. It is interesting to note that many proteins involved in immunological interactions have domain structures: immunoglobulins, T cell receptors, MHC Class I and II molecules to mention only some of them. These molecules were grouped under the same name of immunoglobulin superfamily[70] and it is thought that they all derive from the primitive ancestral domain molecule.

Antibody production is sometimes rapidly terminated. It was in the 70s that Gershon called attention to the suppression of antibody production and hypothesized that not only T helper cells, but also T suppressor cells exist.[71]

---

*See chapter by Maxwell Richter in this volume.

Usually the phenotype of these two cells is different. In the human system the T4 cell is the so-called helper/inducer type, in the mouse the molecule which characterizes this cell is L3T4. The cytotoxic/suppressor T cell (Ts cell) is characterized in humans by the presence of the T8 antigen; in the mouse by the Lyt-2/3 molecule.

Suppression is a most complex phenomenon. In the early 70s it was thought that the T cell responsible for antibody suppression is Lyt-2$^+$ (murine system) or T8$^+$ (human system) cell. Today it is evident that a complex interaction between different types of T cells or their products is necessary to bring about antibody suppression. Tada was the first to show that in the rat a radiosensitive cell can suppress IgE production.[72]

Our experiments were the first to show that in the SJL strain of mice, an Lyt-1 (L3T4) cell must interact with other T cells to produce suppression of IgE production.[73] The great complication is however, that the T cell receptor of the suppressor cells has not yet been identified. It was not easy to identify the T cell receptor of the T helper or cytotoxic cells but the progress in that field was phenomenally fast. Antibody suppression was described more than 15 years ago and we still do not know the structure of the T cell receptor on suppressor T cells.

This opens perhaps different possibilities. The T suppressor cell might use a different recognition system. Below an alternative possibility will also be discussed. In any case, the phenomenon of antibody suppression is a real one and this is not questioned. By what mechanism it is obtained, and are there cells whose only function throughout their lifetime is suppression is open to debate.

The modulation of IgE production is a very complex phenomenon. We had seen that in mice injected with IgE-producing hybridoma cells, as long as the IgE is present in abundance in their sera it is impossible to obtain IgE antibody production by the normal B cells of the host.[74] For example, mice injected with anti-DNP IgE producing hybridoma cells did not produce anti-ovalbumin IgE when injected with ovalbumin. Lyt-2 lymphocytes bearing receptors for IgE were present in these mice.[75] As soon as the hybridoma was eliminated the anti-ovalbumin IgE appeared in their sera. I would like to mention here that we demonstrated that the half-life of the circulating IgE is very short (a few hours) compared to the half-life of IgG1.[76,77] The synthesis of anti-ovalbumin IgE in these mice immunized with ovalbumin after elimination of the anti-dinitrophenyl IgE producing hybridoma is very similar to what we described above concerning the presence of Lyt-2$^+$ cells with receptor for the Fc fragment of IgE mice bearing IgE producing hybridomas.[45]

Potentiation of IgE production by parasitic infections by helminths was studied by Ogilvie,[78] Orr,[79] Jarret[80] in England, and by Bloch,[81] Kojima and myself,[82] Ishizaka,[83] Urban and Katona[84] in this country.

We investigated the allotype of IgE in collaboration with Tomio Tada and his collaborators as we had an anti-DNP IgE producing hybridoma of the a allotype and they had the line from Eshhar, with the b allotype. We described allotype 7, i.e., the allotype of the murine IgE molecule.[85] Using many strains of mice, we found that mice from the SJA/9 strain did not produce anti-DNP IgE antibody when we immunized them using the schedule by which we got anti-dinitrophenyl IgE antibody in the SJL strain. The SJA/9 is congenic with the SJL and both have the same MHC complex. However, using the method of adoptive transfer, we showed that both the B and T cells of the SJA/9 strain can collaborate very well with the SJL T or B cells. This was a puzzle, as we did not understand how could the SJA/9 T or B cell collaborate with the T or B cells from the SJL strain and still not be able to collaborate between themselves. However, when we used SJA/9 mice infected with *Nippostrongylus brasiliensis* as donors of B cells, we got good anti-dinitrophenyl IgE antibody production in adoptive transfers. When the B cell donors from SJA/9 mice were injected one day before priming with SJL T cells we also got good IgE antibody production. From these experiments it was obvious that in ordinary conditions the SJA/9 mice lacked some sort of T cell activity.

We presented a hypothesis based on the above described experiments which postulated that for IgE production intervention of several sequential T cell actions are necessary and IgE antibody is secreted only after the last intervention of T helper cells (and antigen).[86] I could add now: "or the product of T helper cells."

Two great breakthroughs came in the mid-seventies which contributed to shape our thinking and helped to do successful research in the field of immunology. One was the construction of monoclonal antibodies by Kohler and Milstein in 1975 already mentioned,[33] the second was the discovery of the chromosomal organization of the immunoglobulin genes in 1976 by Tonegawa (reviewed in Reference).[87] That the molecule of immunoglobulin is made up from DNA segments (exons) separated by other DNA elements (introns) and that the rearrangement of the "germline" DNA is necessary for the actual protein producing template, or "rearranged" DNA was formidable novelty. These facts opened new horizons for the explanation of antibody diversity and also for the study of the stages of the formation of the immunoglobulins. It turned out that those DNA elements which do not code for the actual amino acid chains of the antibody are nonetheless very important elements as these introns contain the promoters, enhancers and possibly other elements necessary for the production of the antibody molecule.

In 1981 in England, Piper[88] and in Sweden, Samuelsson[89] identified the slow reacting substance of anaphylaxis (SRA-A) as the degradation products by lipooxygenase of arachidonic acid and they were called leukotrienes.

At the same time as these discoveries were made, other, also very important observations showed that different products of lymphocytes and mononuclear cells are necessary for antibody production and immunological reactions. Several of these "factors" were described by different authors. It was not an easy job to keep up to date with the different nomenclatures and the different descriptions of the "factors"! Sometimes the same products were described under different names! These products, synthesized by lymphocytes were called lymphokines and later, when they were cloned the word interleukin was adopted for many of them with a numerical suffix according to the order of definitive identification.

From the several monographs I quote only a few, such as those written by Howard and Paul on B cell growth and differentiation factors,[90] by Kendall Smith on interleukin-2,[91] and its receptor by Green and Leonard,[92] by Durum, Schmidt and Oppenheim on interleukin-1,[93] by Schrader on interleukin-3,[94] by Paul and Ohara on interleukin-4,[95] by Kishimoto and Hirano on interleukin-5 and interleukin-6.[96]

In the mid-eighties it has been seen that IL-4 is essential for production of IgE and IgG1.[97] It was therefore of great interest to study the IL-4 producing T cells. From the DNAX Laboratory, Mossman, Coffman and collaborators[98,99,100] cloned murine L3T4 (T helper) cell lines and showed that there are two different types of cloned L3T4 cells: one which produces among other lymphokines, IL-2 and interferon gamma, but not IL-4 and IL-5. This was called T helper 1, and the other which does not produce IL-2 nor interferon gamma but produces IL-4 and IL-5, was called T helper 2. The T helper 2 is essential for the production of IgE. We had shown that lipopolysaccharide stimulated normal spleen cells from SJA/9 and even from nude mice can produce IgE when IL-4 is added to the cultures.[101] It has been shown long ago that IgE production is absolutely T cell dependent.[102] Our earlier hypothesis was that sequential T cell interventions are necessary for IgE production or the switch to IgE production. These experiments are in line with this hypothesis. Though now we could formulate it in a somewhat modified form. One of the T helper cell (and its product) puts the apparatus of the B cell for antibody production in "motion." This first T cell interactions might be produced by a T helper 1 producing IL-2 or it might be already a T helper 2 producing IL-4. A second interaction, this time certainly by a T helper 2 cell and IL-4 will achieve the work for IgE secretion.

When I wrote above on the works done on antibody suppression, I mentioned that "an alternative possibility" will be discussed. We ourselves had seen that IgE antibody production can be greatly suppressed *in vivo* and that in this suppression an Lyt-1 cell is absolutely necessary.[103] We now have some new experiments, this time IgE suppression *in vitro*. When SJL or BALB/c spleen cells are cultured *in vitro* good IgE production is obtained if IL-4 is added to the cultures. However, if during the entire time of *in vitro* culture, we added also recombinant IL-2, in addition to the recombinant IL-4, IgE production was suppressed. This suppression was not abolished when anti-interferon antibody or normal rabbit serum was added (Hirano et al., submitted). We could postulate, therefore, that to obtain suppression of IgE antibody production it is not necessary to have a special "suppressor" cell. A product of the T helper cell 1 (IL-2, or interferon gamma, for example), if it reaches the cell at the critical time could have a suppressor effect. Suppression may be obtained therefore, without a specialized "suppressor" cell. It is also possible that suppression of antibody production can be obtained by several different mechanisms and the different pathways proposed by different authors are not absolutely exclusive.

We had discussed above antigen processing and the necessity of the processed antigen to be exposed on an Ia molecule. It has also been shown already in the seventies that a virus-infected cell is killed by cytotoxic T cells (CD8 or Lyt2/3) only if both cells have the same MHC[104] and that T cells do not get activated (do not react) against self antigens. To explain these facts a negative and a positive selection was proposed. According to this proposal, in the positive selection: a) progenitors of mature T cells get instructed (educated) in the thymus to recognize "self" MHC molecules; and b) they also get "educated" to recognize antigenic molecules only on a self MHC molecule. In the negative selection three possibilities might be effective: a) inactivation of self-reactive lymphocytes (clonal anergy); b) chronic suppression (clonal suppression); or c) elimination (clonal deletion).[105] However, we had to wait until 1987 when Kappler, Roehm and Marrack showed what T cell tolerance is obtained by clonal elimination.[106] Clonal deletion was confirmed also by other experiments.[107,108]

Quite recently positive selection was also demonstrated.[109,110] Moreover, the selection is operative on very young thymocytes which have both the CD4 and CD8 molecules.[111]

The technique of transgenic mice (reviewed in Reference)[112] is increasingly used to investigate immunological problems.

Discoveries of new facts in immunology developed exponentially in the last 40 years. Complement is an example of this. In 1959 when with Osler we showed that anaphylatoxin is formed from complement[113] there were four components of complement known. We did not even conceive that others might exist. Today not only nine (or eleven) components of the classical pathway have been identified, and 18 including both pathways and the regulatory mechanisms, but many of them have been sequenced and the genes cloned. From the concept of Ir genes (Benacerraf),[114] it was a long way, but rapidly conquered, to identify and sequence the products of these genes and show that they are molecules of the immunoglobulin superfamily.

My remembrances concern only a small portion of immunological research. I tried to restrict myself to the field where I actively worked. Many other, very important fields of immunological research were not even mentioned as I was reluctant to write about things which I really do not know. I kept in mind what I learned from my great former compatriot Selye;[115] "you really know only those things which you discovered yourself or which you have repeatedly experimentally verified."

Addendum

After the completion of this manuscript Metzger and collaborators published the cloning of the cDNA of the gamma chain of the Fc RI and proposed a model for alpha, beta, gamma tetramer which could "account for many of the structural features of the receptor".[116]

REFERENCES

1. **Prausnitz, C. and Kustner, H.,** Studien uber die Ueberempfindlichkeit, *Centralbl. f. Fakteriol.*, 86, 160, 1921.
2. **Heidelberger, M and Kendall, F.E.,** A quantitative study of the precipitin reaction between Type III Pneumococcus polysaccharide and purified hologous antibody, *J. Exp. Med.*, 50, 809, 1929.
3. **Tiselius, A. and Kabat, E.A.,** An electrophoretic study of immune sera and purified antibody preparations, *J. Exp. Med.*, 69, 119, 1939.
4. **Kabat, E.A. and Mayer, M.M.,** Antibodies and their characteristics, in *Experimental Immunochemistry*, Thomas, Springfield, 1961, pp. 326-360.
5. **Schultz, W.H.,** Physiological studies in anaphylaxis. I. The reaction of smooth muscle of guinea pig sensitized with horse serum, *J. Pharmacol. Exp. Therap.*, 1, 549, 1910.
6. **Dale, H.H.,** The anaphylactic reaction of plain muscle in the guinea pig, *J. Pharmacol. Exp. Therap.*, 4, 167, 1913.
7. **Jancso, M.,** Speicherung, Stoffanreicherung im Retikuloendothelial und in der Niere, *Publ. Akademiai Kiado*, Budapest, 1955.
8. **Lewis, Sir Thomas,** Local oedema and various means of producing the triple response, in *The Blood Vessels of the Human Skin and Their Responses*, Shaw and Sons, London, 1927.
9. **Halpern, B.N., Benacerraf, B., Biozzi, G., and Stiffel, C.,** Facteurs regissant la fonction phagocytaire du systeme reticuloendothelial, *Revue d'Hematologie*, 9, 621, 1954.
10. **Chase, M.,** Production of local skin reactivity by passive transfer of anti-protein sera, *Proc. Soc. Exp. Biol. Med.*, 52, 234, 1943.
11. **Ovary, Z.,** Passive cutaneous anaphylaxis, in *Immunological Methods, C.I.O.M.S. Symposium*, J.F. Ackroyd, Ed., Blackwell Scientific Publications, Oxford, 1964, pp. 259-184.

12. **Ovary, Z. and Karush, F.,** Studies on the immunologic mechanism of anaphylaxis. I. Antibody-hapten interactions studied by passive cutaneous anaphylaxis in the guinea pig, *J. Immunology*, 84, 409, 1960.

13. **Ovary, A.,** Activite des substances a faible poids moleculaire dans les reactions antigene-anticorps *in vivo* et *in vitro*, *Comptes Rendus des Seances de l'Academie des Sciences*, 233, 582, 1961.

14. **Ovary, Z.,** The mechanism of passive sensitization in PCA and RPCA in guinea pigs. Proceedings of the 3rd International Pharmacology Meeting, July 24-30, 1966. *Immunopharmacology*, 11, 15, 1968.

15. **Ishizaka, T., Hirata, F., Sterk, A.R., Ishizaka, K. and Axelrod, J.A.,** Bridging of IgE receptors activates phospholipid methylation and adenylate cyclase in mast cell plasma membranes, *Proc. Natl. Acad. Sci. USA*, 78, 6812, 1981.

16. **Porter, R.R.,** The hydrolysis of rabbit gamma globulin and antibodies with crystalline papain, *Biochemical J.*, 73, 119, 1959.

17. **Ovary, Z and Karush, F.,** Studies on the immunologic mechanism of anaphylaxis, II. Sensitizing and combining capacity *in vivo* of fractions separated from papain digests of antihapten antibody, *J. Immunol.*, 86, 146, 1961.

18. **Nisonoff, A., Wissler, F.C., Lipman, L.N. and Woernley, D.L.,** Separation of univalent fragments from the bivalent rabbit antibody molecule by reduction of disulfide bond, *Arch. Biochem. Biophysics*, 89, 230, 1960.

19. **Taranta, A., Franklin, E.C. and Ovary, Z.,** Studies of gamma globulin fragments in C' fixation, immune hemolysis and passive cutaneous anaphylaxis, *Fed. Proc.*, 21, 32, 1962.

20. **Porter, R.R.,** in *Symposium on Basic Problems in Neoplastic Disease*, A. Gellhorn and E. Hirschberg, Eds., Columbia University Press, 1962, pp. 177-194.

21. **Hilschmann, N. and Craig, L.C.,** Amino acid sequence studies with Bence-Jones proteins, *Proc. Natl. Acad. Sci. USA*, 53, 1903, 1965.

22. **Ovary, Z., Saluk, P.H., Quijada, L. and Lamm, M.D.,** Biologic activities of rabbit immunoglobulin G in relation to domains of the Fc region, *J. Immunol.*, 116, 1265, 1976.

23. **Helm, B., Marsh, P., Vercelli, D., Padlan, E., Gould, H. and Geha, R.,** The mast cell binding site on human immunoglobulin E, *Nature*, 331, 180, 1988.

24. **Kebo, D., Glovsky, M.M., Heim, B. and Gould, H.,** Recombinant IgE (301-376) inhibition of passive transfer on reagin and IgE to human basophils, *Fed. Proc.*, 5531, 1988.

25. **Ovary, Z. and Benacerraf, B.,** Separation of skin sensitizing from blocking 7S antibodies in guinea pig sera, *Fed. Proc.*, 21, 32, 1962.

26. **Benacerraf, B., Ovary, Z., Bloch, K. J. and Franklin, E. C.,,** Properties of guinea pig 7S antibodies, *J. Exp. Med.*, 117, 937, 1963.

27. **Ovary, Z., Benacerraf, B. and Bloch, K.J.,** Properties of guinea pig 7S antibodies, II. Identification of antibodies involved in passive cutaneous and systemic anaphylaxis, *J. Exp. Med.*, 117, 951, 1963.

28. **Bloch, K.J., Kourilsky, F.M., Ovary, Z. and Benacerraf, B.,** Properties of guinea pig 7S antibodies, III. Identification of antibodies involved in complement fixation and hemolysis, *J. Exp. Med.* 117, 965, 1963.

29. **Loveless, M.H.,** Reagin production in a healthy male who forms no detectable β_{2A} immunoglobulins, *Fed. Proc.*, 23, 403, 1964.

30. **Ishizaka, K., Ishizaka, T. and Hornbrook, M.,** Physicochemical properties of reaginic antibodies. V. Correlation of reaginic activity with gamma-E-globulin antibody, *J. Immunol.*, 92, 840, 1966.

31. **Ishizaka, K. and Ishizaka, T.,** Identification of E-antibody as a carrier of reaginic activity, *J. Immunol.*, 99, 1187, 1967.

32. **Johansson, S.G.O. and Bennich, H.,** Immunological studies of an atypical (myeloma) immunoglobulin, *Immunology*, 12, 381, 1967.

33. **Kohler, G. and Milstein, C.,** Continuous cultures of fused cells secreting antibody or predefined specificity, *Nature*, 256, 495, 1975.

34. **Bottcher, I., Ulrich, M., Hirayama, N. and Ovary, Z.,** Production of monoclonal mouse IgE antibodies with DNP specificity by hybrid cell lines, *Int. Arch. Allergy Appl. Immunol.*, 61, 248, 1980.

35. Eshhar, Z., Ofarim, M. and Waks, T., Generation of hybridomas secreting murine reaginic antibodies of anti-DNP specificity, *J. Immunol.*, 124, 775, 1980.

36. Liu, F., Goh, J.W., Ferry, E.L., Yamamoto, H., Molinaro, C.A., Sherman, L.A., Klinman, N.R. and Katz, D.H., Monoclonal dinitrophenyl-specific murine IgE antibody: preparation, isolation and characterization, *J. Immunol.*, 124, 2728, 1980.

37. Maekawa, S. and Ovary, Z. Correlation of murine anti-dinitrophenyl antibody content as determined by ELISA, passive cutaneous anaphylaxis and passive hemolysis, *J. Immunol. Meth.*, 71, 229, 1984.

38. Baniyash, M. and Eshhar, Z., Inhibition of IgE binding to mast cells and basophils by monoclonal antibodies to murine IgE, *Eur. J. Immunol.*, 14, 799, 1984.

39. Hirano, T., Miyajima, H., Kitagawa, H., Watanabe, N., Azuma, M., Taniguchi, O., Hashimoto, H., Hirose, S., Yagit, H., Furusawa, S., Ovary, Z. and Okumura, K., Studies of murine IgE with monoclonal antibodies, I. Characterization of rat monoclonal anti-IgE antibodies and the use of these antibodies for determination of serum IgE levels and for anaphylactic reactions, *Int. Arch. Allergy Appl. Immunol.*, 85, 47, 1988.

40. Ishizaka, T., Biochemical analysis of mast cell induced triggering by bridging IgE receptors, in *Structure and Function of Fc Receptors*, A. Froese and P. Paraskevas, Eds., Marcel Dekker, Inc., New York, 1983, pp. 157-176.

41. Metzger, H., Alcaraz, G., Hohman, R., Kinet, J.-P., Pribluda, V., and Quarto, R., The receptor with high affinity for immunoglobulin E, *Ann. Rev. Immunol.*, 4, 419, 1986.

42. Kikutani, H., Inui, S., Sato, R., Barsoumian, E.L., Owaki, H., Yamasuki, K., Kaisho, T., Uchibayashi, N., Hardy, R.R., Hirano, T., Tsunusaura, S., Sakiyama, F., Suemura, M. and Kishimoto, T., Molecular structure of human lymphocyte receptor of immunoglobulin E, *Cell*, 47, 657, 1986.

43. Ikuta, K., Takami, M., Won Kim, C., Honjo, T., Miyoshi, T., Tagaya, Y., Kawabe, T. and Yodoi, J., Human lymphocyte Fc receptor for IgE: Sequence homology of its cloned cDNA with animal lectins, *Proc. Natl. Acad. Sci. USA*, 84, 819, 1987.

44. Yokota, A., Kikutani, H., Tanaka, T., Sato, R., Barsumian, E.L., Suemura, M. and Kishimoto, T., Two species of human Fc receptor II (FC RII/CD23): tissue specific and IL-4 specific regulation of gene expression, *Cell*, 55, 611, 1988.

45. Mathur, A., Makeawa, S., Ovary, Z. and Lynch, R.G., Increased T-cells in BALB/c mice with an IgE secreting hybridoma, *Mol. Immunol.*, 23, 1193, 1986.

46. Mathur, A., Kamat, D.M., Van Ness, B.G. and Lynch, R.G., Thymus-dependent *in vivo* suppression of IgE synthesis in a murine IgE-secreting hybridoma, *J. Immunol.*, 139, 2865, 1987.

47. Ishizaka, K., Regulation of IgE synthesis, *Ann. Rev. Immunol.*, 2, 159, 1984.

48. Marcelletti, J.F. and Katz, D.H., FcR $^+$ lymphocytes and regulation of the IgE antibody system. I. A new class of molecules termed IgE-induced regulants (EIR), which modulate FcR expression by lymphocytes, *J. Immunol.*, 133, 2821, 1984.

49. Spiegelberg, H.L., Structure and function of Fc receptors for IgE on lymphocytes, monocytes and macrophages, *Adv. Immunol.*, 35, 6188, 1984.

50. Boyden, S.V. and Sorkin, E., The adsorption of antibody and antigen by spleen cells *in vitro*, Some further experiments, *Immunology*, 4, 244, 1961.

51. Boyden, S.V., Cytophilic antibody in guinea pigs with delayed type hypersensitivity, *Immunology*, 7, 474, 1964.

52. Berken, A. and Benacerraf, B., Properties of antibodies cytophylic for macrophages, *J. Exp. Med.*, 123, 119, 1966.

53. Tigelaar, R.E., Vaz, N.M. and Ovary, Z., Immunoglobulin receptors on mouse mast cells, *J. Immunol.*, 106, 661, 1971.

54. Unkeles, J.C., Scigliano, E. and Freedman, V., Structure and function of human and murine receptors for IgG, *Ann. Rev. Immunol.*, 6, 251, 1988.

55. Ovary, Z. and Benacerraf, B., Immunological specificity of the secondary response with dinitrophenylated proteins, *Proc. Soc. Exp. Biol. Med.*, 114, 72, 1963.

56. Claman, H.N., Chaperon, E.A. and Triplett, R.F., Incompetence of transferred thymus-marrow cell combinations, *J. Immunol.*, 97, 828, 1966.

57. Miller, J.F.A.P., Mitchell, G.F. and Weiss, N.S., Cellular basis of the immunological defect in thymectomized mice, *Nature*, 214, 292, 1967.

58. Szenberg, A. and Warner, N.L., The role of antibody in delayed hypersensitivity, *Brit. Med. Bull.*, 23, 30, 1967.

59. Mitchison, N.A., The carrier effect in the secondary response to hapten-protein conjugates, II. Cellular cooperation, *Eur. J. Immunol.*, 1, 18, 1971.

60. Rajewsky, K., The carrier effect in the induction of antibodies, *Proc. Roy. Soc. Lond. (Biol.)*, 176, 385, 1971.

61. Hedrick, S.M., Cohen, D.I., Neilsen, E.A. and Davis, M.M., Isolation of CDNA clones encoding T cell-specific membrane-associated proteins, *Nature*, 308, 149, 1984.

62. Shimonkevitz, R., Kappler, J., Marrack, P. and Grey, H.M., Antigen recognition by H-2 restricted T cells, Cell-free antigen processing, *J. Exp. Med.*, 158, 303, 1983.

63. Rock, K.B., Benacerraf, B. and Abbas, A.K., Antigen presentation by hapten-specific B lymphocytes, I. Role of surface immunoglobulin receptors, *J. Exp. Med.*, 160, 1102, 1984.

64. Lanzavecchia, A., Antigen-specific interaction between T and B cells, *Nature*, 314, 537, 1985.

65. Benjamin, D.C., Berzofsky, J.A., East, I.J., Gurd, F.R.N., Hannum, C., Leach, S., Margoliash, E., Michael, J.G., Moller, A., Prager, E.M., Reichlin, M., Sercarz, E.E., Smith-Gill, S.J., Todd, P.A. and Wilson, A.C., The antigenic structure of proteins: a reappraisal, *Ann. Rev. Immunol.*, 2, 67, 1984.

66. Berkower, I., Buckenmeyer, G. K. and Berzofsky, J. A., Molecular mapping of a histocompatibility-restricted immunodominant T cell epitope with synthetic and natural peptides: Implications for T cell antigenic structure, *J. Immunol.*, 136, 2498, 1986.

67. Sette, A., Buus, S., Colon, S., Smith, J.A., Miles, C. and Grey, H.M., Structural characteristics of an antigen required for its interaction with Ia and recognition by T cells, *Nature*, 328, 395, 1987.

68. Allen, P.M., Matsueda, G.M., Evans, R.J., Dunbar, Jr., J.M., Marshall, G.R. and Unanue, E.R., Identification of the T cell and Ia contact residues of a T cell antigenic epitope, *Nature*, 327, 713, 1987.

69. Möller, G., Ed. Antigen processing, *Immunol. Rev.*, 106, 1988.

70. Hood, L., Kronenberg, M. and Hunkapiller, T., T cell antigen receptors and the immunoglobulin supergene family, *Cell*, 40, 225, 1985.

71. Gershon, R.K. and Kondo, K., Cell interaction in the induction of tolerance: the role of thymic lymphocytes, *Immunology*, 18, 723, 1970.

72. Tada, T., Taniguchi, M. and Okumura, K., Regulation of homocytotropic antibody formation in the rat, II. Effect of X-irradiation, *J. Immunol.*, 106, 1012, 1971.

73. Watanabe, N., Kojima, S., Shen, F.W. and Ovary, Z., Suppression of IgE antibody production in SJL mice, II. Expression of Ly-1 antigen on helper and nonspecific suppressor T cells, *J. Immunol.*, 118, 485, 1977.

74. Hirano, T. and Ovary, Z., Studies on immunity in hybridoma-bearing mice. A. Immune response to antigens, I. Role of subcutaneously injected IgE-producing hybridoma on antibody production of different isotypes against immunizing antigen, *Int. Arch. Allergy Appl. Immunol.*, 73, 338, 1984.

75. Hoover, R.G., Gebel, H.M., Dieckgraefe, B.K., Hickman, S., Rebbe, N.F., Hirayama, N., Ovary, Z. and Lynch, R.G., Occurrence and potential significance of increased numbers of T cells with Fc receptors in myeloma, *Immunol. Rev.*, 56, 115, 1981.

76. Hirano, T., Hom, Ch. and Ovary, Z., Half-life of murine IgE antibodies in the mouse, *Int. Arch. Allergy Appl. Immunol.*, 71, 182, 1983.

77. Haba, S., Ovary, Z. and Nisonoff, A., Clearance of IgE from serum of normal and hybridoma-bearing mice, *J. Immunol.*, 134, 3291, 1985.

78. Ogilvie, B.M. and Jones, V.E., Reaginic antibodies and helminth infection. In: *Cellular and Humoral Mechanism of Anaphylaxis and Allergy. Mechanism of Anaphylaxis and Allergy*, H.Z. Movat, Ed., Karger, Basel, 1970, p. 13.

79. Orr, T.S.C. and Blair, A.M.J., Potentiated reagin response to egg-albumin and conalbumin in *N. brasiliensis* infected rat, *Life Sci.*, 8(11), 1073, 1969.

80. Jarrett, E.E.E., Potentiation of reaginic antibody to ovalbumin in rat, *Immunology*, 22, 1099, 1972.

81. Bloch, K.J. and Wilson, R.J.M., Homocytotropic antibody response in the rat infected with the nematode, *Nippostrongylus brasiliensis*, *J. Immunol.*, 100, 629, 1968.

82. Kojima, S. and Ovary, Z., Effect of *Nippostrongylus brasiliensis* infection on anti-hapten IgE antibody response to a heterologous hapten-carrier conjugate, *Cell Immunol.*, 17, 383, 1975.

83. Ishizaka, T., Urban, J.F. and Ishizaka, K., IgE formation in rat following infection with *Nippostrongylus brasiliensis*, Proliferation and differentiation of IgE bearing cells, *Cell. Immunol.*, 22, 248, 1976.

84. Katona, I.M., Urban, J.F., Scher, I., Kanellopoulos-Langevin, C. and Finkelman, F.D., Induction of an IgE response in mice by *Nippostronglylus brasiliensis*: characterization of lymphoid cells with intracellular or surface IgE, *J. Immunol.*, 130, 350, 1983.

85. Borges, M.S., Kumagai, Y., Okumura, K., Hirayama, N., Ovary, Z. and Tada, T., Allelic polymorphism of murine IgE controlled by the seventh immunoglobulin heavy chain allotype locus, *Immunogenetics*, 13, 499, 1981.

86. Hirano, T., Kumagai, Y., Okumura, K. and Ovary, Z., Regulation of murine IgE production: importance of a not-yet described T cell for IgE secretion demonstrated in SJA/9 mice, *Proc. Natl. Acad. Sci. USA*, 80, 3435, 1983.

87. Tonegawa, S., Somatic generation of antibody diversity, *Nature*, 302, 575, 1983.

88. Piper, P.J., Samhoun, M.N., Tippins, J.R., Morris, H.R., Jones, C.M., *Int. Arc. Allergy Appl. Immunol.*, 66(Suppl. 1), 107, 1981.

89. Samuelsson, B., Leukotrienes: mediators of allergic reactions and inflammation, *Int. Arch. Allergy Appl. Immunol.*, 66(Suppl. 1, 98, 1981.

90. Howard, M. and Paul. W.E., Regulation of B cell growth and differentiation by soluble factors, *Ann. Rev. Immunol.*, 1, 307, 1983.

91. Smith, K.A., Interleukin-2, *Ann. Rev. Immunol.*, 2, 319, 1984.

92. Greene, W.C. and Leonard, W.J., The human interleukin-2- receptor, *Ann. Rev. Immunol.*, 4, 69, 1985.

93. Durum, S.K., Schmidt, J.A. and Oppenheim, J.J., Interleukin-1: an immunological perspective, *Ann. Rev. Immunol.*, 3, 263, 1985.

94. Schrader, J.W., The panspecific hemopoietin of activated T lymphocytes (interleukin-3), *Ann. Rev. Immunol.*, 4, 205, 1986.

95. Paul, W.E. and Ohara, J., B cell stimulatory factor 1/interleukin-4, *Ann. Rev. Immunol.*, 5, 429, 1987.

96. Kishimoto, T. and Hirano, T., Molecular regulation of B lymphocyte response, *Ann. Rev. Immunol.*, 6, 485, 1988.

97. Vitetta, E.S., Ohara, J., Myers, C., Layton, J., Kramer, P.H. and Paul, W.E., Serological, biochemical, and functional identity of B cell stimulatory factor 1 and B cell differentiating factor for IgG1, *J. Exp. Med.*, 162, 1726, 1985.

98. Coffman, R.L.., Ohara, J., Bond, M.W., Carty, J., Zlotnick, E. and Paul, W.E., B cell stimulatory factor enhances the IgE response of lipopolysaccharide activated B cells, *J. Immunol.*, 136, 4538, 1968.

99. Coffman, R.L. and Carty, J., A T cell activity that enhances polyclonal IgE production and its inhibition by interferon gamma, *J. Immunol.*, 136, 949, 1986.

100. Mossmann, R.R., Cherwinski, H., Bond, M.W., Giedlin, M.A. and Coffman, R.L., Two types of murine helper T cell clones, I. Definition according to profiles of lymphokine activities and secreted proteins, *J. Immunol.*, 136, 2348, 1986.

101. Azuma, M., Hirano, T., Miyajima, H., Watanabe, N., Yagita, H., Enomoto, S., Furusawa, S., Ovary, Z., Kinashi, T., Honjo, T. and Okumura, K., Regulation of murine IgE production in SJA/9 and in nude mice, Potentiation of IgE production by recombinant interleukin-4, *J. Immunol.*, 139, 2538, 1973.

102. Michael, J.G. and Bernstein, I.L., Thymus dependence of reaginic antibody formation in mice, *J. Immunol.*, 111, 1600, 1973.

103. Itaya, T. and Ovary, Z., Suppression of IgE antibody production in SJL mice. IV. Interaction of primed and unprimed T cells, *J. Exp. Med.*, 507, 1979.

104. Zinkernagel, R.M. and Doherty, P.C., Restriction of *in vitro* T cell-mediated cytotoxicity within a syngeneic or semiallogeneic system, *Nature*, 248, 701, 1974.

105. Robertson, M. Tolerance, restriction and the MLs enigma. Nature 332: 18-19, 1988.

106. Kappler, J.W., Roehm, N. and Marrack, P.C., T cell tolerance by clonal elimination in the thymus, *Cell*, 49, 273, 1987.

107. Kappler, J.W., Staerz, U., White, J. and Marrack, P.C., Self-tolerance eliminates T cell specific for MLs-modified products of the major histocompatibility complex, *Nature*, 332, 35, 1988.

108. MacDonald, H.R., Schnieder, R., Less, R.K., Howe, T.C., Acha-Orbea, H., Festenstein, H., Zinkernagel, R.M. and Hengartner, H., *Nature*, 332, 40, 1988.

109.   **Kisielow, P., Teh, H.S., Bluthmann, H. and von Bohmer, H.,** Positive selection of antigen-specific T cells in thymus by restricting MHC molecules, *Nature*, 335, 730, 1988.

110.   **MacDonald, R.H., Lees, R.K., Schneider, R., Zinkernagel, R.M. and Hengartner, H.,** Positive selection of CD4$^+$ thymocytes controlled by MHC class II gene products, *Nature*, 336, 471, 1988.

111.   **Teh, H.S., Kisielow, P., Scott, B., Kishi, H., Uematsu, Y., Bluthmann, H., and von Bohmer, H.,** Thymic major histocompatibility complex antigens and the T cell receptor determine the CD4/CD8 phenotype of T cells, *Nature*, 335, 229, 1988.

112.   **Palmiter, R.D. and Brinster, R.L.,** Transgenic mice, *Cell*, 41, 343, 1985.

113.   **Osler, A.G, Randall, H.G., Hill, B.M. and Ovary, Z.,** Studies on the mechanism of hypersensitivity phenomena, III. The participation of complement in the formation of anaphylatoxin, *J. Exp. Med. Med.*, 110, 311, 1959.

114.   **Benacerraf, B.,** *The Genetic Control of Specific Immune Responses, The Harvey Lectures*, Academic Press, New York, 1973.

115.   **Selye, H.,** *The Story of the Adaptation Syndrome*, Acta Inc. Medical Publishers, Canada, 1952.

116.   **Blank, U., Ra, C., Miller, L., White, K, Metzger, H. and Kinet, J.-P.,** Complete structure and expression in transferred cells of high affinity IgE receptor, *Nature*, 337, 187, 1989.

Chapter 19

TISSUE ANAPHYLACTIC SENSITIZATION, IMMUNOSUPPRESSIVE PROCESSES AND ANTIBODY PRODUCING CELLS

P. Liacopoulos

The rapid development of immunology in the last two or three decades in deepening the understanding of its own mechanisms as well as in spreading over other areas of biomedical sciences, makes it worthy to undertake a revisiting of the accomplishments and a reevaluation of previous theories attempting to complete gaps of scientific knowledge. Indeed, tendency to formulate a comprehensive image of the surrounding world was always innate to human spirit. Continuous emergence of new findings often invalidated previous theories and replaced them by new concepts more close to the reality not without much fighting between supporters of the older and the newer.

During the one hundred years of immunology, several concepts arose and vanished as confronted by scientifically better established findings, especially after World War II, a period of major progress in all fields of science. This author's work was involved in three areas of immunology where he made his modest contribution; namely, the mechanism of tissue anaphylactic sensitization, the immunosuppressive processes and potentiality of the antibody-producing cell.

TISSUE ANAPHYLACTIC SENSITIZATION

Already before the '40s, the humoral theory of anaphylaxis had become unsupportable because experiments showed that excised and washed muscles of sensitized animals would react *in vitro* to the addition of the specific antigen even when the blood was completely absent. The results of these experiments led to the cellular theory of anaphylaxis. It became, thereafter, unanimously acknowledged that anaphylactic reactions result from the interaction between the antigen and the anaphylactic antibody (IgG_1, IgE) that takes place upon the cells. It was demonstrated, furthermore, that the clinical symptoms of anaphylaxis are caused by mediators such as histamine, serotonin, heparin, leukotrienes and others released by the cells (mast cells, basophils) as a consequence of the antigen-antibody reaction.

In the framework of the cellular theory it was assumed that the main prerequisite for achieving tissue sensitization in order to regularly elicit anaphylactic reactions, was the antibody fixation on the sensitive cells. In an attempt to study the mechanism of this fixation, we undertook in collaboration with B.N. Halpern and R. Binaghi, a systematic investigation of the process of *in vitro* anaphylactic sensitization of guinea pig ileums. This method allowed the study of several parameters of the sensitization. Having first shown that passive *in vitro* sensitization obeys similar rules as *in vivo* sensitization, we moved forward to study its properties.[1] We thus showed that the degree of sensitization increases as antibody concentration rises in the incubating medium or as incubation time is extended when antibody concentration remains constant. However, in order to obtain an equal degree of sensitization, the antibody concentration should vary in relationship to the reciprocal of the square of the time of incubation [$C = f(1/t2)$]. This type of relationship is not an artifact of *in vitro* sensitization. The *in vivo* experiments of Benacerraf and Kabat[2] showed that when the quantity of antibody necessary to obtain a given intensity of reaction (fatal anaphylactic shock in guinea pigs) is plotted against the inverse of the square of the time interval between injections of antibody and antigen, the same linear relationship is found.

Other parameters of anaphylactic sensitization were also found. Thus, lowering the temperature considerably slowed down the process of sensitization. At 38°C, 60 min was required for obtaining a given degree of reaction; at 10°C the necessary time was 420 min. Tissue sensitization was even possible at 5°C by further lengthening the time of incubation. Unlike the temperature correlations, tissue sensitization was similar either at pH 8.0 or 5.6 provided that the incubating medium was acidified.

Pursuing our investigation in this field, we found that a 0.8 M concentration of urea in the incubating medium enhanced the process of sensitization of the ileum strip by about 4 times, regardless of whether this enhancement was measured by the concentration of antibody or by the incubation time necessary to obtain the same anaphylactic reaction.[3] An even greater increase in the intensity of sensitization (about 10 times) was produced when the *in vitro* sensitization of the tissue was performed in media of low electrolytic concentration where the standard Tyrode solution was replaced by an isotonic glucose solution containing 0.0005 M $NaHCO_3/L$.[4] The results of both these types of experiments pointed out the importance of physico-chemical properties of the medium on the process of sensitization. The decrease of the hydrogen bonds between antibody molecules and water caused by the urea and this of interactions between antibody molecules and ions or between antibody and gamma-globulin molecules which depend upon the ionic strength of the medium would either facilitate diffusion of antibody through the tissues or promote interactions between antibody and sensitive cell membranes.

Several publications during the '50s have indicated that the efficacy of antibody in inducing the anaphylactic phenomenon is decreased by the simultaneous presence of non-specific gamma-globulin. These observations favored the idea that nonspecific gamma-globulins compete with antibody for cellular receptors involved in sensitization.[5] Using the same method of *in vitro* sensitization of guinea pig ileum strips, we found that when non-specific gamma-globulins were added to the incubating medium containing rabbit antibody, the inhibition of the passive sensitization of the strip occurred in a quantitative manner. In this type of inhibition the rabbit gamma-globulins were found to be the most active. However, in contrast to what was previously assumed that only gamma-globulins originating from the species of the antibody sensitizing guinea pig tissues, we found that such interactions could occur with gamma-globulins of every animal origin, although higher concentrations were needed. When rabbit antibody was used for sensitization of guinea pig tissues the competitive effect of gamma-globulins of various species decreased in the following order: rabbit > man > dog > guinea pig > rat > horse > cattle > pig > chicken > goat. Although horse, chicken, or goat antibody do not passively sensitize *in vivo* the guinea pig or its organs, gamma-globulins from these species used in adequate concentrations definitely compete with *in vitro* passive sensitization.[6] Moreover, our experiments showed that the competition between antibody and nonspecific gamma-globulins only modify the kinetics of the sensitization process but not the final result. When a sufficient period of incubation is allowed *in vivo* or *in vitro*, tissue sensitization is achieved in spite of the presence of nonspecific gamma-globulins.

Another interesting observation during this study was made with respect to the relationship between antibody concentration in the incubating medium, and the time of incubation for obtaining a given degree of anaphylactic sensitization. We previously mentioned that this antibody concentration is related to the reciprocal of the square of the incubation time ($c = f \ 1/t \ 2$). In this case increased antibody concentration also involved increased non-antibody gamma-globulins since *in vitro* sensitization was performed with dilutions of rabbit immune serum. However, when care was taken to keep constant the total gamma-globulin content of the sensitizing medium this relationship was found to be ($c = f \ 1/t$), i.e., the antibody concentration was proportional to the reciprocal of the incubation time and not to the reciprocal of the square of the incubation time.[6]

The whole body of these observations did not favor the concept of the existence of cellular receptors for anaphylactic gamma-globulins on the membranae of sensitive cells which prevailed in the '50s. Rather, it pointed out the importance of the diffusion process of gamma-globulins into the tissues towards the sensitive cells and especially the quantitative requirements of local antibody concentrations in eliciting the anaphylactic reaction.

While this work was in progress Germuth and McKinnon (1957) showed that soluble antigen-antibody complexes formed in slight to moderate antigen excess were anaphylactogenic. Moreover, Ishizaka et al. (1959) demonstrated that the antigen-antibody complexes are active only when formed in the range from antibody excess to slight or moderate antigen excess ($Ag \ Ab_2$, $Ag_2 \ Ab_2$, $Ag_3 \ Ab_2$). These so-called toxic complexes are most active in triggering anaphylactic reactions, whereas those formed in extreme antigen excess ($Ag_2 \ Ab$) were inactive. Complexes formed in extreme antigen excess are unable to bridge antibodies because both combining sites on each antibody molecule are attached to two different antigen molecules.[7] These findings were consistent with the requirement of antibody fixation on cellular receptors before anaphylactic reactions can be triggered. Immobilization of antibody molecules on a solid support should prevent them from entering into free quantitative relationships with antigen as it happens in precipitin reactions where antigen excess inhibits precipitation. The issue of need of antibody fixation on specific cellular receptors arisen from the aforementioned work, prompted us to undertake further investigations on the effect of antigen excess on the anaphylactic reaction. These experiments showed that antigen excess *in vitro* as well as *in vivo* indeed inhibits anaphylactic reactions provided that the excess is sufficiently large (1,000 x more than optimum amount).[8] Requirement of such an excess can be readily understood if one takes into account the rate of diffusion of antigen into the tissues. As the local antigen concentration gradually increases, as soon as the optimal concentration is reached, the anaphylactic reaction is launched irrespective of the concentration achieved afterwards. Therefore, the large antigen excess is necessary for rapidly reaching a local excess, i.e., to directly form complexes with antibody of the configuration $Ag_2 \ Ab$ which are inactive. The prevalence of active complex formation over antibody fixation was further supported by the demonstration that even in the case of reagins (IgE) which are known to firmly bind to mast cells and basophils, the use of antigen in excess similarly inhibits the allergic reaction.[9]

The better understanding of the quantitative requirements of antigen and antibody concentrations in eliciting anaphylactic reactions allowed us to show that reverse anaphylactic reactions, i.e., first sensitizing the tissues with antigen, even if it is an albumin such as egg albumin, and then adding the antibody, can be regularly produced *in vitro* or *in vivo*,[10,11] although such procedure was considered to be restricted to the use of gamma-globulin as antigen and of the same species of which the antibody was derived for sensitization of guinea pig tissues.[12]

IMMUNOSUPPRESSIVE PROCESSES

Under adequate conditions, administration of an antigen could lead not simply to an epidose of lack of response but to a real unresponsiveness, i.e., a new administration of the same antigen, even associated with adjuvants, fails to elicit an immunological response. This phenomenon has been discovered by Medawar and his associates in the early '50s and called **tolerance**.[13] This type of immunological suppression induced by transfer of lymphoid cells into allogenic fetuses or newborn animals, and these recipients, reaching adulthood, tolerated grafts of donor tissues. Another type of induced unresponsiveness was described ten years earlier by Felton and Ottinger.[14] It was produced in adult mice in injection of large doses of pneumococcal polysaccharides and termed immune paralysis. As both types of unresponsiveness were long lasting and specific, the term tolerance prevailed for designating the inhibition of immunological responses resulting from previous treatment with the same antigen.

Concerning the specificity of tolerance, a number of discrepancies observed by various authors cast some doubt on whether tolerance is as specific as the immunological response. In the early '60s we undertook a systematic study on the specificity of tolerance induced in adult animals by large doses of antigen given for several days. It was found that when an unrelated antigen in an immunizing form was given during the tolerance inducing treatment with a common antigen such as serum albumin or gamma-globulin, the response to the former antigen could be inhibited.[15,16] The degree of inhibition varied according to the day of immunization in relation with the tolerance inducing treatment. When the second antigen was given between the 3rd and 15th day, the response to this second antigen was almost completely suppressed. But when the second antigen was injected after the 20th day of the tolerance inducing treatment, the response to this was again almost normal.[17] This series of experiments pointed out first, that once immunological tolerance was induced it is as specific as the immune response but during the period of its induction the response to unrelated antigens is regularly inhibited. Second, the suppression brought about during the inductive phase of tolerance affects all types of immune responses, i.e., antibody production as well as delayed hypersensitivity,[18] host-vs-graft[19] and graft-vs-host[20] reactions.

This type of immunosuppression was of particular interest since, unlike the known immunosuppressive drugs, it respects the integrity of immunocompetent cells, the inhibition being only functional. As such, it appeared to be very convenient for inhibiting histoincompatibility reactions. However, the inhibition of the unrelated response during the tolerance inducing treatment being of short duration, long-lasting immunological reactions as homograft rejection, were only temporarily inhibited, e.g., the graft survival time was prolonged by 3 to 4 times. Yet, graft-versus-host reactions could be definitely inhibited.[20]   This finding allowed to carry on the following strategy for inducing long-lasting transplantation tolerance: future donor mice were treated for 6 to 8 days with an antigen then their spleen cells harvested and transferred to mid-lethally (500 r) irradiated recipients.   This procedure applied to combination of mice of weak histocompatibility differences such as Balb/c donors to DBA/2 recipients, sharing the same H_2 locus, donor pretreatment with rabbit gamma-globulin resulted in the inhibition of the GVH mortality and also in the permanent survival of donor skin grafts in almost 100% of the experimental recipients as compared to only 16% control recipients which received cells from untreated donors.[21] The results of this first trial have been sufficiently encouraging to apply the same procedure in a mice combination across a stronger histocompatibility barrier, namely CBA (H_2k) used as donors and A/J (H_2a) as recipients (CBA and A/J strains share the K through E loci of MHC but differ at C through D).   In this combination pretreatment of donors with rabbit gamma-globulin resulted in a reduction of GVH mortality from 76.4% in control recipients to 20.6% in experimentals and a permanent tolerance of donor skin grafts in 73.2% of surviving experimental recipients as compared to only 18.6% of surviving controls.[22]

In even stronger histocompatibility barrier combinations [C_{57}B1/6 (H_2b) donors → C_3H/He (H_2k) recipients] the inhibitory effect of donor pretreatment with various antigens was still important.   When recipients were mid-lethally irradiated (500 r) a significant percentage of them (33%) survived the GVH reaction and the others died with a mean survival time of 20 days, while 100% of control recipients died in 10 to 12 days.   Survivors were grafted with donor skin but all of them rejected the graft in 10 to 20 days.[23]   In a new series of experiments the recipients were irradiated with 700 r before receiving pretreatment donor spleen cells.   Survival time of experimental mice was again doubled as compared to that of controls but all experimental mice died from GVH.   Thus, antigen pretreatment of spleen cell donors inhibited to a large extent GVH mortality and regularly induced in surviving recipients transplantation tolerance across weak and medium range histocompatibility barriers and delayed GVH mortality in strong histocompatibility donor/recipient differences.

Among the various antigens used in these treatments some hierarchy could be discerned concerning their activity in inhibiting GVH reactions.   Out of the various serum proteins tested the more active seemed to be the rabbit gamma-globulin.   Somewhat more active was hemocyanin.   Particularly efficient in inhibiting GVH reaction were proved to be bacterial polysaccharides and especially the *Serratia marcescens* LPS modified by treatment with CH_3OK.[24]   Whereas the former needed to be used in mg daily doses, the latter used in μg daily doses proved to be more suppressive.23).

The main observations of this line of investigations, mostly achieved by 1965, raised some interest.   Several authors confirmed and extended the aforementioned findings.   Besides the inhibition of antibody production by previous administration of an unrelated antigen, a phenomenon known as competition of antigens,[25] several authors showed that delayed hypersensitivity can also be inhibited by inclusion of a second antigen in the Freund's mixture that induces this type of hypersensitivity.[26,27,28]   Induction of autoimmune diseases could be prevented by previous or simultaneous injection of unrelated antigens.[29,30]   Prolongation of allograft survival time by unrelated antigen administration was repeatedly shown[31,32,33] and suppression of

GVH reaction with eventually subsequent establishment of transplantation tolerance was reported in several publications.[34,35,36,37]

Concerning the mechanism of the interferences produced in response to two antigens given sequentially or simultaneously, a number of hypothesis have been advanced (for detailed analysis see Liacopoulos and Ben Efraim.[38] Perhaps the more attractive ideas stem from Gershon's discovery of suppressor T cells in 1972[39] which substantiated the previous observation of thymic dependency of antigenic competition.[40]

ANTIBODY PRODUCING CELL MULTIPOTENTIALITY

We have been interested in this topic while the preceding work carried out during the '60s because one of the possible mechanisms of antigenic competition was that antigens compete for a pluripotential immunocompetent cell.[38] Data existing at that time were not all contradictory with such a possibility. The vast majority of authors who studied antibody production at the cellular level during the '60s concluded that individual cells form only one antibody.[41] Nevertheless, a number of authors found that after immunization with two unrelated antigens a low percentage (between 1.5 and 15%) of single cells simultaneously produced antibodies to both antigens.[38] It was thought that if double cells exist they should be looked for at the very early period of the response since maturation of the antibody forming cells towards the plasma cell would involve the restriction to the production of only one type of antibody. Using first the method of rosette formation we found that after immunization of mice with sheep and pigeon erythrocytes double rosettes appeared on the 3rd postimmunization day reached their peak value on the 5th day (13.7% of total rosettes) and disappeared by the 10th day.[42] As these rosettes could be passively formed by cells that bind cytophilic antibodies produced by other cells, we pursued this study using the method of hemolytic plaque forming cells (PFC) which only detects cells actively synthesizing and secreting antibody. With this method we regularly detected double PFC on the 3rd to 5th postimmunization day peaking on the 4th day and reaching according to the pair of antigens used 1.5 to 4.8% out of total PFC.[43] Indeed, these pairs varied in the successive studies from unrelated erythrocytes, hapten substituted erythrocytes up to totally unrelated hapten-carrier conjugates, used for primary or secondary response.[44] Thus in 1970 we got the first evidence that immunization of mice with two unrelated antigens regularly results in the appearance of cells reacting with both antigens, provided that care is taken to elicit a vigorous and rapid response. A number of negative results[41] could be explained by the inappropriate period or the relatively insensitive method used for detecting double cells.

The use of hapten substituted erythrocytes allowed to carry out specific inhibition experiments in order to ascertain that the double cells really secreted two different antibody molecules. In a first series of experiments the mice were immunized with TNP substituted pigeon erythrocytes (TNP-PRBC). On the 4th day their spleen cells plated for PFC detection with native PRBC and TNP-BSA for inhibiting the anti-TNP antibody. Wherein the cells were plated with the antigens alone the usual number of single and double (2.3%) cells was found. Addition of soluble inhibitor (TNP-BSA) provoked a drastic decrease of the number of PFC of the corresponding specificity and the disappearance of the double PFC, without any modification of the number of PFC of the alternate specificity.[45]

More conclusive were the micromanipulation experiments. Double PFC individually transferred from the initial medium to a second medium containing a specific inhibitor, watched for 30 min to observe their lytic activity and then again transferred into a third inhibitor-free medium. Some wasting of the lytic activity of PFC occurred during these successive transfers so that about 50% of the micromanipulated double cells preserved their full activity, the others spontaneously became monospecific or ceased to secrete antibody. Almost all of those cells that exhibited a doubly lytic activity in the third medium lysed in the presence of the soluble inhibitor (2nd medium) only the alternate red cell.[46] Similar results were obtained when hapten-carrier conjugates were used for immunization of mice.[44] In this instance the mice were given the two conjugates in Freund's complete adjuvants and two to three months later they were boosted with the same conjugates in soluble form. Under these conditions the secondary response had an explosive character. The immunization and booster were performed with hapten-carrier conjugates, the lytic activity of the cells was evidenced by erythrocytes substituted with the same haptens and inhibition with substituted proteins different from the initial carriers. Therefore, specific inhibition of the one lytic activity with persistence of the second, should be considered as a proof of simultaneous secretion of two different antibody molecules.

The demonstration of double antibody production by significant proportion of cells during the initial period of immunological response, prompted us to investigate the destiny of these double cells. Two alternatives were conceivable, either that they are in some manner abnormal and hence, terminal cells, or they represent an intermediate step of differentiation and rapidly divide into monospecific daughter PFC. For this study we used the method of Cunningham and Fordham[47] for culturing for 48 hrs individual PFC and looking for their progeny. In these experiments about 20% of individually cultured PFC generate a progeny of two to three times as many daughter PFC, the others cease to function or die. In two series of experiments[44,48] a total of 135 double PFC were cultured and the 31 (23%) that generated a progeny yielded only 6 daughter doubles and 62 monospecific PFC. Thus, double PFC should be considered as representing a transient step of B lymphocyte differentiation, probably very short, before dividing into monospecific daughter PFC.

During these experiments we cultured individual monospecific to scrutinize their progeny, thinking that the monospecific progeny double PFC was definitely committed to produce antibody of the same specificity. However, contrary to what was expected, only about 40% of these monospecific PFC from doubly immunized animals generated nonvariant daughter PFC of the same as the parental cell specificity in a clonal manner. The remaining 60% yielded a variant progeny made up by PFC of either specificity and a few doubles irrespective of the specificity of parental PFC.

In all these experiments the antigens of the pairs used were TD antigens. In a more recent work we examined the relationship between nonvariant versus variant progeny of monospecific PFC after immunization of pairs of TD and TI (type w or 2) antigens[49] the same average proportion of variant versus nonvariant progeny (60% vs 40%) was found when two TD antigens were used either for primary or secondary immunization. However, when mixtures of one TD and one TI-2, one TI-1, and one TI-2 antigens were given to the animals the relationship was reversed, the majority of parental PFC yielding nonvariant progeny (30% variant versus 70% nonvariant). The predominance of nonvariant progeny among cells responding to TI antigens indicate that the B cells responding to these antigens are more differentiated than those responding to TD antigens.

The generation of variant progeny by monospecific PFC from doubly immunized animals suggest that a much higher proportion than the 2-3% of double PFC usually detected, can recognize antigens and react to both of them. Two different pairs of V genes would be activated, but because of the uniqueness of C genes per haploid genome and the allelic exclusion phenomenon, the expression of both antibody specificities issued from successive V-C gene rearrangements could only be transient, probably by means of transcription and translation of one V-C gene pair and translation of the second antibody from a long-lived mRNA. Upon cell division each daughter PFC expresses with equal chance one or the other pair of V genes linked to the unique C genes. Alternatively, simultaneous or successive expression of two V gene pairs could stem from successive activation of both chromosomes, each one of them expressed in each generation while long-lived mRNA inherited from the parental PFC is also expressed in double PFC.

For the generation of variant progeny both antigens must be present in the microculture. If one of them was absent for 48 hrs, only progeny specific to the antigen present in the culture was generated. This suggested that early PFC still bear antigen receptors of specificities unrelated to the antibody produced. So the question arose as to whether spontaneous or early immune PFC secreting antibody of a given specificity, when properly stimulated with an unrelated antigen can generate daughter PFC producing antibody specific for them to this new antigen. Co-cultivation of spontaneous or even immune anti-SRBC PFC with a different antigen (TNP-Horse RBC) for 24 hrs resulted in the generation of only anti-SRBC PFC. However, when this culture was prolonged for 48 hrs about half of so-cultured anti-SRBC PFC generated exclusively anti-SRBC PFC, but the other half generated a variant progeny including both anti-SRBC and anti-TNP daughters.[44] Thus, the new antigen present for 48 hrs in the culture triggered activation and expression of a new V gene pair in not less than half of the individually cultured PFC. Yet, this phenomenon of intraclonal variation is also observed when immune PFC are cultured with their specific antigen, but in a proportion much less than when a different antigen is introduced into the culture (0.025-0.05 vs. 0.565, respectively).[44,47] Thus, presence of antigen drives the naturally occurring intraclonal variation by selecting and activating corresponding V genes, probably through surface Ig molecules (antigen receptors) which also are multiple on each B cell.[50]

These results indicate that the immunological genome is endowed with an important plasticity and flexibility that allow it to quickly and accurately respond to myriads of antigens. This may be due to a rearrangement of V genes in each cell division and a stabilization of V gene pair that met through the expressed surface Ig receptor the specific antigen, until the antigen independent differentiation step (mature plasma cell). Therefore, our findings suggest that in a sense instead of the B cell, the V gene pairs should be considered as the unit for antibody production.

REFERENCES

1. Halpern, B.N., Liacopoulos, P., Liacopoulos-Briot, M., Binaghi, R., and Van Neer, F., *Immunology*, 2, 251, 1959.
2. Benacerraf, B. and Kabat, E., *J. Immunol.*, 62, 517, 1949.
3. Binaghi, R., Halpern, B.N., Liacopoulos, P., and Neveu, T., *Nature*, 184, 1805, 1959.
4. Binaghi, R., Liacopoulos, P., Halpern, B.N., Liacopoulos-Briot, M., and Bloch, C., *J. Immunol.*, 87, 269, 1961.
5. Ovary, Z., *Progr. Allergy*, 5, 459, 1958.
6. Binaghi, R., Liacopoulos, P., Halpern, B.N., and Liacopoulos-Briot, M., *Immunology*, 5, 204, 1962.
7. Ovary, A., *Int. Arch. Allergy*, 14, 18, 1959.
8. Liacopoulos, P., Halpern, B.N., and Frick, O.L., *J. Immunol.*, 90, 165, 1963.
9. Lichtenstein, L.M. Osler, A.G., *Fed. Proc.*, 22, 560, 1963.
10. Liacopoulos-Briot, M., Halpern, B.N., Perramant, M.F., and Liacopoulos, P., *J. Immunol.*, 94, 443, 1965.
11. Liacopoulos, P., Liacopoulos-Briot, M., Halpern, B.N., and Herlem, G., *J. Immunol.*, 94, 456, 1965.
12. Ovary, Z., *Immunology*, 3, 19, 1960.
13. Billingham, R.E., Brent, L., and Medawar, P.B., *Nature*, 172, 603, 1953.
14. Felton, L.D. and Ottinger, B., *J. Bacteriol.*, 43, 94, 1942.
15. Liacopoulos, P., Halpern, B.N., and Perramant, M.F., *Nature*, 195, 1112, 1962.
16. Liacopoulos, P. and Neveu, T., *Immunology*, 7, 26, 1964.
17. Stiffel, C., BenEfraim, S., Perramant, M.F., and Liacopoulos, P., *Ann. Inst. Pasteur*, 111(Suppl.), 94, 1966.
18. Neveu, T., Halpern, B.N., Liacopoulos, P., Biozzi, G., and Branellec, A., *Nature*, 197, 1023, 1963.
19. Halpern, B.N., Liacopoulos, P., Martial-Lasfargues, C., and Aractingi, R., *C.R. Soc. Biol.*, CLVII, 740, 1963.
20. Liacopoulos, P. and Stiffel, C., *Rev. Franc. Etudes Clin. Biol.*, 8, 587, 1963.
21. Liacopoulos, P. and Goode, J.H., *Science*, 146, 1305, 1964.
22. Liacopoulos, P., Herlem, G., and Perramant, M.F., *Ann Inst. Pasteur*, 113, 475, 1967.
23. Liacopoulos, P., Merchant, B., and Harrel, B.E., *Transplantation*, 5, 1423, 1967.
24. Nowotny, A., *Nature*, 197, 721, 1963.
25. Adler, F., *Progress in Allergy*, 8, 41, 1969.
26. Neveu, T., *Ann. Inst. Pasteur*, 107, 320, 1964.
27. Schwartz, M. and Leskowitz, S., *Immunochemistry*, 6, 503, 1969.
28. Ben Efraim, S. and Liacopoulos, P., *Immunology*, 16, 573, 1969.
29. McMaster, P.R.B. and Kyriakos, M., *J. Immunol.*, 105, 1201, 1970.
30. Twarog, F.J. and Rose, N.R., Antigen competition between mouse thyroglobulin and bovine serum albumin demonstrated by adoptive transfer, *J. Immunol.*, 107, 738, 1971.
31. Terrino, E.O., Miller, J. and Glenn, W.W.L., *Surgery*, 56, 256, 1964.
32. Thomas, W.H. and Coppola, E.D., *Transplantation*, 5, 103, 1967.
33. Eidinger, D., Khan, S.A., and Milar, K.G., *J. Exp. Med.*, 128, 1183, 1968.
34. Miller, J. Martinez, C. and Good, R.A., *J. Immunol.*, 93, 331, 1964.
35. Damais, C., Lamensans, A., and Chedid, L., *C.R. Acad. Sci.*, 274, 1113, 1972.
36. Chedid, L., in *Bacterial Lipopolysaccharides*, H.E. Kass, S.M. Wolf, Eds., University of Chicago Press, Chicago, p. 104, 1973.
37. Thomson, P.D., Ramry, P.A., and Jutila, J.W., *J. Immunol.*, 120, 1340, 1978.
38. Liacopoulos, P., and Ben Efraim, S., *Progress in Allergy*, 18, 97, 1975.
39. Gershon, R.K., Cohen, P., Hencin, R., and Liebhaber, S.A., *J. Immunol.*, 108, 586, 1972.
40. Gershon, R.K. and Kondo, K., *J. Immunol.*, 106, 1524, 1971.
41. Mäkelä, O. and Gross, A.M., *Progress in Allergy*, 14, 145, 1970.
42. Liacopoulos, P., Gille, F., and Amstutz, H., *C.R. Acad. Sci.* 70, 1049, 1970.
43. Liacopoulos, P., Couderc, J., Amstutz, H., and Gille, F., *C.R. Acad. Sci.*, 271, 740, 1970.
44. Couderc, J., Bleux, C., Ventura, M., and Liacopoulos, P., *J. Immunol.*, 123, 173, 1979.
45. Couderc, J., Bleux, C., Birrien, J.L., and Liacopoulos, P., *J. Immunol.*, 111, 1155, 1973.

46. Couderc, J., Bleux, C., and Liacopoulos, P., *Immunology*, 29, 665, 1975.
47. Cunningham, A.J. and Fordham, S.A., *Nature*, 250, 669, 1974.
48. Liacopoulos, P., Couderc, J., and Bleux, C., *Ann. Immunol. (Inst. Pasteur)*, 127c, 519, 1976.
49. Fevrier, M., Bleux, C., Bouvet, J.P., Couderc, J., and Liacopoulos, P., *J. Immunogen.*, 13, 361, 1986.
50. DeLuca, D., Miller, A., and Sercazz, E., *Cell Immunol.*, 18, 274, 1975.

Chapter 20

TUMOR IMMUNOLOGY
PERSONAL PEREGRINATIONS AND PERSPECTIVES

David W. Weiss

HOW ONE MAY DRIFT INTO A NON-EXISTING DISCIPLINE
Lace and Loam

Upon completing service in the Regular Army of the United States in 1948, I felt inclined to affect an improvement in the standard of living that a corporal's pay had afforded. I would now cast my lot with capitalism rather than with adventure. The opportunity that presented itself was an apprenticeship in a small family business that traded in gold, platinum, and other precious elements. So as to meet what was then, in New York City's Lower East Side, peer review of social acceptability, I also determined to complete the undergraduate college education interrupted some years earlier by what I diagnosed as fatigue of the gluteal musculature (my elders designated the syndrome in other terms) and curative enlistment in the armed forces.

I enrolled in the night school program offered by Brooklyn College to returning veterans. Not prepared to shoulder a renewed classroom indenture in the interests of higher ideals only, I registered for courses in economics and accounting; I would travel the jungles of commerce equipped. But there was also minimum science requirements to be met on the way to the coveted bachelor's degree. With only a sparse background in basic biology and chemistry, the choices before me were limited. Introductory bacteriology was one. Intelligence provided by fellow veteran scholars impelled the decision: given my inclination to render the least possible that would satisfy the caesarist of the curriculum committee, this subject might afford the optimal compromise between enforced short term expenditure and long term gain. *Mutatis mutandis*, I passed one evening the threshold of the microbiological world guarded by Miss Dorothy Pease, who had dedicated an appreciable number of decades of her life to initiating willing and unwilling students— mostly the latter—to the arcanum of the unseen.

After less than a year in my daytime occupation, I came to realize that I was not made for heavy metal. A sanguine distaste for the role of low man on the totemic hierarchy of a family enterprise undoubtedly had something to do with my now seeking a more rewarding framework for the talents my parents assured me I had inherited.

I answered a newspaper advertisement for the job of assistant to the assistant buyer of ladies' underwear at one of New York's department stores. I was interviewed in the assistant buyers precincts together with several dozen other applicants, and found the ambience of lingerie decidedly congenial. The immediate result of that meeting was refusal of a date by one of the young women who, in an adjacent room, was modeling a particularly instructive set of fashions from Paris. Two weeks later, I also received a refusal by mail from the assistant buyer himself. *Sic transit gloria mundi*. The portals of higher and lower financial endeavor shut behind me, I made my way late that afternoon, downcast, to the unglamorous realm, off Flatbush Avenue, of *Escherichia coli* and *Aerobacter aerogenes* and their differential IMViC exposure.

During the laboratory session, Professor Pease inferred that I might join her for a cup of coffee after the work benches, floors, sinks, and sundry objects in sight had been returned to pristine sterility. Miss Pease had won her own admission to spheres microscopic and submicroscopic under the stern tutelage of Philip Hadley. An aura of reserve and ferocious meticulousness enfolded her. I suppose that went with a life in pursuit of bacterial L-forms and acculturation in lands of New England very distant from Brooklyn. Her students warily kept a distance from the flinty lady. But somehow, for reasons I never plumbed, Miss Pease had seen fit to establish a benevolent predator-prey coexistence with me; somehow, I had stotted my way along the savannah of Petri dishes into her affections. That evening, Miss Pease inquired whether I had given thought to the possibility of graduate school.

I had not. Yet now, captured by a look that held little brief for the vanities of the assistant buyer's quarters from which I had been disbarred, I found myself saying that this was indeed a seriously entertained option. And so I found myself rather peremptorily cramming waking hours during the coming months with courses in biology, chemistry, and physics that were needed to compose a "major" concentration in biological sciences.

Having duly entered the ranks of bachelors of arts, there remained to be overcome the hurdle of Graduate Record examinations. I scored high in what was denoted verbal skills, very likely the patrimony of a rabbinic lineage that on both sides of the family stretched back into centuries only dimly illustrated; in all the natural sciences, my performance was deplorable. With these dire auguries, I promptly applied to graduate programs in bacteriology at several universities. On the strength of Miss Pease's unwavering faith and recommendation, I was accepted.

Two years of subway travel between home in lower Manhattan and academe in Flatbush had not led to an endearment with metropolitan existence. It occurred to me that I could aim for a more sylvan setting to a career in science by training in soil microbiology and then toiling amidst the composts of an experimental farm. I began graduate studies in the Department of Soil Microbiology of Rutgers University's College of Agriculture. There were other reasons for enticement to that seat of higher learning. Fame had brushed the department with the discovery of streptomycin; its students enjoyed a stipendum deriving from royalties of the antibiotic patents. Together with the G.I. Bill of Rights allowance, that made for a living somewhat less ascetic than was the usual graduate student's lot. Alas, I learned that the frivolities of life often come dear and, like many of the research assistants in the department, I learned somewhat too late.

At a brief introductory meeting with Selman Waksman, my thesis supervisor to be, I was handed a sample of barnyard manure and empowered to isolate antibiotic-producing actinomycetales. I would be taught the art of antibiotic screening by the technical staff assembled for invasions of the New Jersey loam intended to extend the antibiotic empire. Graduate students were to take only the minimum number of courses required by the college for the doctorate, and preferably those that would entail the least deflection from our mandate of benefitting mankind and the pharmaceutical industry.

That suited me fine, at the beginning. One was introduced to new techniques and strove toward precisely defined goals, rubbed shoulders with distinguished visitors paying homage to the new panacea and its discoverer, and was firmly enjoined to avoid dusty libraries and the constraints of the classroom. There was also the opportunity of distilling in liberated fermentation units quantities of a lethal liquid, putatively related to applejack, from surplus fruit at the experimental station. When realization dawned that the rare chat with a mentor heavily taxed by the public burdens devolving with glory, and testing culture filtrates for bactericidal potency, did not quite amount to a scientific education, it had also become evident that other schools were not exactly vying for transfer students from New Brunswick.

In what may have been the first student revolutionary movement in America, a group of us plotted to conduct underground research of a more basic nature. We defected nights from our appointed loci on the antibiotic spectrum and, armed with a makeshift Warburg apparatus launched partisan forays into the forbidden territory of microbial physiology. The attempts were, on the whole, abortive. I finished out my term of three years at Rutgers in 1952. The intellectual depth of my dissertation is intimated by its catch-all title, "A Study of Antibiotics Active Against *Mycobacterium tuberculosis*." An ill-assorted medley of descriptive antibiotica and dubious stabs at elucidating modes of neomycin action, it apparently sufficed for the Ph.D.

My graduate years were not, however, wholly without accomplishment. In fact, I acquired something of a reputation in infectious disease circles. After several years of uninterrupted mouth-pipetting virulent, streptomycin-resistant H37Rv cultures, whose nemesis I was to raise from the dung, I had retained a virginal negativity to even the most provocative doses of intradermal PPD.

The White Plague and Others

It may have been this accomplishment that generated an astonishing offer from Rene Dubos for a position in his unit at the Rockefeller Institute. Other explanations were advanced by colleagues there who shared my astonishment. Rene Dubos had earned his doctorate, years earlier, under the same tutelage, and perhaps there was between us an unspoken bond forged of certain shared appreciations. Perhaps, given his scholarly preoccupation with the influence of environment on genotype expression, he found in my innocence of skills and knowledge an illuminating instance of the stunting consequences of sensory deprivation during graduate training; and perhaps if that innocence would shed under more auspicious circumstances, that could make an even stronger point.

The subsequent three years of introduction to scientific research molded many of my future attitudes and perspectives. Through Rene Dubo's eyes I came to see infectious disease as the manifestation of evolutionary—and micro-evolutionary—processes in which the host and environment, ambient and tissue, played determining roles; and to understand that study of the dynamics of pathogenesis and immunogenesis can only be essayed by coordinated analysis at all levels of biological organization. Later, my perspective of neoplasia would perforce be that of progressive, evolutionary host-parasite relationships.[1] Merrill Chase taught me immunology, and provided a model (not very often realized by me) of punctiliousness, skepticism, and fealty to the paradigm of Ecclesiastes, "My son, be admonished: Of making many books there is no end; and much publicity is a weariness of the flesh."

The specific problem proposed to me by Dubos was to investigate the anti-tuberculosis immunizing capacity of a mycobacterial fraction obtained by hot methanol extraction of the killed bacteria. Thirty years earlier, Nègre and Boquet had reported from the Pasteur Institute that such a moiety, *antigène méthylique*, could induce heightened resistance in experimental animals against challenge with virulent strains of tubercle bacilli, and without converting them to tuberculin positivity. Confirmation of their findings would lend support to the principle that non-living vaccines can be as efficacious in protecting against tuberculosis as living preparations, such as the attenuated Bacillus Calmette-Guérin strain of bovine tubercle bacilli, a principle then still hotly disputed. Demonstration anew of the protective efficacy of crude mycobacterial components would also provide further impetus to more precise characterization of the molecular entities differentially responsible for the diverse immunological and adjuvant properties of the organisms, and perhaps also to resolution of a basic question: Is induction of delayed hypersensitivity to tuberculoproteins a requisite or incidental aspect of specifically acquired immunity to infection?

Our studies indicated that a fraction prepared by hot methanol reflux extraction of phenol-killed, acetone-washed tubercle bacilli could indeed afford a degree of protection on intravenously challenged mice equivalent to that induced by optimal BCG vaccination.[2,3,4] It was obvious, however, that tuberculous disease in mice so inoculated bears little semblance to the natural history of tuberculosis in man. Experiments of greater relevance would have to be conducted in guinea pigs, and preferably with animals infected by aerosol inhalation, but neither the required numbers of animals nor the facilities for such work were available at the institute.

I had become fascinated by the recent work of Billingham, Brent, and Medawar on the induction of homograft tolerance, and it occurred to me that here could lie another approach to the study of delayed hypersensitivity and resistance: if guinea pigs could be rendered immunologically unresponsive to tuberculoproteins by prenatal exposure to the antigens, it might be possible to study their reactions to tuberculous infection in adulthood in the absence, or depression, of DTH responses. Apprised of my predilection for escape from urban confinements, Dr. Dubos considered that I try this approach at the Dunn School of Pathology in Oxford. Armed with his blessing and a fellowship, I began in the spring of 1955 what would prove to be, scientifically and personally a rewarding period in the laboratories of A.Q. Wells.

An aristocrat for whom science was an avocation rather than a profession, A.Q. Wells had developed the vole bacillus vaccine and led the British Medical Research Council's program of tuberculosis research at Oxford. Among his many gifts to me was an acquainting with the arts of experimental surgery and the attitudes of *noblesse oblige* that are the hallmark of a gentleman and scholar. He also advised that I fulfill the requirements for a D.Phil. degree in medicine while working in the laboratory. I seized the opportunity of winning letters of greater substance, and in due time was granted what could pass for the colophon of a higher education.

Our experiments did indeed show that guinea pigs injected with tubercle bacillus antigens several weeks before birth have a significant, long-lasting disability at corresponding cell-mediated immunologic responsiveness,[5,6] an observation later confirmed with other bacterial antigens.[7]

In the course of this investigation, the occasion unexpectedly presented itself for repeating the Rockefeller tuberculosis immunization studies, now with guinea pigs infected by aerosols of highly controlled bacterial concentration. The British Ministry of Supplies' superb laboratory facilities at Porton on the Salisbury plains had been opened to general scientific projects, a redirection of the unit's previously clandestine occupations that apparently came as the government's response to public opposition against biological warfare.

Wells and I now conducted extensive immunization experiments with various tubercle bacillus entities. The efficacy of nonliving vaccines was confirmed in these more relevant test systems.[8,9,10,11] It also appeared that our methanol extract was considerably more efficacious when small amounts of the extraction residue were added, and then I made a rather uncomplimentary discovery: carefully prepared methanol extracts that were free of residual bacterial fragments were poorly active, if at all, while extracts carelessly contaminated with the residue proved to have consistent immunizing capacity. My interests in the bacillus had now to turn from the soluble to the insoluble.

However, the winter of 1956-1957 brought my internship in the war against the white plague to an abrupt end.

The guinea pigs at Porton were supplied with a daily ration of fresh cabbage in satisfaction of their vitamin requirements. A British species other than man that also derived major sustenance from that redoubtable plant is the wood pigeon. Wood pigeons in England were in those years endemically infected with *Pasteurella pseudotuberculosis*, a pathogen unrelated to the mycobacteria. Heavily infected birds died in large numbers during the first cold spells of the season, only the more healthy surviving until summer when the cycle of spreading infection and subsequent wintry death recurred. The pigeons roosted at night in the Hampshire cabbage fields. Diseased birds could be distinguished from the healthy by their slow and erratic flight; the gross differentiation was confirmed by autopsy of slow and fast fliers brought down at dusk by shooters at the edges of the fields. That winter, the proportions of disabled pigeons grew steadily, but without a corresponding reduction in the population. The consequence of massive Pasteurella contamination of the cabbages was noted only when most of the Porton guinea pig colony suddenly succumbed to an outbreak of pasteurellosis. Prominent among the survivors were animals that had received injections of tubercle bacillus methanol extraction (MER) in preparation for later tuberculosis challenge.

This fortuitous turn of events aroused our interest, and it came at a moment when decimation of the guinea pig stock brought the tuberculosis immunization project to a standstill. It also coincided with the renascent recognition of the dimension of nonspecificity in immune and immunological phenomena,[12] prompted by the observations of Westphal in Germany, the Dubos group, Elberg and his associates in Berkeley, and others that endotoxin lipopolysaccharides of gram-negative bacteria and various other bacterial constituents can incite states of heterologous anti-microbial resistance. Upon A.Q. Wells' sudden death in 1957, I joined the Department of Bacteriology and Immunology at the University of California in Berkeley and there began a systematic exploration of the abilities of MER to bestow nonspecific protection against microbial disease. The results obtained established MER as a broadly efficacious generator of heterologous immunity.[13,14]

In the summer of 1959 I attended a workshop on nonspecific immunity sponsored by Otto Westphal and Derrick Rowley in Freiburg. Among the distinguished participants were Lewis Thomas and Baruj Benacerraf. Late the last evening of the meeting there unfolded, informally, an unusually unconstrained discussion; the subject waxed daringly teleological. The lack of inhibition may have been fueled by the preceding Schwartzwald dinner. A ceremonial Teutonic institution, the repast consists of a permutation of salted, smoked and pickled pig. I, for religious, and many of the others for gustatory, scruples withstood the temptation and kept caloric intake to the accompanying liquid refreshment, high-proof kirsch.

The central question entertained was, what purpose drove the evolution of the vertebrate lymphoid system and immunological apparatus? Could defense against microbial infection alone explain the requirement of a mechanism that evolved to progressive complexity from the primitive fish upward—a complexity then only dimly appreciated, but already implying large demands on biological economy—when invertebrates effected their resistance against comparable threats of invasion far more frugally and to no lesser avail? Was the vertebrate immunological system perhaps implicated as well in physiological functions entailed by the increasing intricacy of biological organization on the animal phylogenetic ladder? Or, did antibody and cellular immune responsiveness arise to cope with the threat to the organism's integrity that neoplasia posed for vertebrate species?

I had made my acquaintance during the conference with the findings of Benacerraf, Halpern, Old and others that BCG infection can bestow protection on mice against subsequent tumor implantation. That observation seemed compatible with clinical reports appearing early in the century—I had scanned these when writing the historical background of my Oxford thesis— that tuberculosis patients are signally refractory to concurrent or later neoplastic disease (a claim that did not hold up to later epidemiological investigation). The free conversation that night introduced me to thought that came to be known as the theory of immune surveillance against cancer. The conception was elegant and it invited a new approach to elaboration of the nonspecific immunological proclivities of mycobacterial fractions.

Tumor Immunology: A Questionable Undertaking

On returning to Berkeley, I presented myself to Kenneth B. DeOme, director of the University's Cancer Research Genetics Laboratory (CRGL) with an idea and a request. I had a stable, standardized nonliving material— MER—that reliably evoked nonspecific resistance to infection. From all that I had heard in Freiburg, there was reason to assume that would prove active against tumor cells as well. Would Dr. DeOme teach me how to handle murine tumor tissue and provide the animals and growths for an experiment?

DeOme was less than enthusiastic. The suppositions at root of my proposal were flimsy (a flick of association to the assistant buyer's wares!). I had no evidence for an immunological modality of the influence exerted by MER on host defenses. More importantly, there was very little cause to believe that neoplastic cells of autochthonous origin are, in fact, recognized as antigenically distinct by their host. Virtually all preceding work purporting to show acquired immunity against tumors had been conducted with neoplasms of unproven isogenicity with the test subjects, and had to be discarded as demonstrating no more than homograft rejection. Yes, Foley and Prehn and Main had recently reported the immunogenic properties of tumors induced by polycyclic aromatic hydrocarbons in inbred mice of documented isogenicity—but these observations did not dispel the climate of disappointment and suspicion that had descended on immunological endeavors with neoplasms. And even if the immunogenicity of certain experimentally induced tumors should prove incontrovertible, no basis existed for a distinctive immunology of spontaneous neoplasia. The concept of immune surveillance lacked a critical data base. Dr. DeOme surmised that I might do better than bury a reputation before it was made, by rushing in where sober investigators had learned to keep their distance. He also gave a me a cage of BALB/c mice from the rigorously controlled CRGL breeding colony, a uterine sarcoma of spontaneous syngeneic origin, and a lesson in trocar implantation.

To my surprise perhaps no less than his, most of the animals pretreated with MER rejected the tumor isografts while the placebo controls succumbed. Identical results were obtained in repeat experiments. If MER acted by stimulating immunologic reactivity to tumor antigens, the observation and its implications might be worth the further exploring. Several complementary lines of research now seemed at once apt and feasible. I departed the microbial world in their direction.

First and foremost, if I was to work in discipline not yet come to light, I could hardly refrain from making a personal effort to see if it could. The crux of the matter lay with an unequivocal demonstration of the immune recognition of tumors by the autochthonous host or by test animals of undisputed syngenicity with the tumor donor. Then, the range and parameters of MER's prophylactic and possibly therapeutic potency had to be defined in such model systems. And, it was necessary to ascertain whether the fraction does, in fact, function as a promotor of specific immunologic responsiveness to unrelated determinants.

The Mouse Mammary Tumor System

Together with DeOme and a team of co-workers and students, a systematic study was initiated of host responsiveness to mammary adenocarcinomas spontaneously arising in inbred female mice. We chose this model because of the large body of information that had developed at CRGL on the biology of mammary neoplasia and preneoplasia in these animals, and because of a supply of fresh tumors was constantly available from the colony. We viewed the test system as holding greater relevance than experimental models in which the neoplasms were intentionally induced and long-passaged; the impermissibility of regarding these mammary carcinomas, as, in fact, concordant with neoplasia in nature is discussed in a later section.

In a first series of experiments, the primary hosts were of two kinds. One was retired multiparous breeders of strains carrying the milk-transmitted mammary tumor virus (MTV); tumors were detected in these animals at routine periodic inspection. The other host population was young females of genetically identical sublines established by foster-nursing and thereby freed of the MTV—but, as it later emerged, carrying a related, less rapidly tumorigenic agent, the nodule-inducing virus(es), NIV—in which carcinomas arose from syngeneic implants of MTV-free hyperplastic alveolar nodule (HAN) outgrowths; HAN tissue represents an intermediate, preneoplastic stage in mammary tumorigenesis. The tumors appearing were excised surgically, cryopreserved, and after periods of time implanted back into the original hosts and, in parallel, into groups of syngeneic animals. Growth of the challenge tumors was found to be either appreciably retarded or facilitated in most of the primary hosts, relative to growth in the naive control cohorts. Lymph nodes draining the sites of tumor challenge in animals that displayed such resistance or "enhancement" were characterized by marked lymphoid hyperplasia. In reporting these observations,[15,16] we surmised that the acquired changes in resistance could not be attributed to immune responses directed at viral antigens on the neoplastic cells: mice carrying the known, biologically active MTV readily accept a first trocar implant of similarly infected tumor tissue; and, the resistance phenomena were equally discernible in the MTV-free subjects that had been implanted with MTV-free HAN tissue.

So as to extend the scope of the project, most of our further experiments were carried out in syngeneic rather than in autochthonous systems, employing tumors in early transplant generations. We had planned to work with tumors and hosts of the same MTV-carrying strains, but as the supply of these animals was for the time limited we frequently utilized syngeneic mice of corresponding MTV-free sublines as test subjects. We determined that an experimentally terminated prior experience with parent-line neoplastic tissue consistently conferred elevated resistance on MTV-free mice against later tumor challenge; the acquired resistance could be transferred to normal animals by means of lymphoid cells.[17] Analogous immunization of MTV-infected mice bestowed resistance only sporadically, and then often only of a lesser degree.

When we first reported these results at scientific conferences, we found it hard going to prove our innocence of tumor immunology's original sin, a residual heterozygosis of normal isogeneic characteristics between tumor donors and recipients and between MTV-infected and MTV-free sublines of the same strain. On one such occasion, Lloyd Old asked from the audience whether we had routinely conducted second-set skin grafts among randomly chosen animals during the course of the study. To the affirmative reply he expressed a further reservation: establishment of absolute syngeneic purity might demand tertiary testing. Fortunately, an assistant who tended to religiosity in these matters had indeed performed that exercise as well, and I pleaded considerations of mouse welfare and limited body area as our excuse for not proceeding further from there to grafting eternity.

In the course of puzzling over the difference in responsiveness to tumor immunization between MTV-infected and noninfected animals, my attention was called to similar mammary tumor studies then independently carried out by Donald Morton in San Francisco. We met for dinner on neutral territory, Treasure Island. It proved to be a seminal occasion. Morton had recently read a paper at the 1964 annual meeting of the American Association for Cancer Research in which he presented evidence for the acquisition of immunological tolerance to spontaneous mouse mammary carcinomas in consequence of neonatal host infection with the MTV. My brief flirtation with the induction of specific immunological unresponsiveness to microbial antigens in fetal guinea pigs came to mind. Morton's findings suggested that immune response that could be elicited against the neoplasms in virus-free animals are prominently directed at virion or virus-coded determinants. In light of our own first experiments with autochthonous tumors in hosts not infected with the agent, I myself had discounted its role in immunogenesis. Here, however, was an explanation for our subsequent observations in the syngeneic transplantation systems that deserved testing.

We undertook a series of investigations designed to compare the immunogenic capacities of mammary tissues—normal, preneoplastic, and neoplastic—derived from, and implanted into, lines of mice carrying both the MTV and nodule-inducing virus(es), genotypically free of both agents, and selectively freed of or infected with the MTV by appropriate foster nursing. Acquisition of heightened resistance was thus assessed in the various possible combinations, with regard to viral status, of host, immunizing tissues, and challenge tumors. The immunizing ability of purified living and formalinized

MTV preparations, irradiated tumor cells, and inactivated non-mammary tissues was also studied. Additional experiments were performed in autochthonous hosts of spontaneously arising and hormone-impelled carcinomas, and the immunologic nature of induced resistance was tested by passive transfer experiments.

The data accruing during succeeding years left no doubt as to the immunogenicity of the tumors and of preneoplastic mammary parenchyma.[18,19,20,21,22,23,24,25,26,27,28,29,30,31] It also became evident that antigens whose expression on the surface of cells was controlled by the MTV, and perhaps also by the related NIV, account in large part for the immunogenic potency. Thus, virus-free mice exhibited a measure of refractoriness to even first implants of small numbers of infected neoplastic and preneoplastic cells in suspension, whereas infected animals usually offered no such resistance; and, acquisition of immunity to secondary challenge was considerably more consistent and telling when immunization with virus-containing preparations and challenge with infected tissue took place in virus-free rather than in virus-bearing animals.

It was also apparent, however, that virus-associated antigens are not the only immunogens involved. Some virus-containing and some virus-free tumors were clearly immunogenic in syngeneic as well as in autochthonous hosts of equivalent viral status; the immunity induced in such animals was specific for each tumor, unlike the cross-reactivity that characterized acquired resistance in virus-positive virus-negative test combinations.

During these years, comparable transplantation immunity studies were conducted by numerous other investigators with murine neoplasms of diverse etiology. The results attested to the protective immunogenicity of many, although not all, experimentally induced neoplasms in syngeneic test models. Further work by Morton and others documented our observations in the mouse mammary tumor system. And, following the illustration of autochthonous immunogenesis against methylcholanthrene-induced sarcomas by George and Eva Klein and their co-workers at the Karolinska Institute, other workers communicated analogous findings in primary hosts of various neoplasms. By the middle 1960's, tumor immunology had evolved as a legitimate field of immunobiological science.

NONSPECIFIC IMMUNOMODULATION
Effects On Experimental Neoplasia

The parallel program of investigation of MER's impact on tumor resistance disclosed the agent's broadly manifested protective capacities in a variety of test models. Pretreatment enabled mice to reject diverse neoplastic isografts or to slow their growth, inhibited the development of preneoplastic lesions in the mammary glands of females subjected to pituitary hyperstimulation, and, when applied early in life, lowered the incidence of mammary carcinomas in MTV-infected multiparous breeders.[22,32,33,34,35] In inbred guinea pigs, MER afforded complete protection to a significant proportion of the animals against implantation challenge several weeks or months later with hepatoma isografts.[36,37,38] Pretreatment also protected mice infected with a strain of the radiation leukemia virus against the development of progressive leukemia[39] and chickens against that of Rous sarcomas following infection challenge with the Rous sarcoma virus,[40] and retarded the appearance of sarcomas in mice exposed to methylcholanthrene.[41] In extensive further experiments with mice, guinea pigs, and chickens already bearing progressively growing neoplasms, MER was seen to exert therapeutic effects, both with regard to primary tumors and to metastatic dissemination.[42,43,44,45,46,47,48,49,50,51,52,53,54,55,56] Therapeutic efficacy was generally less marked, however, than the often categorical protection that could be elicited prophylactically.

It became clear as these studies progressed that timing, dosage, site, and other parameters of MER pretreatment and treatment are of pivotal importance. Protective action was often restricted to narrowly defined conditions, and these had to be determined empirically in each test system. When optimum conditions were not met, the agent was ineffective or led to an acceleration of the neoplastic process.

A wealth of similar information accumulated simultaneously throughout the world on the ability of a heterogeneous assortment of substances—microorganisms, their fractions and products, polynucleotides, other organic compounds—to provoke nonspecific immunity against neoplastic cells. Our findings with MER were repeated in other laboratories.[55] The body of evidence deriving from these experimental undertakings also focused attention on claims that had long been made by Coley and others that ill-defined bacterial culture preparations could beneficially influence the course of human neoplastic disease. The die was cast, and by the early 1970's extensive clinical trials were under way in cancer patients with living BCG, *Corynebacterium parvum*, levamisole, and a number of other substances that in the laboratory exhibited nonspecific resistance-promoting activity.

Effects on Defined Immunocyte Function

Simultaneously with our efforts to delineate the prophylactic and therapeutic activities of MER, we sought to ascertain its influence on defined immunocyte functionality. We learned that this crude material serves as a potent immunomodulator. Although some of its impact on antibody and cell-mediated responsiveness can perhaps be ascribed to a cross-reactivity between certain of its components and animal cell antigens,[57] there can be little doubt as to its *bona fide* nonspecific effects on immunological reactivity towards a wide spectrum of unrelated epitopes.[58,59,60,61,62,63,64,65,66,67,68,69,70,71,72,73,74,75,76,77,78,79,80,81]

MER can impinge on the functions of all immunocytes, lymphoid and reticuloendothelial. Some of its effects are direct, others mediated via a network of cytokines and soluble specific factors whose release it fosters. Its immunomodulating properties can be shown both *in vivo* and *in vitro*, and its influence is selective. The loci of the effects elicited by MER, and the nature of their consequences, are governed by the parameters of administration, genotype and situation of the organism, and the challenge presented. Under test constellations generally favorable to the augmentation of host resistance against neoplastic and infectious diseases, MER usually also promotes defined immunological reactivities and prevents or reverses congenital and acquired states of immunodeficiency. Conversely, in circumstances under which MER does not facilitate defenses or actually increases susceptibility, it tends to compromise defined immunocyte functionality. A negative input on immunological responsiveness is most likely to result when dosage and frequency of treatment are intensive. Excessive application commonly actuates suppressor functions, specific and nonspecific, whereas MER constrains suppression when the provisions of its administration further host defenses. The large body of information that has accrued on the agents' behavior leaves little doubt that the modalities of its action on host resistance are, to a large part, indeed immunological.

The experience of numerous other investigators with living BCG and various other agents under study was, on the whole, similar. Many, if not all, resistance promoting substances act by immunological channels; and, nonspecific excitation of the immunological apparatus must be regarded as a double-edged scalpel. Recourse to this instrumentality can readily have negative as well as positive import for immunological and immune manifestations.

We have continued to study the range and mechanisms of MER immunomodulation to the present [since 1968 in Jerusalem, to whose environs I found myself transmuted for non-immunological reasons][82] even though a variety of "second and third generation" immunomodulating agents have become available. Chemically defined adjuvants of microbial and other derivation, synthetic analogs of natural products, and an assortment of highly purified and recombinant DNA produced cytokines, some of which appear to be the mediators of effects incited by the crude first generation stimulators, hold the obvious advantage of enabling analyses of structure-function relationships. However, most of the sophisticated BRM have a more confined scope of influence than crude MER; and, although it is of the most dubious propriety to have maintained an involvement with a product deriving not from a gene library but rather from the "Dreckapotheke" (as Otto Westphal put it aptly some years ago), I have not been able to shake off a fascination with the wondrously intricate immunobiological events that devolve from the confrontation of the animal organism with ubiquitous pathogenic bacteria.

The Clinical Adventure

The introduction of living BCG and shortly thereafter of other nonspecific immunomodulators to the cancer clinic took place at a time when modern immunology was only emerging from its neonatal stage, and years before the parameters—not to speak of the mechanism—of BRM action on what was known of immunological responsiveness had been delineated. It is questionable, nonetheless, whether the prevailing ignorance justified the fanfare with which the new therapeutic attempts were launched and the initial impressions greeted. Recognition of the forbidding complexity of the immunological apparatus had already dawned. On more sober reflections, the likelihood of successful intervention in the intricacies of host-tumor interactions by gross, uninformed immunostimulation should have appeared somewhat remote even twenty years ago. Certainly, no encouragement could have been drawn from experience in the analogous realm of host-microbial parasite relationships, immunological intervention in established disease having proven, on the whole, signally ineffective despite the powerful immunogenicity of the pathogenic agents. It can be argued that human and societal pressures to develop new modalities of cancer treatment mitigate the highly unscientific lapse of awareness that the best laid plans of men in mice often go awry when put to the test in patients. Early clinical trials may have been an inevitability. There would seem to be little excuse, however, for the wild optimism at their outset and even less for its stubborn propagation even as the labyrinthine nature of immunological reactivity came fully to light and as the handwritings on laboratory and hospital walls turned increasingly legible: immunomodulators can readily depress immunological capacity rather than promote it, and steer responsiveness into directions of no or negative import for host defenses; treatment must be carefully individualized if the balance of effects is to be favorable; and, the data taken to indicate therapeutic accomplishment weakened progressively with the duration of trials, the number of patients entered, and the rigorousness of the controls.

MER was a late entry into the lists of immunomodulators studied in cancer patients.[83] The experience with the agent proved to be representative of the entire clinical effort at systemic nonspecific immunotherapy.[55] In small, preliminary trials in patients with acute myelocytic leukemia (AML), colorectal carcinomas and several other malignancies, a variety of positive effects were recorded: prolongation of remission and survival times; measurable regression of local and metastatic lesions; improved clinical and immunological status, the latter assessed by a battery of tests of responsiveness to defined mitogenic and antigenic stimulation; and, in a number of instances, apparent cures in persons with progressive disease who had failed on conventional therapy.

The promising intimations of efficacy found their denouement in larger, Phase III randomized-control trials. Although some beneficial effects were noted for MER treatment early in the course of investigation, these benefits almost always proved to be transient, and little if any therapeutic efficacy could be documented statistically at the conclusion of any of the extended studies. There remains, at best, an anecdotal impression of substantial clinical improvement in the occasional patient.

In situ administration of MER, as of BCG and other immunomodulating substances that are themselves immunogenic, can bring about regression or disappearance of tumor foci, and may be of value in the management of certain neoplastic processes that, even while localized, are inaccessible to definitive surgical extirpation (viz., transitional cell carcinoma of the bladder). Such clinical situations, in which there can still be entertained some expectations for nonspecific immunotherapy, are not reflective of the cancer problem as a whole. The verdict on this modality of intervention for the common, systemically manifested syndromes of malignant disease is unmistakable: the effort has so far proven to be largely an exercise in futility, and it provides an illustration of prematurity in clinical science and medicine.

It is the more surprising for the unqualified bleakness of the record that the pattern of attitudes in clinical immunotherapy has not changed appreciably. As newer, refined immunomodulators—the interferons, other cytokines—and other modalities of immunological treatment have been catapulted into the clinic, investigators and physicians have joined institutional administrators and media specimens in symphonies whose preludes are brainless hopefulness, their coda, when the results are in, silence or a dirge of disenchantment. It has not been easy to maintain a balanced perspective in a field unceasingly agitated by the oscillations of an erratic pendulum swinging between heights of precocious hopefulness and disillusionment that, too, is often premature. Precipitous abandonment of effort, and of support, when exaggerated expectations fail to realize is today perhaps no less a danger than untimely undertaking.

It may indeed by of interest to question whether the therapeutic activity seemingly displayed by some immunotherapeutic test agents in small, preliminary trials, and in early stages of larger ones, is wholly illusory or wholly ascribable to artifacts in study design and implementation.[55] Placebo effects are intensified when physicians closely interact with small numbers of patients in a new venture that both believe to hold some promise. Chance and unrecognized bias in patient distribution between experimental and control groups can readily lead to weighted comparisons. The statistical pitfall may be greater still where the controls are "historical" or represented by patients who are current in that institution but not included in the trial and its particular care and ambience. Factors such as these are well recognized to cast a shadow of doubt on the significance of results accruing from any preliminary clinical study, and they are largely excluded in subsequent, large-scale investigations. It is also well known that a considerable proportion of cancer patients, even of those with advanced disease, show temporary or localized responses to a variety of treatments that do not, however, appreciably change the overall picture of pathogenesis or its outcome.

On the other hand, patients in preliminary trials tend to be subject to an individualization of treatment regimen, and this can facilitate genuine therapeutic attainments. Thus, for instance, in the first studies with MER in AML patients, the protocol calling for a given dosage of the agent at given intervals was violated whenever a patient showed decreased immunological responsiveness at periodic testing; treatment was resumed only when immunological reactivity had returned to maximum extent, and was discontinued permanently upon repeated fall. In retrospect, it is not improbable that these patients received MER under conditions making for optimal immunopotentiation and minimal activation of suppressor functions. In addition, careful attention was given to the intercalation of MER administration and chemotherapy, so as to prevent neutralization by the latter of any effects elicited by the immunological arm of treatment. In contrast, routine immunological assessment was not performed in most of the following Phase III trials, dosage and periodicity of MER injection (rather arbitrarily set on the basis of animal experiments and intelligent (?) guessing) remained constant, and chemotherapy was often of an intensity and timing likely to compromise any expression of immunological activation.

It must be said that if faulty design of the earlier immunotherapy trials in general could be laid at the door of an innocence of immunological knowledge, serious errors were introduced into the planning and conduct of later investigations in direct contradiction of information that had accumulated.

Just conceivably, then, nonspecific immunomodulators may have made a better showing in the clinic had the circumstances of their testing been more felicitous. The consideration is academic. There is no realistic prospect of a reexamination of first-generation agents. What is of cardinal importance is that current and future endeavors at immunological intervention—nonspecific and specific, active, adoptive, and passive—be given a fairer chance of evaluation than has been extended to cancer immunotherapy so far. That there are persuasive grounds for continuing with the effort will be discussed in following sections of this article.

TUMOR IMMUNOLOGY AND IMMUNOTHERAPY: WHERE DO WE STAND TODAY?

The body of information now at hand indicates several cardinal points of reference from which my perspective of the field and its likely development in the near future proceeds.

The Question of Human Tumor Immunogenicity

The term immunogenic should properly denote only such antigenic determinants of tumor cells as elicit immunological reactions that are involved in host resistance, whether they are of positive or of negative import.[84] It is however, difficult in practice to discriminate between immunological responses of the autochthonous human tumor host that are inimical to defense and those that do not affect the state of resistance. Accordingly, the designation of immunogenicity shall here be employed in a restricted sense: the ability of tumor antigens to elicit protective responses in course of the natural history of neoplastic disease.

As will be indicated in succeeding paragraphs, the assumption that must be drawn from the available evidence, and that should serve as point of departure of future endeavors at elucidating the dynamics of patient-tumor relationships or at intervening therapeutically by immunological means, is that the great majority of human neoplasms are not, or only poorly, immunogenic. Their immunogenic paucity could indeed have been inferred already some time ago, from the debacle of all forms of immunological therapy: if an appreciable number of human cancers were, in fact, moderately immunogenic but overcome or evade host immune reactions, the bolstering of immunity at a time when tumor burden has been reduced to a minimum by conventional methods would be expected to have proven more efficacious.

Tumor Specific Transplantation Antigen (TSTA)

No convincing evidence has been brought forward for the existence of TSTA—protective antigens unique to the neoplastic state—on the surface or in the cytoplasm of cells of the common human tumors[85] or of "spontaneously" arising tumors of animals.[86] The question of their possible detection in the future is, moreover, theoretical; it cannot be resolved. Any claim of the discovery of such antigens can be countered by the argument that they may represent molecular entities expressed by normal cells as well, but only transiently in ontogeny or to minute extent in other, highly specialized tissues. Point mutations, chromosomal rearrangements, and other genetic changes that are effected by certain carcinogenic stimuli can, in principle, lead to novel antigenicities of neoplastic cells, but the reservation holds with regard to their identification as tumor specific. More importantly, the usual circumstances of carcinogenesis in man do not make for potent tumor immunogenicity, whatever the nature of the deviant antigenicities may be.[87,88] It must be noted that even some, at least, of the putatively specific, strong transplantation antigens of tumors experimentally induced by chemical carcinogens and ionizing radiation have been attributed to the category of transiently expressed or obscure, but nonetheless normally occurring, molecular constituents of the organism.

In addition, formidable methodological difficulties encumber the characterization of human tumor transplantation antigens. Serological techniques may not always reveal epitopes that can incite rejection reactions; this has been found to be the case for the strong transplanation antigens of methylcholanthrene and benzpyrene induced sarcomas of mice. Transplantation experiments with human tumors obviously cannot be performed *in vivo*. It is possible to study the reactivity of patient immunocytes against freshly obtained tumor cells cultured *in vitro*[89] or implanted into athymic, additionally immunosuppressed animal carriers.[90,91] Such work has demonstrated the cytotoxic potential of autochthonous lymphoid cells for some tumors, but it does not confirm the tumor specificity of the inciting and target determinants.

Tumor Associated Transplantation Antigens (TATA)

Many human and animal tumor cells exhibit antigenic profiles that, while not specific to their neoplastic condition, distinguish them from analogous normal cells. Several categories of such tumor-associated antigens have been defined. One may be designated "displacement antigens," i.e., antigens of neoplastic variants that are displaced from the normality of appearance on cells in terms of ontogenic time—the so-called carcinoembryonic and fetal antigens—or tissue localization; such misplaced expression of normal genes may involve not only cellular oncogenes directly involved in oncogenesis but also genes that come to untimely or exaggerated expression late in the course of tumor progression, in consequence of secondary aberrancies that may accompany patterns of disregulated growth. A related category of TATA is that of determinants that characterize stages of normal differentiation in the adult, or of the growth cycle of cells, and that are manifested to abnormal extent by neoplastic variants that are "frozen" at a particular step in the differentiation pathway or prompted into continuous re-entry into the growth cycle. A third category is comprised of epitopes normal to a particular cell type, and not limited to a narrow range of positions along the ladder of differentiation, but expressed to much heightened amounts in consequence of the neoplastic changes. Divergences of cellular antigenic profile that are in essence only quantitative or locational are nonetheless subject to immunologic recognition and reactivity by the organism. In addition to such quantitative deviations from the antigenic character of a tissue, account must be taken of the possible exposure of normally cryptic, masked macromolecules, and of steric rearrangements of normally expressed molecular entities that can occur in the wake of loss of other surface determinants. All these groups of TATA represent departures from normal cell antigenicity that are to be expected from what is known today of the activation and amplification of cellular oncogenes and the deletion of certain differentiation-determining genes ("anti-oncogenes") and their products.[92]

The occurrence of autoimmune pathologies that arise from reactions manifested against normal-self antigens, even if their onset is (sometimes? often?) triggered by qualitative alterations in the structure of the responsible epitopes, and the frequent presence of autoantibodies and T cells with receptors for self-components in healthy individuals, indicate that autoreactivity is not an uncommon aspect of immunological responsiveness. It is also evident, however, that such antigenic divergences from normal do not tend to make for potent cytotoxic responsiveness: evolution of the vertebrate immunological apparatus is based on the operation of homeostatic control mechanisms that prevent prevalent autoimmune disorders. Furthermore, it is improbable that any tumor-associated antigens that can serve as targets for immune attack but that are not an indispensable feature of the neoplastic state of cells are maintained in the antigenic repertoire of a developing population of neoplastic cells; selective pressures exerted by the host are likely to bring about the deletion of clones expressing such epitopes.

Immune Surveillance in Nature

The central premises of the theory of immune surveillance against neoplasia as it was originally formulated—the general immunogenicity of tumors, immunological incompetence as the precipitating cause of neoplastic disease—have proven erroneous: the prevailing clinical tumors apparently are not potently immunogenic, and there is no evidence for an antecedent immunological dyscrasia in most cancer patients. In recent years, many investigators have come to regard the theory as, instead, the "central fallacy" of tumor biology and immunology.[93]

This perception, like so many that erratically wax and wane in this field, is disproportionate. Immune defenses may well be, in fact, definitively efficacious in preventing or halting an appreciable number of neoplastic diseases. The frequency of such diseases is high in individuals suffering from idiopathic, congenital, iatrogenic, and otherwise acquired immunodeficiencies. The incidence of a significant proportion of the neoplasms appearing in these patients may indeed be attributable to immune failure. For at least some of the cancers that arise characteristically in patients with AIDS and in patients intentionally immunosuppressed so as to facilitate retention of an organ implant, a DNA-viral etiology is today postulated. Such tumors may well express immunogenically active antigens that are products of the viral transforming genes and thus essential concomitants of the transformation event (as are, for instance, the TSTA of rodent polyomas). It is of pertinence that tumors of transplant recipients sometimes regress completely at cessation of therapeutic immunosuppression and do not recur even upon further suppressive treatment following a second transplant. It can reasonably be argued that the survival of vertebrate species might be jeopardized by neoplastic diseases whose etiology involves ubiquitous transforming DNA viruses and perhaps other carcinogenic factors that engender immunogenic properties in the neoplastic cells, were it not for effective immune surveillance. A variety of malignancies may not transpire in immunocompetent humans and animals precisely because immunological resistance suffices to halt neoplastic progression at its incipience.

The tumors seen in the usual cancer patient could well represent a minority of potentially occurring neoplasms, those which are characterized by immunogenic paucity or which are able, by one means or another, to evade immune attack.[1] One such means to which we have given considerable attention may be a sequestering of specific humoral and cellular immune reagents by antigenic substances physiologically shed from the surface membrane of cancer cells.[94,95,96,97,98] But immunogenic shortfall does not necessarily imply the immunological inertness of the neoplastic cells that bring about existing disease. The natural history of human neoplastic diseases—their vagaries and discontinuities—suggests that the host, far from being a neutral subject is an active, resisting participant. It also suggests that some, at least, of the defensive riposte is immunological. Thus, for instance, positive prognostic significance is often ascribed to findings—histological, and coming from *in vitro* analyses—of immunocyte activity within tumor foci. Metastatic dissemination probably takes place in many instances before a primary growth is detected and before surgical intervention and other treatment can be effected, yet numerous patients are cured; the seeding of cancer cells by the gloved hands of the surgeon at the time of tumor extirpation has been documented in patients who have remained permanently free of disease.

A measure of immune reactivity in patients suffering from the common forms of neoplasia need not be imputed to the presence of any (still to be distinguished) tumor-specific transplantation antigens. It can be mounted as well against weak, tumor-associated determinants; and, as will be elaborated below, it can be nonspecific. That it is often abortive in the natural course of disease is not surprising: water-tight defenses are not likely to have evolved against a danger that usually materializes in later life and thus does not imperil survival of the species. But even a resistance mechanism that falls short in nature may be subject to therapeutic potentiation.

It might be a truism, then, to say that immune defenses are, in fact, efficacious vis-a-vis neoplastic diseases that do not occur, those that do not progress beyond a certain point, and those whose course is less virulent than would be inferred from the intrinsic neoplastic capacities of the pathogenic cells.

Prospects

These considerations signify the pertinence of continued efforts at immunological intervention in human cancer, for all the failures that have been met, and for all the difficulties to be encountered in any endeavor at interposing in intricate immunological interactions in face of their already manifest shortcoming in the patient.

Tumor-associated antigens provide a handle, albeit a narrow one, for intervention of a specific nature. Such attempts are directed at the induction, recruitment, or potentiation of specific cytotoxic responsiveness against cells expressing TATA. The conceptual framework of such attempts must be the elicitation of a focused autoimmune reactivity. Any therapeutic accomplishment so attained may well be at the cost of generalized autoimmune injury. If the severity of any such pathology can be limited—and there are means at hand for managing autoimmune diseases—the price may not have to be considered unreasonable.

A more promising approach may lie with the activation of nonspecific immunocyte reactivity. In contrast to the many early—and unsuccessful— attempts at nonspecific intervention which were aimed at heightening specific immunological responsiveness by nonspecific adjuvants, the focus now may advisably shift to nonspecificity of the effector arm. It may indeed be that immune defenses against a variety of pathogenic agents are mediated, wholly or in part, by nonspecific reactions that are set in motion by specific interactions between antigens and antibodies or sensitized effector cells. The excitation of macrophages and certain populations of lymphocytes to generalized cytotoxic capacity by cytokines, and the creation of inflammatory tissue microenvironements, are examples of nonspecific resistance mechanisms that are brought about in consequence of specific immunological responses. From an evolutionary perspective, the component of specificity in vertebrate immune defenses may represent, in part, an expedient of archetypic, nonspecific instrumentalities.

Tumor-associated antigens that are inadequately immunogenic or that do not afford the loci for efficacious specific attack may thus nonetheless serve as triggers for a limited specific responsiveness whose broad sequelae can be destructive to the neoplastic invaders. Moreover, TAA can be regarded as indicants of the aberrant growth and deportment of neoplastic cells, and it is not improbable that immunocytes naturally come into play—and can be stimulated to greater participation—in controlling anomalously behaving, displaced cells regardless of their antigenic characteristics. Whether or not the nonspecific defensive activities of lymphoid and reticuloendothelial cells should be considered "immunological" is a question of semantics; the boundaries between the specific and the nonspecific in immunological reactions are labile, and all resistance functions effectuated by cells of the immunocyte family can be properly designated as falling within the scope of immunology.

A plethora of approaches to immunological intervention in human cancer has been delineated[86,99,100] and is today at various stages of clinical investigation. Definitive evidence of success is still awaiting. Some of the recent claims of attainment for several distinct modalities of immunotherapy may be suggestive, but they are as yet far from convincing; the data reported are not, on the whole very much more impressive than those yielded in early phases of the trials with first-generation biological response modifiers (BRM). What can be said now for the current effort is that it is conceptually more solid than the past endeavors, and that study design and conduct are in better keeping with what has been learned of the nature of the immune response. What must also be said is that any prospect of clinical progress in the future is conditioned on the provision of information from relevant test models. A major cause for the uncertainties of tumor immunotherapy until now lies with model irrelevance. The eventuality of immunological treatment remains enigmatic to the present; it is to the future that the tumor immunologist must look. Only future research will tell whether there is, in reality, a place for immunology in the strategy of cancer control; and, the clinical arm of that research cannot be divorced from laboratory experimentation. It is appropriate, accordingly, that the concluding section of this article deal with the question of pertinence of test systems.

Experimental Models

Looming large among the cardinal sins of commission in tumor immunology is the ill-founded extrapolation from laboratory to clinic.[93,101,102] Immunological manipulation can bestow a large measure of protection on laboratory animals against later challenge with neoplastic cells and carcinogenic agents; immunotherapy of already established animal tumors has proven saliently less successful, with the exception, in some instances, where treatment is intralesional and early. Positive findings coming from animal test systems should reasonably not have impelled expectations of accomplishment in the human arena, vis-a-vis advanced, systemic disease. A more serious fault of irrelevance lies with the nature of the overwhelming majority of experimental tumors that have been the subject of study; intentionally induced in inbred strains and long passaged, their correspondence to the cancers of man is exceedingly dubious.

Tumors that appear early after massive experimental exposure to chemical carcinogens or ionizing irradiation tend to be considerably immunogenic. Those that arise late or following only moderate provocation—the prevailing circumstances of chemical and physical carcinogenesis in man—are usually non-immunogenic. Possible reasons for this divergence have been discussed previously.[87,88]

Tumors induced in the laboratory by viral action express novel antigens under control of the viral genome. In the case of DNA viruses, the antigens encoded by the transforming genes are potently immunogenic; definitively efficacious responsiveness has evolved against them. Virion-associated antigens of chronic transforming retroviruses, in permissive systems, are expendable to the neoplastic state of the cells, but they may serve at least temporarily as targets for immune attack of the neoplastic cell population.

Products of the oncogenes carried by acute transforming retroviruses are not unlikely to differ qualitatively from those encoded by corresponding cellular oncogenes, and can thus bestow immunogenic properties on the transformed variants. However, DNA and RNA viruses have been incriminated in the etiology of only a very small proportion of human neoplastic diseases—notably Epstein-Barr, Hepatitis B, and HTLV-I viruses in malignancies largely centered in certain geographic areas, and often associated with immunodeficiency syndromes of environmental, iatrogenic, or congenital origin—and the immunological concomitants of laboratory viral carcinogenesis thus also have no relevant correlates in common human neoplasia.

Neither can tumors that appear "spontaneously" in laboratory animals—that is, without intentional manipulation by the investigator—be considered relevant analogs of cancer in man. The biology and environmental circumstances of the animal hosts differ appreciably from those of the corresponding species in nature and certainly from those of man, and pathogenesis as well as immunogenesis of spontaneous animal neoplasia disaccord with the natural history of clinical neoplastic disease. Inbreeding entails a process of cumulative selections. Selection may be for or against host feedback controls, including those of immunological nature. It is often also for high tumor incidence in the strain; a frequent reason for this is the activity of laboratory-adapted acute transforming retroviruses, some of which bear multiple oncogenes that function in tandem, and for which there seem to be no counterparts in human oncogenesis.

Moreover, selective and adaptive processes invariably entailed by long-maintained passage of cells *in vivo* and *in vitro* seriously impair the comparability of the neoplasms that comprise the investigator's stock in trade with cancers seen in the clinic. Prolonged transfer also raises the specter of tumor immunology's original sin, the uncertain syngenicity of tumor and host; research communications of recent years have not provided assurance that the concern is today unfounded.

Another truism can thus be forwarded: the only relevant experimental models of human tumors are human tumors, freshly derived from the patient. An accurate assessment of immunological responsiveness against them demands that study of their susceptibility to attack be in autochthonous confrontations.[103,104,105] It must also be borne in mind that documentation *in vitro* of autochthonous cellular or humoral reactivity may attest only to the cytotoxic or cytostatic competence of isolated immunologic elements; it does not necessarily afford a portrayal of host resistance. Immunity against cancer can be substantiated with confidence only where immunocytes are shown to effect the destruction of a progressively developing neoplasm, to retard its growth, or to prevent invasiveness and metastatic spread.

A test system that presents itself for this ascertainment, and on which our current efforts at the Lautenberg Center are focused, is the implantation of neoplastic tissue directly form the operating room into athymic animal carriers.[90,91] Additionally immunosuppressed by drugs, irradiation, and monoclonal antibodies directed at interferons and other cytokines, the animals accept a significant proportions of the implants and develop massive pulmonary metastases upon intravenous injection of tumor cell suspensions. Peripheral blood leukocytes are harvested periodically from the patient, before and after surgery, separated into various lymphoid and monocyte populations, and tested for anti-tumor reactivity fresh or after cyropreservation. The immunocytes are stimulated to heightened reactivity by exposure to diverse BRM and by specific tumor sensitization *in vitro*. They are tested for immune capacity by introduction to the tumor hosts bearing first- or second-generation implants, at various stages of the neoplastic process and in conjunction with conventional therapies. For all the patent artificialities of assaying immune capacity in a xenogeneic tumor carrier, a measure of relevant information on autochthonous immune reactivity, before and after stimulation, is provided by such studies. It may be hoped that the data accruing from such model systems will form a more reliable infrastructure for future clinical endeavors.

ACKNOWLEDGMENT

The excellent assistance of Miss Rosaline Cass in the preparation of this manuscript is gratefully acknowledged.

REFERENCES

The references presented are exclusively from among the writer's publications and those of his students and departmental colleagues. The exclusivity of the listing is not prompted by a tendency to megalomania. It is motivated, rather, by the consideration that this is a very individual account, and that it is impossible within the scope of the book to offer an adequate review of the vast literature pertaining to the topic. Many of the references chosen are discursive articles that extensively cite the most relevant work in the areas under discussion.

1.   **Weiss, D.W.** , Neoplastic disease and tumor immunology from the perspective of host-parasite relationships, *Natl. Cancer Inst. Monogr.*, 44, 115, 1976.
2.   **Weiss, D.W. and Dubos, R.J.,** Antituberculous immunity induced in mice by vaccination with killed tubercle bacilli or with a soluble bacillary extract, *J. Exp. Med.*, 101, 313, 1955.
3.   **Weiss, D.W. and Dubos, R.J.,** Antituberculous immunity induced by methanol extracts of tubercle bacilli—its enhancement by adjuvants, *J. Exp. Med.*, 103, 73, 1956.
4.   **Dubos, R.J., Weiss, D.W., and Schaedler, R.W.,** Enhancing effect of adjuvants on the antituberculous immunity elicited in mice by methanol extracts of tubercle bacilli, *Amer. Rev. Tuberc. Pulm. Dis.*, 75, 781, 1956.
5.   **Weiss, D.W. and Wells, A.Q.,** Actively acquired tolerance to tuberculoprotein, *Nature*, 179, 968, 1957.
6.   **Weiss, D.W.,** Inhibition of tuberculin skin hypersensitivity in guinea pigs by injection of tuberculin and intact tubercle bacilli during fetal life, *J. Exp. Med.*, 108, 83, 1958.
7.   **Weiss, D.W. and Main, O.,** The effect of pre- and neo-natally injected diphtheria toxoid on the homologous responsiveness of young guinea pigs—a preliminary report, *Immunology*, 5, 333, 1962.
8.   **Weiss, D.W.,** Antituberculosis vaccination in the guinea pig with non-living vaccines, *Amer. Rev. Tuberc. Pulm. Dis.*, 77, 719, 1958.
9.   **Weiss, D.W.,** Antituberculosis vaccination with non-living vaccines, *Tuberculology*, 17, 63, 1958.
10.   **Weiss, D.W. and Wells, A.Q.,** Vaccination against tuberculosis with non-living vaccines. II. Vaccination of guinea pigs with phenol-killed tubercle bacilli, *Amer. Rev. Resp. Dis.*, 81, 518, 1960.

11. Weiss, D.W. and Wells, A.Q., Vaccination against tuberculosis with non-living vaccines. III. Vaccination of guinea pigs with fractions of phenol-killed tubercle bacilli, *Amer. Rev. Resp. Dis.*, 82, 339, 1960.

12. Weiss, D.W. and Yashphe D.J., Nonspecific stimulation of antimicrobial and antitumor resistance and of immunological responsiveness by the MER fraction of tubercle bacilli, in *Dynamic Aspects of Host-Parasite Relationships*, Vol. I., A. Zuckerman and D.W. Weiss, Eds., Academic Press, New York, 1973, pp. 163-223.

13. Weiss, D.W., Enhanced resistance of mice to infection with *Pasteurella pestis* following vaccination with fractions of phenol-killed tubercle bacilli, *Nature*, 186, 1060, 1960.

14. Weiss, D.W., Bonhag, R.S. and Parks, J.A., Studies on the heterologous immunogenicity of a methanol-insoluble fraction of attenuated tubercle bacilli (BCG). I. Antimicrobial protection, *J. Exp. Med.*, 119, 53, 1964.

15. Weiss, D.W., Faulkin, Jr., L.J. and DeOme, K.B., Acquired resistance to spontaneous mammary carcinomas in autochthonous and isologous mice, *Proc. Amer. Assoc. Cancer Res.*, 4, 71, 1963.

16. Weiss, D.W., Faulkin, Jr., L.J. and DeOme, K.B., Acquisition of heightened resistance and susceptibility to spontaneous mouse mammary carcinomas in the original host, *Cancer Res.*, 24, 732, 1964.

17. Attia, M.A., DeOme, K.B. and Weiss, D.W., Immunology spontaneous mammary carcinomas in mice, II. Resistance to a rapidly and a slowly developing tumor, *Cancer Res.*, 25, 452, 1965.

18. Lavrin, D.H., Blair, P.B. and Weiss, D.W., Immunology of spontaneous mammary carcinomas in mice, III. Immunogenicity of C3H preneoplastic hyperplastic alveolar nodules in C3Hf hosts, *Cancer Res.*, 26, 293, 1966.

19. Lavrin, D.H., Blair, P.B. and Weiss, D.W., Immunology of spontaneous mammary carcinomas in mice, IV. Association of the mammary tumor virus with the immunogenicity of C3H nodules and tumors, *Cancer Res.*, 26, 929, 1966.

20. Attia, M.A.M. and Weiss, D.W., Immunology of spontaneous mammary carcinomas in mice. V. Acquired tumor resistance and enhancement in Strain A mice infected with mammary tumor virus, *Cancer Res.*, 26, 1787, 1966.

21. Weiss, D.W., Lavrin, D.H., Dezfulian, M., Vaage, J. and Blair, P.B., Studies on the immunology of spontaneous mammary carcinomas of mice, in *Viruses Inducing Cancer*, W. J. Burdette, Ed., University of Utah Press, Salt Lake City, 1966, pp. 138-168.

22. Weiss, D.W., Immunology of spontaneous tumors,. in *Proceedings of the Fifth Berkeley Symposium on Mathematical Statistics and Probability*, L. Lecam and J. Neyman, Eds., University of California Press, Berkeley, 1967, pp. 657-706.

23. Dezfulian, M., Lavrin, D.H., Shen, A., Blair, P.B. and Weiss, D.W., Immunology of spontaneous mammary carcinomas in mice, Studies on the nature of the protective antigens, in *Carcinogenesis: A Broad Critique*, Proceedings of the Twentieth Annual Symposium on Fundamental Cancer Research, M.D. Anderson Hospital and Tumor Institute, Williams and Wilkins, Baltimore, 1967, pp. 365-393.

24. Dezfulian, M., Zee, T., DeOme, K.B., Blair, P.B. and Weiss, D.W., Role of the mammary tumor virus in the immunogenicity of spontaneous mammary carcinomas of BALB/c mice and in the responsiveness of the hosts, *Cancer Res.*, 28, 1759, 1968.

25. Burton, D.S., Blair, P.B. and Weiss, D.W., Protection against mammary tumors in mice by immunization with purified mammary tumor virus preparations, *Cancer Res.*, 29, 971, 1969.

26. Weiss, D.W., Immunological parameters of the host-parasite relationship in neoplasia, *Ann. N.Y. Acad. Sci.*, 164, 431, 1969.

27. Vaage, J. and Weiss, D.W., Immunization against spontaneous and autografted mouse mammary carcinomas in the autochthonous C3H/Crgl mouse, *Cancer Res.*, 29, 1920, 1969.

28. Weiss, D.W., Immunological parameters of host-tumor relationships: spontaneous mammary neoplasia of the inbred mouse as a model, *Cancer Res.*, 29, 2368, 1969.

29. Weiss, D.W., Immunity and tolerance in spontaneous mammary neoplasia of the mouse, in *Immunity and Tolerance in Oncogenesis, Proceedings of the IV Perugia Quadrennial International Conference on Cancer*, L. Severi, Ed., Division of Cancer Research, Perugia, 1970, pp. 703-713.

30.   Weiss, D.W., Sulitzeanu, A., Young, L., Adelberg, M. and Segev, Y., Studies on the immunogenicity of preneoplastic and neoplastic mammary tissues of BALB/c mice free of the mammary tumor virus, *Israel J. Med. Sci.*, 7, 187, 1971.

31.   Weiss, D.W., Antigens in preneoplastic tissue during tumorigenesis, *Natl. Cancer Inst. Monogr.*, 35, 89, 1972.

32.   Weiss, D.W., Bonhag, R.S. and DeOme, K.B., Protective activity of fractions of tubercle bacilli against isologous tumors in mice, *Nature*, 190, 889, 1961.

33.   Weiss, D.W., Bonhag, R.S. and Leslie, P., Studies on the heterologous immunogenicity of a methanol-insoluble fraction of attenuated tubercle bacilli (BCG), II. Protection against tumor isografts, *J. Exp. Med.*, 124, 1039, 1966.

34.   Weiss, D.W., Nonspecific stimulation and modulation of the immune response and of states of resistance by the methanol extraction residue fraction of tubercle bacilli, *Natl. Cancer Inst. Monogr.*, 35, 157, 1972.

35.   Weiss, D.W., Discussion: Immunotherapy and immunoprophylaxis of cancer: The application of modulators of immunological responsiveness, in *Seventh Miles International Symposium: The Role of Immunological Factors in Viral and Oncogenic Processes*, Johns Hopkins Journal, Supplement 3, R.F. Beers, Jr., R.C. Tilghman and E.G. Basset, Eds., Johns Hopkins University Press, Baltimore, MD, 1974, pp. 157-169.

36.   Minden, P., Wainberg, M. and Weiss, D.W., Protection against guinea pig hepatomas by pretreatment with subcellular fractions of *Mycobacterium bovis* (BCG), *J. Natl. Cancer Inst.*, 52, 1643, 1974.

37.   Wainberg, M.A., Margolese, R.G. and Weiss, D.W., Tumor immunoprophylaxis and immunotherapy in guinea pigs treated with the methanol extraction residue (MER) of BCG, in *BCG in Cancer Immunotherapy*, G. Lamoureux, R. Turcotte and V. Portelance, Eds., Grune and Stratton, New York, 1976, pp. 39-50.

38.   Wainberg, M.A., Deutsch, V. and Weiss, D.W., Stimulation of antitumor immunity in guinea pigs by methanol extraction residue of BCG, *Brit. J. Cancer*, 34, 500, 1976.

39.   Haran-Ghera, N. and Weiss, D.W., Effect of treatment of C57BL/6 mice with the methanol extraction residue fraction of BCG on leukemogenesis induced by the radiation leukemia virus, *J. Natl. Cancer Inst.*, 50, 229, 1974.

40.   Markson, Y., Doljansky, F. and Weiss, D.W., Effects of prophylactic treatment with the MER tubercle bacillus fraction on the development of Rous sarcomas of chickens following challenge with the Rous sarcoma virus, in *Immunological Parameters of Host-Tumor Relationships*, Vol. V., D.W. Weiss, Ed., Academic Press, New York, 1978, pp. 51-59.

41.   Lavrin, D.H., Rosenberg, S.A., Connor, R.J. and Terry, W.D., Immunoprophylaxis of methylcholanthrene-induced tumors in mice with Bacillus Calmete-Guerin and methanol-extracted residue, *Cancer Res.*, 33, 472, 1973.

42.   Yron, I., Weiss, D.W., Robinson, E., Cohen, D., Adelberg, M.G., Mekori, T. and Haber, M., Immunotherapeutic studies in mice with the methanol extraction residue (MER) fraction of BCG: solid tumors, *Natl. Cancer Inst. Monogr.*, 39, 33, 1973.

43.   Weiss, D.W., Immunological intervention in neoplasia, in *Seventh Miles International Symposium: The Role of Immunological Factors in Viral and Oncogenic Processes*, Johns Hopkins Journal, Supplement 3, R.F. Beers, Jr., R.C. Tilgham and E.G. Basset, Eds., Johns Hopkins University Press, Baltimore, MD, 1974, pp. 131-156.

44.   Yron, I., Cohen, D., Robinson, E., Haber, M. and Weiss, D.W., Effects of methanol extraction residue and therapeutic irradiation against established isografts and simulated local recurrence of mammary carcinomas, *Cancer Res.*, 35, 1779, 1975.

45.   Cohen, D., Yron, I., Haber, M., Robinson, E. and Weiss, D.W., Effect of treatment with the MER tubercle bacilli fraction on the survival of mice carrying mammary tumor isografts: injection of MER at the tumor site or at a distal location, *Brit. J. Cancer*, 32, 483, 1975.

46.   Weiss, D.W., MER and other mycobacterial fractions in the immunotherapy of cancer, in *Medical Clinics Symposium on Immunotherapy in Malignant Disease*, W.D. Terry, Eds., W.B. Saunders Co., Philadelphia, Med. Clinics N. America 60: 473-497, 1976

47.   Treves, A.J., Cohen, I.R., Feldman, M. and Weiss, D.W., Effect of treatment with the methanol extraction residue fraction of killed tubercle bacilli (MER) on the development of spontaneous pulmonary metastases from syngeneic implants of tumor 3LL in C57B1 mice, in *Immunological Parameters of Host-Tumor Relationships*, Vol. IV, D.W. Weiss, Ed., Academic Press, New York, 1976, pp. 104-107.

48. Cohen, D., Yron, I., Grover, N.B. and Weiss, D.W., Chemoimmunotherapy of syngeneic mouse mammary carcinomas employing methanol extraction residue, *Ann. N.Y. Acad. Sci.*, 277, 195, 1976.

49. Wainberg, M.A., Margolese, R.G. and Weiss, D.W., Differential responsiveness of various substrains of inbred Strain 2 guinea pigs to immunotherapy with the methanol extraction residue (MER) to BCG, *Cancer Immunol. Immunother.*, 2, 101, 1977.

50. Wainberg, M.A., Minden, P. and Weiss, D.W., Vertical transmission of tumor resistance in guinea pigs, *Nature*, 259, 213, 1976.

51. Weiss, D.W., Aspects of immunotherapy of cancer with BCG and mycobacterial fractions, *World J. Surgery*, 1, 579, 1977.

52. Weiss, D.W., Host mechanisms for control of tumor growth that can be modulated by nonspecific immunotherapy, in *Immunotherapy of Human Cancer*, Univ. Texas System Cancer Center, 22nd Ann. Clin. Conf. on Cancer, Raven Press, New York, 1978, pp. 41-61.

53. Weiss, D.W., Approaches to "nonspecific" immunotherapy of cancer with microbial immunomodulators, in *The Role of Nonspecific Immunity in the Prevention and Treatment of Cancer*, M. Sela, Ed., Pontificia Academia Scientiarum, Vatican City, 1979, pp. 177-209.

54. Markson, Y. and Weiss, D.W., Effects of therapeutic treatment with the MER tubercle bacillus fraction on Rous sarcomas of chickens induced by the Rous Sarcoma virus, *Cancer Immunol. Immunother.*, 9, 159, 1980.

55. Weiss, D.W., Nonspecific immunity and cancer, in *The Mycobacteria: A Sourcebook, Part B*, G. P. Kubica and L.G. Wayne, Eds., Marcel Dekker, New York, 1984, pp. 863-902.

56. Stupp, Y., Manny, N., Shlomai, Z., Grover, N., Weiss, D.W. and Izak, G., Effect of treatment with the MER tubercle bacillus fraction on syngeneic plasma cell tumors of BALB/c mice, *Cancer Immunol. Immunother.*, 3, 189, 1978.

57. Minden, P., McClatchy, J.K., Wainberg, M., and Weiss, D.W., Shared antigens between *Mycobacterium bovis* (BCG) and neoplastic cells, *J. Natl. Cancer Inst.*, 53, 1325, 1974.

58. Steinkuller, C.B., Krigbaum, L.G. and Weiss, D.W., Studies on the mode of action of the heterologous immunogenicity of a methanol-insoluble fraction of attenuated tubercle bacilli (BCG), *Immunology*, 16, 255, 1969.

59. Yashphe, D.J., Steinkuller, C.B. and Weiss, D.W., Modulation of immunological responsiveness by pretreatment with a methanol-insoluble fraction of killed tubercle bacilli, *Israel J. Med. Sci.*, 5, 259, 1969.

60. Yashphe, D.J. and Weiss, D.W. , Modulation of the immune response by a methanol-insoluble fraction of attenuated tubercle bacilli (BCG), I. Primary and secondary responses to sheep red blood cells and T_2 phage, *Clin. Exp. Immunol.*, 7, 269, 1970

61. Kuperman, O., Yashphe, D.J., Sharf, S., Ben-Efraim, S. and Weiss, D.W., Nonspecific stimulation of cellular immunological responsiveness by a mycobacterial fraction, *Cell. Immunol.*, 3, 277, 1972.

62. Ben-Efraim, S., Constantini-Sourojon, M. and Weiss, D.W., Potentiation and modulation of the immune response of guinea pigs to poorly immunogenic protein-hapten conjugates by pretreatment with the MER fraction of attenuated tubercle bacilli, *Cell. Immunol.*, 7, 370, 1973.

63. Kuperman, O., Feigis, M. and Weiss, D.W., Reversal by the MER tubercle bacillus fraction of the suppressive effects of heterologous anti-lymphocytic serum (ALS) on the allograft reactivity of mice, *Cell Immunol.*, 8, 484, 1973.

64. Ben-Efraim, S., Teitelbaum, R., Ophir, R., Kleinman, R., and Weiss, D. W., Nonspecific modulation of immunological responsiveness in guinea pigs and mice by the tumor protective methanol extraction residue (MER) mycobacterial fraction: Influence of conditions of MER treatment and specific immunization and effect of MER on early stages of the immune response, in *Immunological Parameters of Host-Tumor Relationships*, Vol. III, D. W. Weiss, Ed., Academic Press, New York, 1974, pp. 158-169.

65. Gery, I., Baer, A., Stupp, Y., and Weiss, D. W., Further studies on the effects of the methanol extraction residue fraction of tubercle bacilli on lymphoid cells and macrophages, in *Immunological Parameters of Host-Tumor Relationships*, Vol. III, D. W. Weiss, Ed., Academic Press, New York, 1974, pp. 170-177.

66.   **Yagel, S., Gallily, R., and Weiss, D. W.,** Effect of treatment with the MER fraction of tubercle bacilli on hydrolytic lysosomal enzyme activity of mouse peritoneal macrophages, *Cell Immunol.,* 19, 381, 1975.

67.   **Gallily, R., Yagel, S., and Weiss, D. W.,** Potentiated lysosomal enzyme, bacteriostatic and bactericidal activities of peritoneal macrophages of mice treated with the MER fraction of tubercle bacilli, in *The Reticuloendothelial System in Health and Disease,* S. M. Reichard, M. R. Escobar and H. Friedman, Eds., Plenum Press, New York, 1976, pp. 351-361.

68.   **Weiss, D.W., Kuperman, O., Fathallah, N. and Kedar, E.** Mode of action of mycobacterial fractions in antitumor immunity: Preliminary evidence for a direct nonspecific stimulatory effect of MER on immunologically reactive cells, *Ann. N.Y. Acad. Sci.,* 276, 536, 1976.

69.   **Stupp, Y., Saltoun, R. and Weiss, D.W.,** Prevention by the MER tubercle bacillus fraction of immunosuppression induced by cancer chemotherapeutic agents, I. Antibody response of mice treated with cyclophosphamide, *Cancer Immunol. Immunother.,* 1, 219, 1976.

70.   **Zimber, C., Ben-Efraim, S. and Weiss, D.W.,** Prevention by the MER tubercle bacillus fraction of immunosuppression induced by cancer chemotherapeutic agents, II. Contact hypersensitivity in guinea pigs and mice treated with cyclophosphamide, *Cancer Immunol. Immunother.,* 3, 35, 1977.

71.   **Gallily, R., Douchan, Z. and Weiss, D.W.,** Potentiation of mouse peritoneal macrophage antibacterial functions by treatment of the donor animals with the methanol extraction residue fraction of tubercle bacilli, *Inf. Imm.,* 18, 405, 1977.

72.   **Ben-Efraim, S., Ophir, R., Teitelbaum, R., Zimber, C., Barbash, G. and Weiss, D.W.,** Effect of the MER tubercle bacillus fraction on the responsiveness of mice to T-independent antigens, *Int. Arch. Allergy Appl. Immunol.,* 58, 110, 1979.

73.   **Jacobs, D., Pass, E., Abraham, C. and Weiss, D.W.,** Studies on the influence of the MER tubercle bacillus fraction on immunological responsiveness of mice, Effects on antibody formation to a soluble protein and a T-independent antigen, delayed hypersensitivity to sheep erythrocytes, and numbers of antigen-reactive lymphoid cells, in *Immunological Parameters of Host-Tumor Relationships,* Vol. V, D.W. Weiss, Ed., Academic Press, New York, 1978, pp. 60-74.

74.   **Ben-Efraim, S., Sarir, Ch., Dar, O., Barbash, G., Grover, N.B. and Weiss, D.W.,** Effects of the MER tubercle bacillus fraction on the production of antibodies *in vitro,* I. Effect on the primary response, *Cell. Immunol.,* 50, 314, 1980.

75.   **Gallily, R., Stain, I. and Weiss, D. W.,** Mouse macrophage functions under the influence of factors released by spleen cells preincubated with the methanol extraction residue (MER) tubercle bacillus fraction, *Immunopharmacol.* 3, 221, 1981.

76.   **Zimber, C., Ben-Efraim, S. and Weiss, D.W.** , Variable nonspecific immunopotentiating efficacy of two preparations of MER: Effect on contact hypersensitivity of mice to dinitrofluorobenzene, *Cancer Immunol. Immunother.,* 10, 211, 1981.

77.   **Zimber, C., Ben-Efraim, S., Grover, N.B. and Weiss, D.W.,** Prevention by the MER tubercle bacillus fraction of immunosuppression induced by cancer chemotherapeutic agents, III. Contact hypersensitivity to dinitrofluorobenzene in mice treated with methotrexate, 5-fluorouracil, or cyclophosphamide, or exposed to dinitrobenzenesulfonate, *Cancer Immunol. Immunother.,* 10, 147, 1981.

78.   **Ben Efraim, S., Halperin, D., Reuben, C., Dar, O., and Weiss, D. W.,** Effects of the MER tubercle bacillus fraction on the production of antibodies *in vitro,* II. Effects on macrophage and lymphocyte populations, *Cell. Immunol.,* 86, 33, 1984.

79.   **Zimber, C., Ben-Efraim, S. and Weiss, D.W.,** Effect of methanol extraction residue tubercle bacillus fraction treatment *in vivo* and *in vitro* on the release and activity of suppressor factor inhibiting the efferent phase of contact sensitivity in mice, *Cell. Immunol.,* 95, 443, 1985.

80.   **Halperin, D., Reuben, C., Ben-Efraim, S., Grover, N., and Weiss, D. W.,** Effects of the methanol extraction residue (MER) tubercle bacillus fraction on the production of antibodies *in vitro,* III. Consequence of prior sensitization to MER, *Cell Immunol.,* 92, 404, 1985.

81. Reuben, C., Halperin, D., Ben-Efraim, S. and Weiss, D.W., Induction by an immunogenic immunomodulating agent of nonspecific T cell suppression of lymphocyte responsiveness in MLR but not of antibody production, *Cancer Immunol. Immunother.*, 1987.

82. Weiss, D.W., *The Wings of the Dove*, B'nai B'rith Books, 1987.

83. Izak, G., Stupp, Y., Manny, N., Zajicek, G. and Weiss, D.W., The immune response in acute myelocytic leukemia. Effect of the methanol extraction residue fraction of tubercle bacilli (MER) on T and B cell functions and their relation to the progress of the disease, *Israel J. Med. Sci.*, 13, 677, 1977.

84. Sulitzeanu, D. and Weiss, D.W., Antigen and immunogen - a question of terminology (letter to editor), *Cancer Immunol. Immunother.*, 11, 291, 1981.

85. Sulitzeanu, D., Human cancer-associated antigens: present status and implications for immunodiagnosis, *Adv. Cancer Res.*, 44, 1, 1985.

86. Weiss, D.W., The questionable immunogenicity of certain neoplasms: what then the prospects for immunological intervention in malignant disease? *Cancer Immunol. Immunother.*, 2, 11, 1977.

87. Weiss, D.W., Tumor origin, progression, immunogenicity and immunotherapy, *Transp. Proc.*, 16, 528, 1984.

88. Weiss, D.W., Reflections on tumor origin, immunogenicity and immunotherapy, *Cancer Immunol. Immunother.*, 18, 1, 1984.

89. Vanky, F. et al. as cited Kedar, E. and Weiss, D.W.,, *In vitro* generation of effector lymphocytes and their employment in tumor immunotherapy, *Adv. Cancer Res.*, 38, 171, 1983.

90. Kedar, E., Zeira, E., Lebendiker, Z., Weiss, D.W., Katan, R. and Shouval, D., Human and mouse "LAK" cells expanded in long term cultures: *in vitro* and *in vivo* studies, in *Cellular Immunotherapy of Cancer*, R.L. Truitt, M.M. Bortin and R.P. Gale, Eds., Alan R. Liss, Inc., New York, 1987.

91. Lebendiker, Z., Greenfield, C., Shouval, D., Shiloni, E., Weiss, D.W. and Kedar, E., Human tumors growing in nude mice: an experimental model for studying adoptive cellular immunotherapy, *17th Annual Meeting, Israel Immunological Society, Isr. J. Med. Sci.* 1987.

92. Klein, G. and Klein, E., Evolution of tumors and the impact of molecular oncology, *Nature*, 315, 190, 1985.

93. Weiss, D.W., Animal models of cancer immunotherapy, Questions of relevance, *Cancer Treat. Rpts.*, 64, 481, 1980.

94. Ben-Sasson, Z., Weiss, D.W. and Doljanski, F., Specific binding of factor(s) released by Rous sarcoma virus-transformed cells to splenocytes of chickens with Rous sarcomas, *J. Natl. Cancer Inst.*, 52, 405, 1974.

95. Plesser, Y.M., Weiss, D.W., Markson, Y. and Doljanski, F., Expression and shedding of major histocompatibility complex product and blood group antigens by cells in monolayer cultures, *Cell Immunol.*, 51, 414, 1980.

96. Plesser, Y.M., Markson, Y., Weiss, D.W., Brautbar, D. and Doljanski, F., Shedding of histocompatibility and blood group antigenic determinants from human epithelial cells and fibroblasts in culture, *Cell. Mol. Biol.*, 29, 227, 1983.

97. Friedman, R., Gelfand, T., Weiss, D.W. and Doljanski, F., Patterns of fibronectin disposition in normal and neoplastic fibroblasts and mammary tissue, *Int. J. Tissue Reactions*, 6, 291, 1984.

98. Markson, Y., Weiss, D.W., Weiss, O. and Doljanski, F., Presence of normal human cell surface antigens in plasma of athymic mice bearing a human colon carcinoma and in normal human plasma, *Cancer Immunol. Immunother.*, 20, 129, 1985.

99. Weiss, D.W., Tumor antigenicity and approaches to tumor immunotherapy - an outline, *Curr. Topics Microbiol. Immunol.*, 89, 1, 1980.

100. Kedar, E. and Weiss, D.W., *In vitro* generation of effector lymphocytes and their employment in tumor immunotherapy, *Adv. Cancer Res.*, 38, 171, 1983.

101. Weiss, D.W., Introduction: Do animal models serve as models for human immunotherapy? *Natl. Cancer Inst. Monogr.*, 39, 69, 1973.

102. Weiss, D.W., Animal models of cancer immunotherapy: some considerations. In: *Immunotherapy of Human Cancer*, University of Texas System Cancer Center, *22nd Annual Clinical Conference on Cancer*, Raven Press, New York, 1978, pp. 101-109.

103.   **Wainberg, M.A., Markson, Y., Weiss, D.W. and Doljanski, F.** , Cellular immunity against Rous sarcomas of chickens, Preferential reactivity against autochthonous target cells as determined by lymphocyte adherence and cytotoxicity tests *in vitro*, *Proc. Natl. Acad. Sci. USA*, 71, 3565, 1974.

104.   **Wainberg, M.A., Markson, Y., Doljanski, F. and Weiss, D.W.,** Reactivity of serum from Rous-sarcoma-bearing chickens with autochthonous and with allogeneic tumor cells: preferential autochthonous recognition, *Int. J. Cancer*, 15, 985, 1975.

105.   **Doljanski, F., Markson, Y., Wainberg, M.A. and Weiss, D.W.,** Cellular immunity to Rous sarcomas (RS): preferential autochthonous interactions and application of the immunoadherence technique to mouse tumors, *Transp. Proc. Vol. VII, No. 1, Supp. 1,* M. Schlesinger and R.E. Billingham, Eds., Grune and Stratton, New York, 1975, pp. 519-523.

Chapter 21

THE MACROPHAGE IN IMMUNOBIOLOGY: EXPLORATIONS OF TERRA INCOGNITA

Kurt Stern

Scientific progress may be frequently discerned to pass through three successive phases: exploration, discovery, application. The first stage is encumbered with the highest risk of frustration and failure. To borrow metaphors from geographic exploration, the efforts needed for clearing a path to sites hitherto never entered by a human foot—or a human mind—often end in total disaster: the direction chosen for the approach may turn out to be a hopeless dead end; the intruder may be lured into a morass from which he cannot extricate himself; the newly accessible territory may prove—or erroneously be assumed—to be a barren expanse devoid of any worthwhile assets and, accordingly, it is soon abandoned and forgotten. These considerations are by no means theoretical abstractions as far as I am concerned; rather, I have experienced them more than once during the close to sixty years of undertaking the tantalizing search for answers to critical questions concerning the place in immunobiology of the macrophage (M∅), the flag bearer of the reticuloendothelial system (RES).

In the following, I will attempt to outline the essential aspects of my pertinent research, its motivations, the possible significance of some findings, their place within the broader framework of current knowledge, and, when applicable, the remaining problems that require continued efforts for their resolution. The account will be punctuated by events arising from personal circumstances as well as those reflecting the history of this century, so rich in dramatic developments. The story spans three continents: Europe, where I was born and educated; the United States of America, where I spent most of my professional career; and Israel, where this outline is being written.

I was born in Vienna. After the death of my mother when I was barely four years old, I was brought up by my maternal grandparents in Brünn (Brno) where I lived from 1913 to 1927, completing elementary and high schools. The fact that Brünn is known as the city of Gregor Mendel is not merely a historic association, but it acquired particular significance for me through my high school teacher in biology, Hugo Iltis, who "wrote the definitive biography of Mendel"[1] and who provided me with a strong stimulus for engaging in natural science. While during the early high school years my main scientific interest focused on chemistry, my grandmother's death in 1923 of cancer caused me to commit myself to fight this disease and, therefore, to become a physician. After graduating from high school in 1927, I moved back to Vienna and joined, with my grandfather, the household of my father and his second wife. I entered the faculty of medicine of the University of Vienna from which I obtained the degree of doctor of medicine in January 1933.

---

*Iltis organized the Mendel Museum in Brünn. After immigrating to the United States in 1939, he served as biology professor at the Mary Washington College of the University of Virginia.

In my freshman year I combined courses in chemistry with the medical curriculum. When conflicting schedules in the sophomore year prevented me from continuing this double program, I enrolled as a compromise, in elective courses in biochemistry at the Institute for Medical Chemistry of the university. In due course, I was appointed there as laboratory assistant whose duties included supervision of first year medical students in laboratory exercises and performance of chemical tests on specimens of patients in the teaching hospitals. In addition, I participated in research conducted by Dr. Robert Willheim, a senior staff member of the institute. This was my introduction to cancer research, the specific topic of which may be of interest today only to antiquarians of the field. It concerned the cytolytic, or carcinolytic, reaction, first described by Freund and Kaminer[2] in 1910. Cytolysis of cancer cells occurred and was visually established by counting the cells before and after incubation with sera derived from normal persons or patients without cancer; cytolysis was not observed when the sera were derived from cancer patients.

The phenomenon was assumed to reflect the presence in normal sera of a cytolytic factor, and of an inhibitor of cytolysis in sera of cancer patients. The test was thought to be useful for diagnostic purposes. Having worked with this methodology and some modifications introduced by us, for about ten years, I am convinced of the reality of the phenomenon, although it lacked diagnostic value because false positive and false negative results reached at least 20 %. Without going into details of our findings published in ten papers, I can state retrospectively that two sets of observations decisively influenced my subsequent experimental work. One was the demonstration that the inhibitor of cytolysis appeared in the sera of normal rabbits after their RES was damaged by injections of "blocking" substances, such as India ink, trypan blue, or carmine.[3] Another, possibly even more significant finding was the promotion of growth of transplanted mouse tumors when the inhibitor of carcinolysis was adsorbed to the tumor cells prior to their inoculation. This enhancement of neoplastic growth was expressed in the higher number of takes, shorter latent periods, and increased tumor weights in experimental mice, as compared with controls.[4] We interpreted these results as "...damage of the RES...may bring about changes...preventing lysis of cancer cells and thus promote the growth of cancer"*[5] and "...the carcinolytic phenomenon may be considered to be a functional test of the RES".[6] Admittedly, these were at best educated guesses, but they served as heuristic hypotheses suggesting avenues of further experimental studies. The work with Willheim taught me a number of general lessons: 1) the futility of premature practical application of experimental findings, as exemplified by the failure of the carcinolytic reaction to serve as a reliable diagnostic test; 2) introduction to the use of animal tumors, limited in our laboratory to Ehrlich carcinoma inoculated into random-bred mice, and Brown-Pearce rabbit carcinoma; 3) awareness of the need for functional tests of the RES capable of disclosing depression as well as stimulation of its activities. Indeed, during the ensuing few years before I left Vienna, we utilized a refinement of the Congo Red test[7] for assay of the reticuloendothelial (r.e.) function in rabbits, and we found that injections of carotene emulsions led, in most instances, to accelerated clearance of the dye from circulation, indicative of

---

*This and subsequent quotations translated from German by the author.

increased phagocytosis; the treatment also augmented the carcinolytic activity of the serum.[8]

A fair portion of my time was occupied by authoring with Willheim a monograph published in 1936, entitled, "Die Wege und Ergebnisse Chemischer Krebsforschung" (The Approaches and Results of Chemical Cancer Research).[9] This was an attempt to summarize and analyze the vast body of relevant data gathered by numerous investigators, dispersed in time and space. The book foreshadowed similar efforts I undertook in subsequent years. It seems to me that I was motivated by the conviction that each investigative result could be fully appreciated only within the context of other pertinent information available from studies of the same or related topics. Thus, a particular finding could be viewed as one minute fragment that might be of critical importance for completing the complex and intricate mosaic representing biomedical knowledge. Hence, we tried to establish associations between observations made in our cancer research and those derived from other studies which involved an ever increasing number of disciplines and more and more sophisticated methods. This, we thought, should enable us to disclose similarities as well as discrepancies, with the latter in need for explanations of the conflicting findings. The coverage of the monograph extended beyond the strict limits of biochemistry suggested in the title, inasmuch as it included a fairly long chapter on immunobiology, a part of which dealt with the relationship between cancer and the RES.

Ominous clouds had gathered on the political horizon of Austria. Soon after my graduation from medical school, Jews were barred from internships and residencies in state and municipal hospitals, forcing me to obtain my clinical training as a volunteer. The anti-Jewish discrimination worsened after the establishment of an authoritarian government in 1934 by Dollfus, who was murdered in an unsuccessful Nazi revolt less than half a year later. In March 1938 any semblance of normal Jewish life in Vienna ceased, with Austria becoming a part of the German Nazi Reich. Having been aware much earlier of the threat of total disenfranchisement of Jews in Austria, as were many others, I spent two months in Palestine in 1935 trying to secure an academic appointment. After I failed in these efforts, I returned to Vienna and combined private practice of medicine with continued research at the Institute for Medical Chemistry of the university. Soon after the Nazi takeover, I had to stop this work. Emigration remained the only solution for me as it did for the rest of Viennese Jewry. For me luckily, my father's sister and her family had settled in the United States before World War I and a cousin sent me the affidavit which enabled me to enter the United States in September 1938, a few days before the Munich pact postponed the already then feared outbreak of World War II for nearly one year.

In the baggage which I transported across the ocean, there were concealed (and hence safe from customs examination) the notion I had nurtured for some years about experimental studies of the interactions between the RES and cancer. It would take many years before I could put them to the test. My first year in the "new world," though difficult, brought some progress. Through the helpfulness of Dr. Ira I. Kaplan, I obtained a fellowship at the New York City Division of Cancer headed by him. I met and married my helpmate for life. I passed the State Board examination and received the license to practice medicine in the State of New York. The fellowship enabled me to resume experimental studies, though within narrow limits. First, I worked at the New York City Cancer Hospital, then located on

Welfare Island. Later, I was appointed postgraduate observer at the New York University Medical School where I was fortunate to enjoy the hospitality of the laboratory of Dr. Anna Goldfeder. We became life-long friends, and in later years we collaborated on scientific topics of shared interest. A few modest results ensued from my work. Assisted by the availability of cancer patients hospitalized in the city hospital, I evaluated their r.e. function by means of the Congo Red test.[8] Delayed clearance of the dye, i.e., impaired phagocytic function, was demonstrated in 86 out of 100 patients suffering from a variety of advanced malignant tumors, whereas normal values were obtained in 49 patients with noncancerous diseases. Moreover, the degree of r.e. inadequacy seemed to possess some prognostic significance: 70% of patients with most severe impairment died within 6 to 9 months after the test was performed, as compared with only 30% of those with the least degree of r.e. damage.[10] I also published a review of the relationship between cancer and the RES[11] in which I included data obtained before I left Vienna concerning stimulation of the RES in rabbits injected with carotene and uracil, and preliminary observations on slight retardation of the growth of rabbit Pearce carcinoma by these substances. The article also proposed and presaged, experimental approaches that might be useful for elucidation of the role of the RES in development of neoplasia: "...experiments with animal strains exhibiting a high percentage of hereditary spontaneous cancer would be especially interesting...It would be extremely desirable to study the reticuloendothelial system in these animals before the appearance of neoplasms and to compare (them with) findings in control animals."

In 1939, Dr. Willheim spent a few months in New York City on the way to Manila where he had accepted an appointment at the University of the Philippines. At this time, we found a publisher for a revised and updated English edition of the monograph published in German (9). The book, *The Biochemistry of Malignant Tumors*[12] appeared in 1943. It was almost double the size of the earlier version; it contained a separate chapter on tumor origin and tumor growth which dealt with heredity, growth-promoting and growth-inhibiting factors, and viral tumors. The chapter on immunology included a discussion of the role of the RES in cancer, expanded to nearly 100 pages with citation of 250 references.

In the meantime, World War II had broken out in Europe in September 1939 and the United States was brought into the conflict by the Japanese attack on Pearl Harbor in December 1941. These "fateful events cut off all possibilities of collaboration"[13] on the book by Willheim and me. I had to carry out the work alone.

After termination of the fellowship, I tried to find an academic or research position but to no avail. **Faute de mieux**, I practiced general medicine and conducted a private clinical laboratory. After the United States entered the war, I applied for, but failed to get, a medical commission in the armed forces. Being subject to placement by the Man Power Commission, I was offered several choices of which I elected to accept a position as junior physician at the New York State Institute for the Study and Treatment of Malignant Diseases (now Roswell Park Memorial Institute) in Buffalo. I held this position for two years, until the end of the war.

As far as experimental work was concerned, my first decade in America could be considered a period of suspended animation, reflecting either hibernation or, at best, incubation. This time span was essential for my acquiring the basic understanding of the prerequisites and additional qualifications necessary for my locating a niche where I could develop opportunities for research. In this context, the Buffalo experience was of considerable help. One, I gained a valuable background and insight into diagnosis, treatment and clinical course of cancer; this equipped me with a realistic appreciation of the human disease, which investigators exclusively concerned with animal models sometime lack. Two, I became well acquainted with the breeding, properties, and utilization of inbred strains of mice, which were to be the mainstay of much of my future work. Three, close contact with the department of pathology and the day-to-day instruction I received from its head, Dr. A.A. Thibaudeau and his staff, contributed significantly not only to my knowledge of the discipline, but also to the realization that specialization in pathology would probably be the most efficient way for my gaining access to medical research. Thus, when the war ended, I was most receptive to an offer to serve as assistant pathologist at the Mount Sinai Hospital in Chicago, where I remained, in various capacities, for 15 years and was closely associated with Dr. Israel Davidsohn, head of the department. I was charged with assisting him in the daily conduct of the active laboratory, and he guided and supervised my formal training in pathology. Davidsohn was no easy taskmaster, but he was an outstanding teacher to whom I owe the major part of my understanding of pathology and laboratory administration. In 1948, I passed the examination of the American Board of Pathology in pathologic anatomy, and in 1950 in clinical pathology. In the same year, I was appointed assistant professor of pathology at the Chicago Medical School, serving under Davidsohn's chairmanship.

In parallel with carrying out my duties in hospital pathology, laboratory administration, and academic teaching, I gradually developed a program for experimental work, much of it in collaboration with Davidsohn. One area of research was immunohematology, a field in which Davidsohn pioneered from the early days of his career. Accordingly, I benefitted greatly from his experience and ideas. On the other hand, I contributed methods and approaches, not previously employed in the department, to another field, viz., cancer research, by introducing the use of animals of inbred strains, chemical carcinogenesis, and work with spontaneous, induced, transplanted tumors. The opportunities for research increased considerably in 1949 with the establishment of the Mount Sinai Medical Research Foundation, of which I became associate director. In addition, in 1950, I assumed an active role in blood transfusion therapy when I was appointed director of the blood center affiliated with the Research Foundation, and charged with the tasks of serving the wider community as well as engaging in pertinent research.

During the final year in Buffalo, at least subconsciously influenced by growing involvement in, and familiarity with, tissue morphology, I changed my approach to the assay of r.e. function: in place of the indirect techniques of determining the clearance from the circulation of injected substances, such as Congo Red, I utilized direct visual observation in tissue sections of phagocytosis of macromolecular compounds, such as lithium carmine. In fact, this represented a return to the original methodology by means of which Metchnikoff[14] discovered and described the activity of the MØ (literal translation: "big eater"), and it reflected as well the criteria used by Aschoff[15] for defining the components of the RES. In Buffalo I began a pilot study of the program I had proposed in 1941[11] by comparing the phagocytic activity of Kupffer cells in the liver and splenic MØs in healthy mice of the low-tumor strain C57BL and the high-mammary tumor strain Marsh-Albino.

In Chicago I supplemented these preliminary experiments by testing larger numbers of healthy C57BL mice and mice of the high-mammary tumor strain C3H. Hepatic and splenic phagocytosis of carmine was significantly greater in animals of the low-tumor strain than in those of the high-tumor strains. At that time I cautioned that "it would be premature to speculate on a possible relationship between susceptibility or resistance to spontaneous cancer development...and the reticuloendothelial activity of the strain, as expressed in the dye storage...".[16]

During the four decades that have elapsed from the time I expressed these thoughts until my writing these comments, I endeavored to find answers to three basic questions concerning the interactions between the RES and the neoplastic process: (1) It is possible to demonstrate some deviations from the norm in r.e. functions that are associated with higher risks for development of cancer? (2) What effects does presence of cancer have on r.e. functions? (3) To what extent can one interfere with, or even reverse, development and progression of neoplasia by modifying specific functions of the RES?

In connection with the first question, data obtained in our further work, and subsequently supported by results reported by other investigators, gave strong evidence for genetic factors being one of the determinants of phagocytic activity. Proliferation of Kupffer cells induced by injection of the sulfonated azo dye cloth red B was greater in C57BL than C3H mice.[17] Storage in M∅ of another sulfonated azo dye, Erie Fast Rubin (EFR) was considerably heavier in C57BL than C3H mice, whereas accumulation of the synthetic polymer polyvinylpyrrolidone (PVP) was more pronounced in spleen and liver of C3H than C57BL mice,[18] and PVP-induced splenomegaly in C3H, CBA, and AKR mice was shown to exceed that occurring in C57BL and C57L mice.[19] Larger amounts of the orally administered rimino dye B.663 were stored in livers and spleens of C57BL than in comparably treated animals of strains BALB/c and AKR.[20] When radioisotopes became available, we utilized in place of the microscopic determination of phagocytosed matter, radioassays of livers and spleens of animals that had been injected with colloidal radiogold (^{198}Au). This made it possible to test more accurately and more efficiently larger numbers of animals of additional inbred strains with known incidence of spontaneous tumors and leukemias. Results so obtained showed that phagocytic activity, in general, was greater in healthy mice of low-cancer, low-leukemia strains (C57BL, C57L) than in those of high-cancer or high-leukemia strains (C3H, CBA, AKR).[21,22]

Considerable weight was added to the importance of these interstrain differences established for an essential r.e. function, by results of parallel studies that we carried out on humoral hemoantibodies in normal mice of similar provenience. While presence of natural agglutinins for sheep erythrocytes appeared to be limited to sera of C57BL mice,[23,24,25] mean titers of natural agglutinins for chicken erythrocytes were significantly higher in six low-tumor strains than in five out of six high-cancer or high-leukemia strains.[26] Likewise, immunization with sheep or chicken red cells produced higher titers of agglutinins and hemolysins in animals of six low-tumor strains as compared with findings in five out of six high-cancer or high-leukemia strains.[27] Direct proof for genetic regulation of humoral antibodies was derived from experiments in which natural agglutinins for sheep erythrocytes were compared in mice of strains C57BL, C3H, their F_1 offspring, and backcrosses of F_1 to parent strains.[28] In one of the earlier studies, we interpreted the interstrain differences in immune responses to red cell antigens as indicating "that mice of strain C57BL have a more responsive agglutinin-producing RES than the other five strains".[24] More conclusive evidence for a correlation between overloading of the RES and depression of immune responses was obtained by comparing titers of hemolysins for sheep red cells (SRC) in control mice and in mice injected with high-molecular PVP prior to immunization. Significant depression of hemolysins was noted in mice of strains C3H, CBA, and AKR, but not in those of strains C57BL and C57L.[29] As stated previously, administration of PVP caused considerably greater splenomegaly and PVP accumulation in animals of the three first-named strains than in those of the two latter strains.[19]

What does all this add up to? It would be tempting to propose that malfunction of the RES, as expressed in defective phagocytosis, represents a risk factor for development of cancer. However, this assumption must be hedged by several reservations. One, it may not be permissible to extrapolate observations made with one particular model, viz., mice of inbred strains, to other systems. Two, phagocytosis is only one of the many r.e. functions that may be relevant to neoplasia. Three, phagocytosis *per se* is by no means a uniform process; rather, it is critically dependent on variables that include nature, size, and route of administration of the particulate or macromolecular substrate employed in the assay. A good example for the disparate behavior of different substrates in the same host surfaced in our studies to which I have previously referred: PVP was much more heavily stored in C3H than C57BL mice,[19] whereas the opposite held true for carmine,[16] sulfonated azo dyes,[17] and colloidal radiogold.[21]

When the results of our investigations of r.e. phagocytosis and immune responses are viewed within the context of current knowledge, it must be emphasized that our work was done prior to the availability of such basic information as the critical role of MØ fulfills in the immune response by engaging in uptake, processing, and presentation of antigen (cf. References)[30,31,32] and the operation of the immune response genes that are closely linked to the major histocompatibility complex (see Ref.).[33] On the other hand, our observations of impaired r.e. activity and immune responsiveness in cancer-prone hosts obviously is reminiscent of the theory of immune surveillance of cancer, as it was proposed and developed toward the end of the 1950's.[34] In a survey published in 1983[35] I summarized data reported by other investigators who compared phagocytosis as well as cytostatic and cytotoxic activities of MØ in mice of inbred strains; in general, the results were in accord with our findings. One study deserves special mention since it may be considered to be a veritable mirror image of our approach. Biozzi and his associates,[36] instead of testing available inbred strains with known incidence of spontaneous tumors as we did, developed by suitable matings and inbreeding, two lines of mice; one of them was characterized by high immune responses to SRC and numerous other antigens, whereas the other line consistently produced low immune responses. Significantly, after administration of the carcinogen benzopyrene, mice of the "high antibody" line were most resistant to induction of tumors than those of the "low antibody" line, and tumor growth was more rapid in the latter than the former.[37]

More definitive answers, as well as some new insights, emerged from our attempts to determine the effects on the RES of the presence of neoplasia. In Lewis rats bearing transplanted syngeneic lymphomas, radioassay of liver and spleen performed 24 hrs after intraperitoneal injection of [198]Au revealed a significant increase of phagocytosed colloid per gram of liver, but a significant decrease per gram of spleen, when compared with findings in tumor-free controls.   Because of the considerable hepatomegaly and splenomegaly in tumor bearers, the differences in uptake were even more marked for the entire liver, but less for the whole spleen. These effects were clearly the result of progressive tumor growth since they were less pronounced in rats with small tumors than in those with large, metastasizing ones.[38]   In interpreting these observations, we concluded: "It is obvious that to speak of hyperfunction or hypofunction of the reticuloendothelial system in neoplasia... would be a misleading oversimplification" in light of the changes in the opposite directions of phagocytosis in hepatic and splenic MØ, as well as in view of the inverse correlation between hepatic phagocytosis and immune response to sheep red cells, with the latter associated with diminished splenic phagocytosis. In order to make experimental conditions for testing phagocytosis more similar to those used for examining immune responses, in subsequent work we employed xenogeneic or allogeneic cells labeled with radiochromium. Thus we compared splenic and hepatic uptakes of ^{51}Cr-labeled sheep red cells (^{51}Cr-SRC) in tumor-free control mice and in mice with transplanted tumors. In 12 experiments carried out with animals of five inbred strains, inoculated either with syngeneic tumors or with sarcoma 180, splenic phagocytosis of ^{51}Cr-SRC was decreased consistently and significantly, while hepatic phagocytosis was diminished in some experiments, unchanged, or even increased, in others. Also, in this model the depression of splenic phagocytosis reflected the tumor load, becoming more marked with the time elapsed between inoculation of tumor and assay.[39]   Additional evidence for the discordant behavior of splenic and hepatic MØ was provided by the response of control and tumor bearing mice to injection of polylysine (PL).   This synthetic polyamino acid was shown in previous work to suppress levels of immune hemolysin for SRC[40] and to interfere with phagocytosis of ^{51}Cr-SRC.[41] Administration of PL to tumor-bearing mice depressed phagocytosis much more severely in the spleen than in the liver.[36] It must be also kept in mind that splenomegaly and hepatomegaly, commonly occurring in tumor-bearing rodents are to a large extent the expression of proliferation of splenic MM and Kupfer cells in the liver. Thus, in these models of neoplasia, morphologic and functional changes in the RES do not run parallel. In line with the interstrain differences in r.e. activity discussed previously, dissimilar effects of presence of tumors were encountered in mice of particular strains: transplanted tumors lowered phagocytic uptake of the rimino dye B.663 to a lesser extent in C57BL than BALB/c and AKR mice.[20] Similarly, in X/Gf mice—a strain highly resistant to induction of tumors by x-irradiation and some chemical carcinogens—presence of syngeneic transplanted tumors failed to inhibit phagocytosis, by contrast with tumor-bearing C3H mice tested in parallel experiments.[42]

Spontaneous tumors are undoubtedly a model more germane to the clinical disease than are transplanted tumors. For this reason, we invested considerable effort in testing the phagocytic function of mice with spontaneous mammary carcinoma of strains C3H, DBA, A/Sn, and BALB/cf (the latter having acquired the mammary tumor virus by foster nursing to C3H females), and mice with spontaneous lymphoma of strains AKR and SJL. Tumor-free litter mates served as controls. Again, splenic phagocytosis of ^{51}Cr-SRC was significantly impaired in tumor bearers. Hepatic phagocytosis was less frequently affected and, when observed, the decrease was limited to the radioactivity assayed per g of liver, but not for the whole organ because of the hepatomegaly. After intravenous injection of chromic radiophosphate, blood clearance of the radiolabel was delayed in C3H and BALB/cf mice with mammary carcinoma when compared with tumor-free litter mates.[43] We supplemented the use of the models of transplanted and spontaneous tumors by studying the effect of chemical carcinogens. "A progressive decrease in splenic phagocytosis occurred in mice injected with methylcholanthrene (MCA), prior to manifestation of induced tumors".[44] In the final part of the essay, further elaboration of this work will be described.

In parallel with investigating the effects on r.e. phagocytosis of the presence of tumor, we examined immune responses of tumor-bearing hosts. As compared with suitable controls, lower titers of immune hemolysin for sheep and chicken erythrocytes were found in AKR and DBA mice inoculated with syngeneic lymphoma and C57BL mice with syngeneic myeloid leukemia.[45] After primary immunization of rats with human red cells of group A, they were divided into two groups with similar distribution of antibody levels; one served as control while rats of the other were transplanted with Walker tumor. Secondary immunization with human group A red cells given to rats of both groups when the average diameter of tumors reached 2 cm, produced significantly lower titers of hemolysin in tumor-bearing than tumor-free rats.[46] In extensive experiments with mice of five strains, inoculated with 13 different tumors (syngeneic carcinomas, sarcomas, and lymphomas, or sarcoma 180), we found varying degrees of depression of the secondary immune response to xenogeneic red cells in tumor-bearing animals, with the exception of a single tumor. The interference with the immune response was more pronounced in mice with lymphoma than in those with carcinoma or sarcoma. In the latter animals, antibodies were more markedly lowered after challenge with a single large dose than after multiple injections of smaller amounts of antigen. We attributed this differential effect to the fact that the spleen is primarily involved in the immune response to a single large dose of antigen, whereas extrasplenic sites become more active after repeated antigenic stimulation.[47] Immune responses to red cell antigens were also decreased after percutaneous application of MCA to DBA/2 mice which developed leukemia, but this did not occur in DBA/1 mice, not susceptible to this form of leukemogenesis. Likewise, fractionated x-irradiation induced leukemia and diminished formation of antibodies in young C57BL mice, but not in old ones which are refractory to radiation-induced leukemia.[48]

In the survey mentioned previously,[35] we included some investigations by other workers who recorded defective splenic and enhanced hepatic phagocytosis in tumor-bearing animals and cancer patients. Observations of accelerated clearance from the blood stream of intravenously injected substrate was documented in a number of studies; this would be viewed as reflecting augmented phagocytosis by Kupffer cells which rapidly remove circulating macromolecular and particulate matter. Another important r.e. function, demonstrated to be impaired in animals and patients with cancer, is the chemotactic response of monocytes and MØ (see Refs.).[49,50,51]

Juxtaposition of the observations made in the host prior to, and after, development of neoplasia, fragmentary though they may be, raise the intriguing albeit hardly encouraging possibility of the operation of a vicious cycle: impairment of defensive functions, such as phagocytosis and immune responsiveness, may facilitate appearance of cancer, and this is followed by the manifest disease inflicting additional damage to these mechanisms of resistance. Obviously, such a sequence of events does not bode well for the success of measures that might counteract the neoplastic process by improving the efficiency of the RES, a potential goal considered in the third question about the interactions between the RES and cancer, which we attempted to answer. Indeed, experience gained not only in our own limited work, but also in endeavors made by numerous other investigators, confirms this unfavorable expectation. Thus, prolonged administration of the sulfonated azo dye EFR produced proliferation of hepatic and splenic MØ, but it succeeded in inhibiting the growth in C3H mice of transplanted mammary carcinoma only transiently. Similarly, in C57BL mice injected with MCA, treatment with the dye delayed appearance of induced tumors up to 17 wks, but there was no significant difference between control and experimental groups in the cumulative incidence and the rate of growth of tumors.[17] Feeding of the rimino dye B.663 to C57BL, BALB/c, and AKR mice bearing syngeneic sarcomas, caused only moderate inhibition of tumor growth.[20] Approximately ten years were to elapse before I searched for new approaches that might demonstrate antineoplastic effects of the MØ and its products more convincingly.

As far as the essential nature of cancer is concerned, there is general agreement that malignant tumors cannot be placed into any of the categories of degenerative, inflammatory, or metabolic disorders, regardless of the specific etiologic factor(s) suspected or proven to be responsible for the genesis of one or the other particular type of neoplasm. Shortly after my arrival in the U.S. I read and was much impressed by the report published by a committee appointed by the Surgeon General and assigned the task of formulating guidelines for research to be conducted and fostered by the recently established National Cancer Institute.[52] One of the conclusions reached by the committee—in my opinion, as valid today as it was fifty years ago—stated: whatever the etiology of cancer may be, "the end result is the same - a cell with a capacity for unlimited and uncontrolled growth. Have they become "fast" to the conditions which normally control cell growth in the body, or is there a break in the internal control of cell activity? ...The investigation of characteristics of the cancer cell belongs in the field of cell physiology, and the understanding of the process must be dependent upon the advance in the understanding of growth and differentiation of normal cell." I included the last sentence of the statement in a review published in 1941 (11). In view of these considerations, it is not surprising that I was eager to study a model of noncancerous growth that would permit evaluation of the possible role of the MØ in its regulation. The obvious choice for such an experimental design was the phenomenon of regeneration or, more correctly, restoration of liver tissue after partial hepatectomy. The results were clear cut: when phagocytosis was assayed in Lewis and Wistar rats three to eight days after two-thirds hepatectomy, uptake of colloidal radiogold was significantly higher in liver and spleen of hepatectomized than sham-operated animals. No such differences were noted on day 16 post-hepatectomy, at which time restoration of liver tissue was complete. An increase in the spleen/body weight ratio attested to splenic proliferation resulting from the intervention.[53] In a subsequent publication[54] we remarked that "the maximal increase in phagocytic activity coincides with maximal mitotic activity...This may be more than coincidental." By means of preoperative injection of [198]Au into the rats, we developed an isotopic dilution technique which permitted quantitation of restoration of liver tissue by comparing the concentration of the radiolabel in the hepatectomized tissue with that found in the liver tissue present at specified intervals after the operation. While the data so obtained agreed, in principle, with that recorded in the literature and based on the assumption that in the standard technique actually two-thirds of the organ has been removed, our more accurate estimation disclosed two important details: 1) considerable individual variations in the rate of restoration between animals of the same sex; 2) an apparently faster rate of restoration in female than male rats.[54] An even more remarkable sexual dimorphism was observed in the experiments with hepatectomized as well as tumor-bearing rats;[38] the phagocytic activity was significantly higher in liver and spleen of female than male normal rats. In this connection, it is pertinent to refer to the previously documented parallelism between r.e. phagocytosis and immune responses, inasmuch as we also demonstrated sex- and strain-dependent differences in mice immunized with xenogeneic red cells. Higher titers of immune hemolysin for SRC were found in normal female than male C57BL mice, whereas this was not the case in C3H mice. Moreover, pretreatment with estrogen markedly elevated the level of hemolysin in immunized C57BL, but not in C3H mice. By contrast, administration of cortisone was much more effective in reducing the immune response of C3H than C57BL mice.[55] In view of the report that estrogen induced proliferation of r.e. tissues,[56] we speculated that "stimulation of macrophage activity may be the mechanism responsible for the enhancement of antibody formation".[55] Returning to the primary objective of our study, viz., the inquiry into the possible participation of the MØ in homeostasis of growth, we were impressed by the changes in opposite directions of phagocytic activity accompanying the noncancerous, limited growth following partial hepatectomy, on the one hand, and, on the other, those associated with uncontrolled neoplastic growth. This encouraged us, in spite of the scant direct evidence available then, to assign at least heuristic value "to the hypothetical assumption that normal and pathologic r.e. functions may be involved in growth processes".[54] Attempting to test this hypothesis, we employed an experimental design intended to simulate "cellular events associated with processes of physiologic or pathologic tissue breakdown, and subsequent repair and regeneration." For this purpose, we examined the effects in mice of injections of subcellular fractions prepared from normal syngeneic organs (liver, spleen, kidney) on hepatic and splenic uptakes of ^{51}Cr-SRC. Microsomal fractions proved to be most effective in significantly reducing hepatic and splenic phagocytosis, assayed six hrs after the last of three injections of the material. The depressed uptake persisted for approximately 48 hrs; prolonged administration of microsomes during 11 wks produced "waxing and waning" changes. Analogous findings were obtained in rats treated with subcellular fractions.[57] In extension of this work we observed that ribosomes were more potent in affecting phagocytosis than were microsomes, with the activity of the fractions correlated with their RNA rather than protein count. The ability of reducing phagocytosis was diminished, or absent, in subcellular fractions prepared from 8 months, as compared with 6 wks old donors; from liver collected six hrs after partial hepatectomy; and from transplanted syngeneic tumors,[58] findings that suggest that some modifications in the subcellular machinery brought about by age, enhanced DNA synthesis, and neoplastic growth. Although these observations provided only circumstantial evidence for participation of the RES in regulation of growth, their significance has risen in the light of solid data presented within the last two decades by several investigators who furnished proof for the cytostatic activity of the MØ and for secretion by MØ of growth-inhibiting and growth-promoting factors. Nevertheless, much remains to be learned and elucidated in order to fully comprehend the role of the RES in homeostasis of growth and, particularly, to pinpoint mechanisms that could be exploited for counteracting development and progression of cancer.

The account so far presented dealt with our studies of the RES in cancer and in regulation of growth. This work utilized animal models exclusively; it had *a priori* defined goals—even though they were not always reached; and it was initiated and pursued on the basis of previous experimental observations, certain hypothetical assumptions and, admittedly, some preconceived ideas. By contrast, research in the third area of our major interest—immunization to red cell antigens—originated from clinical medicine, and only in later stages did we attempt to devise animal models that would permit better controlled conditions than clinical studies. Unanticipated findings in the animal experiments first brought to our attention the possibility that the MØ may play a significant role in phenomena of inhibition and suppression of alloimmunization. My responsibility for the blood transfusion service and the work of the Rh laboratory of Mount Sinai Hospital shared a common denominator: alloimmunization to red cell antigens. In selecting compatible blood for transfusions, it was essential to prevent alloimmunization by all possible means and, if present, to avoid administration of red cells subject to destruction by antibodies present in the recipient. In parallel, prenatal and neonatal laboratory tests demonstrating alloimmunization are critical for diagnosis, prognosis, and treatment of hemolytic disease of the newborn (HDN; previously called fetal erythroblastosis). In the introduction to a paper on "Experimental Studies on Rh Immunization",[59] we commented: "Solutions to problems in biology almost invariably lead to as many, and sometimes more, new questions that are left unanswered...The discovery that maternal isosensitization to the Rh factor is the most frequent cause of hemolytic disease of the newborn was no exception to this maxim. Although the etiology and pathogenesis of more than 90% of cases of this disease are now explained by the typical triad of an Rh-negative mother carrying an Rh-positive fetus that is exposed to Rh antibodies, it is still a mystery why only 1 of 20 to 25 Rh-negative women actually develops Rh antibody...it is still not known why it does not occur...in apparently identical situations." Parenthetically, the figure of 5% for the risk of pregnancy-induced alloimmunization is too low and should be at least doubled. However, this numerical change does not lessen the validity of the question raised above. Levine,[60] the immuno-hematologist who first identified the etiology of HDN, pointed to an unexpected clinical observation: Rh immunization was significantly less frequent in Rh-negative women whose Rh-positive fetus was ABO incompatible with the mother than when ABO compatible; in other words, Rh immunization was inhibited when maternal anti-A or anti-B antibodies were reactive with the fetal red cells. Subsequently, numerous surveys, including one conducted in our laboratory,[61] confirmed this finding. Not being satisfied with explanations offered for this phenomenon, we studied alloimmunization to the Rho (D) blood factor in Rh-negative (rh) men injected with Rh-positive blood. This work was done with the help of inmates of the Illinois State Penitentiary, Joliet, Illinois, who volunteered for participation in the project. We complied with all rules required for experiments on human subjects, including obtaining written informed consent from each subject, and using all safeguards needed for protection of the participants from harmful effects of the injections of blood. The experimental results were in unequivocal agreement with the clinical data: 10 out of 17 Rh men injected with ABO compatible blood developed Rh antibodies, whereas only two out of 22 men injected with ABO-incompatible blood did so In subsequent work,[62] we expanded the number of subjects to 24 Rh men immunized with ABO compatible blood of whom 17 developed antibodies, as contrasted with only five out of 32 immunized with ABO incompatible blood. In addition, we showed that ABO incompatible blood was an inferior stimulus for secondary immune responses in subjects already immunized to the Rh antigen. In order to rule out the possibility that by chance a higher percentage of constitutional "nonresponders" may have been present in the group injected with ABO incompatible blood, we injected, after unsuccessful exposure to ABO incompatible blood, ten such subjects with ABO compatible blood, a treatment that induced Rh antibodies in six of them. We also wanted to test the potential inhibitory effect on Rh immunogenicity of anti-A or anti-B attached to the red cell surface carrying the corresponding antigens. For this purpose, we coated A Rh-positive red cells *in vitro* with anti-A prior to injection into eight A Rh men, six of whom developed Rh antibodies, thus ruling out any inhibitory activity of anti-A antibodies *per se* on Rh immunization. Following up the use of red cells coated with anti-A, we treated group O Rh-positive red cells *in vitro* with Rh antibody before using them for immunization. Remarkably, none of the 16 rh men formed Rh antibodies after receiving four to five injections of the antibody-coated red cells, whereas subsequent administration of untreated Rh-positive blood induced Rh immunization in five out of ten subjects so tested. Work initiated about the same time by investigators in New York[63] and in England[64] demonstrated that anti-Rh immunoglobulin injected separately from Rh-positive blood into rh recipients also prevented formation of Rh antibodies. This important achievement led to the development of prevention of Rh alloimmunization by administration, within 72 hrs *post partum*, of anti-Rh immunoglobulin to rh women giving birth to Rh-positive infants. The effectiveness of this measure has been amply proven during the past twenty years.

Concerning the mechanism responsible for the interference with Rh immunization of concomitant ABO incompatibility, we proposed the "hypothesis of 'clonal competition for antigen', namely, that presence of large numbers of antibody forming cells for one red cell factor may interfere with antibody response to another blood factor contained in the same red cell".[62] In other words, when a group O rh subject is exposed to A Rh-positive red cells, these would be diverted to immune cells already equipped for the anti-A response and thus be prevented from reaching cells with the potential for forming Rh antibodies. A modified version of the hypothesis, applicable to ABO incompatible blood as well as to red cells coated with Rh antibody, will be outlined in the final portion of this account.

At this point of the narration, it is appropriate to point to the year 1960 as a watershed in my career: for a variety of reasons, the most important of which was a change in the policies of the Mount Sinai Medical Research Foundation, I decided to leave the positions at Mount Sinai Medical Center and Chicago Medical School, and I accepted an appointment as professor of pathology at the University of Illinois College of Medicine. While this relocation involved a physical move of barely a few miles, it did bring about far reaching changes in professional duties and conduct of research. My primary assignments were participation in the teaching of pathology to medical students; rotation in the services of the department (surgical and autopsy pathology; cytology); and pursuit of my research. A smooth transition from the old to the new job was facilitated by several factors. From the beginning and throughout the ensuing nine years, I enjoyed greatly the association with Cecil A. Krakower, chairman of the department, not only because of his high professional standards, but also because of the supportive attitude he consistently showed to the staff, including myself, actively encouraging the specific interests of each member. The cordial relationship prevailing among the staff of the department soon gave me the feeling of being an integral part. The proximity between the University of Illinois and Mount Sinai made it easy to maintain contact with associates there, needed for completing and reporting work that had been started prior to my changing positions.

In general, I continued with the investigations into the relationship between the RES and cancer, and the possible role of the MØ in homeostasis of growth. In fact, most of this work carried out at the University of Illinois has already been dealt with in the preceding account in order to preserve its continuity. This applies to studies cited in References.[20,39,42-44,57,58] However, by necessity, a profound change had to take place in the investigation concerned with the mechanism(s) of interference with Rh alloimmunization by simultaneous ABO incompatibility. As a matter of fact, even before I ceased to direct the blood transfusion service and discontinued the experimental immunization to red cell antigens of human subjects, I realized the essential need for developing an animal model capable of simulating the conditions encountered in man. Before leaving Mount Sinai Medical Center, I attempted to do so by immunizing rabbits with the human red cell antigens M and N, taking advantage of the fact that some rabbits are genetically equipped to develop antibodies for the human red cell antigen A. This enabled us to compare formation of anti-M and anti-N in rabbits possessing anti-A and injected with either OM(ON) or with AM(AN) red cells. The results indeed conformed to expectations: e.g., titers of anti-N were significantly lower in rabbits possessing anti-A and immunized with AN red cells, as compared with rabbits immunized with ON red cells.[65] However, this experimental design suffered from several disadvantages: the effect on the immune response was quantitative rather than qualitative, i.e., it was expressed as difference in antibody titers and not as suppression of antibody formation. Moreover, because of unavailability of inbred rabbits, there was considerable animal-to-animal variability, necessitating the testing of large numbers of rabbits in order to obtain statistically significant results. In searching for another more suitable model, we exploited the fact that rats immunized with SRC exhibit a two-fold immune response by developing, in addition to isophilic antibodies reactive exclusively with SRC, heterophilic antibodies, so designated because they react not only with SRC, but also with heterophilic antigen (HA) present in tissues of certain species, such as the guinea-pig and the mouse. Examination of the effect on the immune response to SRC of preceding immunization of rats with HA revealed a marked reduction in hemolysin, with nearly complete suppression of formation of isophilic antibodies.[66] For the purpose of detailed analysis of this phenomenon, rats of four inbred strains were immunized with HA, given in the form of boiled homogenates of guinea pig kidney (GPK) prior to injection with SRC; rats injected with SRC only, served as controls. Comparison of units of

50% hemolysis in the sera showed uniformly and significantly lower values in experimental than control rats. This held true for the total hemolysin made up of heterophilic and isophilic antibodies. Absorption of the serum with GPK removed the heterophilic antibody so that the remaining isophilic antibody could be determined separately; the latter was reduced to trace amounts in sera of rats preimmunized with HA. By contrast, secondary immune response to HA, administered after immunization with SRC, yielded higher levels of heterophilic hemolysin in rats preimmunized with HA than in controls. In order to test the kinetics of antibody formation, hemolysin was assayed in sera sampled 1, 3, 6, 9 and 14 days after injection of SRC; in experimental as well as control rats, peak levels of hemolysin were present six days after immunization, but at all time intervals antibodies were lower in experimental than control rats. Important clues concerning the mechanism of the inhibition of formation of antibodies by preimmunization with HA became available from two sets of experiments. A negative clue was provided by passive immunization of rats with large amounts of heterophilic antibodies or mixtures of heterophilic and isophilic antibodies. Although this treatment inhibited the immune response to subsequently injected SRC, the fact that in HA-immunized rats tested prior to challenge with SRC the sera contained either no or low levels of anti-HA antibodies contradicts the assumption that circulating antibodies were responsible for the observed inhibition of the immune response. On the other hand, a positive clue was furnished by experiments in which rats were splenectomized 24 hrs before the injection of SRC; this intervention considerably lowered antibody levels in controls, but not in rats preimmunized with HA, supporting the conclusion that in the latter animals antibody formation should be assigned to extrasplenic sites. On the basis of these findings, we proposed that the phenomenon of interference with the immune response "appears to be more compatible with cellular than exclusively humoral mechanisms....possible candidates for this role include macrophages engaged in uptake of particulate antigens, immunologically competent cells in various stages of development, or any of these cells invested with cytophilic antibody".[67] The validity of these arguments was strengthened by results of two additional experimental approaches: neonatal administration of antigen.[68,69] and uptake of radiolabeled antigen by liver and spleen.[70,71] Administration to newborn inbred rats of HA during the first week of life caused profound depression of the immune response to SRC injected 10 to 18 wks later; litter mates injected neonatally with saline served as controls. On the other hand, challenge with HA at the age of 12 to 18 wks induced significant amounts of heterophilic hemolysin in rats treated neonatally with Ha, whereas only traces of such antibodies appeared in controls. This finding ruled out neonatally-induced tolerance as causing the interference with the immune response to SRC in adulthood. Moreover, it was unlikely that humoral mechanisms were involved, since sera tested prior to immunization with SRC contained no circulating antibodies or only small amounts. Accordingly, we interpreted these observations "as resulting from imprinting of large numbers of cells with receptors for heterophilic antigen after neonatal exposure to the antigen, and **cellular diversion of antigen** upon challenge of adult animals with sheep red cells".[71] Even stronger evidence for cellular mediation of the phenomenon under study was obtained from the localization in spleen and liver of radiolabeled antigens.[70,71] Administration to adult or neonatal rats of HA significantly depressed hepatic and splenic uptakes of subsequently injected ^{51}Cr-SRC, as shown by comparing experimental and control animals. Uptake of ^{51}Cr-HA was not affected by preceding exposure to HA. On the basis of these findings, we suggested that "the changes in phagocytosis and immune responses may be attributable to imprinting of numerous macrophages with receptors specific for HA. Subsequently-introduced SRC may thus be diverted to HA-specific macrophages and be prevented from contact with macrophages better equipped to phagocytose and process this substrate containing both heterophilic and isophilic antigens".[71]

During the Ninth International Cancer Congress in Tokyo in 1966, I met and discussed with, Professor Jack Gross, chairman of the Department of Experimental Medicine and Cancer Research, Hebrew University, Hadassah Medical School, Jerusalem, the possibility of spending a sabbatical period with him. These plans came to fruition and from February to August 1968, we and his staff collaborated in studying phagocytosis of ^{51}Cr-SRC in mice, viz., the kinetics of storage and elimination of the radiolabel up to 60 days after injection,[72] and the effects on these events and on plasma hemopexin levels of administration of lipopolysaccharide.[73]   On the personal level, we benefitted from the sabbatical leave not only by enjoying the company of our daughter and her husband living in Israel but, as a rare example of planned grandparenthood, we arrived just in time for the birth of our first grandson. Moreover, it was a source of particular satisfaction that, as a spin off of my scientific interest, our Rh-negative daughter was fortunate to receive, after birth of an Rh-positive baby, the preventive treatment with anti-Rh immunoglobulin, at that time still an investigative drug. Finally, the stay in Israel led to a major turning point in my personal and professional life when I was offered an appointment at the Department of Life Sciences at Bar-Ilan University. After returning to Chicago in the fall of 1968, I resumed my activities at the University of Illinois during the academic year 1968/69 and the fall quarter of 1969/70. During that time, mutual agreement was reached concerning my joining Bar-Ilan University. In November 1969, we immigrated to Israel, and I took up the position at Bar-Ilan University which I was to occupy for approximately ten years. The first year was a period of adjustment to the new conditions, including preparation of lectures in Hebrew, a language I was familiar with, albeit not within the scientific framework. Throughout the following years, I taught undergraduate courses in basic biology, histology, immunology and mammalian genetics, and graduate courses in immunohematology and experimental cancer research. Regrettably, and notwithstanding assurances given to me in advance of my arrival, adequate laboratory facilities for my research did not become available until approximately two years later when I could resume the experimental studies.

From 1972 to 1979, my work was directed toward two main areas: 1) study of the mechanism(s) operative in the interference with the immune response of rats to SRC after immunization with HA, an animal model simulating the interaction of ABO incompatibility with Rh alloimmunization in man; 2) investigation of the role of host factors in neoplasia, as represented by immune responsiveness and phagocytic activity in inbred mice during chemical carcinogenesis. Each of these topics formed the subject of the dissertation of a doctoral student.

Before I left the University of Illinois, we began to utilize the technique of splenic plaque-forming cells (PFC) for assay in rats of the immune response to SRC. This method, developed by Jerne and Nordin,[74] is based on the fact that each splenic cell producing hemolysin, is surrounded by a clear plaque visible in the opaque agar medium containing evenly distributed SRC. For our particular purposes, it was helpful that we succeeded in neutralizing splenic cells secreting heterophilic antibody by incubating the cell suspension with HA before they were plated on agar; this procedure left only PFC-forming isophilic antibody observable. On the other hand, plating, in parallel with untreated splenic cells yielded PFC corresponding to cells producing heterophilic as well as those producing isophilic antibody; hence they were designated "total PFC." With Aliena Hellering Zaidman, this methodology was applied to a detailed analysis of the phenomenon under study, supplementing the information on humoral antibodies gained in previous studies.[66-69] When rats were injected with HA two to four days before receiving SRC, maximal suppression of total PFC was noted, with almost complete absence of isophilic PFC. When the interval between HA and SRC was extended to six days, the suppression abated, and SRC given 18 days after HA elicited immune responses indistinguishable from those of untreated rats.[75] Pretreatment with HA significantly impaired the secondary immune response to SRC as well, suggesting interference with formation of memory cells. Having established these effects of immunization with HA on the immune response to SRC *in vivo*, we studied the *in vitro* response. When splenic cells were prepared from rats three days after administration of HA, culture with SRC completely failed to induce PFC, by contrast with splenic cells from untreated rats which showed peak responses of PFC after four days of culture with SRC. The *in vitro* system permitted separation of adherent (A) and nonadherent (NA) splenic cells, and examination of mixtures of A and NA cells, prepared from either control animals or rats injected with HA at specified time intervals before the assay. Testing of such combinations of A and NA cells for the formation of PFC after culture with SRC showed that A cells exert the strongest inhibitory effect when they were derived from rats given HA 4 to 6 days prior to the assay; this activity was lost at longer intervals after HA administration. On the other hand, NA cells became inhibitory when examined 14 to 18 days after rats had received HA. Thus, a sequence of two inhibitory mechanisms of the immune response to SRC operated in rats after exposure to HA: in the early phase, the inhibition was mediated by MØ and, later on, by T suppressor cells.[76] In a further attempt to elucidate the phenomenon of alloimmunization induced by pregnancy, I analyzed data recorded in the literature for 175 families with maternal immunization to red cell antigens, exclusive of A, B and Rho. In less than 5% of instances, ABO-incompatible fetal red cells were responsible for immunization of the mother, in accordance with previously discussed inhibition by ABO incompatibility of Rh antibody formation in rh subjects. Furthermore, documentation was available for 20 families in which preceding immunization of the mother to a variety of unrelated red cell antigens prevented subsequent immunization to potent immunogens, such as Rh_o (10 families), hr' (8 families), and K (2 families).[77] As already stated, both in connection with alloimmunization in man and in the context of the animal models studied by us, we offered the interpretation of "diversion of antigen" as explanation for the inhibitory effects of immune responses to one antigen (Rh; SRC) exerted by preceding immunization to another antigen (A, B; HA). In the light of current knowledge, I propose that, at least in relation to Rh alloimmunization, a common denominator can be found for the two seemingly distinct forms of inhibition, or suppression, represented by ABO incompatibility and administration of anti-Rh immunoglobulin. In the first case, numerous immunocompetent cells can be assumed to carry anti-A and/or anti-B immunoglobulin molecules that are capable of intercepting the ABO incompatible red cells, thus preventing them from reaching sites equipped for mounting efficient responses to the Rh antigen. In the second situation, anti-Rh immunoglobulin introduced into the rh recipient can be expected to be bound to the Fc receptors widely distributed on MØ and immunocompetent cells. Rh-positive red cells circulating in the recipient are attracted indiscriminately to the cell-bound anti-Rh antibody. This produces a "dilution effect" which again interferes with the red cells reaching suitable effector cells required for eliciting the Rh antibody response. Obviously, these propositions are speculative and in need of critical experimental testing.

The role of host factors in carcinogenesis was investigated by Rahel Schreiber and the author.[78,79,80] The basic experimental design consisted of subcutaneous injection of 600 µg in oil of methylcholanthrene (MCA) to male and female mice of strains C57BL/6 and C3H/eB; control mice were injected with oil only. One series of experiments was concerned with changes in phagocytic activity, assayed by splenic and hepatic uptakes of ^{51}Cr-SRC at specified intervals after administration of the carcinogen. Groups of 10 to 30 experimental and control mice were tested from 2 to 13 wks after MCA. In line with previously reported results,[44] significant depression of splenic phagocytosis was observed in all strain-sex combinations of MCA-injected animals, except for female C57BL/6 mice. Hepatic phagocytosis was less frequently and less severely impaired. Confirming our earlier observations, the phagocytic activity of untreated C57/BL mice exceeded that of untreated C3H/eB mice, and it was greater in female than male C3H/eB mice. We concluded that "while the manifestation of chemically induced tumors was preceded ....by impaired phagocytic function ...this phenomenon cannot be causally related to carcinogenesis." "....phagocytosis may be an imperfect measure of functional activity of MØ inasmuch as the assay determines only ingestion, but not digestion, of metabolizable material".[79]

The target of the second series of experiments was the effect on the immune responsiveness of exposure of the host to carcinogen.[78,80] The fact that most chemicals, and many other carcinogenic agents, induce immunosuppression has been demonstrated in numerous investigations. However, the majority of these studies, including one reported from our laboratory in 1956,[48] provided merely statistical evidence for this phenomenon. Our aim was to examine as to whether there was a correlation in the individual animal between the degree of immunodepression and the manifestation of the induced tumor. In order to find an answer to this question, surgical splenectomy was done four days after immunization with SRC, and times at specific intervals after MCA administration. Splenic PFC were assayed and compared with those found in suitable controls. The splenectomized mice were observed for appearance of tumors up to 52 wks following MCA injection. By means of this technique, we tested male and female C57BL/6 and C3H/eB mice, with each group comprising from 80 to 120 animals. Strong correlation between severity of immunodepression and rapidity of tumor appearance were noted in male C57Bl/6 mice tested 4, 6, and 11 wks and female C57BL/6 mice tested 4, 6, 8 wks after MCA. In C3H/eB mice this correlation was found only in the group of male mice tested 8 wks after MCA, but in none of the female mice. Another discordant finding was that MCA administration was followed by more pronounced immunodepression in C3H/eB than C57BL/6 mice, whereas the incidence of tumors was higher in the latter than the former strain. Thus, these results still leave open the question of the exact role played by immunodepression in the etiology and pathogenesis of carcinogenesis. We commented that "it may not be coincidental that superior phagocytic activity is characteristic of strain C57BL/6 in which the degree of immunodepression is correlated with the carcinogenic process. One may speculate that impaired processing of antigen by splenic macrophages may be responsible for defective immune response in carcinogen-treated mice".[80]

It felt both like coming home and leaving home when, after six years in Israel, I took a sabbatical in the United States. For the first part of it, I worked in Dr. Herman Friedman's laboratory in the Albert Einstein Medical Center, Philadelphia. Our friendship, continuing to this day, dates back to frequent joint attendance of scientific meetings and mutual visits. Our studies were concerned with the *in vitro* immune response to SRC of splenic cells derived from carcinogen-treated mice. The rest of the period I spent in the cancer research laboratory of Dr. Anna Goldfeder at the Francis Delafield Hospital, New York City. We examined the effect on tumor growth exerted by MØ collected from mice of inbred strains after they had rejected semiallogeneic F_1 tumors. While the time available was insufficient for completing this study, it provided the baseline for experiments carried out several years later.

After returning to Israel, I resumed my work at Bar-Ilan University during the academic years 1976/77 and 1977/78 when I reached academic retirement age. After pursuing experimental work there for another year, I realized that funding difficulties made it impossible to continue with this activity. Since I was not yet ready to relinquish my involvement in research, I considered it a stroke of good fortune—and consider it so to this day—when Professor David W. Weiss responded affirmatively to my request for being given the opportunity to do research in the department chaired by him, the Lautenberg Center for General and Tumor Immunology, The Hebrew University, Hadassah Medical School, Jerusalem. During the past eight years, I have appreciated the support given to my work, and I have been stimulated by the intellectual atmosphere of the Center reflecting the wide ranging research interests of the chairman and the staff.

The primary goal of my own efforts during the past years was to search for strategies permitting analysis of the antineoplastic effects of the MØ and its products. The basic experimental design employed consisted of inoculation of mice of the inbred strains X/Gf and C3H with tumors induced by MCA in F_1 mice derived from the two inbred strains. As a rule, these semiallogeneic tumors do not grow in the parent strains, and thus it is possible to immunize them by repeated transfer of the F_1 tumors. Peritoneal MØ are elicited by thioglycollate and collected from the immunized mice. After inoculation of F_1 tumor cells together with immune MØ into F_1 recipients, growth of tumors was either prevented, inhibited, or delayed. Similar results were obtained in experiments in which X/Gf mice were repeatedly immunized with irradiated syngeneic tumor cells until they were resistant to challenge with live tumor cells; admixture of peritoneal MØ of immunized mice to syngeneic tumor inocula interfered with tumor growth. Peritoneal MØ from untreated mice, used in similar fashion, did not possess antitumor activity. Injections of immune MØ at sites remote from the tumor inoculum were ineffective. Incubation *in vitro* of immune MØ with tumor cells yielded supernatant fluid which, when used for suspending tumor cell inocula, inhibited, in some instances, tumor growth in suitable recipients.[81]   Work along these lines continues. This appears to be the appropriate point in time to stop the story: accounts of unfinished work in progress, in my opinion, are of little value, except possibly when offered in support of grant applications.

EPILOGUE

I harbor no illusions about my explorations having led to the discovery of a new continent or fabulous treasure troves. Nor do I wish to cover up for my failures by hiding behind the alibi of extraneous circumstances that more than once placed serious obstacles in the path of my professional career. Rather, I blame the lack of success of some endeavors on inadequate scientific knowledge available to me while pursuing a particular research topic. With this in mind, I have compared my situation "to that of a shipwrecked person who tries to gather suitable material for building a raft that may carry him across an uncharted body of water to a settlement or place of rescue".[54] In retrospect, I cannot help but marvel at the tremendous progress which has been achieved in our understanding of the M∅ system, thanks to the contributions of scores investigators. Many of us recall the discussions concerning the best way of characterizing the biologic role of the RES. Does it mainly serve as a garbage disposal by means of which the body rids itself of effete and dead cells and harmful waste? Should we consider it an integral component of the defense factory which attempts to protect the organism against foreign invaders and deviant autochthonous cells through humoral and cellular immune mechanisms? Or, does it function as a homeostat which critically regulates processes of growth, repair, and regeneration? It is, perhaps, charged with all these tasks? Turning away from this anthropomorphic imagery, we cannot fail to be profoundly impressed by the solid evidence that has emerged during the past decades for the astounding complexity of the M∅ as a cell synthesizing and secreting dozens of biologically active substances, including enzymes, components of complement, cytokines, prostaglandins; a cell that is involved in coagulation and angiogenesis; a cell that emits, and receives, signals to and from widely dispersed tissues and organs. To this must be added what we have learned about the intricate phenomena of maturation and activation to which the M∅ is subject, and the effects on the M∅ its and specialized functions of the microenvironment in which it is located. And yet, we must also acknowledge the many gaps in our understanding of the activities of the RES, their regulation, and how one may exploit these insights for combatting serious threats to the organism, such as neoplasia. Being inclined to an optimistic outlook, I would like to believe that "the best is yet to come."

ACKNOWLEDGMENT

Grateful appreciation is expressed, for partial financial support of the work performed by the author and described in this article, to the following sources (listed alphabetically): American Cancer Society; Dr. Anna Goldfeder Fund; Illinois Division of the American Cancer Society; Israel Cancer Society; Lautenberg Center for General and Tumor Immunology; Hebrew University-Hadassah Medical School, Jerusalem, Israel; Leukemia Research Foundation, USA; Mount Sinai Medical Research Foundation, Chicago, Illinois; National Cancer Institute, US Science Foundation, USA; Otto and Marianne Wolman

Philanthropic Fund, Los Angeles, California; Research Authority of Bar-Ilan University, Ramat-Gan, Israel; Stanley Johnson Foundation, Switzerland; US Atomic Energy Foundation.

REFERENCES

1. Dunn, L.C., Hugo Iltis: 1882-1952, *Science*, 117, 3, 1953.
2. Freund, E. and Kaminer, G., Die biochemischen Grundlagen der Karzinomdisposition, *Biochem. Z.* 26, 312, 1910, Springer-Verlag, Wien, 1925.
3. Willheim, R. and Stern, K., *Z. Krebsforsch.*, 38, 502, 1933.
4. Willheim, R. and Stern, K., *Z. Kerbsforsch.* 39, 54, 1933.
5. Willheim, R. and Stern, K., First International Cancer Congress, Madrid, 1933, p. 353.
6. Stern, K. and Willheim, R., *Z. Krebsforsch.*, 46, 379, 1937.
7. Adler, H. and Reimann, F., *Z. Ges. Exp. Med.*, 47, 617, 1925.
8. Stern, K. and Willheim, R., *Z. Ges. Exp. Med.*, 97, 354, 1935.
9. Willheim, R. and Stern, K., *Die Wege und Ergebnisse Chemischer Krebsforschung*, Aeskulap-Verlag, Wien, 1936, 473 pp.
10. Stern, K. , *J. Lab Clin. Med.*, 26, 809, 1941.
11. Stern, K., *New Internatl. Clinics*, Vol. III, Ser. 4, p. 111, 1941.
12. Stern, K. and Willheim, R., *The Biochemistry of Malignant Tumors*, Chemical Publishing Co., Inc., Brooklyn, NY, 1943, 931 pp.
13. Stern, K. and Willheim, R., *The Biochemistry of Malignant Tumors*, Chemical Publishing Co., Inc., Brooklyn, NY, 1943, preface page VII.
14. Metchnikoff, E., *Immunity in Infectious Diseases*, Cambridge University Press, London, 1905.
15. Aschoff, L., *Ergeb. Inn. Med. Kinderheilk.*, 26, 1, 1927.
16. Stern, K., *Proc. Soc. Exp. Biol. Med.*, 67, 315, 1948.
17. Stern, K., *Cancer Research*, 10, 565, 1950.
18. Stern, K., *Proc. Soc. Exp. Biol. Med.*, 79, 618, 1952.
19. Stern, K., Spencer, K. and Farquhar, M., *Proc. Soc. Exp. Biol. Med.*, 89, 126, 1955.
20. Stern, K., *J. Reticuloendothelial Soc.*, 6, 24, 1969.
21. Stern, K., *Proc. Amer. Assoc. Cancer Res.*, 2, 48, 1955.
22. Stern, K., The reticuloendothelial system and neoplasia, in *Reticuloendothelial Structure and Function*, J.H. Heller, Ed., The Ronald Press Company, New York, 1960, p. 233.
23. Davidsohn, I. and Stern, K., *Proc. Soc. Exp. Biol. Med.*, 70, 142, 1949
24. Davidsohn, I. and Stern, K., *Cancer Research*, 9, 426, 1949.
25. Davidsohn, I. and Stern, K., *Cancer Research*, 10, 571, 1950.
26. Stern, K. and Davidsohn, I., *J. Immunol.*, 72, 209, 1954.
27. Davidsohn, I. and Stern, K., *J. Immunol.*, 72, 216, 1954.
28. Stern, K., Brown, K.S. and Davidsohn, I., *Genetics*, 41, 517, 1956.
29. Stern, K., Spencer, K. and Farquhar, M., *Proc. Soc. Exp. Biol. Med.*, 89, 126, 1955.
30. Unanue, E.R. and Askonas, B.A., *J. Exp. Med.*, 127, 915, 1968.
31. Unanue, E.R., *Adv. Immunol.*, 15, 95, 1972.
32. Unanue, E.R., *Adv. Immunol.*, 31, 1, 1981.
33. Benacerraf, B., *Science*, 212, 1221, 1981.
34. Burnet, M.F., *Prog. Exper. Tumor Research*, 13, 1, 1970.
35. Stern, K., Control of tumors by the RES, in *The Reticuloendothelial System. A Comprehensive Treatise*, Vol. 5, Cancer, R.B. Herberman and H. Friedman, Eds., Plenum Press, New York, 1983, p. 64.
36. Biozzi, G., Stiffel, C., Mouton, D., Bouthillier, Y. and Decreusefond, C., *Ann. Inst. Pasteur (Paris)*, 115, 465, 1968.
37. Biozzi, Stiffel, C., Mouton, D., Bouthillier, Y. and Decreusefond, C., *Transplant. Proc.*, 3, 1333, 1971.
38. Stern, K. and Duwelius, A., *Cancer Research*, 20, 587, 1960.
39. Stern, K., *Cancer Research*, 24, 1063, 1964.
40. Stern, K., *J. Immunol.*, 84, 295, 1960.

41.   Stern, K., *Proc. Exp. Biol. Med.*, 114, 321, 1963.
42.   Stern, K. and Goldfeder, A., *Israel J. Med. Sci.*, 7, 42, 1971.
43.   Stern, K., Bartizal, C.A. and Divshony, S., *J. Natl. Cancer Inst.*, 38, 169, 1967.
44.   Stern, K., *Ninth International Cancer Congress*, Tokyo, 1966, p. 59.
45.   Davidsohn, I. and Stern, K., *Cancer Research*, 12, 257, 1952.
46.   Stern, K. and Davidsohn, I., *Proc. Amer. Assoc. Cancer Research*, 1, 46, 1954.
47.   Taliaferro, W.H. and Taliaferro, G., *J. Infect. Dis.*, 98, 205, 1952.
48.   Davidsohn, I., Stern, K., Sabet, L., *Proc. Amer. Assoc. Cancer Res.*, 2, 102, 1956.
49.   Snyderman, R., Pike, M. C., Meadowns, L., Hemstreet, G. and Wells, S., *Clin. Research*, 23, 297A, 1975.
50.   Stevenson, M. M. and Meltzer, M. S., *Fed. Proc.*, 34, 991, 1975.
51.   Norman, S. J. and Sorkin, S., *J. Natl. Cancer Inst.* 57, 135, 1976.
52.   Experimental Cancer Research, Report of a Committee Appointed by the Surgeon General, *Pub. Health Rep.*, 53, 2121, 1938.
53.   Stern, K. and Duwelius, A., *Proc. Soc. Exp. Biol. Med.*, 100, 546, 1959.
54.   Stern, K., *Ann. N.Y. Acad. Sci.*, 88, 252, 1960.
55.   Stern, K. and Davidsohn, I., *J. Immunol.*, 74, 479, 1955.
56.   Nicol, T. and Helmy, I.D., *Nature*, 167, 201, 1951.
57.   Stern, K. and Matsumoto, H., *Proc. Soc. Exp. Biol. Med.*, 120, 843, 1965.
58.   Stern, Titchener, E.B. and Duwelius, A., *Life Sciences*, 8, 821, 1969.
59.   Stern, K., Davidsohn, I., and Masaitis, L., *Am. J. Clin. Path.*, 26, 833, 1956.
60.   Levine, P., *J. Hered.*, 34, 833, 1956.
61.   Davidsohn, I., Stern, K. and Mackeviciute, M., *Bib. Haematol*, 7, 1, 1958.
62.   Stern, K., Goodman, H.S. and Berger, M., *J. Immunol.*, 87, 189, 1961.
63.   Freda, V.J., Gorman, J.G. and Pollack, W., *Transfusion*, 4, 26, 1964.
64.   Clarke, C.A., Donohoe, W.T.A., McConnel, R.B., Woodrow, J.C., Finn, R., Krevans, J.R., Kulke, W., Lehane, D. and Sheppard, R.M., *Brit. Med. J.*, 1, 979, 1963.
65.   Stern, K., *Fed. Proc.*, 19, 200, 1960.
66.   Stern, K., *Fed. Proc.*, 24, 179, 1965.
67.   Stern, K., *Clin. Exp. Immunol.*, 4, 253, 1969.
68.   Stern, K., *Fed. Proc.*, 26, 700, 1967.
69.   Stern, K., *Vox Sanguinis*, 18, 481, 1970.
70.   Rhone, D.P. and Stern, K., *Fed. Proc.*, 27, 491, 1968.
71.   Rhone, D.P. and Stern, K., *Proc. Soc. Exp. Biol. Med.*, 133, 1297, 1970.
72.   Markus, R., Carmel, N., Gross, J., and Stern, K., *Israel J. Med. Sci.*, 8, 1775, 1972.
73.   Carmel, N., Markus, R., Gross, J., Stern, K., *Israel J. Med. Sci.*, 8, 1783, 1972.
74.   Jerne, N.K. and Nordin, A.A., *Science*, 140, 405, 1963.
75.   Stern, K., *Transfusion*, 15, 179, 1975.
76.   Hellering, I. and Stern, K., *Eur. J. Immunol.*, 5, 705, 1975.
77.   Stern, K., *Transfusion*, 15, 179, 1975.
78.   Stern, K. and Schreiber, R., *Proc. Am. Assoc. Cancer Res.*, 17, 85, 1976.
79.   Schreiber, R. and Stern, K., *Oncology*, 41, 431, 1985.
80.   Schreiber, R. and Stern, K., Oncology 41: 436, 1985.
81.   Stern, K., Sharir, C.H. and Gabay, A., *Seventh European Immunology Meeting*, Jerusalem, 1985, p. 165.

Chapter 22

THE IMMUNE-NEUROENDOCRINE CIRCUITRY: A GENERATION OF PROGRESS

Andor Szentivanyi

Of the various evolving views on immunologic inflammation, immunity, and hypersensitivity, this chapter discusses the irrevocable shift and turnabout in our concepts of immunoregulation as connected with our growing understanding of the immune-neuroendocrine circuitry. This network, which is powerful enough both conceptually and in **de facto** functioning to bring about a radical change in our perceptions of the human immune, endocrine, and nervous systems, has already enlisted the minds and resources of a large number of leading laboratories in many areas of life sciences on an international scale.

The Discovery of the Immune-Neuroendocrine Circuitry and the Concepts of Prevailing Immunologic Thought that Impeded the Timely Recognition of its Role in Immune Homeostasis

The integrative center of this awesome edifice is the hypothalamus. The hypothalamus is a small, anatomically complex region of the diencephalon, which in a variety of ways contributes to a large number of regulatory systems. The functional and anatomic complexity of the hypothalamus results in part from its role as a nodal region for 1) convergence of input from the limbic system, which contributes to an association between visceral and behavioral functions, 2) bidirectional bundles of nerve fibers with their cell bodies (perikarya) in the telencephalon or brain stem, and 3) local neurons coordinating distant organ system activities through the effector functions of the endocrine and autonomic nervous systems.

The role of hypothalamic influences in the induction and expression of immunologic inflammation, immunity, and hypersensitivity was first discovered in my laboratory in the fall of 1951 at the University of Debrecen School of Medicine in Hungary. The rationale behind the decision for a systematic exploration of the hypothalamus was as follows. Historically, the interpretation of the symptomatology and the underlying reaction sequence of human asthma was patterned after those of the anaphylactic guinea pig. However, the range of atopic responsiveness in asthma includes a variety of stimuli that are non-immunologic in nature. Foremost among these are a broad range of pharmacologically active mediators that today could be considered as the chemical organizers of central and peripheral autonomic regulation. Therefore, I believed that anaphylaxis could not be used as a model for the investigation of the constitutional basis of atopy in asthma. It was postulated that such a model, if it was to be meaningful, must be able to imitate both the immunologic and autonomic abnormalities of the disease. Since at that early time (1951) none of the current neuroactive agents (agonists, antagonists, etc.) that one could conceivably use as an experimental tool to induce an autonomic imbalance were in existence, it was concluded that the best chance to develop such a condition would be through various manipulations at the neuroendocrine regulatory level of the hypothalamus. Consequently, hypothalamically imbalanced anaphylactic animals were used. These were produced by the electrolytic lesion, and conversely, the electrical stimula-

0-8493-4722-X/94/$0.00 + $.50
© 1994 by CRC Press, Inc.

tion of various nuclear groupings in the hypothalamus through permanently implanted depth electrodes placed stereotaxically into the hypothalamus. The resulting cumulative findings obtained with such a model indicated that the hypothalamus has a modulatory influence on all cellular and humoral immune reactivities and that both neural as well as endocrine pathways are required for hypothalamic modulation of immune responses.[1,2,3,4,5,6,7,8,9,10,11,12,13,14,15,16,17,18,19,20-,21,22,23,24,25,26,27,28,29,30,31,32,33,34,35,36,37,38,39]

Concurrently with these developments, however, an unparalleled expansion of information on the basic aspects of immunology in general and on the nature of antibody diversity in particular started to occupy the center stage of immunologic interest. Most importantly, the new perceptions surrounding the nature of antibody diversity began to surface in the late 1950s with the first conclusive genetic studies having been completed and a new set of concepts defined. These circumstances led to a total transformation of prevailing immunologic thought, ultimately leading to the replacement of instructionist theories by the selective theories as advanced by D.W. Talmage in the spring of 1957 and M Burnet in the fall of 1957.

Three major postulates were implicit in these theories of heritable cellular commitment: 1) the antigen receptor site and the antibody combining site whose synthesis that cell controls are identical and are derived at least partially from the same structural gene; 2) the condition guaranteeing the correspondence of the immunoglobulin (Ig) synthesized with the antigen is that they are limited to the same cell that is the cell specialized for the synthesis of a single antibody; and 3) the cell specialization stipulated in item 2 is inherited and therefore clonal (the clonal selection theory of acquired immunity). Subsequently, it became established that virtually all antibody diversity and specificity encoded in the immune system can be accounted for in genetic terms and thus the controls for the antibody response must reside largely within the major histocompatibility complex (MHC) where different genes appear to code for immune response, suppression, and cell interaction.[40] An impediment in the timely recognition of the significance of the immune-neuroendocrine circuitry in immune homeostasis was the ability to have immune reactivities to proceed *in vitro*. This further supported the concept that the immune system is a totally autonomous and self-regulating unit (this view overlooked the rich neurohormonal milieu in which most *in vitro* immune responses occur). Sporadic refutations of these postulates have occurred and continue to surface in the literature, but the great bulk of the evidence is supportive of the clonal selection theory. The theory's sheer eloquence, however, has probably been most responsible for its dominant role in immunologic thought and its acceptance as dogma since the early 1960s. In any case, these concepts and the large body of supportive evidence have so permeated the field that it became difficult, if not impossible, to think of immunology outside of this framework.[41]

In the late 1950s and throughout the 1960s the two conceptual centers of these ideas were under the leadership of Talmage at the University of Chicago and later at Colorado, and the group at Walter and Eliza Hall Institute in Australia under Burnet. Because of the close association with Talmage, extending over a period of ten years, I was very much under the influence of these views and developed reservations against the significance of our hypothalamic findings in immunoregulation. Nevertheless, by 1966 in a chapter of a German text (*Pathogenese und Therapie allergischer Reactionen.*

Grundlagenforschung und Klinik, Ferdinand Enke Verlag, Stuttgart, Germany, 1966), through an extensive analysis of our findings and the dominant immunologic concepts, I came to articulate the following conclusions: 1) the significance of the immunopharmacologic mediators of immune manifestations in normal mammalian physiology is that they are the chemical organizers of central and peripheral autonomic action; 2) the preceding suggests the inseparability of the immune response system from the neuroendocrine system; 3) such inseparability indicates the *de facto* existence of immune-neuroendocrine circuits and the necessity for a bidirectional flow of information between the two systems; 4) one must distinguish between the concepts of autoregulation as one that primarily revolves around one effector molecule of immunity, the antibody, and satisfies the requirements of antibody diversity and specificity, in contrast to the more complex requirements of immune homeostasis; 5) in contrast to autoregulation that is always self-contained, homeostatic control is always beyond the constraints of one single cell or tissue system; and 6) thus, immune homeostasis must represent a far more sophisticated level of control than autoregulation, and is based on immune-neuroendocrine circuits. Indeed, as Schechter[42] pointed out, no bodily system is as simple, sacred, or singular as once thought. Instead, as in any good relationship, the separate components strive for sensitivity, synchrony, and synergy. Recognition and communication among the immune, endocrine, and nervous systems exemplify the formula for harmony and homeostasis.

While the manifold similarities between the immune and nervous systems are fully realized (see below), the immune system has a major additional level of complexity over that of the nervous system. Although the nervous system with its spectacular masses of much-revealing and well-defined projection patterns is well moored in the body in a static web of axons, dendrites, and synapses, the elements of the immune system are in a continuously mobile phase, incessantly scouring over and percolating through the body tissues, returning via an intricate system of lymphatic channels, and then blending again in the blood. This dynamism is relieved only by scattered concentrations called lymphoid organs. These circumstances would appear to indicate that the functional plasticity of the immune system is far greater than that of the nervous system, and consequently, its regulation must require a more complex and sophisticated level of control. For these reasons, in the 1966 text I raised the frivolous question in the 1966 text, whether the immune system is more "intelligent" than the brain.

When these conclusions were reached (in the 1960s), our understandings of cellular immunology were in an early phase. The 1970s saw the discovery of the lymphokines, monokines, and a broad range of other effector molecules of immunologic inflammation, immunity, and hypersensitivity, but it was only in the 1980s that we recognized that the cells of the immune system, primarily the lymphocytes, synthesize, store, and release neurotransmitters, hypo-thalamohypophyseal hormones, and so on, and by all criteria serve as neuroendocrine cells "par excellence".[16,18,19,40,43]

Developmental Interrelationships Among the Cellular and Humoral Components of the Immune-Neuroendocrine Circuitry

The developmental interrelationships among the cellular and humoral components may be briefly stated through a discussion of 1) the cells involved in the synthesis, storage, secretion, and/or release of the effector molecules of immunologic reactivities; 2) neural crest interactions in the development of the immune system; 3) cerebral dominance or lateralization and the immune system; (4) the ancient superfamily of immune recognition molecules and the neural cell adhesion molecule (N-CAM); 5) the immune system and the nervous system sharing the capacity to remember; and 6) the unique recognition and communication powers of the immune and nervous systems as shared characteristics.

The Cells Involved in the Synthesis, Storage, Secretion, and/or Release of the Effector Molecules of Immunologic Reactivities.

The functions of the immune system are the properties of cells distributed throughout the body. They include 1) free or circulating cells of the blood, lymph, and intravascular spaces; 2) similar cells collected into units that allow for close interaction with lymph or circulating blood—lymph nodes, spleen, liver, and bone marrow; and 3) two major control organs for the system, the thymus gland and the hypothalamic-pituitary-adrenal complex.

The cells involved in the synthesis, storage, secretion, and/or release of the effector molecules of immunologic inflammation, immunity, and immunologically based hypersensitivity (allergy) represent a continuous spectrum of related cell types specialized in the production and storage of various physiopharmacologically active effector substances in variable proportions, that is, of cells that have a common developmental origin, with differentiation being determined by the specific requirements of the local neurohumoral regulation [40]. Accounting only for those effector molecules for which the cell type has been identified, this incomplete spectrum of cells and effector substances includes macrophages and lymphocytes (interleukins (IL) 1-11, interferons (IFN), tumor necrosis factors (TNF), lysosome and complement components, prostaglandins, leukotrienes, acid hydrolases, neutral proteinases, arginase, nucleotide metabolites, various neuroactive immunoregulatory peptides including corticotropin (ACTH), corticotropin-releasing factor (CRF)-like activity, bombesin, endorphins, enkephalins, thyrotropin (TSH), growth hormone, prolactin, neurotensin, chorionic gonadotropin, vasoactive intestinal peptide (VIP), tachykinin neuropeptides including substance P (SP), substance K, neuromedin K, somatostatins, mast cell growth factor, suppressin, etc.); neutrophil leukocytes (slow-reacting substance of anaphylaxis [SRS-A], eosinophilic chemotactic factors of anaphylaxis [ECF-A], enzymes, platelet-activating factor [PAF] and other vascular permeability factors, kinin-generating substances, a complement-activating factor, histamine releasers, a neutrophil inhibitory factor, VIP, 5-hydroxyeicosatetraenoic acid [5-HETE], etc.); basophilic leukocytes (histamine, SRS-A, ECF-A, neutrophil chemotactic factor [NCF], PAF, SP, somatostatins [SOMs], etc.); murine basophilic leukocytes (the same as in humans plus serotonin); eosinophilic leukocytes (PAF, 8,15-diHETE, SRS-A, eosinophil peroxidase, major basic protein, etc.); serosal, connective tissue or TC mast cells (histamine, SRS-A, ECF-A, NCF, PAF, VIP, SP, SOMs, etc.); mucosal or T mast cells (histamine, SRS-A, ECF-A, NCF, PAF, VIP, SP, SOMs, etc.); "chromaffin positive" mast cells (dopamine in ruminants; in other species possibly norepinephrine and neuropeptide Y); the so-called P-cells (histamine, serotonin); enterochromaffin cells (serotonin); chromaffin cells (epinephrine, norepinephrine, dopamine, neuropeptide Y, IL-1α, etc.); platelets (depending on species, histamine, serotonin, catecholamines, prostaglandins, 12-HETE); neurosecretory cells (histamine, serotonin, catecholamines, acetylcholine, prostaglandins, and other eicosanoids, kinins, the various hypothalamic substances that release or inhibit the release of the anterior pituitary hormones, and the group of neuroactive immunoregulatory peptides including ACTH, bombesin, neurotensin, endorphins, enkephalins, TSH, growth hormone, prolactin, luteinizing hormone [LH], LH-releasing hormone [LHRH], chorionic gonadotropin, VIP, the tachykinin neuropeptides, somatostatins, neuropeptide Y, ILs 1-6, suppressin, etc.); the medullary thymic epithelial cells and the Hassal corpuscles (thymosins and other thymic factors, oxytocin, vasopressin, etc); the serum inhibitory factor (SIF) cells (dopamine); and other nerve cells including essentially all the effector molecules listed under the neurosecretory cells. These various cells produce their effector molecules either constitutively or on induction. For more detailed information on all the foregoing cell types and effector molecules see other publications.[16,18,19,40,44]

Many of these cell types possess different morphologic, physicochemical, and general biologic characteristics. Nevertheless, in passing from one member of this cell spectrum to another, obvious transitions are seen in all these characteristics. Furthermore, when one surveys their properties and their probable physiologic function in the higher organism, significant cohesive features become apparent and set them apart from other body constituents as a distinct single class of cells that must be included in current concepts of neurosecretion.

Some workers postulated that the cellular components of the immune-neuroendocrine circuitry and their effector molecules could be viewed as two different divisions of this network. The two major divisions according to these workers may be defined as involved in neurovascular immunology and neuroendocrine immunology. Neurovascular immunology is concerned with immune response-related actions of vasoactive neurotransmitter substances that function as potent, short-lived local "hormones," first identified and studied as mediators of immunologic inflammation and hypersensitivity. They also play important roles in blood flow, vascular permeability, and pain transmission. These soluble effector molecules are simple compounds (i.e., amine mediators), short-chain peptides (i.e., kinins, SP, etc.), and short-chain lipids (i.e., prostaglandins, leukotrienes) and have a long evolutionary history in biologic defense. They use paracrine and synaptic signaling on their effector cells. The second major division, defined above as involved in neuroendocrine immunology, represents all the immune response-related hypothalamic, pituitary, and other hormones that use endocrine signaling and are primarily immunomodulatory in character. This perhaps convenient but arbitrary functional separation of these two divisions is intrinsically incorrect, as discussed in Szentivanyi et al.[44]

Neural Crest Interactions in the Development of the Immune System

In discussing neural crest interactions in the development of the immune system, first I must briefly characterize the developmental biology of this structure. The neural crest is produced from ectodermal cells which are released from the apical portions of the neural folds at about the time fusion occurs to form the neural tube and a separate overlying ectodermal layer. The basement membrane underlying the neural crest cells breaks down, the cellular characteristics change, and they become separated from the other components of the neural fold. There is a change in relative spatial relationship, or migration, of the neural crest cells to varied associations and destinies.[45]

The portion of the neural crest pertinent to this discussion is that which is closely associated with the developing brain, specifically, the hind brain. Crest cells in this cranial portion (anterior to the fifth somite) differentiate into mesenchyme, in addition to other connective tissue, muscular and nervous components. Neural crest cells migrate ventrolaterally through the bronchial arches and contribute mesenchymal cells to a number of structures. It is this mesenchyme that forms the layers around the epithelial primordia of the thymus.[46]

The full significance of the foregoing will be even more appreciated when viewed in the context of three additional considerations: 1) the thymus is formed by contributions from different sources that must interact in a precisely timed sequence for proper development; 2) ablation of small portions of the neural crest prevents or alters the development of the thymus; and 3) formation of the thymus precedes that of the more secondary, peripheral lymphoid tissues, reflecting a critical thymic role already in the early development of the immune system. Taken together, development of the immune system is inherently linked to the neural crest and any aberration in this link results in defective immune development such as that seen for instance in DiGeorge's syndrome.

Cerebral Dominance or Lateralization and Immune Disorders

The recognition of cerebral lateralization grew out of the discovery in the last century of cerebral dominance, that is, the superior capacity of each side of the brain to acquire particular skills. Over the past 120 years, it was believed that hemispheric dominance was based on functional asymmetry, on the differences in function of the two sides of the brain and of specific regions within them. In the face of the prevalent belief that cerebral dominance lacked an anatomic correlate, work over the past three decades has conclusively established that cerebral dominance is based on asymmetries of structure. An early example of this is the early detectable asymmetry in the human brain that involves the upper surface of the posterior portion of the left temporal lobe, the *planum temporale*. The larger size of the left *planum temporale* reflects the greater extent of a particular temporoparietal cytoarchitectonic area on the left. There are other asymmetries in the human brain and the same applies to the findings throughout the animal kingdom. In addition to genetic, several other factors in the course of development, both prenatal and postnatal, influence the direction and extent of these structural differences.[47]

Associations of anomalous cerebral dominance include not only developmental disorders such as dyslexia, autism, stuttering, mental retardation, and learning disorders, as well as some extraordinary musical, mathematic, athletic and other talents,* but also alterations in many bodily systems including the immune system. In these situations, the same influences that modify structural asymmetry in the brain also modify other systems such as the immune system. The suspected molecular mechanisms involved in the influence of structural asymmetry on the development of immune reactivities are discussed in more detail in two larger reviews.[48,49] Here I shall only mention that there is good evidence that left-handedness more frequently occurs in persons with diseases of atopic allergy (asthma, allergic rhinitis,

---

*It is difficult to speak in some of these cases of extraordinary talents as the "pathology of superiority" but that is what the evidence dictates.

atopic dermatitis), and that animal experiments in the past ten years provided some insight into the nature of the association between anomalous hemispheric dominance and immune reactivities.

Thus, beginning in 1980 and continuing throughout the decade, Renoux and coworkers showed in a series of studies that immunomodulation of the T-cell lineage in rodents can be a phenomenon of hemispheric lateralization. In 1980, the initial observation presented data indicating that lesioning the left cerebral neocortex depresses T-cell mediated responses in mice without affecting B-cell responses. These observations were extended in experiments where animals with a right cortical lesion served as controls for animals with a left cortical ablation. The findings demonstrated a balanced brain asymmetry in which the right hemisphere controls the inductive influence on T-cells of signals emitted by the left hemisphere. In addition, most recent studies found that ditiocarb sodium (Imuthiol), an immunostimulant specifically active on the T-cell lineage, can replace the signals emitted by the left neocortex, since mice without a left neocortex were stimulated to increased T-cell-dependent responses by treatment with ditiocarb sodium, whereas the agent did not modify the responses already increased in right decorticates. B-cell-dependent and some macrophage-dependent responses are not affected by either neocortical ablation or ditiocarb sodium. This lateralization of cortical influences on immune function in rodents is likely to be predictive of an even greater influence in humans with more profound and complex cortical functions.[50]

The Ancient Superfamily of Immune Recognition Molecules and the Neural Cell Adhesion Molecule

The ancient superfamily of immune recognition molecules and the N-CAM represent another aspect of the interrelationships among the cellular and molecular components of the immune-neuroendocrine circuitry. Most of the glycoproteins that mediate cell-cell recognition or antigen recognition in the immune system contain related structural elements, suggesting that the genes that encode them have a common evolutionary history. Included in this Ig superfamily are antibodies, T-cell receptors, MHC glycoproteins, the CD2, CD4, and CD8 cell-cell adhesion proteins, some of the polypeptide chains of the CD3 complex associated with T cell receptors and the various Fc receptors on lymphocytes and other white blood cells—all of which contain one or more Ig-like domains (Ig homology units). Each Ig homology unit is usually encoded by a separate exon, and it seems likely that the entire supergene family evolved from a gene coding for a single Ig homology unit similar to that encoding Thy-1 or β_2-microglobulin which may have been involved in mediating cell-cell interactions. Since a Thy-1-like molecule has been isolated from the brain of squids, it is probable that such a primordial gene arose before vertebrates diverged from their invertebrate ancestors some 400 million years ago. New family members presumably arose by exon and gene duplications, and similar duplication events probably gave rise to the multiple gene segments that encode antibodies and T cell receptors.[51]

An increasing number of cell-surface glycoproteins that mediate Ca^{2+}-independent cell-cell adhesion in vertebrates are being discovered to belong to the Ig superfamily. One of these is the so-called N-CAM, which is a large, single-pass transmembrane glycoprotein (about 1,000 amino acid residues long). N-CAM is expressed on the surface of nerve cells and glial cells and causes them to stick together by a Ca^{2+}-independent mechanisms. When these membrane proteins are purified and inserted into synthetic phospholipid vesicles, the vesicles bind to one another, as well as to cells that have N-CAM on their surface; the binding is blocked if the cells are pretreated with monovalent anti-N-CAM antibodies. Thus, N-CAM binds cells together by a homophilic interaction that directly joins two N-CAM molecules.[52]

Anti-N-CAM antibodies disrupt the orderly pattern of retinal development in tissue culture and when injected into the developing chick eye, disturb the normal growth pattern of retinal nerve cell axons. These observations suggest that N-CAM plays an important part in the development of the central nervous system by promoting cell-cell adhesion. In addition, the neural crest cells that form the peripheral nervous system have large amounts of N-CAM on their surface when they are associated with the neural tube, lose it while they are migrating, and then re-express it when they aggregate to form a ganglion suggesting that N-CAM plays a part in the assembly of the ganglion.

There are several forms of N-CAM, each encoded by a distinct messenger RNA (mRNA). The different mRNAs are generated by alternative splicing of an RNA transcript produced from a single large gene. The large extracellular post of the polypeptide chain ($\sim$ 680 amino acid residues) is identical in most forms of N-CAM and is folded into five domains characteristic of antibody molecules. Thus, N-CAM belongs to the same ancient superfamily of recognition proteins to which antibodies belong.[53]

I have mentioned earlier the guidance provided by the neural crest in the development of the thymus, that is, a central regulatory organ for the immune system. The converse also appears to be true: the immune system has a special role in the development of the nervous system. In this context, the most critical feature of the immune system is its tremendous polymorphism so that lymphocytes that are produced can recognize enormous numbers of different antigens. For this reason, the immune system is ideally suited to provide markers or "anchoring sites" that enable developing structures to be built up in precisely the correct form. In no organ system is this type of detailed anchorage mechanism as important as in the developing nervous system in which many millions of nerve fibers traverse great distances and establish connections with particular groups of target cells. Marking by means of histocompatibility antigens provides exactly such a system, as indeed the original function of the MHC antigens has been defined already in the 1970s as the general plasma membrane anchorage site of organogenesis-directing proteins.[54]

The Immune System and the Nervous System Sharing the Capacity to Remember.

The immune system and the nervous system possess short- or long-term memory, or both. The latter may be defined as the recording of experiences that can modify behavior. This general definition encompasses a broad spectrum of phenomena from the bacterial capacity of sensing chemical gradients to cognitive learning in humans.

The clonal selection theory of acquired immunity provides a useful conceptual framework for understanding the cellular basis of immunologic memory. According to this scheme, immunologic memory is generated during the primary immune response because 1) the proliferation of antigen-triggered virgin cells creates a large number of memory cells—a process known as clonal expansion; 2) the memory cells have a much longer life span than do virgin cells and recirculate between the blood and secondary lymphoid organs; and

3) each memory cell is able to respond more readily to antigen than does a virgin cell.

One reason, if not the most important reason, for the increased responsiveness of memory B-cells is the higher affinity (avidity) of their antibody receptors for the homologous antigen. Thus, with the passage of time after immunization, there is a progressive increase in the affinity of antibodies produced against the immunizing antigen. This phenomenon is known as affinity maturation, and it is due to the accumulation of somatic mutations in variable (V)-region coding sequences after antigen stimulation of B-lymphocytes. The rate of somatic mutation in these sequences is estimated to be 10^{-3} per nucleotide pair per cell generation, which is about a million times greater than the spontaneous mutation rate in other genes [41]. This process is called somatic hypermutation. Since B-cells are stimulated to proliferate by the binding of antigen, any mutation occurring during the course of an immune response that increases the affinity of a cell surface antibody molecule will cause the preferential proliferation of the B-cell making the antibody, especially when antigen concentration decreases with increasing time after immunization. Thus, affinity maturation is the consequence of repeated cycles of somatic hypermutation followed by antigen-driven selection in the course of an antibody response.

Research in the field of neuronal memory is still in an early phase, primarily because of methodologic difficulties and the validity of approaches currently used. The human brain is extraordinarily complex (10^{12} neurons) and intricate (an average neuron may have 10,000 dendrites interacting with other neurons), dictating the use of reductionist approaches which always require a correlation with the whole organism to verify the conclusions reached at the molecular level. Such relationship emphasizes the importance relating the biochemical events in single cells to the more complex organisms such as Aplysia, Drosophila, rodents, cats, and humans. The fact, however, that adjacent neurons are practically never identical means that the quantity of material needed to biochemical analysis necessitates a cell line approach. Both bacteria and neural cell lines provide a homogeneous population of cells that can be studied biochemically. Bacteria detect chemical gradients using a memory obtained by the combination of a fast excitation process and a slow adaptation process. This model system, which has the advantages of extensive genetic and biochemical information, shows no features of long-term memory.

To study long-term memory, other biologic systems that exhibit two phenomena associated with learning and memory, habituation and potentiation, must be used. Habituation is defined as the decreased responsiveness to a stimulus when it is presented repetitively over time. Potentiation, on the other hand, is defined as the increased responsiveness to a stimulus when that stimulus is presented repetitively over time. In the mammalian brain, the hippocampus plays a special role in learning: when it is destroyed on both sides of the brain, the ability to form new memories is largely lost, although previous long established memories remain. The evidence obtained on hippocampal slices indicates that the biochemical changes in the synapse represent the molecular bases for long-term memory[55,56] Despite the wealth of information provided by investigations in mammalian brain slices, it became increasingly clear that the study of cultured neural cells is more desirable because only in such a system could one be certain that the complete biochemical pathway, that is, the complete signal transduction pathway from stimulatory input to a behavioral output, could be analyzed. To study memory, however, some modifiable behavior needs to be observed. Because neurons communicate with each other chemically through the release of a neurotransmitter, the secretion of neurotransmitters (the output) evoked by various chemical stimuli (the input) could be used to monitor the responsiveness of the cell. This experimental system was used to study the input-output properties of a particular neuron, and both habituation and potentiation could be demonstrated in neuronal cell lines, indicating that they can serve as good model systems for the memory process, except that they do not possess synaptic connections. In the early phase of these studies the absence of synaptic connections posed a substantial problem for two major reasons: 1) as stated before, current evidence favors (in more organized neural tissue such as brain slices) the idea that the biochemical changes in the synapse are the molecular basis of long-term memory, and 2) the synapse is a unique anatomic association of two cells that occurs only in the nervous system and therefore represents a special *sui generis* neuronal feature.

Whether memories however, are generally recorded in presynaptic changes or in postsynaptic changes, in synaptic chemistry or in synaptic structure, or indeed in synapses at all, are still open questions. Regardless of the validity of any of these questions, it appears that the biochemical features of all memory-forming processes (i.e., habituation, potentiation, and associative learning in invertebrates, mammalian brain slices, and cultured clonal neural cell lines) are highly similar (the PC 12 cells[57,58] and HT4 cells).[59,60] They can be characterized as follows: 1) a monoamine (primarily serotonin) and a glutamate receptor (known as NMDA receptor because it is selectively activated by the artificial glutamate analog N-methyl-D-aspartate) are involved; 2) binding of the neurotransmitter (serotonin, glutamate) by these receptors initiates a cascade of enzymatic reactions; 3) the first step in this cascade is the activation of a G-protein, which may either interact directly with ion channels or control the production of cyclic adenosine monophosphate (AMP) or Ca^{2+}; 4) the two second messengers in turn regulate ion channels directly or activate kinases that phosphorylate various proteins including ion channels; 5) at many synapses both channel-linked and non-channel-linked receptors are present, responding either to the same or to different neurotransmitters; 6) responses mediated by non-channel-linked receptors (serotonin) have a slow onset and long duration, and modulate the efficacy of subsequent synaptic transmission providing the basis for memory formation; 7) channel-linked receptors that allow Ca^{2+} to enter the cell (NMDA receptor) also mediate long-term memory effects; and 8) either too much or too little cyclic AMP can interfere with memory formation.[61]

In all these processes, the interaction between serotonin and glutamate and their respective receptor systems can be illustrated by the studies carried out on the HT4 neural cell line.[61] The HT4 cells do not habituate to repetitive membrane depolarization, but after exposure of these cells to various neurotransmitters, serotonin has the capacity to potentiate cellular responsiveness. Depending on the strength of the serotonin stimulus, both short- and long-term potentiation can be induced. For instance, a 2 minute exposure to serotonin results in the transient increase in cellular responsiveness, where a 5 minute presentation gives rise to a more permanent potentiation, the difference between the two involving the activation of NMDA receptors. Thus, the stronger (5 min) serotonin stimulus results in the endogenous release of excitatory amino acids with activation of NMDA receptors. Consistent with this mechanism, long-term secretory potentiation can also be produced with a 2 min stimulus of serotonin only if glutamate or NMDA is given simultaneously.

As I now begin a comparison of immunologic versus neuronal memory, I have to return to an earlier statement that immunologic memory is due to clonal selection and lymphocyte maturation. Although this is correct in cellular terms, in molecular terms the problem of clonal selection and expansion reduces to the issue of affinity maturation of the antibody on the surface of the lymphocyte. In other words, the entire antigen-driven selection of antibody-producing lymphocytes is based on the strength of the antibody-antigen interaction, which depends on both the affinity and the number of binding sites. The affinity of an antibody reflects the strength of binding of an antigenic determinant to a single antigen-binding site, and it is independent of the number of sites. However, the total avidity of an antibody for a multivalent antigen, such as a polymer with repeating subunits, is defined as the total binding strength of all of its binding sites together. When a multivalent antigen combines with more than one antigen binding site on an antibody, the binding strength is greatly increased because all the antigen-antibody bonds must be broken simultaneously before the antigen and antibody can dissociate. Thus, a typical IgG molecule will bind at least 1,000 times more strongly to a multivalent antigen if both antigen-binding sites are engaged than if only one site is involved. For the same reason, if the affinity of the antigen-binding sites in an IgG and an IgM molecule is the same, the IgM molecule (with ten binding sites) will have a much greater avidity for a multivalent antigen than an IgG molecule (which has twosites). This difference in avidity, often 10^4-fold or more, is important because antibodies produced early in an immune response usually have much lower affinities than those produced later. Because of its high total avidity, IgM—the major IG class produced early in immune responses—can function effectively even when each of its binding sites has only a low affinity.[41]

In the late 1950S, an excellent correlation was shown between the body temperature of rabbits and the affinity and avidity of the antibody produced against the radiolabeled antigen as tested in equilibrium dialysis experiments.[62] The higher the body temperature was, the greater the affinity and avidity were. In the beginning of these studies commercially available *E. coli* endotoxin was used, but later the rise in temperature was reproduced by electrical stimulation of the posterior hypothalamus or hippocampus through stereotaxically implanted permanent depth electrodes in studies without endotoxin administration.[63] Discovery of the peptidoglycan and its derivatives as powerful immunologic adjuvants opened up a new window for the consideration of the relationship between immunologic and neuronal memory. The peptidoglycan, which is the basal layer of the bacterial cell wall, is a rigid macromolecule surrounding the cytoplasmic membrane. It is formed by the polymerization of a disaccharide tetrapeptide subunit; in the intact peptidoglycan, disaccharides form linear chains whereas peptides are linked by interpeptide linkages.[44] The recognition of the immunomodulating properties of peptidoglycans and peptidoglycan fragments is the result of the work aimed at identifying the structure responsible for the adjuvant activity of the mycobacterial cells in Freund's adjuvant.[64] Simple active molecules were soon produced by organic synthesis followed by a vast array of analogs and derivatives that can be classified into several categories. The one that is most pertinent to this discussion is the group of "simple muramyl peptides." Of these the smallest immunoactive synthetic muramyl peptide is N-acetyl-muramyl-L-alanyl-D-isoglutamine (MDP).[65,66] This substance has a pyrogenic effect that originally was attributed to its ability to induce the release of endogenous pyrogen from mononuclear phagocytes. However, a direct central nervous system action could not be excluded since MDP was found to be active by the intracerebroventricular route (MDP was shown to cross the blood-brain barrier,[67] and in rabbits made leukopenic by nitrogen mustard treatment.[44] In addition, it was subsequently shown that MDP can also induce sleep, and the somnogenic effect can be separated from its pyrogenic activity. MDP's pyrogenic activity does not affect brain temperature changes that are tightly coupled to sleep states.[68] More importantly, with respect to the direct central nervous system neuronal effects of MDP, this substance is capable of specific binding to serotonin receptors of synaptosomal membranes of brain tissue and competes with serotonin for these binding sites, and the kinetics of serotonin binding to brain homogenates is altered after sleep deprivation.[69] Additional findings on the capacity of MDP to act directly and specifically on central neurons include the following: MDP alters neuronal firing rates in different regions of the brain,[70] humoral antibody responses are enhanced by lowering serotonin levels in the brain,[71] administration of para-chlorophenylalamine which markedly decreases the level of brain serotonin completely abolishes the MDP-induced rise in body temperature as well as the somnogenic effect.[72] Finally, it has been established that immunization decreases the concentration of serotonin in the hypothalamus and the hippocampus.[73]

Although the foregoing evidence is fragmentary, it does establish a set of future reference points to begin to undertake a more informed comparison of the molecular mechanisms involved in immune and neuronal memory.

The Unique Recognition and Communication Powers of the Immune and Neuroendocrine Systems as Shared Characteristics.

Earlier I cited Schechter, pointing out that a good relationship between two biologic systems must be sensitive, synchronized, and synergistic [43]. There are no two biologic systems where such characterization of an ideal relationship would be more valid than in case of the immune and neuroendocrine systems, as reflected by their unique recognition and communication powers as shared characteristics. The latter are based on four critical features shared by both: 1) They are composed of extraordinarily large numbers of phenotypically distinct cells organized into intricate networks. Moreover, the size of this extensive cellular arsenal continuously increases as new sequence information becomes available and enormous numbers of new members of the Ig supergene family surface each year. Within these cell networks, the individual cells can interact either positively or negatively, and the response of one cell reverberates through the system by affecting many other cells; 2) cells of both systems synthesize, secrete and/or release the same effector molecules; 3) recognition of these effector molecules is realized by the same cellular receptors and second messenger mechanisms of both cell systems; and 4) these cellular and molecular determinants make a continuous, bilateral flow of information, the *sine qua non* of the unique interactions within the immune-neuroendocrine circuitry, possible.

A more amplified view on the basic biochemistry and molecular biology of receptor-effector coupling by G-proteins (i.e., the fundamental mechanism used by hormones, neurotransmitters, and the immunomodulatory cytokines for signal transmission by G-proteins) is presented by Szentivanyi[49] and by Lochrie and Simon,[74] and Birnbaumer and Brown.[75] HereI shall only mention that about 80% of all known neurohormones, neurotransmitters, immunomodulatory lymphokines and other autocrine and paracrine factors that regulate cellular interactions in the immune-neuroendocrine circuitry, called "primary" messengers, elicit cellular responses by combining with specific receptors that are coupled to effector functions by G-proteins. Although the primary messengers are many, the number of physicochemically and biologically distinct receptors that mediate their action is even larger. So far about 80 distinct receptors that recognize 40 hormones, neurotransmitters, and so on, can be identified. It is reasonable to assume that the total number of distinct receptors coupled by G-proteins will be 100 to 150. In contrast to receptors, the number of final effector functions regulated by these receptors and the number of G-proteins that provide for receptor-effector coupling are much lower, probably not much more than 15 each.

At the time of writing, receptors for simple substances, such as the amine mediators, and short-chain peptides as well as lipids, and for more than 20 different hypothalamopituitary peptides have been identified in the cells of the immune system, essentially in lymphocytes. In addition, to the hypothalamo-pituitary hormones, lymphocytes also express receptors for peptides secreted from neurons together with other neurotransmitters. These neuropeptides take on added significance as immunomodulators, since it is now known that lymphoid organs are directly innervated with nerves secreting these agents. From the standpoint of the integration of information in the immune-neuroendocrine circuitry, future studies will have to examine these parallel signaling pathways in isolation. In other words, it will be necessary to determine how an individual cell completely processes and integrates information from these individual pathways. This is all the more remarkable because the cell is faced with the task of balancing the need to communicate with other cells with the need for growth and maintenance of the differentiated state while preserving adequate flexibility to support regulation, sensitivity, and gain. One early result of such inquiries is the demonstration of cross-regulation (cross-talk) between the various G-protein mediated signaling pathways. Thus, it was shown that in the cross-regulation between α_1 and β_2-adrenergic receptor-mediated pathways, activation of β_2-adrenergic receptors increased α_1-adrenergic receptor mRNA levels.[76] Conversely, activation of the $G_{1\alpha}$-mediated inhibitory pathway of adenylate cyclase cross-regulates the stimulatory ($G_{s\alpha}$-mediated) ß-adrenergic-sensitive adenylate cyclase system by 1) upregulating β_2-adrenergic receptors and enhancing the activation of the stimulatory ($G_{s\alpha}$-mediated) adenylate cyclase pathway, and 2) downregulating elements of the inhibitory adenylate cyclase pathway, $G_{1\alpha2}$ and A_1-adenosine receptor binding, respectively.[77] It may be added that cross-regulation is also observed between signaling pathways that do not share the same effectors. Although much more work remains to be done to unravel the complexities of the coordinated regulation of information processing and integration by the cell, it is already possible to state that there is cross-regulation between neurally derived substances and lymphokines.

In the foregoing sections, discussions of the reciprocal, regulatory interplay between the immune and neuroendocrine systems have mainly covered the peripheral pathways by which the neuroendocrine influences are able to affect immune functions. However, as stated earlier, the flow of information in the immune-neuroendocrine circuitry is bidirectional, and there is conclusive evidence that products of the immune system are capable of modulating neuroendocrine processes. There are two lines of evidence indicating that the products of the immune system can influence the brain or the pituitary gland, or both. The first is provided by correlational studies, which show that changes occur in the brain during the course of an immune response. Along this line, Korneva and Klimenko[78] recorded single unit activity in the hypothalamus showing significant changes in the neuronal firing patterns in the posterior, ventromedial, and supramaxillary nuclei during the course of an immune response. These observations were independently confirmed by Besedovsky and coworkers[79] who found a considerable increase in the firing rate of neurons in the ventromedial hypothalamus 1 to 5 days following sensitization to trinitrophenol (TNP)-hemocyanin. Srebro and associates[80] found a significant increase in the nuclear volume of neurosecretory cells in the supraoptic nucleus during skin allograft rejection. Changes in the serotonin levels occur in the hypothalamus and hippocampus following immunization with typhoid antigen,[74] whereas increases in dopamine-stimulated adenylate cyclase activity in caudate homogenates are found following bacille Calmette-Guérin (BCG) antigen administration.[81] In recent years, these observations have been expanded by the findings on the effects of Newcastle disease virus on the metabolism of cerebral biogenic amine,[82] and similar changes have also been observed with influenza virus.

The second line of evidence implicating the immune system in regulating physiologic processes at the level of the brain or the pituitary gland, or both, is derived from studies in which products of the cells of the immune system were administered to experimental animals or added to cultured neuronal or pituitary cells. IL-1 stimulation of ACTH secretion was first shown in a mouse pituitary cell line, AtT-20 cells[83] and subsequently confirmed on primary pituitary cells.[84,85] In addition, IL-1 alters the release of TSH, growth hormones, and prolactin;[86] stimulates astroglial proliferation following brain injury;[87] stimulates somatostatin synthesis in the fetal brain;[88] inhibits progesterone secretion in cultures of granulosa cells;[89] and elicits the production of CRF by the hypothalamus.[90,91] In these neuronal interactions IL-1 acts on specific receptors in the brain.[92] IL-1 shows complex, multi-targeted effects on insulin secretion: 1) it has direct glucose-dependent inhibitory and stimulatory effects on pancreatic B-cell function [[93]]; 2) IL-1 induces hyperinsulinemia by a central action;[94] and 3) it acts as a hypoglycemic agent independently from effects on insulin release.[95] Other lymphokines also have effects on the neuroendocrine system. IL-2 stimulates oligodendroglial proliferation and maturation[96] and also induces ACTH secretion in pituitary cells.[97] TNF-α and IL-6 augment ACTH secretion *in vivo* together with numerous other effects on the neuroendocrine system,[93,98,99,100,101] and the thymic hormone, thymosin fraction 5, stimulates prolactin and growth hormone release from anterior pituitary cells.[102]

THE FUTURE

The immune-neuroendocrine circuitry represents an immensely complex, powerful and wide-ranging charter of human physiologic and pathologic possibilities, which among others is working its way to the creation of a new kind of immunology is based on a vastly enlarged vision of immunologic potential in health and disease. The emergence of this new interdisciplinary field will require a critical re-examination of some of our basic current views on the pathophysiologic and immunopharmacologic realities surrounding the problems of human asthma.

REFERENCES

1. **Szentivanyi, A, Filipp, G, and Legeza, I.**, Investigations on tobacco sensitivity, *Act. med. hung. Tomus III, Fasciculus*, 2, 175, 1952
2. **Filipp, G, and Szentivanyi, A.**, Zur Frage der Organlokalisation der allergischen Reaktion, *Wierner klin. Wschr.*, 65, 620, 1953.
3. **Filipp, G, and Szentivanyi, A.**, Experimentelle Data zur regulativen Rolle des Neuro-endokriniums in experimenteller Anaphylaxie I. Relazioni e Communicazioni, *Rome II Pansiero Scientifico*, 229, 1, 1956.
4. **Szentivanyi, A.**, *Allergie und Zentralnervensystem. Acta. Allergologica*, 6, 27, 1953.
5. **Szentivanyi, A, and Filipp, G.**, Experimentelle Data zur regulativen Rolle des Neuro-endokriniums in experimenteller Anaphylaxie, II. Relazionie e Communicazioni, *Rome II Pansiero Scientifico*, 237, 1, 1956.
6. **Szentivanyi, A and Szekely, J.**, Effect of injury to, and electrical stimulation of hypothalamic areas on the anaphylactic and histamine shock of guinea pig, *Ann. Allergy*, 14, 259, 1956.
7. **Filipp, G, and Szentivanyi, A.**, Die Wirkung von Hypothalamuslasionen auf den anaphylaktischen Schock des Meerschweinchens, *Allergie und Asthmaforschung Bd.*, 1, 12, 1957.
8. **Szentivanyi, A, and Szekely, J.**, Uber den Effekt der Schadigung und der elektrischen Reizung der hypothalamischen Gegenden auf den anaphylaktischen und Histamin-Schock des Meerschweinchens, *Allergie und Asthmaforschung Bd.*, 1, 28, 1957.
9. **Szentivanyi, A. and Szekely, J.**, Wirkung der konstanten Reizung hypothalamischer Strukturen durch Tiefenelektroden auf den histaminbedingten und anaphylaktischen Schock des Meerschweinchens, *Acta. Physiol. Hung. Suppl. V*, 11, 41, 1957
10. **Szentivanyi, A, and Filipp, G.**, Anaphylaxis and the nervous system, Part II, *Ann. Allergy*, 16, 143, 1958.
11. **Filipp, G, and Szentivanyi, A.**, Anaphylaxis and the nervous system, Part III, *Ann. Allergy*, 16, 306, 1958.
12. **Szentivanyi, A, and Szekely, J.**, Anaphylaxis and the nervous system, Part IV, *Ann. Allergy*, 16, 389, 1958
13. **Szentivanyi, A.**, Hypothalamic Influences on Antibody Formation and on Bronchial Responses to Histamine, in *Proc. of the Fourth Aspen Conf. on Res. in Emphysema and Asthma*, Aspen, Colorado, 1961, p. 78.
14. **Szentivanyi, A. and Fishel, C. W.**, Effect of Bacterial Products on Responses to the Allergic Mediators, in *Immunological Diseases*, M. Samter, Ed, Boston: Little, Brown and Company, 1965, pp. 226-241.
15. **Szentivanyi, A. and Fishel, C. W.**, Die Amin-Mediatorstoffe der allergischen Reaktion und die Reaktionsfahiegkeit ihrer Erfolgeszellen, in *Pathogenese und Therapie allergischer Reaktionen, Grundlagenforschung und Klinik*, G. Filipp and A .Szentivanyi, Eds, Stuttgart, Germany: Ferdinand Enke Verlag, 1966, pp. 588-683.
16. **Szentivanyi, A, Krzanowski, J. J, and Polson, J. B.**, The Autonomic Nervous System: Structure, Function, and Altered Effector Responses, in E Middleton, CE Reed, and EF Ellis (Eds), Allergy: Principles and Practice, St. Louis: The CV Mosby Company, 1978, pp. 256-300.
17. **Szentivanyi, A, Polson, J.B, and Krzanowski, J.J.**, The Altered Reactivity of the Effector Cells to Antigenic and Pharmacological Influences and its Relation to Cyclic Nucleotides. I. Effector Reactivities in the Efferent Loop of the Immune Response, in G Filipp (ed), Pathomechanismus und Pathogenese allergischer Reaktionen, Munich: Werk-Verlag Dr. Edmund Banachewski, 1980, pp. 460-510.

18. **Szentivanyi, A. and Fitzpatrick, D.F.,** The Altered Reactivity of the Effector Cells to Antigenic and Pharmacological Influences and its Relation to Cyclic Nucleotides. II. Effector Reactivities in the Efferent Loop of the Immune Response, in G Filipp (Ed), Pathomechanismus und Pathogenese allergischer Reaktionen. Munich: Werk-Verlag Dr. Edmund Banachewski, 1980, pp. 511-580.

19. **Szentivanyi A, and Szentivanyi, J.,** Immunomodulatory Effects of Central and Peripheral Autonomic Mechanisms Mediated by Neuroeffector Molecules, in *Proc. of Internatl. Symp. on Biological Resp. Modifiers in Clin. Oncol. and Immunol.*, New York: Plenum, 1982, p. 8.

20. **Szentivanyi A. and Szentivanyi, J.,** The Emergence of Neuroendocrine Disorders as a New Group of Autoimmune Diseases, in *Proceedings of Symposium on Clinical Laboratory Immunology*, New York: Plenum, 1982, p. 3.

21. **Filipp, G, and Szentivanyi, A.,** Anaphylaxis and the Nervous System, Part III, in S Locke, R Ader, HO Besedovsky, NR Hall, G Solomon and T Strom (Eds), *Foundations of Psychoneuroimmunology*, Hawthorne, NY: Aldine Publishing, 1985, pp. 1-12.

22. **Szentivanyi, A. and Szentivanyi, J.** Immune-neuroendocrine circuits in antibiotic-bacterial interactions, in *Proc. of Third Internatl. Symp. on the Influence of Antibiotics on the Host-Parasite Relationship, Heidelberg*: Springer Verlag, 1987.

23. **Szentivanyi, A, Reiner, S, Filipp, G, and Heim, O.,** The Influence of Anterior Hypothalamic Lesions on the Kinetic Parameters of ^{125}I-VIP (vasoactive intestinal peptide) Binding to Murine Mononuclear Cells, in Proc. of Workshop 12 on Mediators in Asthma, XII World Congress of Asthmology. Madrid: Editorial Garsi, 1987, p. 41.

24. **Szentivanyi, A., Krzanowski, J.J, and Polson, J.B.,** The Autonomic Nervous System and Altered Effector Responses, in E Middleton, CE Reed, and EF Ellis, Eds. Allergy: Principles and Practice (3rd ed). St. Louis: The CV Mosby Company, 1988, pp. 461-493.

25. **Szentivanyi, A., Szentivanyi, J., Haberman, K. and Heim, O.,** Nonantibiotic properties of antibiotics in relationship to immune-neuroendocrine influences, *Clin. Pharmacol. Therap.*, 43, 166, 1988.

26. **Szentivanyi, A, Haberman, K., Heim, O., Schultze, P., Filipp, G. and Reiner, S.,** Hypothalamic and Other Central Influences on Antibiosis and Host Immunity, in Proc. of the Fourth Internatl. Conf. on Immunopharmacol., Oxford: Pergamon, 1988, Abstract 510129.

27. **Szentivanyi, A., Reiner, S., Heim, O., Filipp, G. and Abarca, C.M.,** Some Biochemical and Cellular Features of Adrenergic Mechanisms Induced by Bacterial Lipopolysaccharide Endotoxin in Rats With or Without Chemical Sympathetic Ablation Achieved by 6-Hydroxydopamine Hydrobromide (6-OHDA), in Proc. of Internatl. Symp. on Endotoxin, Tochigi, Japan: Jichi Medical School, 1988, Abstract SV-8.

28. **Szentivanyi, A., Reiner, S., Heim, O., Filipp, G. and Abarca, C.M.,** The Effect of 6-Hydroxydopamine Hydrobromide on Endotoxin-Induced Adrenergic Mechanisms, in Proc. of Second Internatl. Mtg. on Resp. Allergy, Rome: Pythagora Press, 1988, Abstract 311.

29. **Szentivanyi, J., Szentivanyi, A., Schultze, P., Filipp, G. and Heim, O.,** Influences of hypothalamic and extrahypothalamic brain structures on the immunogenicity of antibiotic-pretreated bacteria, in *Proc. of An. Mtg. of the Internatl. Soc. for Interferon Res.*, Kanagawa, Japan: Japanese Society for Interferon Research, 1988, Abstract 5-30.

30. **Schwartz, M.E., Reiner, S., Heim, O., Abarca, C. and Szentivanyi, A.,** Further Observations on the Cellular and Molecular Mechanisms Involved in the Reciprocal Histamine-Catecholamine Counterregulatory Interplay in Relation to Induction of Histidine Decarboxylase Synthesis by Interleukin-3 and Granulocyte-Macrophage Colony Stimulating Factor, in Proc. of XIII Internatl. Cong. of Allergol. and Clin. Immunol. St. Louis: Mosby-Yearbook, 1988, Abs. 64.

31. **Szentivanyi, A.,** The Discovery of Immune-Neuroendocrine Circuits and the Concepts of Prevailing Immunologic Thought that Impeded the Timely Recognition of Their role in Immune-Homeostasis, in Proc. of the Internatl. Symp. on Interactions Between the Neuroendocrine and Immune Systems, Rome: Pythagora Press, 1988, pp. 23-24.

32. Szentivanyi, A., Plenary Lecture: Natural Neuropeptides in the Immunologic Inflammation of the Airways in Asthma, in Proc. of XIV World Cong. of Natural Med., Malaga, Spain, 1988, p. 1.

33. Szentivanyi, A. and Szentivanyi, J., Antibiotic-Bacterial Interactions in Relation to Immune-Neuroendocrine Circuits, in Proc. of XIII Internatl. Cong. of Allergology and Clin. Immunol. St. Louis: Mosby-Yearbook, 1988, Abstract 986.

34. Szentivanyi, J., Szentivanyi, A., Schultze, P., Filipp, G. and Heim, O., Changes in the Immune Parameters of Antibiotic-Bacterial Interactions Induced by Hypothalamic and Other Electrolytic Brain Lesions Produced Through Stereotaxically Implanted Depth Electrodes, in G Gillissen, W Opferkuch, G Peters, and G Pulverer, Eds., The Influence of Antibiotics on the Host-Parasite Relationship. Heidelberg, Germany: Springer-Verlag, 1989, pp. 237-244.

35. Szentivanyi, A., Reiner, S., Heim, O., Filipp, G., and Abarca, C., The effect of sympathetic ablation [6-hydroxydopamine hydrobromide (6-OHDA); axotomy] on endotoxin induced adrenergic mechanisms, *The Pharmacologist*, 31, 118, 1989.

36. Szentivanyi, J., Schultz, P., Heim, O., Abarca, A., and Szentivanyi, A., Hypothalamic and other central influences on antibiotic modulated bacterial immunogenicity, *The Pharmacologist*, 31, 193, 1989.

37. Szentivanyi, J., Schultze, P., Heim, O., Reiner, S., Robicsek, S., Abarca, C. and Szentivanyi, A., The effect of hypothalamic and extrahypothalamic nuclear groupings on the antibiotic modulated bacterial immunogenicity and production of IL-1, IFN and TNF, *Cytokine*, 1, 364, 1989

38. Szentivanyi, A., Reiner, S., Schwartz, M.E., Heim, O., Szentivanyi, J. and Robicsek, S., Restoration of normal beta adrenoceptor concentrations in A549 lung adenocarcinoma cells by leukocyte protein factors and recombinant interleukin-1α, *Cytokine*, 1, 118, 1989.

39. Szentivanyi, A., Krzanowski, J.J., Polson, J.B., and Abarca, C.M., The pharmacology of microbial modulation in the induction and expression of immune reactivities, I. The pharmacologically active effector molecules of immunologic inflammation, immunity, and hypersensitivity, *Immunopharmacol. Rev.*, 1, 159, 1990.

40. Szentivanyi, A., Maurer, P. and Janicki, B.W., Eds. Antibodies: Structure, Synthesis, Function, and Immunologic Intervention in Disease, New York: Plenum Press, 1987.

41. Szentivanyi, A., The Discovery of Immune-Neuroendocrine Circuits in the Fall of 1951, in J.W. Hadden, G. Nistico, and K. Masek, Eds, Interactions Among the Central Nervous System, Neuroendocrine and Immune Systems, Rome, Italy: Pythagora Press, 1989, pp. 1-5

42. Schechter, G., A good relationship: sensitive, synchronized and synergistic, *Prog. Neuro-Endocrine Immunol.*, 2, 35, 1989.

43. Hadden, J.W. and Szentivanyi, A., Eds, The Pharmacology of the Reticuloendothelial System, New York: Plenum Press, 1985.

44. Szentivanyi, A., Szentivanyi, J., Middleton, E., Jr, Friedman, H. and Abarca, C.M., The pharmacology of microbial modulation in the induction and expression of immune reactivities, II. Effector mechanisms in the afferent and efferent limbs of the immune response, *Immunopharmacology Rev.*, 1993 (in press).

45. Goodman C.S. and Pearson, K.G., Neuronal development: cellular approaches in invertebrates, *Neurosci. Res. Program Bull.*, 20, 777, 1982

46. LeDouarin, N., The Neural Crest, Cambridge, England: Cambridge University Press, 1982.

47. Geschwind N. and Galaburda, A.M., Cerebral lateralization: biological mechanisms, associations, and pathology, Parts I-III, *Arch Neurol.*, 42, 428 1985.

48. Szentivanyi, A., Immune-Neurodendocrine Circuitry and Its Relation to Bronchial Asthma, in *Bronchial Asthma - Mechanisms and Therapeutics* (3rd ed). EB Weiss and M. Stein, Eds, Boston: Little, Brown and Company, 1993, pp. 421-438.

49. Szentivanyi, A., Beta-adrenergic subsensitivity in asthma and atopic dermatitis: A status report, *Acta. Biomed. Hung. Amer.*, 1, 1, 1991.

50. Renoux G., Biziere, K., Renoux, M., Bardos, P. and Degenne, D., Consequences of Bilateral Brain Neocortical Ablation on Imuthiol-Induced Immunostimulation in *Mice*, in *Neuroimmune Interactions: Proc. of the Second Internatl. Workshop on Neuro- immunomodulation*, B.D. Jankovic, B.M. Markovic and N.H. Spector, Eds, *Ann. NY Acad. Sci.*, 496, 346, 1987

51.   **Cunningham, B.A., Hemperley, J.J., Murray, B.A., Prediger, E.A., Brackenbury, R., and Edelman, G.M.**, Neural, cell adhesion molecule: structure, immunoglobulin-like domains, cell surface modulation, and alternative RNA splicing, *Science*, 236, 799, 1987.

52.   **Milner, R.J., Lai, C., Sutcliffe, J.G. and Bloom, F.E.**, Expression of Immunoglobulin-Like Proteins in the Nervous System: Properties of the Neural Protein 1B236/MAG, in *Neuroimmune Networks: Physiology and Diseases,* E.J. Goetzl and N.H. Spector, Eds, . New York: Alan R. Liss, Inc., 1989, pp. 9-15.

53.   **Williams, A.F. and Barclay, A.N.**, The immunoglobulin superfamily - domains for cell surface recognition, *Ann. Rev. Immunol.*, 6, 381, 1988.

54.   **Edelman, G.M.**, Neural Darwinism, New York: Basic Book, Inc., 1987.

55.   **Malinow, R. and Tsien, R. W.**, Presynaptic enhancement shown by whole-cell recordings of long-term potentiation in hippocampal slices, *Nature*, 346(6290), 177, 1990.

56.   **Bekkers, J. M. and Stevens, C. F.**, Presynaptic mechanism for long-term potentiation in the hippocampus, *Nature*, 346(6286), 724, 1990.

57.   **McFadden, P. N. and Koshland, D. E., Jr.**, Habituation in the single cell: diminished secretion of norepinephrine with repetitive depolarization in PC12 cells, *Proc. Natl. Acad. Sci.*, USA 87, 2031, 1990.

58.   **McFadden, P. N. and Koshland, D. E., Jr.**, Parallel pathways for habituation in repetitively stimulated P12 cells, *Neuron*, 4, 615, 1990.

59.   **Morimoto, B. H. and Koshland, D. E., Jr.**, Excitatory amino acid uptake and N-methyl-D-aspartate-mediated secretion in a neural cell line, *Proc. Natl. Acad. Sci. USA*, 87, 3518, 1990.

60.   **Morimoto, B. H. and Koshland, D. E., Jr.**, Induction and expression of long- and short-term neurosecretory potentiation in a neural cell line, *Neuron*, 5, 875, 1990.

61.   **Dudai, Y.**, Neurogenetic dissection of learning and short-term memory in Drosophila, *Ann. Rev. Neurosci.*, 11, 537, 1988.

62.   **Szentivanyi, A. and Filipp, G.**, Propriètès Immuno-Chimiques et Physico-Chimiques des Anticorps, Paris, France: Editions Mèdicales Flammarion, 1962

63.   **Szentivanyi, J., Szentivanyi, A., Williams, J.F. and Friedman, H.**, Virus Associated Immune and Pharmacologic Mechanisms in Disorders of Respiratory and Cutaneous Atopy, in A. Szentivanyi and H. Friedman, Eds., *Viruses, Immunity and Immunodeficiency*, New York: Plenum Press, 1986, pp. 211-244.

64.   **Friedman, H., Klein, T. W. and Szentivanyi, A.**, Eds., *Immunomodulation by Bacteria and Their Products*, New York: Plenum Press, 1981.

65.   **Szentivanyi, A., Middleton, E., Williams, J. F. and Friedman, H.**, Effect of Microbial Agents on the Immune Network and Associated Pharmacologic Reactivities, in E Middleton, C. E. Reed and E. F. Ellis, Eds, *Allergy: Principles and Practice*, St. Louis: The CV Mosby Company, 1983, pp. 211-236.

66.   **Klein, T. W., Specter, S., Friedman, H. and Szentivanyi, A.**, Eds, *Biological Response Modifiers in Human Oncology and Immunology*, New York: Plenum Press, 1983.

67.   **Krueger, J. M., Obal, F. Jr., Johannsen, L., Cady, A. B. and Toth, L.**, Endogenous Slow-Wave Sleep Substances, A Review, in C. Dugsovic and A. Wauquier, Eds, *Current Trends in Slow-Wave Sleep Research*, New York: Raven Press, 1988.

68.   **Krueger, J. M., Obal, F. Jr., Opp., M., Johannsen, L., Cady, A. B. and Toth, L.**, Immune Response Modifiers and Sleep, in J. W. Hadden, K. Masek and G. Nistico, Eds, *Interactions Among Central Nervous System, Neuroendocrine and Immune Systems*, Rome, Italy: Pythagora Press, 1989, pp. 323-350.

69.   **Fillion, M. P., Prudhomme, N., Haour, F., Fillion, G., Bonnet, M., Lespinats, G., Masek, K., Flegel, M., Corvaia, N. and Launay, J. M.**, Hypothetical Role of the Serotonergic System in Neuroimmunomodulation: Preliminary Molecular Studies, in J. W. Hadden, K. Masek and G. Nistico, Eds, *Interactions Among Central Nervous System, Neuroendocrine and Immune Systems*, Rome, Italy: Pythagora Press, 1989, pp. 235-250.

70.   **Dougherty, P. M. and Dafny, N.**, Central opioid systems are differentially affected by products of the immune response, *Soc. Neurosci. Abstr.*, 13, 1437, 1987.

71.   **Eremina, O. F. and Devoino, L. V.**, Production of humoral antibodies in rabbits following destruction of the nucleus of the midbrain raphe, *Byull. Eksp. Biol. Med.*, 74. 258, 1973.

72. **Masek, K., Horak, P., Kadlec, O. and Flegel, M.,** The Interactions Between Neuroendocrine and Immune Systems at the Receptor Level, The Possible Role of Serotonergic System, in *Interactions Among Central Nervous System, Neuroendocrine and Immune Systems,* J. W. Hadden, K. Masek and G. Nistico, Eds, Rome, Italy: Pythagora Press, 1989, pp. 225-234.

73. **Vekshina, N. and Magaeva, S. V.,** Changes in the serotonin concentration in the limbic structures of the brain during immunization, *Bull. Exp. Biol. Med.,* 77, 625, 1974.

74. **Lochrie, M. A. and Simon, M. I.,** G protein multiplicity in eukaryotic signal transduction systems, *Biochemistry,* 17, 4957, 1988.

75. **Birnbaumer, L. and Brown, A. M.,** G proteins and the mechanism of action of hormones, neurotransmitters, and autocrine and paracrine regulatory factors, *Am. Rev. Respir. Dis.,* 141, S106, 1990.

76. **Morris, G. M., Hadcock, J. R. and Malbon, C. C.,** Cross-regulation between G-protein-coupled receptors, Activation of ß$_2$-adrenergic receptors increases α1-adrenergic receptor mRNA levels, *J. Biol. Chem.,* 266(4), 2233, 1991.

77. **Hadcock, J. R., Port, J. D. and Malbon, C. C.,** Cross-regulation between G-protein mediated pathways. Activation of the inhibitory pathway of adenylyl/cyclase increases the expression of ß$_2$-adrenergic receptors, *J. Biol Chem.,* 266(18), 11915, 1991.

78. **Korneva, E. A. and Klimenko, V. M.,** Neuronale hypothalamusaktivitt und homoostatische rektionen, *Ergebn. Exp. Med.,* 23, 373, 1976.

79. **Besedovsky H. O., Sorkin, E., Felix, D. and Haas, H.,** Hypothalamic changes during the immune response, *Eur. J. Immunol.,* 7, 325, 1977.

80. **Srebro, Z., Spisak-Plonka, I. and Szirmai, E.,** Neurosecretion in mice during skin allograft rejection, *Agressologie,* 15, 125, 1974.

81. **Cotzias, G. C. and Tang, L. C.,** Adenylate cyclase of brain reflects propensity for breast cancer in mice, *Science,* 197, 1094, 1977.

82. **Dunn, A. J., Powell, M. L., Moreshead, W. V., Gaskin, J. M. and Hall, N. R.,** Effects of Newcastle Disease virus administration to mice on the metabolism of cerebral biogenic amines, plasma corticosterone, and lymphocyte proliferation, *Brain Behav. Evol.,* 1, 216, 1987.

83. **Woloski, B. M. R. N. J., Smith, E. M, Meyer, W. J., Fuller, G. M. and Blalock, J. E.,** Corticotropin-releasing activity of monokines, *Science,* 230, 1035, 1985.

84. **Bernton, E. W., Beach, J. E., Holaday, J. W., Smallridge, R. C. and Fein, H. G.,** Release of multiple hormones by direct action of interleukin-1 on pituitary cells, *Science,* 238, 519, 1987.

85. **Kehrer, P., Turnill, D., Dayer, J-M., Muller, A. F. and Gaillard, R. C.,** Human recombinant interleukin-1ß and -α, but not recombinant tumor necrosis factor-α stimulate ACTH release from rat anterior pituitary cells *in vitro* in a prostaglandin E$_2$ and cAMP independent manner, *Neuroendocrin.,* 48, 160, 1988.

86. **Rettori, V., Jurcovicova, J. and McCann, S. M.,** Central action of interleukin-1 in altering the release of TSH, growth hormone and prolactin in the male rat, *J. Neurosci. Res.,* 18, 179, 1987.

87. **Giulian, D. and Lachman, L. B.,** Interleukin-1 stimulation of astroglial proliferation after brain injury, *Science,* 228, 497, 1985.

88. **Scarborough, D. E., Leo, S. L., Dinarello, C. A. and Roichlin, S.,** Interleukin-1ß stimulates somatostatin biosynthesis in primary cultures of fetal rat brain, *Endocrinol.,* 124, 549, 1989.

89. **Fukuoka, M., Yasuda, K., Taii, S., Takakura, K. and Mori, T.,** Interleukin-1 stimulates growth and inhibits progesterone secretion in cultures of porcine granulosa cells, *Endocrinology,* 124, 884, 1989.

90. **Sapolsky, R., Rivier, C., Yamamoto, G., Plotsky, P. and Vale, W.,** Corticotropin-releasing factor-producing neurons in the rat activated by interleukin-1, *Science,* 238, 522, 1987.

91. **Berkenbosch, F., van Oers, J., Del Rey, A, Tilders, F, and Besedovsky, H.,** Corticotropin-releasing factor producing neurons in the rat activated by interleukin-1, *Science,* 238, 524, 1987.

92. **Farrar, W. L., Kilian, P. L., Ruff, M. R., Hill, J. M. and Pert, C. B.,** Visualization and characterization of interleukin-1 receptors in brain, *J. Immunol.,* 139, 459, 1987.

93. **Zawalich, W. S., Zawalich, K. C. and Rasmussen, H.,** Interleukin-1α exerts glucose-dependent stimulatory and inhibitory effects on islet cell phosphoinositide hydrolysis and insulin secretion, *Endocrinology,* 124, 2350, 1989

94. **Cornell, R. P.,** Central interleukin-1 elicited hyperinsulinemia is mediated by prostaglandin but not autonomics, *Am. J. Physiol.,* 257, R839, 1989.

95. **Del Rey, A. and Besedovsky, H.,** Antidiabetic effects of interleukin-1, *Proc. Natl. Acad. Sci. USA,* 86, 5943, 1989.

96. **Benveniste, E. N. and Merrill, J. E.,** Stimulation of oligodendroglial proliferation and maturation by interleukin-2, *Nature,* 321, 610, 1986.

97. **Smith, L. R., Brown, S. L. and Blalock, J. E.,** Interleukin-2 induction of ACTH secretion: presence of an interleukin-2 receptor α-chain-like molecule on pituitary cells, *J. Neuroimmunol.,* 21, 249, 1989.

98. **Sherry, B. and Cerami, A.,** Cachectin/tumor necrosis factor exerts endocrine, paracrine, and autocrine control of inflammatory responses, *J. Cell Biol.,* 107, 1269, 1988.

99. **Naitoh, Y., Fukata, J., Tominaga, T., Nakai, Y., Tami, S., Mori, K. and Imura, H.,** Interleukin-6 stimulates the secretion of adrenocorticotropic hormone in conscious, freely-moving rats, *Biochem. Biophys. Res. Commun.,* 155, 1459, 1988.

100. **Sternberg, E. M.,** Monokines, Lymphokines and the Brain, in J. M. Cruse and J. E. Lewis, Eds, *The Year in Immunology* (vol. 5), Basel: Karger, 1989, pp. 205-217.

101. **Mealy, K., Robinson, B. G., Majzoub, J. A. and Wilmore, D. W.,** Hypothalamic-pituitary-adrenal (HPL) axis regulation by tumor necrosis factor, *Prog. Leukocyte Biol.,* 10B, 225, 1990.

102. **Spangelo, B. L., Judd, A. M, Ross, P. C., Login, I. S., Jarvis, W. D., Badamchian, M., Goldstein, A. L. and MacLeod, R. M.,** Thymosin fraction 5 stimulates prolactin and growth hormone release from anterior pituitary cells *in vitro, Endocrinology,* 121, 2035, 1987.

Chapter 23

THYROID AUTOIMMUNITY: A VOYAGE OF DISCOVERY

Noel R. Rose

This chapter consists of two sections. The first describes the discovery of thyroid autoimmunity as seen through the eyes of one of the original investigators. Under the general title of "Immunology Yesterday", it was published in *Immunology Today* (Vol. 12, #5, 1991, pp. 167-168) and is reprinted here with the kind permission of the editor, Dr. Richard Gallagher. The second section traces the evolution of thought with respect to self-nonself discrimination and autoimmunity, using autoimmune thyroiditis as a paradigm. This section is based on a lecture given during a symposium, entitled "From Immunity to Cellular and Molecular Immunology", held on the island of Ischia, (Naples) Italy, in June 1992).

THE DISCOVERY OF THYROID AUTOIMMUNITY

In 1951 there were not many places where a newly minted Ph.D. could go to learn immunology. Michael Heidelberger was at Columbia working on the immunochemistry of polysaccharides and Ernest Witebsky in Buffalo was engaged mostly in studying human blood groups and isolating the blood group substances. Having just completed a Ph.D. in Stuart Mudd's department at the University of Pennsylvania, I decided to make my future in immunology and was seeking a suitable training position. Most of my colleagues thought that I was quite made, since it seemed that the major problems in immunology had all been solved. The instructive template theories accounted for the formation of antibodies, and immunochemical studies by Landsteiner taught us all there was to know about antibody specificity. A number of useful diagnostic tests and a few vaccines had been developed. However, the biological basis of the immune response was entirely obscure and intrigued me sufficiently to want to learn more about immunology. After some discussion, Witebsky was kind enough to offer me an instructorship in his department together with the opportunity to complete my medical studies. Thus my wife and I packed all our belongings into the back of an ancient Oldsmobile and journeyed from Philadelphia to Buffalo in September 1951. A few months after I settled at the University of Buffalo, Witebsky suggested that I look into the problem that had intrigued him since his own student days, organ specificity. He considered that normal tissues and cancers contained alcohol-soluble constituents (called 'lipoids' in the alcoholic extracts of brain and suggested that I might want to look at thyroglobulin, the principal antigen of the thyroid gland. Thyroglobulin, he thought, was a unique example of an organ-specific protein.

Witebsky had studied thyroglobulin during his tenure at Heidelberg and had found that it is both thyroid-specific and crossreactive among thyroids of other mammalian species. However, he feared that these crossreactions were artifacts due to the inevitable denaturation of thyroglobulin during preparation. He challenged me, therefore, to prepare a native thyroglobulin to determine conclusively organ specificity and crossreactivity.

Working with a skilled protein chemist, Sidney Shulman, I developed a simple method of stepwise ammonium sulfate precipitation for the preparation of a relatively pure thyroglobulin product from bovine and other thyroid

0-8493-4722-X/94/$0.00 + $.50

glands. I then made the appropriate antisera in rabbits and showed a considerable degree of organ specificity and crossreactivity. "Ah, ha!" said Witebsky, "you must have denatured the material". Greatly deflated by this reaction on the part of my new boss, I sought a way of proving that the material was still in its native state. I hit upon the idea of preparing thyroglobulin from rabbit thyroid glands and injecting the material into rabbits. It seemed obvious that a native protein would not induce a response in the same species, whereas a denatured product might well do so. I made a batch of rabbit thyroglobulin, injected it intravenously into rabbits and was gratified to find that no immune response followed.

As was often the case, Witebsky and I discussed these results in the Serology Laboratory of the Buffalo General Hospital while he was reviewing the day's Wassermann tests. We began to speculate about why the rabbit was incapable of producing antibodies to its own thyroglobulin. Nothing in the instructive theories of antibody formation could explain it, unless we assumed that a surplus of antigen in the blood stream was causing a kind of immunological paralysis. I then suggested the perfect experiment. Why not remove the thyroids from some rabbits, since we could then be certain that all of the organ-specific thyroglobulin would be eliminated? We would then immunize the rabbit with rabbit thyroglobulin and produce a response. Because of Witebsky's long experience with blood groups, he pointed out the possible importance of individual differences and suggested that I immunize each rabbit with an extract of its own gland. The appropriate control was the extract prepared from the single lobe of a hemithyroidectomized rabbit. With the help of John Paine (Professor of Surgery) and Richard Egan (Assistant Professor of Surgery), I performed the necessary thyroidectomies and hemi-thyroidectomies, and made up individual thyroid extracts. Since the available antigen was in such short supply, I needed the most cost-effective method of immunization.   I, therefore, visited Jules Freund at the Public Health Research Institute in New York City, where I learned to emulsify the thyroid antigen in complete adjuvant. We then injected three groups of rabbits with this antigen-adjuvant mixture, namely, completely thyroidectomized, hemi-thyroidectomized and sham-thyroidectomized rabbits.   The results were completely unexpected. All three groups of rabbits produced antibodies that by complement fixation tests were found to be specific for thyroglobulin! (Incidentally, we later learned that injecting thyroglobulin with adjuvant, or in repeated small doses, is critical for eliciting an autoimmune response. Intravenous injection of a large bolus often enhances self tolerance.)

When we examined the thyroids of the immunized rabbits, we were even more astonished to find that they were extensively infiltrated with mononucle-ar cells. At this juncture, we repeated the experiment again and again with additional controls using adjuvant alone or adjuvant plus a number of their organ extracts to show the specificity of the phenomenon. The results proved to be consistent. Immunization of rabbits with rabbit thyroglobulin or even crude thyroid extract resulted in the production of thyroglobulin-specific antibodies. The antibodies could be demonstrated by complement fixation and even by direct precipitation. We were forced to conclude that we had actually produced an autoimmune response and, even more exciting, an autoimmune disease, by this method of experimental immunization. As we reviewed the histological material with our surgical collaborator, Paine remarked that the glands reminded him of Hashimoto's thyroiditis. Following this lead, we contacted several endocrinologists in Buffalo, requesting that they send us samples of serum from their Hashimoto patients. All of the endocrinologists affirmed that Hashimoto's disease occurs very rarely and they hardly expected to find a case. In fact, it took us three years to collect 12 sera. During this period, however, we were fortunate enough to be visited by Robin Coombs and his wife, Ann, who taught us the proper way to perform the tanned cell hemagglutination test. Using this very sensitive technique, we tested the precious thyroiditis patients' sera and found that all 12 of them contained thyroglobulin-specific autoantibodies.

Next, the question of what to do with these findings arise. I presented a ten-minute paper on the experimental immunization of rabbits at the annual meeting of the American Association of Immunologists (AAI) in March 1956. At the same time, we prepared the detailed findings for publication in a prestigious journal. A lengthy article was submitted by Witebsky accompanied by a letter pointing out the significance of the experimental observations and relating them to our, as yet unpublished, human findings. The paper was promptly returned by the journal with comments from the editor to the effect that it was common knowledge that such autoimmunization, as discussed in our paper, was impossible and the findings must be artifactual. Witebsky was very upset by this response and insisted that the entire body of experiments was repeated one final time. We then prepared a send series of two brief articles and submitted them to the *Journal of Immunology* where they were eventually published in June 1956.[1,2] The impact of these papers can be seen from the fact that they were included among the "Citation Classics" by E. Garfield of the Institute for Scientific Information in Current Contents (February 11, 1991).

Witebsky decided that the human studies should be published separately in the *Journal of the American Medical Association*. John Talbot, a close colleague of Witebsky's and former chairman of medicine at Buffalo, had just become editor of this journal and Witebsky was anxious that important new scientific findings be communicated there. We spent a long time working on the paper that related the experimental observations to our human studies. Since we anticipated that these findings might stimulate other investigators to search for autoimmune etiologies of enigmatic human disease, we also used the occasion to outline the four steps that we considered were appropriate to assign an autoimmune etiology to a human disease. These steps are now widely referred to as 'Witebsky postulates'. The paper eventually appeared in the *Journal of the American Medical Association* in June 1957[3] and was declared a 'landmark paper' by E. Garfield in Volume 257 of the *Journal of the American Medical Association* in 1987.

While we were preparing the *Journal of the American Medical Association* paper, I received a letter from Deborah Doniach from London. She told us that she had seen our AAI abstract and that, together with a 'young immunochemist' (as she called him), she had tested some sera from Hashimoto patients. They had found that several of the sera gave positive precipitation reactions with human thyroglobulin. Ivan Roitt and Deborah Doniach, together with Peter Campbell and Ralph Vaughan Hudson, presented these findings in preliminary form in the *Lancet* in late 1956 and published a definitive landmark article in the *Journal of Clinical Endocrinology and Metabolism* in 1957. Not long after this, we had the pleasure of having Deborah Doniach and Ivan Roitt visit our laboratory so that we could compare results of their precipitation tests with our tanned cell hemagglutination methods. The visit established a friendship that remains to the present day.

Looking back, I find it most fortunate that his work was carried out in Ernest Witebsky's laboratory. As the inheritor of the Paul Ehrlich mantel, Witebsky was well known as a proponent of the 'horror autotoxicus' doctrine and a great skeptic with respect to the autoimmune etiology of human disease. Only because of his well known skepticism and his reputation for rigorous investigation were the findings of thyroid autoimmunity finally accepted. They opened new vistas of research in the clinical applications of immunology and helped to trigger a rethinking of the instructional theories of antibody production that has contributed significantly to our current understanding of the clonal selection basis of the immune response.

THE RENAISSANCE OF AUTOIMMUNITY

A word of explanation is in order concerning the title of this section. The notion that autoimmunity could cause human disease was quite popular in the early days of the twentieth century. The concept lost popularity as immunologists learned that animals do not usually develop immune responses to constituents of their own bodies. There were, nevertheless, well-recognized exceptions. Certain tissues and organs appear to be isolated from the immune system and therefore are treated as foreign invaders when introduced into the body proper. The outstanding examples were the lens of the eye, the sperm of the testes, and the brain. Extracts of these suggested tissues injected into the same animal give rise to autoantibodies and, in some instances, to actual disease of the respective organ. Experimental allergic encephalomyelitis, autoimmune orchitis, and autoimmune uveitis can be cited as examples of experimentally induced autoimmune diseases elicited by introduction of sequestered antigens.

Autoimmunity to Non-Sequestered Antigens

The discovery of thyroid autoimmunity in 1956 required a rethinking of the theory of sequestered antigens.[1,2,3] It was difficult to believe that the thyroid gland is sequestered when it has such a rich vascular supply. In fact, thyroglobulin was known already in 1956 to be circulating in the blood stream, although in very low amounts. The real significance of the discovery of autoimmune thyroiditis was the realization that many tissues of the body elicit autoimmune responses when injected with a potent adjuvant. Autoimmune responses to antigens of self can result in autoimmune disease. Subsequently, there was a rush to examine human diseases of unknown origin to see if there were associated autoimmune responses. Many such examples were reported. It turned out to be difficult, however, to prove that autoimmunity is the cause rather than the consequence of disease.

During the years since 1956, valuable lessons concerning the curative role of autoimmunity in disease have been learned. In a few instances, the new knowledge arose initially from studies of thyroiditis in experimental animals or in human subjects. In other cases, different examples of autoimmune disease led the way, but investigations of autoimmune thyroiditis served for confirmation and solidification of the finding. It is possible, therefore, to trace the evolution of thought with respect to autoimmunity and self/non-self discrimination by recounting briefly the major landmarks that have led to our current understanding of thyroid autoimmunity.

Molecular Mimicry

Thyroglobulin occupies a special place among tissue antigens because many of the antigenic determinants are shared with thyroglobulins of foreign species. We showed that thyroiditis can be produced in rabbits by injections of bovine thyroglobulin, rather than homologous rabbit thyroglobulin.[4] If repeated injections are given, it was not necessary to use complete Freund's adjuvant. However, the lesions developed by animals immunized with foreign thyroglobulins were much milder than those produced by immunization with thyroglobulin of the same species. These studies showed that autoimmunity can be induced by cross-reactive foreign antigens as well as by autologous constituents, a phenomenon now referred to as molecular mimicry.

Roles of T Cells and B Cells in Autoimmune Disease

During the decade of the 1960's the emphasis in the study of immuno-pathological phenomena shifted from humoral antibody to immunocompetent cells. In the case of thyroiditis, it has been difficult to demonstrate a role for antibody in producing lesions of the disease.[5] On the other hand, it is possible to transfer experimental thyroiditis between genetically compatible animals by transfer of lymphocyte populations.[6] Although transfer experiments strongly implicate cell-mediated immunity, they should not be regarded as excluding a role for antibody, since the transferred cells are capable of initiating antibody production in recipient mice.[7] Since T cells are required for induction of thyroiditis, it was possible to demonstrate directly that T cells responsive to thyroglobulin are present even in normal mice of certain strains.[8,9] During immunization of mice, T cells are important in regulating the vigor of the autoimmune response.[8] T cells are also capable of directly injuring thyroid epithelium in cell culture.[10]

The involvement of B cells cannot be demonstrated in some species. In the spontaneous form of thyroiditis occurring in the OS chicken, removal of the bursa greatly diminishes the severity of thyroid disease.[11] Readministration of bursa cells restores autoimmune thyroiditis in bursectomized OS chickens.[12] Both T cells and B cells are required, it seems, to produce the full picture of spontaneous autoimmune thyroiditis in chickens.

Association of Autoimmune Disease with Major
Histocompatibility Complex MHC)

The association of autoimmune disease with the MHC has had an enormous impact on research in the field. The first evidence of such an association arose from investigations carried out on experimental thyroiditis in collaboration with Adian Vladutiu.[13] We examined a large number of inbred mouse strains and found that they differ greatly in their susceptibility to experimentally induced thyroiditis. By using congenic strains, we were able to show that the major site of control resides within the MHC. Later investigations showed two levels of MHC regulation of autoimmune thyroiditis in the mouse. The induction of disease depends largely upon class II MHC genes located at I-A.[14,15] The severity of disease, on the other hand, is modulated by genes at the K or D locus, representing class I genes.[16] These initial discoveries of the importance of MHC in experimental disease in mice were followed by the demonstration of the importance of the MHC in spontaneously occurring thyroiditis in OS chickens.[17] Shortly afterwards, the association of HLA in the human MHC with thyroiditis and other autoimmune disease in humans was published.[18]

Non-MHC Associations

Important as it is, MHC is not the only determinant of susceptibility to autoimmune disease. In contrast to inbred mice, for example, inbred rats initially showed little association of susceptibility with MHC.[19] Only by more detailed analysis was subtle MHC regulation detectable. Presumably, the MHC regulation was overshadowed by non-MHC genetic traits. The same principal findings were demonstrated using inbred mice that are matched at the MHC, but differing in non-MHC (background) genes.[20]

In the spontaneous form of thyroiditis in the OS chicken more information about the non-MHC regulation of autoimmune thyroiditis was educed. Two major categories of non-MHC genes were recognized. One set of genes influenced the maturation of the thymus and controlled the balance of various sub-populations generated there.[21] A second set of genes regulated the function of the thyroid epithelial cell, particularly regarding its ability to take up iodine and incorporate it into thyroglobulin.[22,23] The OS chicken is highly susceptible to autoimmune thyroiditis because it bears all three of these diverse genetic traits. Animals with only two of these three properties are less likely to develop the disease spontaneously, even though it can be induced by experimental immunization.

Other non-MHC influences were identified later. Females are generally more susceptible to autoimmune disease than males. Sex hormones have a profound effect on the development of experimental thyroiditis in mice as well as on spontaneous disease in OS chickens.[24,25] Secondly, environmental agents play a role. Even in genetically identical BUF rats, the prevalence of spontaneously developing autoimmune thyroiditis increased greatly following administration of the drug methylcholanthrene.[26] In addition to the well-documented effects of drugs, infection, diet, irradiation and even stress are all possible factors in determining the actual severity of autoimmune disease.

Autoimmune Escalation

A striking phenomenon, first demonstrated with autoimmune thyroiditis, is the sequential occurrence of multiple autoimmune reactions affecting the same organ. In studies of experimental thyroiditis in the rhesus monkey, it was possible to show that initial immunization with thyroglobulin led to the subsequent induction of autoimmune response to the thyroid microsomal antigen.[27] The initial autoimmune response triggered response to a second, unrelated antigen of the thyroid. Although the presence of antibodies to microsomal antigen (thyroid peroxidase) is an excellent indicator of clinical disease, it should be remembered that thyroglobulin was the initiator of the original autoimmune response.

V Gene Usage

In recent years, a great deal of attention has been devoted to the question of whether autoimmune responses arise from a restricted repertoire of variable region (V) genes of the B cell or T cell. Early studies suggested that autoantibodies were encoded by V genes of particular V_H families, especially those that are closest to the site of V-J recombination.[28] Latre, more detailed studies by Rudolph Kuppers and his colleagues, however, have shown that this association does not occur in experimentally induced thyroid autoantibodies.[29] In fact, the V-region genes seem to be mobilized in random order. In addition, Kuppers' studies showed that most autoantibodies are not the result of somatic mutation, finally putting to rest Burnet's concept of "forbidden clones" as the investigators of autoimmune diseases.

Pathogenic Epitopes

Results of current investigations suggest that autoimmune diseases result from the recognition of particular antigenic determinants on the autoantigenic molecule. To investigate the question, studies of thyroglobulin are well suited because thyroglobulin is a large molecule with many potential determinants. Our group has been using two approaches to analyze this question. One depends upon splitting the thyroglobulin molecule by chemical or enzymatic means and testing each peptide fragment for its ability to induce an autoimmune response.[30,31,32,33] Parallel studies are carried out of human thyroglobulin using peptide fragments.[31,32,33] This second approach is necessary because many of the determinants recognized by antibodies are conformational in nature and therefore disrupted by degradation. In order to detect conformational antigens, monoclonal antibodies were prepared to cover a large portion of the surface of the thyroglobulin molecule.[34,35] The ability of a monoclonal to interfere with the binding of human patients' sera provides a method to identify the determinants recognized.[36] Based on this approach, we have been able to distinguish two types of antigenic determinants on thyroglobulin. Some determinants are widely shared among mammalian species. Many normal people have low levels of antibody to these shared determinants. Other determinants are relatively species restricted as shown by the lack of cross-reaction on the part of the respective monoclonal antibodies. It is to the species-restricted determinants that most thyroiditis patients produce autoantibodies.

Specific Therapies of the Future

Presently, autoimmune diseases are treated by global suppression of the immune response, or by life-long replacement of a lost physiological function of a damaged target organ. The eventual goal in studies of autoimmune disease is to develop a means for specifically arresting or for even preventing the harmful effects of autoimmunity without suppressing the overall immune capabilities of the patient. The genetic studies described previously offer the opportunity of recognizing individuals at greatest risk of developing particular autoimmune diseases. While that goal is not yet attainable in random human populations, it is already possible to predict with a fairly high degree of accuracy the eventual development of autoimmune thyroiditis in children in families where one child already has been diagnosed with clinically evident disease.[37,38,39]

Specific therapy depends upon recognizing the particular peptide or peptides responsible for pathogenic responses. Identifying the class II MHC determinants necessary to present that peptide or sorting out the particular V gene specificities of the T-cell receptor required for recognition of the peptide-MHC-class-II-complex then becomes possible. The goal is to develop blocking peptides or monoclonal antibodies to the cellular receptors. These approaches are presently being investigated. In the case of experimental thyroiditis, it has already been shown that antibodies to the MHC determinant and to the peptide can block the *in vitro* cytotoxic effects of T lymphocytes on thyroid monolayers.[10]

The most promising long range strategy is to prevent the onset of autoimmune disease before tissue damage can occur. A prototype for this approach was described in collaboration with David Silverman a number of years ago.[40] We employed inbred BUF rats which are genetically predisposed to develop autoimmune thyroiditis after they attain 12-18 wks of age. The onset of disease was inhibited by intravenous injection of intact thyroglobulin.

Intravenous injection of thyroglobulin unaccompanied by adjuvant leads to a state of unresponsiveness, so that experimental thyroiditis cannot be induced.[41] The unresponsive state can be transferred to naive recipients using T cells from the spleen. With Eyal Talor, we have recently identified a population of T cells arising in the thymus which is able to pre vent autoantibody production by splenic B cells.[42] Although the basis of the refractory state of animals produced by injection of aqueous antigen is not yet well understood, the experiments suggest that it is possible to use natural regulatory mechanisms in order to prevent the onset of autoimmune disease. The potential value of early recognition of individuals predisposed to the onset of autoimmunity, therefore, becomes dramatically evident.

EPILOGUE

Studies of autoimmune thyroiditis have been a true voyage of discovery. Through this model, it has been possible to originate or evaluate many of the key concepts that underlie contemporary immunology. At the same time, a whole new area of immunology, clinical immunology, has emerged. The diagnosis and treatment of autoimmune disease is now a major component of medical practice. It is difficult to imagine a more versatile vessel upon which to set sail on a voyage of scientific discovery. And the end of the journey is not in sight!

REFERENCES

1. **Witebsky, E. and Rose N. R.,** Studies on organ specificity, IV. Production or rabbit thyroid antibodies in the rabbit, *J. Immunol.,* 76, 408, 1956.
2. **Rose, N. R. and Witebsky, E.,** Studies on organ specificity, V. Changes in the thyroid glands of rabbits following active immunization with rabbit thyroid extracts, *J. Immunol.,* 76, 417, 1956.
3. **Witebsky, E., Rose N. R., Terplan, K., Paine, J. R. and Egan, R. W.,** Chronic thyroiditis and autoimmunization, *J. Am. Med. Assoc.,* 164, 1439, 1957.
4. **Witebsky, E. and Rose, N. R.,** Studies on organ specificity, VII. Production of antibodies to rabbit thyroid by injection of foreign thyroid extracts, *J. Immunol.,* 83, 41, 1959.
5. **Terplan, K. L., Witebsky, E.,Rose, N. R., Paine, J. R. and Egan, R. W.,** Experimental thyroiditis in rabbits, guinea pigs and dogs, following immunization with thyroid extracts of their own and of heterologous species, *Am. J. Pathol.,* 36, 213, 1960.
6. **Twarog, F. J. and Rose, N. R.,** Transfer of autoimmune thyroiditis of the rat with lymph node cells, *J. Immunol.,* 104, 1467, 1970.
7. **Twarog, F. J. and Rose, N. R.,** The refractory period in adoptive immunization following secondary stimulation of mice, *J. Immunol.,* 102, 375, 1969.
8. **Vladutiu, A. O. and Rose, N. R.,** Cellular basis of the genetic control of immune responsiveness to murine thyroglobulin in mice, *Cell Immunol.,* 17, 106, 1975.
9. **Esquivel, P. S., Kong, Y. M. and Rose, N. R.,** Evidence for thyroglobulin-reactive T cells in good responder mice, *Cell Immunol.,* 37, 14, 1978.

10. **Creemers, P., Rose N. R. and Kong, Y. M.,** Experimental autoimmune thyroiditis: *In vitro* cytotoxic effects of T lymphocytes on thyroid monoloayers, *J. Exp. Med.*, 157, 559, 1983.

11. **Welch, P., Rose, N. R. and Kite, J. H., Jr.,** Neonatal thymectomy increases spontaneous autoimmune thyroiditis, *J. Immunol.*, 110, 575, 1973.

12. **Nilsson, L-Å and Rose, N. R.,** Restoration of autoimmune thyroiditis in bursectomized-irradiated OS chickens by bursa cells, *Immunol.*, 22, 13, 1972.

13. **Vladutiu, A. O. and Rose, N. R.,** Autoimmune murine thyroiditis, Relation to histocompatibility (H-2) type, *Science*, 174, 1137, 1971.

14. **Tomazic, V., Rose, N. R. and Shreffler, D.C.,** Autoimmune murine thyroiditis. IV. Localization of genetic control of the immune response, *J. Immunol.*, 112, 965, 1974.

15. **Beisel, K. W., David, C. S., Giraldo, A. A., Kong, Y. M. and Rose, N. R.,** Regulation of experimental autoimmune thyroiditis: Mapping of susceptibility to the I-A subregion of the mouse H-2, *Immunogenetics*, 15, 427, 1982.

16. **Kong, Y. M., David C. S., Giraldo, A. A., ElRehewy, M. and Rose, N. R.,** Regulation of autoimmune response to mouse thyroglobulin: Influence of H-2D-end genes, *J. Immunol.*, 123, 15, 1979.

17. **Bacon, L. D., Kite, J. H., Jr., and Rose, N. R.,** Relation between the major histocompatibility (B) locus and autoimmune thyroiditis in obese chickens, *Science*, 186:274, 1974.

18. **Vladutiu, A. O. and Rose, N. R.,** HL-A antigens: Association with disease, *Immunogenetics*, 1, 305, 1974.

19. **Rose, N. R.,** Differing responses of inbred rat strains in experimental autoimmune thyroiditis, *Cell Immunol.*, 18, 360, 1975.

20. **Beisel, K. W., Kong, Y. M., Babu, K. S. J., David, C. S. and Rose, N. R.,** Regulation of experimental autoimmune thyroiditis: Influence of non-H-2 genes, *J. Immunogenetics*, 9, 257, 1982.

21. **Jakobisiak, M., Sundick, R. and Rose, N. R.,** Abnormal response to minor histocompatibility antigens in obese strain chickens, *Proc. Natl. Acad. Sci.* 73, 2877, 1976.

22. **Wlodarski, K., Sundick, R. and Rose, N. R.,** ^{131}I-uptake by obese strain and Reaseheath Line R chicken thyroid and thymic epithelium cultured *in vitro*, *Folia Biol.*, 27, 85, 1979.

23. **Truden, J. L., Sundick, R. S., Levine, S. and Rose, N. R.,** The decreased growth rate of obese strain chicken thyroid cells provides *in vitro* evidence for a primary target organ abnormality in chickens susceptible to autoimmune thyroiditis, *Clin. Immunol. Immunopathol.*, 29, 294, 1983.

24. **Okayasu, I., Kong, Y. M. and Rose, N. R.,** Effect of castration and sex hormones on experimental autoimmune thyroiditis, *Clin. Immunol. Immunopathol.*, 20, 240, 1981.

25. **Bacon, L. D. and Rose, N. R.,** Influence of major histocompatibility haplotype on autoimmune disease varies in different inbred families of chickens, *Proc. Natl. Acad. Sci.*, 76, 1435, 1979.

26. **Silverman, D. A. and Rose, N. R.,** Spontaneous and methylcholanthrene-enhanced thyroiditis in BUF rats, I. The incidence and severity of the disease, and the genetics of susceptibility, *J. Immunol.*, 114, 145, 1975.

27. **Andrada, J. A., Rose, N. R. and Kite, J. H., Jr.,** Experimental thyroiditis in the rhesus monkey, IV. The role of thyroglobulin and cellular antigens, *Clin. Exp. Immunol.* 3, 133, 1968.

28. **Monestier, M., Bonin, B., Migliorini, P., Dang, H., Datta, S., Kuppers, R., Rose, N., Maurer, P., Talal, N. and Bona, C.,** Autoantibodies of various specificities encoded by genes from the V_H J558 family bind to foreign antigens and share idiotypes of antibodies specific for self and foreign antigens, *J. Exp. Med.*, 166, 1109, 1987.

29. **Gleason, S. L., Gearhart, P., Rose, N. R. and Kuppers, R. C.,** Autoantibodies to thyroglobulin are encoded by diverse V-gene segments and recognize restricted epitopes, *J. Immunol.*, 145, 1768, 1990.

30. **Anderson, C. L. and Rose, N. R.,** Induction of thyroiditis in the rabbit by intravenous injection of papain-treated rabbit thyroglobulin, *J. Immunol.*, 107, 1341, 1971.

31. **Rose, N. R. and Stylos, W. A.,** Splitting of human thyroglobulin. I. Reduction and alkylation, *Clin. Exp. Immunol.*, 5, 129, 1969.

32. **Stylos, W. A. and Rose, N. R.,** Splitting of human thyroglobulin. II. Enzymatic digestion, *Clin. Exp. Immunol.* 5, 285, 1969.

33.   **Mehta, P. D. and Rose, N. R.,** Splitting of human thyroglobulin, III. Comparison of fragments obtained during enzymatic digestion and by reduction and alkylation, *Clin. Exp. Immunol.,* 17, 267, 1974.

34.   **Rose, N. R., Accavitti, M., Pydyn, E. F., Leon, M. A. and Brown, R. K.,** The Use of Hybridoma Antibodies to Probe the Antigenic Determinants of Thyroglobulin, in *Immunobiology of Proteins and Peptides-II,* Chapter 2, M. Z. Atassi, Ed., Plenum Publishing Corp., NY, 1982.

35.   **Bresler, H. S., Burek, C. L. and Rose, N. R.,** Autoantigenic determinants on human thyroglobulin, I. Determinant specificities of murine monoclonal antibodies, *Clin. Immunol. Immunopathol.,* 54, 64, 1990.

36.   **Bresler, H. S., Burek, C. L., Hoffman, W. H. and Rose, N. R.,** Autoantigenic determinants on human thyroglobulin, II. Determinants recognized by autoantibodies from patients with chronic autoimmune thyroiditis compared to autoantibodies from healthy subjects, *Clin. Immunol. Immunopathol.,* 54, 76, 1990.

37.   **Burek, C. L., Hoffman, W. H. and Rose, N. R.,** The presence of thyroid autoantibodies in children and adolescents with autoimmune thyroid disease and in their siblings and parents, *Clin. Immunol. Immunopathol.,* 25, 395, 1982.

38.   **Burek, C. L., Rose, N. R., Najar, G. M., Hoffman, W. H., Gimelfarb, A., Zmijewski, C. M., Polesky, H. F. and Hoffman, W. M.,** Autoimmune Thyroid Disease, in *Immunogenetics,* Chapter 9, G. S. Panayi, C. S. David, Eds., Butterworths, London, 1984.

39.   **Rose, N. R. and Burek, C. L.,** The interaction of basic science and population-based research: Autoimmune thyroiditis as a case history, *Am. J. Epidemiol.,* 134, 1073, 1991.

40.   **Silverman, D. A. and Rose, N. R.,** Inhibition of genetically determined autoimmune disease by organ specific antigen, *Lancet,* 1, 1257, 1974.

41.   **Kong, Y. M., Okayasu, I., Giraldo, A. A., Beisel, K. W., Sundick, R. S., Rose, N. R., David, C. S., Audibert, F. and Chedid, L.,** Tolerance to thyroglobulin by activating suppressor mechanisms, *Ann. N. Y. Acad. Sci.,* 392, 191, 1982.

42.   **Rose, N. R. and Talor, E.,** Antigen-specific immunoregulation and autoimmune thyroiditis, *Ann. N.Y. Acad. Sci.,* 636, 306, 1991.

INDEX